PSYCHOLOGY RESEARCH PROGRESS

Additional books in this series can be found on Nova's website under the Series tab.

Additional e-books in this series can be found on Nova's website under the e-books tab.

PSYCHOLOGY RESEARCH PROGRESS

COGNITIVE DEFICIT IN MENTAL AND NEUROLOGICAL DISORDERS

HANA KUCEROVA
AND
MAREK PREISS
EDITORS

nova publishers
New York

Library of Congress Cataloging-in-Publication Data

ISBN: 978-1-60741-957-0

Published by Nova Science Publishers, Inc. † New York

Contents

Preface

Clinical neuropsychology is a sub-specialty of clinical psychology that specializes in the diagnostic assessment and treatment of patients with brain injury or neurocognitive deficits. This book comprises contributions from different clinical domains /in particular neurology, psychology and psychiatry/ and summarizes significant theoretical and above all practically usable information regarding a variety of disorders that a clinical neuropsychologist can come across in practice the most. This book explores etiology of cognitive deficit, history of its examination, variables that are concerned with cognitive functions and rehabilitation possibilities. All chapters were written by experienced clinicians who are used to prevailing, typical problems of their patients that overlap cognitive functions to domains such as emotions and everyday difficulties problem solving. We assume this book to be useful for individuals interested in neuropsychological diagnostics and rehabilitation, students of psychology and alike-oriented professions.

Chapter I - This chapter aims to offer an overview, based on our experiences as well as on evidence presented in the literature, concerning cognitive functioning of patients with unipolar depressive disorders during remission. This is a topic rarely focused on by medical and/or psychiatric care research. Neuropsychological study of depressive disorders in remission represents a fringe, yet interesting area, which interconnects possible qualitative and quantitative psychological investigations. It seems likely that future assessments of remission in depressive disorders will be multi-dimensional. Furthermore, it is possible that future multifactor assessment of remission will include the patients´ subjective views as to their quality of life. According to the statistics, approximately one-third of the depressed patients show, during the periods of remission, a significant impairment of cognition, which most likely reflects a real functional deficit. Neuropsychological deficits can, however, be fairly subtle and may not even be detected during usual psychological assessments. It seems sensible that, in this respect, we may better rely more on the patients' subjective impressions of their own abilities and performances. Older patients are in greater danger of cognitive impairment, and the clinical approach might, thus, offer a refinement of methods, enabling repeated testing of cognitive functioning during old age. It has been already established that depression with psychotic symptoms, chronic depression or onset of depression in advanced age all tend to entail more severe weakening of cognitive functions. It has, however, not been conclusively shown that neuropsychological impairment follows an increased frequency of depressive episodes or hospitalizations. It may be recommended that for the purposes of assessing cognitive functioning during remission, the patient stays in his home.

Some factors complicating objective measurement of cognitive deficit during remission are: methodologically, the Flynn effect, and from the viewpoint of the patient's actual ability, influence of the so-called brain reserve (hypothesis) or the increased performance fluctuation during episodes of illness.

At present, there is no generally accepted formal testing procedure oriented towards the neuropsychological functioning and performance of patients in remission or, for that matter, during the course of depressive episodes. By gradually refining and honing the existing psychological testing norms, and by an inclusion of demographic indicators such as age, gender and education, we can make the diagnostic procedures more sensitive to detecting an impaired and/or enhanced cognitive functioning during remission. Attempts, which suggest some directions and possibilities of cognitive rehabilitation during remission, indicate a growing interest in caring for patients during remission and not just during a period of hospitalization. Rehabilitation attempts include variety of approaches (e.g., meditation, neuropsychological rehabilitation, different versions of cognitive-behavioral therapy (CBT), approaches based on exploring brain plasticity, direct training of cognitive functions). The present state of research does not allow us to select a specific preferred approach. Future studies will increasingly explore links between cognition and neuropsychological tests. Most likely, there will be more longitudinal follow-up studies, focusing on patients´ everyday functioning and performance. There still is an unanswered question as to the premorbid performance of patients with unipolar depressive disorder. This gap contrasts with such evidence as studies concerning bipolar affective disorders or schizophrenia. One can assume that in comparison to schizophrenia, establishing a clear relationship between depressive illness in adulthood and premorbid cognitive functioning might be more problematic.

Chapter II - Eating disorders include mainly anorexia nervosa (AN) and bulimia nervosa (BN) and their atypical forms. The spectrum of eating disorders also includes psychogenic overeating and night overeating connected with obesity. Lifelong prevalence in women is 0.5 to 3.7% in AN, and 1.1 to 4.2% in BN according to the selected criteria. The results of studies dealing with the impairment of cognitive functions in patients suffering from eating disorders differ depending on the studied subdiagnosis, phase of the disease (severely affected patients in acute phase of the disease, chronic patients, patients in remission) and on specific functions that are in the centre of authors‘ attention and selected tests. Patients with eating disorders have manifested slowed reaction time and disorders of short-term visual memory and recollection-based long-term memory. Particularly female AN patients have disrupted capacity to solve three-dimensional tasks where they are supposed to reproduce a complex figure, supplement missing parts of the picture and analyze spatial disposition. Vigilance and memory are focused on a narrow areas of eating and body proportions. One of the specific characteristics of patients with eating disorders is the distorted body perception (it is the most significant in patients with AN) connected with the disorder of interoception. As consistently described in the literature, patients suffering from eating disorders have also manifested the change in pain perception. The research focuses on connections between these changes and lower hormone levels and also specific cognitive features that are responsible for impaired perception of inner feelings and body scheme. Based on the combination of neuropsychological tests and magnetic resonance, several studies investigated relations between structural changes and cognitive deficits. In anorexia nervosa, the brain atrophy can be detected by imaging methods as soon as a few months after the onset of the disease. However, correlations between structural and the described functional disorders were weak.

The studies using functional imaging methods (SPET, PET and fMRI) have shown that there is a lower blood flow in patient's brain, neurons consume less glucose and electric response to standard impulses is slowed down. The reduced perception and cognitive flexibility is described in patients with AN. It is very difficult for these patients to use alternately various cognitive strategies, to perceive various impulses and to do various tasks at a time (the so-called multitasking). Also observed was an excessive focus on detail upon concurrent insufficient perception of the whole. In recent years, batteries of test have been used that are specifically focused on this type of damage, and there exists a system of tasks used in patients' rehabilitation. The questions remain to what extent structural and functional disorders in patients with eating disorders disappear after the patients regain weight, or to what extent they persist even after their recovery, or whether these characteristics are connected with the disease or whether they are permanent features of such patients. The examination of cognitive functions should be first of all a part of clinical assessment of the disease prognosis and one of the criteria upon decision-making whether to recommend the patient for work or invalidity.

Chapter III - Schizophrenia is often associated with cognitive deficits, particularly within the domains of attention, memory, executive functions, and language skills. Specific cognitive deficits have recently been linked to psychotic phenomena, including verbal hallucinations and disorganized speech. Impairments of working and semantic memory are primarily due to dysfunction of the frontal cortex, temporal cortex, and hippocampus.

Examination of cognitive functions in patients with schizophrenia is complicated for many reasons. So far neither a unified examination battery nor a terminological consensus exists, which causes problems in the acquisition and interpretation of data (proposal of MATRICS initiative).

Cognitive skills in schizophrenia predict social functioning and may serve as outcome measures in the development of effective treatment strategies. There are extensive possibilities to therapeutically influence cognitive dysfunction; however, so far, their effects have not been investigated in detail. An integrated approach, including pharmacotherapy, social skills training and cognitive training, seems to be the optimal solution.

Chapter IV - The chapter is divided into groups by different types of addictive substances with particular respect to specific features pertaining to the potential risks of the development of cognitive deficits associated with the use thereof. Considerably greater attention is paid to some of the substances, as the users of such substances and the consequences of using them are encountered more frequently in practice. For example, this emphasis was applied for cannabis and MDMA ("ecstasy"), as these are substances that have become very popular among adolescents and young adults, and there are no signs of any major reversal of this tendency. Significant attention was also paid to the group of stimulants whose risk in terms of cognitive deficits is unfortunately often underestimated in practice, as opposed to the risk associated with opioid use, which, conversely, is overestimated. A separate area of concern involves volatile substances whose significant risks, including those to cognitive functions, are well known—the professional community has been pointing this issue out—but these facts are not adequately reflected in writings published in professional journals, nor in other messages. Finally, the concluding section of the chapter deals with assessment methods and recommended procedures for the identification and proposal of treatment and rehabilitation interventions aimed at addressing cognitive deficits caused by addictive substance use.

Chapter V - Antidepressants globally belong to the most frequently prescribed medicinal products. This is supported by the fact that the depressive condition is one of the five most frequent diseases that significantly decrease working abilities of the patients, disable them or lead to their untimely death (Látalová et al., 2004).

Chapter VI - The subject of cognitive dysfunction in schizophrenia patients is discussed at large in other sections of the book; this chapter reviews both currently available and experimental options of pharmacological treatment. It has been postulated that a cognitive deficit represents the core impairment of schizophrenia with considerable negative impact on the course and functional outcome of the illness (Sharma a Harvey, 2000; Harvey et al., 2004). The deficit, presumably generalized, thus interferes with basic everyday functioning, including integration into the community, ability to cope with social problems, or acquisition of psychosocial skills. Effective remediation of a cognitive dysfunction is one of the unmet needs in the complex schizophrenia treatment. The schematic relationship between real (functional) outcome and various therapeutic interventions is depicted in the Figure 1.1 (adapted from Green and Nuechterlein, 1999). The scheme illustrates the fact that psychotic symptoms have little impact on outcome, which largely depends on cognitive performance and can be affected by pharmacotherapy mostly indirectly.

Chapter VII - Training of cognitive functions has become so popular recently that the British newspaper *The Guardian* is offering aides for the improvement of basic cognitive abilities via their online interactive brain training games, including memory and processing speed (www.lumosity.com/guardian). As these and other training methods become more popular, the training of cognitive functions continues to be developed in both a scientific and professional framework.

Chapter VIII - The neuropsychological examination should support a correct and early diagnosis of Alzheimer's disease by fulfilling the international criteria of the disease. A comprehensive neuropsychological assessment includes examination of global cognitive ability, memory, verbal abilities and language, executive functions and visuospatial functions. These cognitive domains may be examined by physicians using simple and concise tests and by psychologists using more complex methods. Their basic description and appropriate usage in diagnosing Alzheimer's disease and related diseases are given.

Chapter IX - Not only one disease is concerned but a number of markedly various syndromes. It is better to talk about epilepsies rather than about epilepsy itself. There is no uniform profile of cognitive functions. On the one hand, there are special disorders that occur, especially in early childhood, and that cause severe cognitive deficits. On the other hand, there are a considerable number of people with compensated disease who are well adapted to work and social life.

A summary of classifications of seizure disorders, neuropsychological impacts of localization and epileptogenic factors, impacts of ethiological factors and EEG abnormalities on neuropsychological performance is provided.

The prevalence in the population is 0.5 to 1%. Compared to the current prevalence, the lifetime prevalence is higher (2 to 5%), which means that most patients have a chance for long-term remission.

Characteristics of changes in the main domains of measurable cognitive functions are provided. Important factors include etiology, heredity, disposition, age of disease onset, duration of disease, type and intensity of seizures, frequency of seizures, pharmacotherapy and status epilepticus. The most common subjective complaints and objective finding in adults include memory disorders, mental retardation and attention disorders. In children, cognitive disorders cause speech difficulties, learning disorders, poor school results, behavioral problems, and unfavorable social and vocational prognosis. Except for cognitive disorders, the following disorders are common: behavioral disorders, mental difficulties in adults—especially depressions, dysphorias and increased anxiety—and, according to some authors, personal specificities, and learning disorders in children. Cognitive performance can especially be affected by depressive disorders and anxiety.

Neuropsychological methods designed especially for epilepsy, such as the Neuropsychological Battery for Epilepsies (NBE), FePsy Battery, Washington Psychosocial Seizure Inventory (WPSI), memory test as a part of the Wada Test, Quality of Life in Epilepsy Inventory (QOLIE-89) and others are described.

The course of cognitive deficits is described in subsections of the longitudinal follow-up and includes the question of dementia, monitoring of concomitant factors, effects of neurosurgery, prediction of surgical results, quality of life, and antiepileptic medication.

The proposal for a standardized examination of cognitive functions is divided into examinations performed at the standard clinics and at specialized clinics for the treatment of epilepsy. Detailed examinations are performed in relation to brain surgeries in response to pharmacoresistant epilepsy. Except for cognitive areas, neuropsychological examinations should also describe psychosocial problems of patients, personality, disease adaptation, subjective quality of life, possible psychopathology, or suicidal tendencies.

Methods of psychotherapy and rehabilitation of cognitive deficits are subdivided according to the type of intervention and the declared target for psychological-educative, relaxation, behavioral and methods aimed at social psychological adaptation and cognitive rehabilitation.

The main emphasis is transferred from diagnostics and localization to the description of weak and strong cognitive features and to cognitive and psychosocial rehabilitation.

Chapter X - Huntington's disease (HD) is an autosomal dominantly inherited neurodegenerative disease caused by gene mutation on a short arm of the 4th chromosome, with incidence of about 1: 10-15,000. The mutation consists in expansion of CAG triplet with critical limit of about 40 repeats. HD is manifested by combination of motor symptoms (especially, the choreatic dyskinesias are characteristic), neuropsychiatric disorders (depression, anxiety, irritability or apathy, obsession and compulsion, psychotic symptoms) and progressing dementia. Typically, HD begins between the 35th and 50th year of age, however, juvenile and late forms also exist.

The progression of HD cannot be substantially therapeutically influenced, but some of the symptoms may be at least temporarily effectively confronted using pharmacological and psychosocial interventions. However, the course of HD leads unevitably to the total dependency on the neighbourhood and patients die in uncontrollable marasmus.

The diagnosis of HD is confirmed by a genetic test. In persons at risk (the offspring of the ill or positively tested person) who want to know their genetic state, presymptomatic DNA testing is performed using a specific protocol. Prenatal testing is also possible.

Chapter XI - Normal Pressure Hydrocephalus (NPH) in adults is a disease with varied etiology. In typical examples, it is manifested by a triad of symptoms—gait disorders, incontinence and cognitive functions disorders or even dementia. It develops most often with an, as yet, unexplained etiology (idiopathic hydrocephalus, iNPH) or less often as a result of another disease or injury. Normal pressure hydrocephalus occurs in all age groups, but most cases occur in the over those over 60. Both forms of NPH—Normal Pressure Hydrocephalus— cause 3 to 6% of all dementia and may be very effectively treated by shunting. In cases with a timely diagnosis, the cognitive abilities may be restored to premorbid levels—it is an extraordinary form of reversible dementia. Other forms of hydrocephalus occurring in the adulthood include diagnoses of slowly developing obstruction hydrocephalus and atrophic hydrocephalus. Within differential diagnostics, neuropsychology primarily deals with NPH. A significant problem in NPH involves making the correct diagnosis in patients over 60. A suspicion of NPH can be confirmed using imaging methods such as CT and MRI.

The loss of cognitive functions is especially related to memory, attention and executive functions. The cognitive deficit develops concomitantly with gait disorders and is not apparent to those around them, since no changes in personality or behavior occur. Left untreated, progression of the NPH will begin to affect cognitive abilities; manifesting as orientation disorders and significant memory/attention disorders, additionally qualitative consciousness disorders also begin to appear. These stages are accompanied by a loss of mobility and self-reliance. However, in cases with an early NPH diagnosis, coupled with timely surgery, improvement or even full recovery can occur or, at the very least, the progression of the clinical symptoms can be stopped.

Chapter XII - Parkinson's disease (PD) is a serious neurodegenerative disease affecting one to two persons out of every 1,000 in the general population. In addition to being a movement disorder characterized by progressive hypokinesia, rigidity, tremor at rest, and stance/gait disorders, PD is also often associated with mental changes. Cognitive disorders, especially executive dysfunction, affect up to 90% of patients. Subcortical-type dementia develops in at least 20% of these patients. Over the course of the disease, at least 50% of patients experience depression, which is often combined with anxiety. Psychotic complications of drug therapy affect relatively few patients, although patients with cognitive defects are at an increased risk.

In addition to the crucial deficit of dopamine, disturbances in other neurotransmitters that participate in basal ganglia circuits and ascending pathways constitute the neurobiological background of the mental symptoms associated with PD. Consequently, not all of these disorders can be managed pharmacologically through dopamine replacement therapy.

Neuropsychological examinations help in the diagnosis and determination of the severity of various components of mental problems associated with PD. The recommended tests help in evaluation and long-term monitoring of global cognitive deficits, cognitive disorders (especially executive dysfunction), and depression.

Chapter XIII - Subarachnoid hemorrhage (SAH) from aneurysms of the cerebral arteries (AN) is a medical term referring to the bleeding in the subarachnoid space. The bleeding mostly occurs in the region of the basal cisterns, which is in close relation to the arterial circle of Willis. The occurrence of SAH is 6 to 12 cases/100.000 inhabitants every year. SAH is often fatal and represents a significant cause of invalidity in a young and otherwise healthy population. The natural course leads to death in 25 to 30% of cases within a 24-hour period. Without treatment, another 30% of patients die within the next four weeks.

The aetiology of the aneurysm formation is a defect of elastic tissues, genetically based and specifically evolved during embryonal development. The exact pathophysiology is not certain. There are several risk factors for rupture, such as hypertension, alcohol abuse, smoking and physical/psychical stress. The signs of the rupture include headache, nausea, vomiting and loss of consciousness.

During the acute phase, the patient is endangered by increased intracranial pressure and a limited amount of oxygen blood to the brain. SAH can be diagnosed by a lumbar tap (bloody cerebrospinal fluid); the next step is a CT scan of the brain, showing characteristic blood clots in the area of the basal cisterns. Further investigations depict the exact location, size and shape of the aneurysm—a CT angiography or digital subtraction angiography are used.

The choice of adequate treatment is based on the results of a radiological examination and the condition of the patient. A surgical solution is traditional and uses clips to exclude the aneurysm from the circulation (clipping). A more modern method is the endovascular solution by filling of the aneurysm with platinum coils (coiling).

It is impossible to influence the acute phase of the SAH. The solution of the primary source of the SAH is chosen and performed. Even after successful treatment, there are still delayed and very serious complications of SAH. Most often seen are cerebral vasospasms, mineral metabolism disbalances and a development of hydrocephalus. The management of these complications is challenging, since they often produce delayed cerebral ischemia with subsequent neuropsychological impairments. The most often are disorders of speech, movement, memory, and there are also emotional and social disturbances, personality changes, or drop in IQ.

Personality changes and cognitive changes, if present, have a significant influence to everyday life of the patients. Patients after SAH thus require not only rehabilitation of motor and speech deficits, but also extensive and systematic neuropsychological care. Postoperative cognitive rehabilitation as well as crisis interventions (if needed) should start as soon as possible, and the patients should be followed in long-term aspect. The role of the neuropsychologist is of major importance in both diagnostics and postoperative care.

Chapter XIV - Cognitive functions impairment as a consequence of a head/brain injury represents a wide-ranging and heterogeneous spectrum of disorders. Seriousness of such disorders, as well as their duration and extent of recovery, depend on both the severity of the trauma itself (i.e., on a primary process) and consequent events inside the skull (i.e., on a secondary impact). In general taxonomy, severe, moderate, and mild forms of traumatic impairment are described. The severe head injuries have their structural correlates visible on CT (Computed Tomography) or MRI (Magnetic Resonance Imaging) – —it is an impaired parenchyma. The moderate and mild forms, as well as a so-called diffuse axonal impairment (DAI), do not need to have a structural finding. They can be thus even more dangerous, since such sufferers are only rarely neuropsychologically explored. Moreover, they are often not medically examined at all or they are considered as healthy and without any damage when leaving a medical institution. Incidence of mild brain injuries is ever more frequent as a result of increasing popularity of sports activities of all kinds (especially of the adrenaline ones preferred by the young generation, in which the health hazard is even higher), as well as of strong pressure of media, which emphasize that sport contributes to health maintenance. Neuropsychological evaluation of a person with a head/brain traumatic impairment usually finds deficiencies in the following areas: attention/concentration, memory/learning, and executive functions. Furthermore, also cognitive domains, such as thinking, language, visuospatial abilities, mathematics, etc., may be affected. Additional problems in emotional living and behavior (irritability, impulsiveness, apathy, loss of motivation, lack of interest in the others) can even lead tdo psychotic disorders (mania, touchiness, delusions) in some cases. Depressions and suicidal thoughts are not rare. The neuropsychological examination itself begins with a detailed interview – —with a patient, their relatives or a partner, or with their friends – —and should lead to a "holistically integrated neuropsychological evaluation" (Klonoff, Dawson, 2004). Collection of such an amount of data is necessary especially in mild forms of head and brain impairments, since a relevant medical resource may be absolutely absent (actually, from a medical point of view, the person in question does not have any damage). Subsequently, the data collection leads to a choice of diagnostic tools and a plan of neurocognitive retraining (see chapter on neuropsychological rehabilitation). Since the supply of neuropsychological tests is extensive, their selection is based mainly on the previously defined areas of cognitive functions, emotions, behavior, and personality. Responsibility for a proper diagnosis of a mild form of head impairment tends to be emphasized, for instance, in forensic proceedings regarding injury consequences, compensation of treatment expenses, etc. The examination of a person in question must be carried out by an experienced neuropsychologist, who is familiar with the subject, since a sole clinically psychological examination is only rarely sufficient and its later revision is usually very problematic. However, this domain does not tend to be properly regulated in the forensic practice.

Chapter XV - Vascular dementia (VaD) is the second most common type of dementia in elderly people, just after Alzheimer's disease (AN). Nevertheless, it is often underestimated or even neglected. However, physicians still more often draw attention to the possible increase of incidence of this disease in the future—especially due to the growing incidence of cardiovascular diseases.

Generally, vascular dementia is defined as a cognitive deficit on the basis of vascular brain disease. In order to consider such a diagnosis, we need the following evidence: reduction of cognitive abilities (neuropsychological examination), signs of vascular brain disease (imaging methods) and a causal relationship. Other etiologies must also be excluded.

In contrast to Alzheimer's disease, VaD is not a disease with a uniform clinical picture and course. The term "vascular dementia" needs to be perceived as a broad spectrum of cognitive disorders associated with vascular brain disease, of which only a part meets the general criteria of dementia. Therefore, the current effort is to replace this term with a more comprehensive name *"vascular cognitive impairment"* (VCI).

Vascular cognitive impairment is a disease that is potentially "causally" curable if diagnosed in the early stages. Hence, the principle is the *causal* approach—focused on the cause of the disease. The anti-aggregation therapy, completed with a consistent therapy of underlying vascular risk factors (especially arterial hypertension, diabetes mellitus, and hypercholesterolemia), is mainly concerned.

The role of a psychologist, except for mapping the cognitive abilities and possible personality changes, will consist of psychotherapeutic and cognitive-rehabilitation care (in cooperation with other specialists, as needed).

Chapter XVI - The aim of a medical stay of patients after traumatic head and brain injuries is their complex rehabilitation (a so-called integrative model). One of the components of such rehabilitation is represented by treatment of impaired cognitive functions. A structure of the model is situationally conditioned mainly by the size of a rehabilitation institution (here, situation in a particular institution—Army Rehabilitation Institute in Slapy nad Vltavou, Prague-West—is being described). The clinic is not primarily oriented only to the patients in question. The rehabilitation treatment is offered also to patients after other brain lesions, such as strokes, and to patients after brain operations due to various causes (tumors, aneurysms). However, the main portion of patients is represented by persons after orthopedic operations (joint replacements) and other skeleton injuries that require subsequent treatment.

Part 1. Neuropsychology in Psychiatry

In: Cognitive Deficit in Mental and Neurological Disorders ISBN: 978-1-60741-957-0
Editors: H. Kucerova, M. Preiss

Chapter I

Depression and Performance - Cognitive Performance During the Periods of Remission of Depressive Illness

Marek Preiss

Abstract

This chapter aims to offer an overview, based on our experiences as well as on evidence presented in the literature, concerning cognitive functioning of patients with unipolar depressive disorders during remission. This is a topic rarely focused on by medical and/or psychiatric care research. Neuropsychological study of depressive disorders in remission represents a fringe, yet interesting area, which interconnects possible qualitative and quantitative psychological investigations. It seems likely that future assessments of remission in depressive disorders will be multi-dimensional. Furthermore, it is possible that future multifactor assessment of remission will include the patients´ subjective views as to their quality of life. According to the statistics, approximately one-third of the depressed patients show, during the periods of remission, a significant impairment of cognition, which most likely reflects a real functional deficit. Neuropsychological deficits can, however, be fairly subtle and may not even be detected during usual psychological assessments. It seems sensible that, in this respect, we may better rely more on the patients' subjective impressions of their own abilities and performances. Older patients are in greater danger of cognitive impairment, and the clinical approach might, thus, offer a refinement of methods, enabling repeated testing of cognitive functioning during old age. It has been already established that depression with psychotic symptoms, chronic depression or onset of depression in advanced age all tend to entail more severe weakening of cognitive functions. It has, however, not been conclusively shown that neuropsychological impairment follows an increased frequency of depressive episodes or hospitalizations. It may be recommended that for the purposes of assessing cognitive functioning during remission, the patient stays in his home.

Some factors complicating objective measurement of cognitive deficit during remission are: methodologically, the Flynn effect, and from the viewpoint of the patient's actual ability, influence of the so-called brain reserve (hypothesis) or the increased performance fluctuation during episodes of illness.

At present, there is no generally accepted formal testing procedure oriented towards the neuropsychological functioning and performance of patients in remission or, for that matter, during the course of depressive episodes. By gradually refining and honing the existing psychological testing norms, and by an inclusion of demographic indicators such as age, gender and education, we can make the diagnostic procedures more sensitive to detecting an impaired and/or enhanced cognitive functioning during remission. Attempts, which suggest some directions and possibilities of cognitive rehabilitation during remission, indicate a growing interest in caring for patients during remission and not just during a period of hospitalization. Rehabilitation attempts include variety of approaches (e.g., meditation, neuropsychological rehabilitation, different versions of cognitive-behavioral therapy (CBT), approaches based on exploring brain plasticity, direct training of cognitive functions). The present state of research does not allow us to select a specific preferred approach. Future studies will increasingly explore links between cognition and neuropsychological tests. Most likely, there will be more longitudinal follow-up studies, focusing on patients´ everyday functioning and performance. There still is an unanswered question as to the premorbid performance of patients with unipolar depressive disorder. This gap contrasts with such evidence as studies concerning bipolar affective disorders or schizophrenia. One can assume that in comparison to schizophrenia, establishing a clear relationship between depressive illness in adulthood and premorbid cognitive functioning might be more problematic.

Introduction

Psychologists are used to measuring cognitive functions, which forms one of the contributions of their work within health care services. The possibility of quantification of mental/psychological capacity is important and has a number of practical implications, for example, in the evaluation of patients´ prognosis, life options, plans and ambitions. On the other end of the spectrum, it is used in making applications for disability pension and decisions as to the ending of patients' productive period of life. The degree of quantification can, however, be such that the patient may rightly feel that he is a mere object of measurements, rather than a real person, in whose inner life a psychologist has a human interest. Nevertheless, measuring plays without a doubt an important part and enables one to avoid mistakes or make unfounded assumptions about a long-term deterioration of cognitive functioning.

Perhaps the simplest method to ascertain abilities of depressive patients in remission is to simply ask them. Thus, we have asked three questions during focus group of six hospitalized patients with depressive illness: 1. How do they feel when the illness is in remission? 2. How would they evaluate their performance when they are not suffering from depression? and 3. Do feel that during the remission, some aspects of their performance are either better or worse than before the first onset of depression?

To the first question (how do they feel when the illness is in remission), we received answers such as the passing of depressive episode is perceived as a kind of liberation, if only for a while; the end of a depressive episode enables them to return to work; and that everything tends to return to a normal way of functioning. However, with the ending of depression, there also appeared to be worries about a return of the illness and other unpleasant thoughts. Answering the second question (how they perceive their performance when they are free of depression), the patients said that their performance may be completely normal, even better than usual, but also worse than before in some cases. To the third question (do they perceive that during the remission some aspects of their performance are either better or worse than before the first onset of depression), they answered that they are aware of a diminished interest from other people, that their performance compared to the time before the onset of illness has decreased, even deteriorated permanently; yet they also mention some benefits stemming from their depression—particularly a greater appreciation of their own health. The answers were, on the whole, highly idiosyncratic, and it is almost impossible to draw general conclusions on their basis. We can only hope that the following sections of this chapter will better illuminate the question of performance during remission, although the individual and subjective view will, at least for a clinical psychologist, remain more significant than any group results and their statistical analysis.

The aim of this chapter is to summarize existing knowledge and data concerning cognitive functioning of depressive patients in remission—an area in which medical and psychiatric care research has so far shown very little interest. To begin with, we wanted to examine whether there exist cognitive deficits during the period of remission (and our answer is YES), and whether an eventual cognitive impairment is not only a subjective symptom of this frequently occurring illness (and the answer is NO). The standard treatment of depression has until now shown only mild and temporary benefits (Fava et al., 2007). Yet it has become clear that depression represents a serious illness, which disrupts work capacity and performance, and that cognitive impairments are its integral part. As compared to other mental disorders (e.g., schizophrenia), it affects a much greater percentage of the population (5 to 19%). For all the people suffering from depression in the USA, the loss of working capacity has been estimated at 44 billion dollars, which is 31 billion more than for people not suffering from depression (Stewart et. al., 2003).

Average Lost Productive Time (LPT), in Hours per Week, Among US Workers With Depression and Expected LPT in the Absence of Depression, by Type of LPT and Presence of Physical Symptoms (Stewart et al., 2003; Absenteeism=sum of hours per week absent from work for a health-related reasons; Presenteeism=sum of hours per week of health-related reduce performance on workdays)

	Any Depression Mean (SE)	Major Depression	Dysthymia	Partial Remission of Recurrence of Major Depression	Expected Mean LPT in the Absence of Depression
Absenteeism	1.0	1.2	0.5	1.5	0.4
Presenteeism	4.6	7,2	3.3	5.3	1.5
Total LPT	5.6	8,4	3.3	5.3	1.5

This study ascertained the loss of work performance as a result of depression. Persons suffering from depression showed 3.7 greater estimated loss of productive work time, as compared to people not suffering from depression (on average 5.6 hours per week as compared to 1.5 hours). There was a noticeably greater prevalence of impaired work performance due to medical reasons, as opposed to work absenteeism for the same reasons.

Although the subtitle of this chapter is “Cognitive Performance during the Periods of Remission of Depressive Illness,” we will often consider also depression during its acute phase; sometimes for the sake of maintaining continuity, sometimes because the data on remission are missing. During the course of writing this book, we have considered most and foremost the possibilities of helping patients with depressive disorder (see, for example, the chapter on rehabilitation), an area that is both expanding and multifaceted. If the chapter would result in a growing interest in the period of remission following depressive episodes, we would consider our purpose to be fulfilled.

Review Studies

Three studies dealing with cognitive deficits as related to depression and its remission have been published since the beginning of this millennium: Austin et al. (2001) *Cognitive Deficits in Depression*; Marvel and Paradiso (2004) *Cognitive and Neurological Impairment in Mood Disorders*, and Roiser et al. (2006) *Neuropsychology of Mood Disorders*. Austin et al. (2001) state that their work is based on earlier assumptions—namely, that an impairment of mood, movements and cognition is merely an epiphenomenon of depressive disorder. They conclude their overview by an assertion that memory and performance impairments are a mere epiphenomenon of depressive disorder. Focusing on the relationship among motivation, affective and cognitive functions may facilitate our better understanding of links between key aspects of dorsal and ventral areas of the prefrontal cortex in the case of depressive disorders. The authors have found only very few studies focusing on the remission of depressive disorder (they name only nine such studies). They conclude that “… a residual deficit in mnemonic and executive functions appears to be seen in some patients with a history of depression.” They suggest that correlations with basic epidemiological variables, such as age, treatment methods, duration, chronic parameters of illness and number of episodes should be established with a greater degree of certainty. In a section dealing with the depth/severity and type of depression and their effects on cognitive functions, the authors quote studies in which correlations between HAMD and cognition were investigated. Eleven of these studies confirm such a relationship, but nine studies do not. Melancholic features and severity of depression correlated positively with the degree of cognitive deficit.

Marvel and Paradiso (2004) pinpoint three major categories of deficits as related to depressive disorders: attention, executive functions and memory. In the section on attention, they summarize it as follows: “…patients with mood disorders can experience measurable deficit of attention during euthymic and disturbed mood states. Because attention and working memory are cognitive functions that are integral to many types of neuropsychological tests, the interpretation of studies showing deficit in a broad range of cognitive abilities should take into account the role of poor attention /working memory capacity/ in these patients.” Their view is similar as far as executive functions are concerned. In the case of memory, they point to unimpaired abilities of depressive patients in the area of implicit memory. In their view, the impairment of attention is also supported by structural abnormalities in the dorsolateral prefrontal cortex, functional abnormality and post-mortem evidence in the same area.

Symptoms of mood disorders can be classified into three areas: psychological and vegetative, neurocognitive, and neurological. The authors emphasize their efforts to discuss state and trait changes. State characteristics, such as cognitive and neurological symptoms, can, according to them, facilitate insight into core brain abnormalities. Types of cognitive deficits are similar in bipolar and unipolar depression, and there could, thus, exist a common substrate of neuro-cognition; although the two groups of patients suffer from the clinical perspective from rather different kinds of problems.

Roiser et al. (2002) offer an overview of the cognitive function (impairments) area as related to unipolar and bipolar disorders. They state that due to progress in theoretically based cognitive tests, we can now assess various cognitive deficits with a greater sensitivity and precision. They quote as an example the Cambridge Neuropsychological Test Automated Battery (CANTAB), which allows researcher to gain better understanding of the neural basis of cognitive dysfunction through comparative manner. For unipolar depression, the profile indicates temporal and frontal dysfunctions. They recommend the use of so-called "hot" or emotion-dependent processing and "cold," or emotion-independent, processing. Cognitive impairments are good candidates for endophenotypes because they are easy to assess without the use of invasive procedures, and they fulfill many of the criteria for endophenotypes like specificity, state-independence, heritability, family association, etc.

Comparison of unipolar depressed, bipolar depressed, frontal lobe lesions and temporal lesions patients (Roiser, Rubinsztein and Sahakian, 2006)

Test	Unipolar	Bipolar	Frontal	Temporal
Pattern recognition	+	+	-	+
Spatial recognition	+	+	+	-
Simultaneous match to sample	+	-	-	-
Delayed match to sample	+	+	-	+
Tower of London	+	-	+	-
Attentional set-shifting	+	+	+	-

+, impairment, -, no impairment

On the whole, only few studies provide relatively robust evidence as to the existence of a long-term cognitive deficit during periods of remission, as compared to healthy samples of volunteers, when various aspects of cognitive functioning are compared. Furthermore, considerable methodological problems are obvious in such comparative studies, e.g., definition of remission itself, or controlling for the effects of medication; and further questions of influence of variables concerning the length and manner of assessments need to be explored, e.g., in what location they took place (during a visit in a clinic, at home or during hospitalization), or what is the effect of patient's sex on the interpretation of results. Findings related to the reversibility of eventual cognitive deficit in depression are also controversial.

Some authors have found a mild improvement of cognitive performance, others have not. Even when such improvements during remission were noted, they did not, on all parameters, reach the levels of healthy controls or those of normative standards. Moreover, questions as to the most suitable research design arise in these types of studies. The best so far appears to be a repeated testing over time (these studies usually select the beginning and the end of hospitalization period, or even measure during its course and after discharge) and a comparison with control subjects. A parallel version method in such repeated assessments seems most suitable. Further studies in this area are required. Majority opinion calls for investigation of causal relationships and for a combined use of psychological and neuroimaging methods.

The Definition of Remission

According to the International Classification of Diseases (ICD-10), a depressive condition is considered to be in remission when the patient's present state neither fulfills the criteria for depressive episode of whatever severity, nor for any other condition listed under F30-F39. In practical terms, this means that patients may suffer from sleep disturbance, loss of self-confidence and self esteem, changes in appetite for food or an unjustified sense of guilt and self-blame, lowered capacity for thinking and concentration, and recurring thoughts about death or suicide, and still be considered to be "in remission."

Full remission is defined as a relatively brief period during which an individual is asymptomatic. Asymptomatic state does not, however, mean a complete absence of symptoms, but instead, it is a condition with no more than minimal symptoms. Asymptomatic condition is defined operationally as a particular score on the depression scale (Zimmermann et al., 2006). Other constructs are also sometimes used in defining remission, such as the capacity to cope with stress, well-being, quality of life or sense of normality. Psychometrically, remission is most frequently defined in terms of a score of seven or less on the HAM-D scale (the same as HDRS-Hamilton Depression rating Scale). The HDRS scale is considered to be the "gold standard" of clinical studies (O´Donovan, 2004).

Remission and Residual Symptoms

The presence of residual symptoms during remission has, during the last decades, attracted increasing professional attention (Fava et. al., 2007). For example, Paykel and Weissman found already in 1973, interpersonal difficulties (e.g., increased tension and diminished interpersonal communication) in the case of recovered depressive patients when compared to control subjects. Other studies have shown impaired social adaptability in spite of a remission, e.g., dysfunctional attitudes and negative attribution. Residual symptoms correlate with adverse long-term course of illness and can be found even after undergoing psychotherapeutic interventions. It also appears that such residual symptoms are probably the most usual cause of relapse. Thus, improving the quality of remission may play a key role in enhancing the quality of treatment as a whole. The usual treatment of depression has so far brought only temporary and partial results. Not all the residual symptoms have, however, the same significance. The authors propose a following new *definition of cure:*

- The patient remains in full remission even after the end of treatment.
- If sub clinical signs persist, they do not constitute a significant obstacle to daily life and social adaptation.
- The patient perceives his own psychological well-being at least in one area, as specified by Ryff.
- Biological markers should be within a normal range.

The two following assumptions have been crucial in our work:

1. Quality of remission is different in the case of ambulatory as opposed to hospital treatment. Hospitalization can in itself create stress—the patient is mostly under a treatment regime, receives a range of new information about himself, and changes in medication treatment are greater.
2. In comparison, the remission achieved during the course of usual living, i.e., outside a hospital environment, is significantly more akin to the usual coping processes—the patient is usually working, living in his natural environment, which he knows, and maintains contact with his family and friends. As far as he is able to cope under such normal conditions, and the level of depressive symptoms remains under a manageable level, the quality of remission is quite different from that achieved in a hospital setting.

Our opinion in this matter has found support also among other authors. For example, Hamilton and Abramson (1983) wrote in a discussion to a study carried out already 24 years ago, which reported the absence of deviations in thinking of patients during hospital discharge, that: "we strongly recommend that future investigators assess remitted depressive's cognitive styles not only when the patients are discharged from the hospital but also after these individuals have returned to their natural environments. It is possible that the negative cognitive styles exhibited during the depressive episode may reappear as the former patients experience the stresses of life outside the hospital." Also, Haeffel et al. (2005) put forward a similar view: "In the typical remitted depression study, post episode cognitive style is measured at discharge from an inpatient setting and temporarily may be reflecting the therapeutic environment. That is, it is possible that the effects of therapy (or even the underlying causes of spontaneous remission) may suppress or deactivate participants' usual maladaptive cognitive patterns for a limited amount of time." Zimmermann et al. (2006) talked with patients about their remission, and as a result of such interviews, compiled a list of 16 potentially important items. Patients were then asked to judge the items' significance. Of the 16 items, they considered those related to mental/ psychological health (e.g., optimism, energy, self-confidence), feeling of being normal, and "being as usual," as the most important with regards to their remission.

Sources of Cognitive Deficit in Unipolar Depressive Disorder

Robert Burton (1850) wrote with regards to the treatment of melancholia: "... when its causes could not be found to begin with, the treatment was imperfect, weak and had not lead to its goal...but when the cause is removed the consequences/symptoms disappears also. I admit, nevertheless, that it is most difficult to recognize the causes and their origin, since they are so many and so varied, that we can hardly know which was the original one."

Causes of cognitive deficit are in the existing research literature treated in the form of tentative suggestions or possibilities rather than facts. We find, for example, suggestions such as, "we need a synthesis of cognitive, clinical, developmental, neurological and social-psychological knowledge and research" and/or challenges, bringing attention to the insufficient state of knowledge in this area and a need to accumulate findings over a longer period of time.

Circumplex model of depression according to Heller (1993; In: Shenal, Harrison and Demaree, 2003) divides the brain into four quadrants defined by the valenxe axis (pleasant or unpleasant) and the arousal axis (high or low). Activation/deactivation in the particular quadrants then represents/reflects different dysfunctions—left frontal, right frontal, right posterior, left posterior. Left frontal dysfunction can cause a scarcity of negative affect, right frontal emotional disregulation, lability, right posterior dysfunction a poor affect perception. There is no specific hypothesis as to the left posterior quadrant. Neurocognitive performance has been shown to be related to emotional functioning. According to these authors, the model suggests that a number of activation/deactivation patterns may result in depressive symptoms; it is suspected that many different patterns of cognitive impairment may be evidenced in depressed patients. For example, left frontal dysfunction can, apart from disturbing positive emotions, also weaken verbal fluency and planning or sequencing of more complex information. Right frontal dysfunction can disturb nonverbal fluency. These different brain regions/domains should then be, according to this model, related to specific cognitive impairments.

Schotte et al. (2006) emphasize that contemporary models of depression (e.g., the biological, cognitive, interpersonal, etc.) belong to the category of diathesis-stress model, which is based on the hypothesis that specific genetic dispositions or other characteristics, such as a particular cognitive style, biological dysfunction or problems in social skills area, can constitute a vulnerability towards depression, if the patients are confronted with a specific and stressful life situation the initial judgment processing "embark" on a course of quarrelsome, paranoid behavior.

Protective factors, such as material prosperity, adopting a less hectic or stressful lifestyle, being in good health, being raised in a warm and loving home, and having loved ones, a functioning and supportive social network, social solidarity, well-developed social skills and meaningful activities, can buffer or diminish the vulnerability to depression. Related depressive episodes are a burden for the psychobiological substrate and increase the vulnerability to depression.

Marvel and Paradiso (2004) claim that they have found that cognitive deficits can develop in the course of depressive illness and point to a study, during which the researchers followed up older patients over a period of seven years. The participants who did not have any symptoms of depression at the beginning of the study showed each consecutive year a mild weakening of cognitive functions, which seemed to be due to their natural aging. However, with each depressive symptom recorded at the onset of the study, a yearly increase of cognitive deterioration was 24%, as compared to the symptom-free subjects. Depressive symptoms at beginning of the study were also associated with a greater risk for Alzheimer's dementia. Similarly, Chamberlain and Sahakian (2004) considered only those deficits that emerged during the course of illness: "With patients with a history of affective disorders, there appear to be residual cognitive deficits, which persist even after the patients are considered clinically to have been cured." The most common residual cognitive deficits are psychomotor deceleration, disturbed visual discrimination, and impaired maintenance of attention. Such residual cognitive deficits may, in the case of patients with affective disorders, constitute the greatest obstacle to rehabilitation, similarly as has been found to be the case with schizophrenics.

Marvel and Paradiso (2004) assume a reduction of the structural and functional integrity in some areas of the brain and consider it to be a factor in the cognitive impairments in unipolar depression. They further suggest that cognitive deficits in remission are as yet not susceptible to existing forms of treatment.

Is Performance Impaired Already before the Onset of Illness?

Knowledge about the possible premorbid performance of patients with unipolar depressive disorder has a considerable significance for our better understanding of the causes of depressive illness and for clinical work. We are not certain, as yet, whether cognitive deficits develop during the course of illness or are present already before its onset.

A number of research teams have been trying to answer this question, and there exist several hypotheses, among them the following two.

- Long-lasting stress, imbalance of neurotransmitters and a whole range of other factors influence the brain of a predisposed/susceptible individual, which can disturb his brain plasticity and can, in turn, lead to a whole number of functional brain disturbances. Among them are not only cognitive impairments, but also emotional ones. Depression is thus seen as a result of brain impairment.
- Depression itself leads to brain impairment, which then causes dysfunctions of the cognitive and executive abilities.

Which of the two above hypotheses is the correct one? It would seem that they both are. While this problem has not yet been satisfactorily solved, the real life appears to be too complex to be reduced in the way that theoretical and research paradigms would attempt to do. A number of factors that influence the premorbid patient-to-be, the most powerful of which seems to be long-lasting stress, systematically weaken the brain at several levels (unbalancing neurotransmitters, causing structural and cellular changes), already before the first symptoms of depression become noticed and/or enter awareness (Sheline, 2004). The fully developed depressive illness then exerts a further destructive influence and exacerbates even more the pathological processes leading to the genesis of cognitive deficits. An additional influence, that of innate factors, needs to be added to these, since these can also cause a greater susceptibility of the brain toward the development of depression; and last but not least, the important influence of comorbid disorders can further deepen the depression, as well as the already existing cognitive problems.

While in the case of other disorders, e.g., schizophrenia, a number of studies have investigated the question of premorbid cognitive functioning (e.g., Müller et al. 2004), establishing the cognitive dysfunctions as a possible precursor of the illness, such research is still lacking in the case of the depressive disorder. A number of studies have already focused on the cognitive functioning of close relatives in the case of patients with bipolar affective disorder. Christensen et al. (2006) mention nine such studies, while stating that no such research has been published for close relatives of patients with unipolar depression. It is, however, clear that studies of this kind are important for a better understanding of biological vulnerability, both in the unipolar and bipolar depression. As far as we know, there is also no study investigating cognitive functions of persons at risk for unipolar or bipolar disorders, which would, at the same time, involve brain-imaging methods.

Christensen et. al (2006) made use of the Danish data base register, which identifies every person and utilizes also other registers, including the national psychiatric records, with information about every hospitalization and every outpatient hospital visit. The researchers used also the records of twins. From such a database, they selected a group of monozygotic twins of the same sex with a high risk for pathology, only one of whom has already been hospitalized because of affective disorder, but not the other one. The participants of this study were interviewed using a structured interview schedule designed to detect psychiatric pre-morbidity (Schedule for Clinical Assessment in Neuropsychiatry, SCAN) and were subjected to self-assessment, as well as objective assessment of depression, cognitive battery assessment (CAMCOG) and further neuropsychological tests. Hospitalizations for unipolar and/or bipolar depression during the period between 1968 and 2005 were also followed up. The monozygotic control twins had no history of hospitalization for psychiatric problems and were paired to the high-risk target twin for age, sex and zygozicisity. The results showed that the high-risk control twins had the worst cognitive performance outcomes. Regression analysis after adjustment for age, gender, education and score in BDI (Beck Depression Inventory) showed significant correlations for neuropsychological test (Trail Making Test) and the CAMCOG battery. Healthy twins who were discordant for unipolar depressive disorder had lower performance scores in virtually all the tests of cognitive functioning: selective attention and its maintenance, executive functions, speech processing, declarative memory; and when controlled for demographic variables, they also showed higher levels of sub clinical symptoms and mild pathology. The authors' interpretation of these results views the cognitive dysfunction as a non-specific marker for affective disorders as a whole. They explain the cognitive deficit by relating performance to the integrity of the white brain matter and a disturbed HPA, particularly due to the effects of cortisol on cognitive functions.

Airaksinen et al. (2007) investigated depression over a three-year period in a normal population sample (N=708), ranging between 20 and 64 years of age. Their first data collection measured episodic memory, demographic and socioeconomic variables, abuse of alcohol, anxiety and depression. The results showed that participants who scored up to the 25th percentile range on three memory parameters had an increased risk for depressive illness three years later (after controlling for differences in demographics, socioeconomics, alcohol use and anxiety level). The authors considered episodic memory as a premorbid marker of depression.

Zammit et al. (2008) studied the role played by premorbid intellectual ability in later incidence of severe psychological disorders—such as schizophrenia, bipolar disorders (meaning the depressive type and manic-depressive psychosis) and other psychotic illnesses. They used a group of 50,087 Swedish men conscripted for compulsory military training at the ages of 18 to 20. The conscripts underwent a psychological assessment that measured intelligence using a non-standardized test battery, which consisted of four subtests (verbal IQ, visuospatial ability, general knowledge and mechanical ability) and which enabled a location of IQ scores along a nine-point scale, representing nine levels of intelligence. Twenty-seven years later, these authors used the Swedish national census to examine all cases of recorded psychiatric hospitalizations occurring during the intervening years within the original conscript sample. This showed that 113 participants had been hospitalized for depression (manic-depressive psychoses, depressive type ICD 8: 296.0, 296.2, 298.0; ICD-9: 296.1, 298.0) during those 27 years. One hundred and seventeen participants had been hospitalized for severe depressive disorder, and low IQ increased the likelihood of this disorder to 1.19. In addition to severe depression, premorbid IQ was also associated with a risk for schizophrenia (OR 1.26), schizoaffective disorders and other psychotic conditions but not with bipolar disorders. This is the first longitudinal study concerned with severe depression. The authors emphasize that the performance IQ is more strongly associated with the risk for depression than verbal IQ. One comment made in the discussion referred to the possibility that people with lower IQ are more likely to be hospitalized (with the exception of patients with bipolar disorders, in whom the opposite seems to be the case). The results suggest that the causes of bipolar and other affective disorders may be of different kind. This study did not, however, explore the unipolar depressive disorder. In a longitudinal study, Block et. al (1991) investigated the relationship between developmental measures (measured by the CES-D-Centre for Epidemiological Studies Depression Scale) and proclivity to depression in a sample of 88 (46 girls) adolescents; the measures were taken at 3, 4, 5, 7,11, 14 and 18 years of age. Wechsler Preschool and Primary Scale of Intelligence (WPPSI) was administered to the children at four years of age. The total WPPSI scores did not correlate significantly with subjectively assessed depressive symptoms at 18 years of age for girls (0.25, n.s.), but this correlation was statistically significant for boys (-0.36, p=0.04). The gender correlation difference suggests that lower IQ poses an increased danger for depression in boys but not in girls. However, the authors point out that such an indication, i.e., that more intelligent girls on the one hand and the less clever boys on the other hand tend to be at a greater risk for depression, is still rather speculative. Most likely, the explanation could lie in the difference between the boys' and the girls' gender roles and perceptions—such as e.g., that more intelligent girls become increasingly aware of potential problems, which they may encounter in future life as well as the various criteria by which they may be judged. Less intelligent boys are likely to receive relatively more negative feedback, may try to better themselves, yet not effectively enough, which in turn could lead to increasing anger and frustration. There were also found significant positive correlations between the girls' cognitive measures, such as fluency of expression, ability to concentrate, attention and negative reaction to stress (a tendency to become unproductive and immobilized) at three to four years of age, and their disposition towards depression when 18 years old. The boys' measures of competitiveness at three to four years of age, transience of their relationships and a poor ability to admit their own feelings or excessive reactions to frustration, showed significant correlations with depressive tendencies at the age of 18 years.

Cui et al. (2007) published an article entitled *Does Depression Precede or Follow Executive Dysfunction? Outcomes in Order Primary Care Patients.* The authors argue that the understanding of the cognitive dysfunctions in depression is important in both elucidating the pathogenesis of this illness and in enabling more specifically focused interventions. Cognitive impairment can contribute to depression and/or the depression may precede cognitive deficits as an early sign of brain impairment. Research findings so far have supported the first hypothesis, i.e., that cognition, and particularly executive functions, plays a crucial role in the genesis of geriatric depression. The authors focused on the area of primary care, since a large number of old people do not seek out psychiatric help. They put forward two hypotheses: (1) depressive disorder and symptoms predict subsequent decline in selected components of executive functioning (measured by Mattis Dementia Rating Scale and other tests), and (2) executive dysfunction predicts subsequent depressive outcome. In a prospective study, the authors examined several hundred people aged 65 years or more and followed this sample over a period of two years. No cognitive measure was significantly independently associated with depression diagnosis.

Ormel et al. (2004) studied psychosocial deficits in a large sample of normal population (N=4796). Structured interview (CIDI) was administered to these participants, designed to identify a majority of neurotic symptoms, including depression. A great advantage of this study was that the authors were able to carry out three assessments on one part of this large sample still in their premorbid period, i.e., before the onset of the first episode of depression. The identification of the psychosocial disabilities by means of the interview focused on four areas: partner relationships, employment, housework and leisure time. In the interview, the participants were asked to evaluate their own behavior in a way in which they imagined a person close to them would do. Participants who later developed depression were compared to the ones who had not. The results pointed to:

1. "Trait Effect"—i.e., the participants who later became ill with depression showed significantly higher psychosocial disability scores during the premorbid assessment than those not touched by depression (effect size 0.42 to 0.47; effect size 0.2 is indicative of a small effect, 0.5 a medium and 0.8 a large effect size).
2. "State Effect"—subjects who had depression but were presently in remission had higher psychosocial disability scores than the depression-free participants.
3. "Scare Effect"—disability that was not present before the MDE but developed during the episode and lasted beyond recovery was, however, not confirmed by this study.

The authors interpret the results in terms of two independent processes: the influence of psychosocial disability during the premorbidity period on the development of depression and the concurrent effect of the relationship between depressive symptoms and the psychosocial disability. According to this study, psychosocial impairments can be found and recognized already long before the onset of depression and long after its genesis.

Judd et al. (2008) followed a group of 371 patients with unipolar depressive disorder over a period of 10 years. Trained observers evaluated the patients at half-yearly intervals, using the LIFE (Longitudinal Interval Follow-up Evaluation). Two basic dimensions were assessed: work and partner relationship. The authors interpreted the results with reference to enduring and chronic course of illness, which nevertheless changes when the patient is symptom free. The work-related scale had the following six values: 1—no impairment, high level of functioning; 2—no impairment, satisfactory level; 3—mild impairment; 4—moderate impairment; 5—severe impairment; 6—did not do this all during the period because of depressive psychopathology. The average score level of the asymptomatic patients was 1.7; of those with sub clinical signs, it was 2.6; of those with mild depressive symptoms, it was 2.5; and the average of patients with unipolar disorder was 4.7. The authors also explored the influence of the patients' state ("state effect"). The results show the differences between the premorbid stage and during an episode, as obtained within a group of patients with the first depressive episode (N=85) and show clearly that the homework performance is relatively least affected, while the ability to utilize leisure time is affected the most.

Study of Christensen et al. (2006), Zammit et al. (2008) and Airaksinen et al. (2007) point to an impairment of executive functions/performance (the healthy twin sample), to premorbid impairment of intelligence (the conscript sample) and to the weakening of episodic memory (normal population), as being risk factors in the genesis of depressive disorders. Three studies, looking at this area from different points of view, have demonstrated that cognitive impairment can appear already before the first onset of the illness. The authors of the first study interpret their results by suggesting that the cognitive impairment can be a nonspecific marker for affective disorders. Block et al. (1991), however, question the possibility of premorbid impairment by pointing to the findings of different characteristics of boys and girls, where the assumption of the impairment of cognitive functions holds only for boys; while for girls, the higher intelligence scores correlate positively with depressive symptoms. The study by Block et al. (1991) is not based on a diagnosis, but on a tendency towards depressive symptoms (as measured by a self-assessment scale) and is thus more remote from the direct and objective measurements of cognitive deficit. Similarly, the study by Ormel et al., (2007) discovered, in addition to a loss of productive time during a period of partial remission, also a psychosocial disability (not measured by neuropsychological tests) present prior to the onset of depressive illness. Study of older depressive patients by Cui et al. (2007), which utilized a direct measurement of cognitive functions, did not find a relationship between patients in primary care and a later depression. It seems likely that for investigating the levels of performance (not only loss of productive work time or psychosocial disability) studies using neuropsychological methods will be required.

Clinical Factors, which Influence Cognitive Performance of Patients with Depression

Influence of Mood on Cognitive Functions

The question whether cognitive functions are related to mood have been repeatedly investigated in the case of the Alzheimer's disease. However, there seems to be no consensus as to the strength of the relationship between cognitive impairments and mood states (anxiety, depression), and information and understanding of this relationship is important to clinicians, as well as for personnel care. Bierman et al. (2007) studied a large sample (N=1562) of older subjects from the normal population as a part of a Longitudinal Aging Study Amsterdam

(LASA) and a sample of individuals with Alzheimer's diagnosis (N=66). The researchers controlled for the occurrence of depressive disorders in these two groups of participants who were also assessed by MMSE and categorized into quartiles according to the level of the longitudinal measures/functions, defined as good (N = 395), average (N = 394), moderate (N = 389) or poor (N = 384). Concurrently, the researchers were tracking the participants' mood by means of self-reports concerning depression (measured by CES-D) and anxiety (measured by HADS-A). The authors noted that MMSE is extremely sensitive to age and education, and thus, they used MMSE that was adjusted for both of these two variables. The results showed that depression and anxiety increased with the level of cognitive impairment. The anxiety symptom measures of individuals whose cognitive functioning fell into the first quartile were 8.6%; of those in the second quartile, 8.1%; of those in the third quartile, 11.8%; and of those in the fourth quartile, 10.7%. The anxiety symptoms measure was 6% in the Alzheimer's group. While the between-group differences on the anxiety measures were not significant, the prevalence of depressive symptoms differed significantly. Participants whose cognitive measures were within the first quartile had depressive symptom score of 8.9%; those in the second quartile, 11.4%' those in the third, 22.1%; and those in the fourth 21.1%. The depression score of the Alzheimer's patients was 16.7%. The authors of the study concluded that a weakening of cognitive functions follows a trend towards a growing prevalence of anxiety, comorbiding with anxiety and depression, and towards the depressive symptoms proper.

With depressive patients in remission, Kessing (1988) found the following correlations: between BDI-21 and MMSE - 0.16, between BDI-21 and CAMCOG –0.13, and between BDI-21 and Mattis Dementia Scale -.07. Porter et al. (2003) found correlations between HRSD-17 and various parameters of RAVLT between -0.30 and - 0.38. Gallagher et al. (2007) correlated HDRS-17 with several domains of cognitive functioning, but found no significant relationships for either patients in remission or the others who were not in remission (-0.220 and 0.057). Our own study (Preiss et al., 2009) showed also only non-significant correlations between various neuropsychological measures and mood. It is conceivable that under certain circumstances, higher cognitive processes and emotions involve completely distinct systems. On the other hand, some research studies have suggested a rather close relationship between emotional and cognitive functioning. The fairly low, yet statistically significant, correlations obtained in some studies go some way to support the latter hypothesis.

Types of Depression and Cognitive Deficits

In the *Anatomy of Melancholy*, Robert Burton writes that "it matters only little what doctors say in their books about the various kinds, since in the patient's body are all these kinds thoroughly mixed…and it is extremely unclear how to distinguish the various types and to reach some clarity in this thicket of circumstances and variations, since only rarely do we find two patients who will suffer with the same disease per omni, that is in all its facets….but at last I will somehow extricate myself from this labyrinth of doubts and errors and penetrate to the very causes of melancholia."

Fairly little is still known about the influence of various subtypes of depression on the cognitive performance. Attempts at comparing endogenous and exogenous types of depression have encountered theoretical, methodological and practical problems. With the endogenous depression, findings point to rather serious deficits of cognitive functioning. Also successful were studies looking at differences in cognitive functioning/performance, comparing depressive patients with and without psychotic symptoms. These showed that the patients with psychotic symptoms reach significantly poorer cognitive performance than those without psychotic signs in all the assessed areas, e.g., verbal and non-verbal memory, attention/vigilance and cognitive flexibility (Basso and Bornstein, 1999; Schatzberg et al., 2000). Most frequently, the differences appeared on tests concerned with vigilance/attention and psychomotor speed (e.g., in the Trail Making Test, Continuous Performance Test or in Stroop Test). Psychotic depression lasts usually longer, does not respond as well to treatment and is often accompanied by structural abnormalities of the brain, as well as by a greater atrophy of the cortex. Fleming et al. (2004) arrived at interesting findings as a result of their meta-analysis of studies, comparing the cognitive performance of depressive and schizophrenic patients. Depressive patients with psychotic symptoms tended to have the same profile of cognitive functioning as the patients with schizophrenia, while the depressed patients without psychotic comorbidity scored significantly higher on neuropsychological tests.

Patients with chronic depressive illness have shown more severe deficits in cognitive functions (Riso et. al, 2003); the difference is to be found in the degree of the impairment rather than in its kind. It is assumed that the impairments in judgment functions could lead to the formation of maladaptive mental constructs, which in turn lead to maladaptive thinking and beliefs. A theme in its own right could also be the cognitive performance of patients with the bipolar illness. Unipolar depression has been in recent years often compared to the depressive phase of the bipolar condition. It has been shown that patients with the bipolar depression exhibit poorer results on neuropsychological tests, especially on those measures that are sensitive to the impairment of frontal cortical lobes (Chowdhury et al. 2003). It is also of interest that such cognitive deficits correlate with the duration of illness only in the patients with unipolar depression. It could be that this reflects different genetic as well as developmental mechanisms of these two illnesses. Neuropsychological deficit was occasionally observed also in some bipolar patients during the manic phase of the illness (Clark et. al., 2001). However, in view of the fact that, for example, intentional impairments are directly related to manic symptoms, it is impossible to draw any meaningful conclusions from such findings, at least without further research. Studies show, nevertheless, that it makes sense to investigate cognitive performance of patients with bipolar affective dysfunction, since it has been shown that while about 97% of these patients improve in the clinical sense as a result of treatment, only 37% reach a full functional recovery (Tohen et. al, 2000).

Medication

An important factor, which affects the results of neuropsychological studies, is medication. It is precisely the use of antidepressants that constitutes one of the limits in the interpretation of neuropsychological test findings. The question arises as to what extent is the measured cognitive deficit caused by the illness itself, and to what extent is it due to the medication used in the treatment? The influence of medication is generally considered to be an intervening variable. Since many antidepressants contain an anticholinergic substance, which can influence cognitive functions, comparisons and interpretations of studies that include patients on medication, or not, should be done with great care (Tancer et. al, 1989). Antidepressant medication tends to improve cognitive functioning. The two mechanisms considered to be responsible for this are: 1) the pharmacological effect on the receptor system and 2) secondary effect due to the improvement of the depression itself (Kopecek, 2006). It is generally assumed that the traditional tricyclic antidepressants disturb cognitive functions, especially memory and psychomotor tempo, more than the new generation of antidepressants (IMAO, SSRI). Depressive patients are often, besides antidepressants, given also an additional medication from the benzodiazepine group, in order to improve their sleep and attenuate anxiety. Benzodiazepine medication can, as a consequence of its sedative effect, cause memory impairment and slow down the cognitive performance in particular. While several studies have investigated the effects of antidepressants on cognitive performance of patients with depression, such effects with regard to the benzodiazepines remain rather unclear. Several studies have investigated the effects of antidepressant treatment on cognitive performance of depressive patients, in order to better understand the parameters of such influence. For example, Ravnkilde et. al (2002) attempted to minimize the influence of medication on cognitive performance profiles of depressive patients by comparing a sample of patients who were on medication only for a short period with patients who used medication for prolonged periods. Their results showed no significant difference between the two groups, from which the authors concluded that the influence of treatment with antidepressants on cognitive performance is negligible.

In order to entirely eliminate the possible influence of medication on cognitive functioning, Porter et al. (2003) carried out a study in which they explored differences between a sample of non-medicated depressive patients and a group of comparable healthy volunteers. The research found a number of neuropsychological deficits in various areas of functioning of the depressive patients, as compared to the healthy participants. Especially, they showed impairments of memory, executive functions and visual-spatial abilities, as well as of attention. Their motor and psychomotor functions remained, however, unimpaired. Severity of depression correlated with the patients´ ability to learn and performance on memory tests, but not with their executive functions. The authors speculated that the executive deficit may be seen as a stable trait marker, while memory functions appear to depend on the patient's clinical condition. A study by Weiland-Friedler (2004) showed similar results with non-medicated patients in remission. On the other hand, Pardo et al. (2006) didn't find any differences between non-medicated patients and controls, but their sample was very small (N=9). It would seem that despite the generally recognized influence of antidepressants on cognitive functioning, signs of impaired cognitive functioning appear also in patients who are not taking medication.

Hospitalization

It seems that hospitalization is an important factor in determining performance on neuropsychological tests. Studies in general conclude that differences exist between groups of inpatients and outpatients. We might think that impaired cognitive performance in hospitalized patients relates to the fact that people with more severe symptomathology are hospitalized. Nevertheless, Elliot et al. (1998) found a significant difference in the performance of hospitalized patients and outpatients, despite the fact that the groups did not differ in levels of depressive symptomatology. Purcell et al. (1997) used the same test battery in a group of inpatients and found less global impairment than Elliot. It was interesting to find that patients with a history of hospitalization had worse results than those without such a history. We suggest two possible explanations for these results. The first is that neuropsychological impairment is an important indicator for the need of hospitalization. Secondly, factors related to hospitalization affect cognitive deficits. One of such factors could be differences in treatment regimens. This might cause a wide range of impacts. Neuropsychological assessment is an ideal strategy for obtaining collaborative data in a psychiatric population due to the presumed absence of self-report bias (Fleming, Blasey and Schatzberg, 2004).

Aging

Robert Burton in *Anatomy of Melancholy* writes that "natural melancholia is an almost inseparable accompaniment of old age, but a pathological melancholia is much more common in middle-aged individuals…and thus nobody is safe and it makes no exception, no matter what temperament, life condition, age or gender." The greatest frequency of psychopathology, such as neurosis, addictions, schizophrenia, is found in the young to middle age bracket, while after the 45 years of age, prevail affective disorders, and among them the most frequent is depressive illness. Psychotic episodes of unipolar and also bipolar depression only very rarely appear for the first time after 65 year of age (Bastecky et. al., 1994). All forms of affective disorders in seniors can be complicated by somatic illnesses. Such complications affect not only the course of illness, but also change its clinical picture. It would appear that depressive symptoms do not worsen during old age. And if depression persists, it tends to be experienced increasingly through various somatic symptoms. A precondition for a positive prognosis of depression in old age is a good physical health and an absence of pronounced neurotic features in a patient's history (Bastecký et al., 1994)

Generally, it seems safe to assume that the depressive patients' cognitive performance will deteriorate with growing age. Yet foremost, it is important to differentiate between individuals, who have been suffering from depression most of their lives and those whose depressive illness appeared first at a later age. With the former group of patients, cognitive performance is most strongly influenced by the length of the illness duration, apart from other factors and the patient's chronological age. With the latter group, a whole range of possible comorbiding conditions have an effect, as already mentioned above. Most prominent among these seem to be brain disorders and circulatory disease. These have been shown as frequent comorbidity factors in depression, but they can also lead to impairments of cognition in their own right.

In view of the relatively short history of cognitive performance research with depressive patients, we are not as yet in a position to state precisely whether the fact that a person has suffered from depression all his life has had a significant influence on his cognitive functioning in the old age. We can assume this to be the case, but without longitudinal studies lasting many years, we cannot make conclusive claims. It has been shown that long-lasting stress impairs brain plasticity; on the other hand, it can be assumed that treatment of depression leads to a recovery of the lost plasticity (Vavrusová, 2004). However, we do not as yet know enough about the effects of such repeated fluctuations during repeated episodes of depression.

Differences in the cognitive functioning of chronic and acute patients have been demonstrated by Riso et. al (2003), but the factor of aging had not been controlled for in this research. So far, it has been established that chronic patients do significantly worse on neuropsychological tests. The longest lasting longitudinal study so far has investigated, over a period of 12 years, the relationships between depression and later cognitive functioning (Cervilla et. al, 2000). It showed that a significant correlation between depression and the impairment of cognition can be seen only in male participants. A weakness of this study was its failure to account for other possible factors, which could have influenced the final results. The possibility that this was not a true causal relationship cannot be, however, excluded, since men suffer much more often with illnesses, which themselves can impair their cognitive functioning (e.g., vascular). This possibility is supported by the fact that the mean age of participants included in the study was almost 70 years. Yet, this, at the same time, devalues the conclusions, which we would have liked to draw about the influence of depression on cognitive performance and by implication about the effects of aging.

In old age, there is a growing number of possible etiopathological factors related to depression. Among the most prominent—apart from the loss of sense of life's meaning, loneliness and grieving—belong a number of diseases, which not only increase the risk of depression, but often actually cause it. Both clinically and through research findings, an organic depressive condition has already been established in patients with vascular brain stroke, Parkinson's disease, or epilepsy (Anders et al., 2001). This is also the reason why for old people a connection is often drawn between their cognitive deficit in depression and other serious illnesses. Research has most frequently been focused on the mutual influence between depression and dementia. And it has shown that depression represents a risk factor in the genesis of dementia and has a significant effect on poor prognosis of patients with dementia (Butters et. al., 2000).

The progress of mild cognitive deficit in older depressive patients has also been investigated. O'Brien et al. (2004) tracked changes in cognitive functioning, using a detailed battery of tests on a sample of 40 healthy individuals and in a sample of 40 subjects with a depressive impairment diagnosis, during the acute period of illness and after six months of treatment. In addition, a subgroup of depressive patients (N=26) who were in remission (remission being defined here by a score of less than 8 on MADRS) was also investigated. The healthy and the depressive participants were matched on age, sex, social class and education. The results revealed a significantly poorer cognitive performance in the depressed patients at the onset of illness, as compared to the normal controls, on a number of neuropsychological measures. At the same time, only slight differences were found between the patients examined after six months in remission (despite the fact that their level of depression decreased significantly) and those who were not in remission. A lasting cognitive impairment was found in a number of parameters, but the depressive patients improved after the six months on some parameters (which was interpreted as a combination of the effects of practice and familiarity with the assessment procedures). The authors found that 41 % of the depressive participants fulfilled the criteria for a mild cognitive impairment (according to Petersen et al., 2002, mild cognitive impairment = performance on the Auditory Verbal

Learning Test that is lower than 1.5 SD bellow the norm). Further findings showed that the depressed patients suffered form *hypercortisolemia,* as measured by a heightened level of cortisol in the patients' saliva. These levels returned back to normal after six months. Finally, the depressive patients had also, according to MRI examination, smaller right hippocampus.

Number of Depressive Episodes and the Duration of Illness

Paelecke-Habermann et al. (2005) refer to a study by Kessing (1998), suggesting that repeated episodes of depression lead to a greater cognitive impairment, as compared to patients who suffered only one episode. In their own study, they found that patients who suffered three episodes of depression showed a greater impairment of cognitive functions, as measured by a number of tests, than patients who had only one to two such episodes. Kessing (1988) found that euthymic unipolar and bipolar patients showed a greater impairment than patients, who had only one episode, or control participants. In this study, the subgroup of unipolar and bipolar patients with more than one episode, scored lower on MMSE than 24 points in 16.2 % and 14.3.% respectively, while the sample of patients with one episode only in 4% of cases. All controls had MMSE scores within the norm, i.e., above 24 points. The duration of the illness, however, showed no correlation with the cognitive measures in this study. Oldenhinkel et. al (2003) found no differences between persons with one or more episodes, and their results, thus, do not support the hypothesis concerning cumulative effects of increasing vulnerability. Their sample contained 26 older participants in remission and 96 controls. Neu et al. (2005), in a study with 27 patients, found no correlation between performance on cognitive tests, number of hospitalizations, age at the onset of illness and the number of episodes.

Severity of Cognitive Deficits

Biringer et al. (2005) found among the very few researchers, who report a recovery to premorbid levels of cognitive functioning, where z-scores of the patients (based on a comparison with control subjects) ranged from +0.3 to -0.61. The worst results came on the Stroop test and the best on non-preservative scores of WCST. After the treatment, the patients´ average z-score was –0.24, while before the treatment it was –0.55. Paelecke-Habermann et al. (2005) found a significant deficit in the area of attention, as compared to control participants (Cohen d = 0.42–0.97) and of executive functions (maximum -1.4, minimum 0.15). According to Kessing (1998), the cognitive deficit becomes more severe with every consecutive episode by 0.2 units on CAMCOG and MATTIS. According to Paradiso et al. (1997), z-scores of patients with unipolar depression in remission, as compared to controls, ranged from -0.7 to 0.1. As is clear from the above findings, in no case were the deficits greater than 1 SD bellow the norm, while the 1 SD mark is considered to be clinically significant.

Christensen et al. (1997) pooled 154 studies with depressive patients and utilized 172 separate comparisons with control participants (831 effect sizes). Effect size was calculated according to the outcomes of the depressive patients, as compared to the controls. Positive values represent comparisons, in which the controls did better than the patients. This paper summarizes the influence of depressive illness on performances on the most commonly used psychological tests.

Clinical Problems in Assessing and Interpreting Cognitive Functions of Remitted Depressive Disturbances

The measurement of cognitive deficit in depressive impairments in remission is complicated by several factors. Comparisons usually involve mean values of the samples of patients and often reach a given level of significance, yet their practical implications and use are highly problematic.

One of the limitations in assessing individuals is the fact that even a relatively small deficit can be significant (e.g., 0.2 SD).

Psychologists are usually satisfied with an interpretation of performance within the norm according to age (+/- 1SD), and as long as the performance is within normal range, the tendency is also to describe them as being "normal". Subtle deviations, especially decreases in performance, may thus not be recognized.

When no quantitatively impaired performance is found, psychologists may have a tendency to interpret results of the assessment as objectively normal, while judging an eventual inconsistent and negative self-perception of the patient as being exaggerated or inappropriate. Nevertheless, this may not correspond to the real condition and state of the patient. For a more objective assessment, tests measuring basic cognitive functions, such as attention/vigilance or working memory, as well as instruments for ascertaining qualitative aspects of performance, would be appropriate.

According to the Flynn effect (Flynn, 1987) IQ increases on average by 0.3 points per year, which means by three points in a decade. This has an influence on the normative criteria of psychological tests, and Flynn also points out that this implies a need to repeatedly review such test norms. The Flynn effect can have a considerable impact on the interpretation of cognitive test results. In particular, it makes it more difficult to establish cognitive impairments in the more educated and intelligent individuals. The Brain Reserve Hypothesis (Christensen et al., 2008) is an influential hypothesis in neurology and cognitive science. Briefly stated, the hypothesis is that high premorbid intelligence, education, an active, stimulating lifestyle, or a physically larger brain provide reserve capacity that protects the individual from the negative effects of aging and disease of brain function.

By the term "inconsistency" (Hultsch et al., 2005) are meant fluctuations (increased variability) in the context of an individual's performance during one session, or over several measurements (hours, days, weeks). The phenomenon "inconsistency" is commonly related to the reliability of measuring instruments, but it can also represent a constant feature of an individual, as reflected in various cognitive or somatic variables. It is calculated by means of standard deviation, sometimes by transforming it to weighted scores, and methodologically also by limiting the effects of practice (i.e., by repeated practice until the performance over the successive repetitions does no longer increase). Hutsch et. al (2005) found that the inconsistency in cognitive and physical performance is greater in older, as compared to younger individuals; and that it is also greater in patients with neurological impairments, even during the period of preclinical signs of the depressive illness, as compared to individuals with no neurological impairments. Such differences among individuals in the level of inconsistency rate are "consistent and stable" and are observed across number of cognitive and somatic domains. According to these authors, a heightened inconsistency is related to the more impaired levels of performance on cognitive and intelligence tests, and also to an approaching death in patients with cardiovascular disorders. It is possible that patients with depressive disorder in remission perform less consistently than their healthy peers, and that precisely such fluctuations, though relatively small, are a particular marker of their disorder.

Measurement of Cognitive Deficits

There are many ways of measuring cognitive performance, and it is primarily up to the examining clinical psychologists, which test they choose. As far as we know, there is no obligatory or even preferred method for assessing depressive patients. Individual researchers (Reppermund et al., 2007; Gallagher et al., 2007; Williams et al., 2000; Deuschle et al., 2004; Clark et al., 2005; Pardo et al., 2006; Weiland-Fiedler et al., 2004; Neu et al., 2005; Marcos et al., 2005; Ravnkvilde et al., 2002; Fleming et al., 2004; Basso et al., 1999; Paradiso et al., 1997; Porter et al., 2003; Kessing et al., 1998; Paelecke-Habermann et al., 2005; Airaksinen et al., 2006; Fennig et al., 2002; Biringer et al., 2005) have used many different kinds of psychological tests.

Nevertheless, during the selection of tests and the interpretation of their results, several rules need to be adhered to:

1. Tests should be relatively short and not too demanding/exhausting for the patient. For example, classical Bourdon test can generally reveal interesting information about error-making and psychomotor speed, but for a person suffering from depression, it is far too demanding.
2. The tests should cover at least the following domains: attention/vigilance, learning capacity and memory. It is often not possible to carry out a complex neuropsychological assessment due to the patient's state, yet it is necessary to ascertain the state of the most frequently impaired functions. Apart from the affected attention, memory and learning functions, a reason for the poorer performance can be also a slower psychomotor speed; this needs to be taken into account when interpreting results.
3. It is also important to evaluate the assessment procedures qualitatively. A considerable level of fluctuation during the course of assessment is typical for depressive patients. In the beginning, they often perform within a normal range, but gradually, their performance shows a considerable deterioration and/or fluctuation.
4. Results need to be interpreted very carefully, as the patients´ performance has a tendency towards pronounced fluctuation resulting from a number of factors, such as immediate mental state, fatigue, motivation, etc. Thus, it is desirable to make such assessments over a longer period of time. Although the existing research frequently

confirms impaired cognitive performance during the period of remission, it would be premature to draw any definitive conclusions as to the patients´ prognosis.

Which specific tests should then be considered in a view of the above criteria? They should certainly include methods currently used in neuropsychological diagnostics, in order to make comparisons with reference groups possible. We should also give priority to tests that have a verified/validated alternative form (Reischies and Neu, 2000).

Rehabilitation and Psychotherapy

Mundt (2002) emphasized the growing importance of health psychology and adaptation in the treatment of depression and its residual symptoms, which are considered to be a significant predictor of relapse. At present, there are, however, no specific neuropsychological rehabilitation procedures for treating cognitive deficits in depression. Most attention has been focused on psychotherapeutic approaches. During the rehabilitation using neuropsychological methods, it is possible to proceed in the three following steps:

1. To find out, best by means of repeated assessments, whether the cognitive deficit in depression exists also on the neuropsychological level; that is on the level measurable by neuropsychological tests. And, thus, to establish whether one is dealing with an objective/measurable phenomenon or merely a subjective impression of an impaired performance. Nevertheless, even the latter alternative should be considered important.
2. In case that a cognitive deficit has been found, efforts should be made to find ways how best to compensate for the impaired capacity (e.g., patient, suffering even during remission with minor problems in the area of verbal memory, can be encouraged to use various notes).
3. To adjust psychotherapy to the patient's cognitive deficits, which can then be repeatedly assessed.

The Mindfulness-Based Stress Reduction (MBSR) (Smith et al., 2007) is a combination of cognitive-behavioral therapy and a modification of Buddhist meditation, and is suitable for older people. This therapeutic approach has been developed by Kabat-Zinn (the original reference with the title *Full Catastrophe Living: How to Cope with Stress, Pain and Illness Using Mindfulness Meditation* is from 1990) in the Massachusetts General Hospital, in the form of eight sessions directed towards enhancing attention/mindfulness and awareness of one's own psychic processes by means of repeated mediation exercises.

Paelecke-Habermann et al. (2006) advocate the use of "neurocognitive training" with depressive patients, similarly as in the case of other groups of patients, e.g., schizophrenics. They propose an extension of antidepressant therapy or CBT by training of attention and executive functions, especially for patients with diagnosed impairments in relation to their premorbid state. A need for such training is based on results of their own study with depressive patients during the period of remission. The actual nature/content of their training is, however, not described.

The idea of a training program for aging populations, which exploit our knowledge of brain functioning, is presented by Mahncke et al. (2006). The authors present the initial results of a study with 41 participants (active training for 60 minutes a day, 5x week, over eight weeks period) in comparison with a control group (N=16). The controls, who followed educational materials presented through the same computers, were contacted at the onset of the study, but underwent no direct education or training. The first results look promising.

In: Cognitive Deficit in Mental and Neurological Disorders ISBN: 978-1-60741-957-0
Editors: H. Kucerova, M. Preiss

Chapter II

Eating Disorders

Hana Papezova and Svetlana Zuchova
Supported by VZ 0021620816

Abstract

Eating disorders include mainly anorexia nervosa (AN) and bulimia nervosa (BN) and their atypical forms. The spectrum of eating disorders also includes psychogenic overeating and night overeating connected with obesity. Lifelong prevalence in women is 0.5 to 3.7% in AN, and 1.1 to 4.2% in BN according to the selected criteria. The results of studies dealing with the impairment of cognitive functions in patients suffering from eating disorders differ depending on the studied subdiagnosis, phase of the disease (severely affected patients in acute phase of the disease, chronic patients, patients in remission) and on specific functions that are in the centre of authors‘ attention and selected tests. Patients with eating disorders have manifested slowed reaction time and disorders of short-term visual memory and recollection-based long-term memory. Particularly female AN patients have disrupted capacity to solve three-dimensional tasks where they are supposed to reproduce a complex figure, supplement missing parts of the picture and analyze spatial disposition. Vigilance and memory are focused on a narrow areas of eating and body proportions. One of the specific characteristics of patients with eating disorders is the distorted body perception (it is the most significant in patients with AN) connected with the disorder of interoception. As consistently described in the literature, patients suffering from eating disorders have also manifested the change in pain perception. The research focuses on connections between these changes and lower hormone levels and also specific cognitive features that are responsible for impaired perception of inner feelings and body scheme. Based on the combination of neuropsychological tests and magnetic resonance, several studies investigated relations between structural changes and cognitive deficits. In anorexia nervosa, the brain atrophy can be detected by imaging methods as soon as a few months after the onset of the disease. However, correlations between structural and the described functional disorders were weak. The studies using functional imaging methods (SPET, PET and fMRI) have shown that there is a lower blood flow in patient's brain, neurons consume less glucose and electric response to standard impulses is slowed down. The reduced perception and cognitive flexibility is described in patients with AN. It is very difficult for these patients to use alternately various cognitive strategies, to perceive various impulses and to do various tasks at a time (the so-called multitasking). Also observed was an excessive focus on detail upon concurrent insufficient perception of the whole. In recent years, batteries of test have been used that are specifically focused on this type of damage, and there exists a system of tasks used in patients' rehabilitation. The questions remain to what extent structural and functional disorders in patients with eating disorders disappear after the patients regain weight, or to what extent they persist even after their recovery, or whether these characteristics are connected with the disease or whether they are permanent features of such patients. The examination of cognitive functions should be first of all a part of clinical assessment of the disease prognosis and one of the criteria upon decision-making whether to recommend the patient for work or invalidity.

1. Introduction

Eating disorders are described as a continuum of pathological eating behavior that is conditioned biologically, psychologically and socially as well as multifactorially. The most significant nosological units are anorexia nervosa (AN) and bulimia nervosa (BN), their atypical forms. The spectrum of eating disorders includes atypical forms of AN and BN, psychogenic overeating and night overeating often connected with obesity. Development, psychological, social and biological factors affect the origin, course and end of the disease to a different extent. AN is characterized by intentional self-starvation and inability to maintain healthy body weight. It is defined by body weight and BMI (body mass index in kg/m^2) reduced to 17.5 and less. The patients are at the same time intensively concerned about food, their body shapes and their weight.

Amenorrhea caused centrally by sex hormones deficiency is an integral part of AN symptomatics, but it is often covered by hormonal substitution. BN patients are also intensively concerned about food, dissatisfied with their own body shape and weight; however they are not significantly underweight like patients with AN, despite the fact that they also long for lower weight than their healthy weight is. They suffer from overeating episodes (the so-called binge eating—consumption of large amounts of high-caloric food that they otherwise resist) and subsequently, they struggle to get rid of such calories in various manners (the so-called purging-vomiting, excessive training, diuretics, laxatives). There also exists purgative AN. Both AN and BN have many psychological, social and somatic consequences. Bulimic patients have tendencies toward behavioral and cognitive impulsivity, and they have disorganized, narcissistic and higher suggestibility. BN is often connected with other addictions (alcohol, drugs), depressions, self-injury and impulsive behavior such as thefts. Very frequent are atypical forms under MKN-10, or EDNOS (Eating Disorders Not Otherwise Specified) under DSM-IV that are defined as diagnostic units, which in certain aspects do not achieve the intensity of AN or BN or lack any of their symptoms.

The results of studies focused on cognitive functions in patients with eating disorders are not unequivocal. Significant is mainly the disorder of patient's perception of his/her own body, which has been included in diagnostic criteria. Also described have been slowed reaction time, deterioration of short-term visual memory and recollection-based long-term memory. Compared to intentional learning in control groups, deterioration applies mainly to automatic processing of information. In recent years, attention has been paid to reduced flexibility in problem-solving, increased focus on detail and reduced capacity to perceive the whole.

2. Epidemiology

Incidence and prevalence of eating disorders were generally on the rise in the second half of the 20th century, in our country about one or two decades later. They are significantly affected by the modern cult of bodily beauty, extreme slenderness and performance ("fitness"). Promotion of these ideals is supported by media and commercialization of this area (e.g., dietary food and preparations, cosmetic surgery). Patient's dissatisfaction with his/her own body and inappropriate dietary behavior are on the rise, particularly in risk population of adolescents and immature juveniles. The increase of the problem requires searching for new and more effective forms of treatment (e.g., self-supporting programs and manuals), where the knowledge of cognitive impairment can play a significant role. The lifelong prevalence in women is stated as 0.5 to 3.7% in AN, and as 1.1 to 4.2% in BN according to the selected criteria. The disease appears mainly (90 to 95%) in adolescent girls and young women, rarely in young boys and men. However, it has been extending to other, originally atypical age groups and social and economic classes. In recent years, the occurrence of the disease has been increasing in younger pre-pubescent children and in older women. Origin of eating disorders in women above 35 years of age is usually connected with stress from loss of loved ones, divorce or fear of aging. According to clinical experience symptomatics, treatment and course of the disease are not significantly different (Papežová, 1999, 2004).

As far as the prevalence of cognitive impairment in patients with eating disorders is concerned, the literature has been providing inconsistent information. It is not clear to what extent these changes result from eating disorders symptomatology and to what extent they belong to permanent features of the respective patient ("trait marker"). Several studies have shown that cognitive deficit persists even in recovered patients, based on the used criteria of recovery. In addition, some types of cognitive deficits are specific just for certain sub-diagnosis, while the others are connected with both AN and BN.

3. Czech and Foreign Studies of the Neuropsychology of Eating Disorders

A mere significant weight decrease by 35% of previous body weight (of military prisoners) resulted in impaired vigilance, concentration and memory. An acute 24-hour starving of women who were not on diets has not resulted in any significant changes in cognitive functions (just psychomotoric slowdown), while the impaired level of vigilance, slower reactions, worse recollection of words without psychomotoric slowdown and decreased vigilance have been described in women with normal body weigh who were on diets (Green and Rogers, 1995). Cognitive changes may be caused by both inadequate caloric intake and food composition (Lauer, 1999). Changes in neuropsychological tests in acute AN were described by Hamsher et al. already in 1981. The patients most often manifested slowed reaction time and worse results in mental arithmetic test, short-term visual memory and long-term memory recollection. Strupp et al. (1986) pointed out impaired automatic (unintentional) processing of information in contrast to intentional learning. The difference has been ascribed to the increased arousal (anxiety, increased concern about weight and food), narrowed attention and decreased overall cognitive capacity. The focus of attention and memory to the narrow area of food and body proportions impairs certain types of learning in other areas (Murphy, 2002).

The later studied, more complex cognitive functions (capacity to solve problems, categorization and abstraction, visual and tactile spatial orientation) have again not arrived at consistent conclusions. It has seemed that in AN, only some executive functions are deteriorated, which is ascribed to prefrontal circuits. Relevant for the clinical practice is insufficient flexibility in the strategy of problem solution, first of all in situations with uncertain results (Tchanturia, 2001, 2002). The cognitive deficit in AN is in many aspects similar to findings in the obsessive-compulsive disorder (Cavedini, 2002; Murphy, 2002).

The deficit in executive functions was in AN demonstrated in tests focused on problem solutions (Lauer et al., 1999; Szmukler et al., 1992), working memory (Green et al., 1996) and cognitive and perception flexibility (Kingston et al., 1996; Tchanturia et al., 2001). Some authors point out impaired working memory (Green et al., 1996), while they have not confirmed this deficit (Lauer et al., 1999). While the capacity to solve problems improves with weight gain (Lauer et al., 1999), perception flexibility of attention (set shifting) remains reduced even after a long-term remission (Tchanturia et al., 2001). The results indicate that rigidity and impaired flexibility may be permanent characteristic features connected with a predisposition for anorexia (the so-called trait markers).

Eating disorders are connected with complications during pregnancy and childbirth. The highest risk represents the hypoxic brain injury. The first study carried out in Sweden (Cnattingius et al., 1999) used the register of perinatal complications in the period between 1973 and 1984. Out of 781 girls and young women hospitalized for AN in the period from 1987 to 1994, a significantly higher percentage had a history of premature childbirth and childbirth trauma than a comparable population. The study has demonstrated that perinatal complications represent a risk factor for the development of severe forms of AN, but the measured factors have explained only about 5% of all AN cases.

The second study based on the twin register in American Virginia (Foley et al., 2001) has identified that complications during pregnancy and childbirth are connected with a higher risk of the development of AN and BN, while the risk of development of anxious disorders, depression and addictions has not been significantly increased. A premature childbirth was connected with the risk of AN but not with risk of BN. The absolute increase of risk was lower than in the Swedish study, which is probably an artifact caused by different severity of included cases: the Swedish study included patients hospitalized for severe forms of anorexia, while the American study mostly included less serious subclinical cases.

Uher and Treasure (2004) summarized comparatively rare cases of causal association between brain impairment and the syndrome of eating disorder, which provided valuable information about neurobiology of eating disorders. In a literature search, they have identified 54 case reports referring about patients whose brain impairment was connected with changes in food intake (increase, reduction and change in taste preferences). Some cases also demonstrated psychopathology that is typical of eating disorders (for example unsubstantiated fear of obesity, distorted perception of patient's own body, hyperactivity and obsessive-compulsive thinking and behavior). Ten of these cases manifested diffusion or disseminated impairment; in the remaining 44 cases, the impairment was localized into a certain brain structure. The correlation between impairment location and the symptom of eating disorders was obvious. Most often, it was the damage of hypothalamus, when the majority of cases manifested atypical disorders of eating behavior without characteristic psychopathology. As far as brain stem damage is concerned, there were fewer case reports and fewer clear connections. The damage of cortex of cerebral hemispheres more often resulted in typical presentation of the syndrome of eating disorders (AN more often than BN); it was localized particularly in the right frontal cortex areas of frontal and temporal lobes, and in five cases, a causal connection was quite obvious. The most important from the clinical viewpoint were the cases of long-term and treatment-resistant eating disorders, which disappeared after successful surgical treatment or medication treatment of epilepsy (Levine et al., 2003; Trummer et al., 2002).

4. Principal Domains of Measured Cognitive Functions

The enumeration of neuropsychological impairments in AN is not complete, despite the fact that the research has already brought quite a lot of information (Cnattingius, 1999; Katzman, 2001; Uher, 2002; Kaye, 2000). The studies focused on AN are less frequent than those focusing on other psychiatric disorders. They differ in the performance, selection of patients (case-control, cross-sectional or longitudinal) and methodology (various tests for the same functions), small sets and severity of the disease. The methodology has been gradually improved, and the studies have included larger sets, longitudinal data and clearer definitions of diagnoses and outcome of the disease. The recent research has shifted from broad test batteries to narrow-focus studies testing individual hypotheses, e.g., observation of AN with high "harm avoidance" score, deteriorated flexibility of thinking and rigidity of eating behavior and high perfectionism (Bulik, 2003).

4.1. Cognitive Flexibility in Anorexia Nervosa- Set Shifting

The studies started with a simple perception test—The Haptic Illusion Task (Tchanturia, 2001, see below)—and continued in mapping the ability of a change in the area of perception (Grunwald, 2001). The problems with flexibility are not limited to the area of perception, and they even persist in the long-term recovered anorexic patients (Tchanturia, 2002). A broader battery for "set-shift" testing was later developed and used in a larger sample of women suffering from eating disorders (see Chapter 6.4.8). Impairment of perception and cognitive flexibility was described in acute anorexia, after weight gain (Tchanturia, 2004) and also in healthy twins of girls suffering from AN that pointed out the genetic background of observed changes (Holliday, 2004).

The authors have also tested hypotheses that (in)flexibility is connected with rigid features of personality in AN. Premorbid features of rigidity in childhood they explained by 40% variability (Tchanturia, 2004). Out of the temperament scale TCIr (Holliday, 2004), it was only "harm avoidance" (12%) that had a slight effect on neuropsychological performances. (In)flexibility in childhood had the greatest effect on tested variables. Tchanturia (2005) describes identically neuropsychological characteristics of patients suffering from AN—rigidity in thinking, high degree of harm avoidance and perfectionism.

The therapeutic program of cognitive remediation issues from findings of cognitive rigidity. The first case reports and studies show that feedback and cognitive remediation can be applied in AN in serious stages of the disease (Davies and Tchanturia, 2005). The question to what extent the cognitive functions deficit persists after recovery is not yet consistently answered (Tchanturia et al., 2005).

Kaye (2008) states that patients suffering from anorexia have obsessive and rigid cognitive style and problems with set shifting. They find difficult to use feedback and to modify their behavior upon its basis. They are unable to efficiently recognize affective and social impulses and to incorporate them in the environment. Patients suffering from AN pay an above-average attention to the processing of details, and they use logic and an analytical approach, but they fail in tasks that require consideration of the whole and global solution strategies. Tchanturia (2005) includes into main neuropsychological characteristics of patients with AN a rigidity of thinking, high level of harm-avoiding behavior and perfectionism.

4.2. Central Coherence

The term central coherence originates from the autism research, and Uta Frith was the first to describe it (in 1989). Weak central coherence defines the cognitive style with dominating tendency to local detail-oriented processing of information and reduced capacity to integrate information into the context (Lopez et al., 2008). The tendency to focus on detail is reflected, for example, in an above-average performance in the sub-test of color cubes puzzle, which is a part of the Wechsler Intelligence Test, when the tested person's task is to arrange cubes with white, red and red and white sides according to the pattern, and in a below-average performance in the sub-test consisting in the object set-up, when the tested person's task is to analyze the object and then put individual parts together. Weak central coherence is also connected with a low score in the picture arrangement test created by Silvan Tomkins (1957), when the tested person is shown a picture of the man with various facial expressions. The tested person is supposed to make up the story based on such pictures. Lopez (2008) measured central coherence in patients with AN through some neuropsychological tests used in the investigation of persons with autistic spectrum disorders. These were in the centre of focus particularly of Francesca Happé. Lopez has issued from the assumption of Gillberg (1996) who states that AN can be considered a part of autistic spectrum disorders. The central coherence tests include the following:

Rey-Osterrieth Complex Figure

Qualitative mistakes when redrawing complex geometric configurations, e.g., Rey-Osterrieth Complex Figure, often reflects patient's incapacity to perceive the whole (*gestalt*) or global characteristics of the whole (it is similar in patients with lateralized impairment of the right hemisphere). The Rey-Osterrieth Complex Figure is a neuropsychological test used for measuring visual and spatial memory (reproduction of a geometric figure based on a pattern and reproduction by memory after a three-minute interval). However, many psychologists stress that neuropsychological understanding of the deficit does not depend only on the final score in the test, but also on the qualitative description of the type of mistakes (Swanda a Haaland, 2005). Thus, this test can evaluate not only the component of memory, but also the tested person's focus on the whole or on a detail.

The tested person is redrawing the picture with colored pencils according to a pattern. He/she always completes one element ("lifts the pencil from paper") and the testing person changes the color pencil (Lopez, 2008). This way it is possible to retrospectively reconstruct the order in which the tested person recorded individual elements of the figure. The testing person's work can be supported by a video recording. The tested person's reproduction is assessed from the viewpoint of accuracy, and the total of 18 elements are evaluated. Each element can bring the tested person from zero to two points (one point for the position and one point for the correct number of its components). The Savage's score system evaluates the organization strategy. It assesses five main elements of the figure, while the tested person can achieve from zero to six points for each element (a higher score represents better organization strategy). The Booth's score system has been developed mainly for quantification of central coherence and besides the continuity of drawing, it pays attention also to the tested person's procedure upon the figure reproduction—from the whole to a detail or vice versa. The result is the so-called *coherence index*. A higher score in the coherence index proves more coherent cognitive style. It means that the tested person started with global elements (Lopez, 2008).

The Embedded Figure Test

The complex color pictures in this test include twelve simple shapes. The tested person's task is to find these simple shapes in the complex picture, and the time the tested person needs is measured. Lopez (2008) submitted to the tested persons a complex picture together with a simple shape, whereby she did not pay regard to memory component of the test. The tested persons had 60 seconds to identify the simple shape inside the complex picture. Score for one task can range between 1 and 60. The total score is an average score from all (twelve) pictures. A shorter time and fewer mistakes prove a greater extent of local processing of information; the tested person concentrates just on the detail and does not take into consideration the context (color picture).

Completing the Sentences

In this version of the test modified by F. Happé (2001) and Lopéz (2008), the task of the tested person is to supplement sentences on a tape recording. Eighteen from the total of 25 sentences end with the word that is often associated with another word (e.g., "up" and "down:" "In the morning the sun came up and ..."). This word is understood as an expression of local processing of information and in the context of the whole sentence is incorrect. Measured are the answer and the reaction time. The tested person gets two points for the answer indicating local processing of information, one point for the answer provided after more than 10 seconds, for an incorrect answer that cannot be assessed as local processing of information or for a missing answer, and 0 points for a meaningful answer provided within the time limit of 10 seconds. This proves that the higher score indicates local processing of information or difficulties in global processing of information. The tested person has the maximum of 20 seconds for one answer.

The Geometric Figure Style

The tested person is submitted a certain geometric picture together with the instruction to describe the figure to the testing person in such manner that he/she will be able to draw it. When describing the geometric picture, the patients suffering from AN focus on details, and therefore, for the testing person drawing the figure according to such description the description becomes incomprehensible. The patient's focus on detail at the same time prevents him/her to subsequently draw the picture correctly from memory.

Lopez (2008) demonstrated that in the Rey-Osterrieth Complex Figure, individuals suffering from AN have had lower scores in organization strategy and lower coherence index, however they do not differ from a healthy control group in accuracy of reproduction. In the *Embedded Figure Test,* the patients with AN recognize simple shapes in complicated pictures faster and with fewer incorrect answers compared to a healthy control group. In the test consisting of completing the sentences, individuals with the diagnosis of AN had worse results compared to a healthy control group. These facts indicate that persons suffering from AN have a tendency to focus on detail and fail to perceive the whole (in common speech this cognitive style is well described by phrase "can't see the woods for the trees").

4.3. Specific Cognitive Impairment and Estrogen Levels

The loss of menstruation with continuously decreasing level of estrogens is one of the basic diagnostic criteria for AN. Attention has been paid in literature to relations between changes in the levels of estrogen and cognitive functions in Alzheimer's disease (Monk and Brodaty, 2000). As far as AN is concerned, such studies were missing despite the fact that in recent years, the specific cognitive deficits have been reliably described. In various conditions connected with estrogen insufficiency (after ovarectomy, in the event of Turner syndrome, after physiological menopause), a subtle but specific cognitive impairment was described in correlation with estrogen levels (Hampson, 1995; Duff and Hampson, 2000). Following the estrogen substitution, the impairment was reversible. Since the hormone substitution with estrogen is used quite often in AN patients, the research of the impact on cognitive processes is still relevant, particularly in cases of their dysfunction. The impairment of visual and tactile spatial processes and attention disorders have been described in several studies (Fox, 1981; Maxwell et al., 1984; Hamsher at al., 1981; Rovet et al., 1988; Kingston et al., 1996; Lauer et al., 1999; and Szmukler et al., 1992). Patients suffering from AN have difficulties in spatial tasks, reproduction of complex figures, supplementing the missing parts of the picture and analysis of spatial arrangement. According to some authors, the attention disorder usually disappears with weight gain (Fox, 1981, Hamsher et al., 1981, Kingston et al., 1996 and Szmukler et al., 1992), but the impaired visual and tactile spatial orientation may persist even after recovery (Grunwald et al., 2001; Szmukler et al., 1992; Kingston et al., 1996). Some studies have also described improvement of spatial orientation following the recovery (Jones et al., 1991; Szmukler et al., 1992). According to some authors, the right parietal association cortex that is considered the centre of visual and spatial processes and attention has been injured in AN (Braun and Chouinard, 1992; Maxwell et al., 1984; Neumarker et al., 2000). The predominating impairment of the right hemisphere is indicated in the works dealing with larger impairment of non-verbal and numerical processes in AN in contrast with comparatively maintained verbal functions and often excellent study performances based on them (Fox, 1981; Maxwell et al.,1984, Neumarker et al., 2000). However, some studies have not confirmed these findings (Jones et al., 1991; Kingston et al., 1996). The first results of the study of substitution with androgens in AN indicate normalization of the brain metabolism (Miller et al., 2004). However, the impact on cognitive capacities in eating disorders has yet not been tested.

4.4. Cognitive Dysfunction, Body Perception and Dissociation

The body perception disturbance represents the basic characteristic of eating disorders, particularly AN. It is connected with changed interoception, which is necessary for identification of own emotions and emotions of other people. The deficit in cognitive processing of emotions-alexithymia was described by Sifneos (1973). The perception of body scheme (spatial aspects of perception of size, shape and position) and "body image" (emotional and cognitive attitudes towards one's own body) depend on sensor perceptions of multiple modalities, including proprioception and visual and tactile feelings (Cumming, 1988; Damasio, 1999; Smeets and Kosslyn, 2001). In contrast with original concept of body representation by homunculus in the brain, the current perception of one's own body is considered a complex function including the structures of brain stem and association areas of cerebral cortex (Damasio, 1999). The lesion of parietal association cortex—particularly on the right side—and its connection with thalamus leads to asomatognosia and anosognosia (Cumming, 1988; McGlynn and Schacter, 1989, Uher, 2004). Anosognosia is common in many neurological injuries and is often connected with personality disorder or personality changes. The area of right parietal cortex and proximal frontal area are important for body scheme representation, for its cognitive processing and recognition. Affection of this function appears, for example, in epilepsy. In eating disorders, we search for cognitive mechanisms responsible for changes in the body perception. An example is dissociation that leads to insufficient integration of complex perceptions of the body scheme and their insufficient or incorrect processing. Our study demonstrated positive correlations between BAT II (scale II from the Body Attitude Test, which is mapping dissociation of one's own body expressed e.g., by item "My own body appears to me like an object without feelings."), and somatoform dissociation evaluated on the basis of the SDQ (Somatoform Dissociation Questionnaire) (Uher et al., 2004).

Stroop's Test and its Modification for Eating Disorders

One of the cognitive processes that is paid considerable attention in connection with eating disorders is selective attention. Individuals suffering from eating disorders have negative attitudes toward food and their own body proportions. Compared to the healthy control group, they pay more attention to these stimuli. The selective attention processes are studied on the basis of modified tasks of the Stroop's Test. The standard Stroop's Test investigates basic processes of attention and processing of information. It is based on the presentation of words designating colors written in incongruent colors (the word "red" is written in green). The tested person is asked to "read" either colors or words. The testing person measures time in ms. For the purposes of investigation of selective attention in patients with eating disorders, there exist the so-called "*food Stroop*" a "*body Stroop*" (which include words that apply to food or body shapes). It has turned out that patients suffering from eating disorders identify colors more slowly, when the respective word applies to body weight, body shapes or food (Johansson et al., 2005, Dobson and Rozpis, 2004). Patients with AN identify more slowly the words that apply to food, but not the words that apply to body shapes or body weight (Johansson et al., 2005, Dobson and Rozpis, 2004).

4.5. Cognitive Dysfunction and Perception of Pain

The disrupted perception of pain has been also consistently described in AN and other types of eating disorders. However, the mechanism of increased pain threshold is not known yet. The causes are discussed in many contexts (sensitivity of nocisensors, neuromediators of pain transfer, sensory fibers, antinociceptive mechanisms, central processing of pain impulses) with affective-motivational and cognitive factors (anxiety, depression, subjective unpleasant feeling of pain and the context of pain perception). The pain perception is associated with estrogen levels during the menstrual cycle in healthy women and with the intensity of experimental stress. In eating disorders, the change in pain perception can reflect lower hormone levels, but also specific cognitive features that result in completely disrupted perception of inner feelings and body scheme (Yamamotová and Papežová, 2001; Papežová et al., 2005; Yamamotová et al., 2005).

5. Neuropsychological Tests

As early as in 1973, Hilde Bruch described the basic specific features of AN: impaired recognition of inner feelings (interoceptive perception disorder), body scheme (body perception, body image) and feelings of inner inefficiency. These components create the EDI (Eating Disorder Inventory) scale, which has been most often used for the detection of specific psychopathology of both AN and BN (Garner, Olmsted and Polivy, 1983). The original scale includes eight partial subscales, which are focused on specific personality and behavioral features. They are used in studies concentrated on the detection of risk individuals in the population. Individual scales are focused as follows:

- urge to be slim (extreme effort to slim down and focus on diets),
- bulimia,
- bodily dissatisfaction,
- inefficiency (feeling of the overall uncertainty and worthlessness),
- perfectionism,
- interpersonal distrust (feeling of dissociation and aversion to create close relationships, reduction of positive emotions towards other people),
- impaired interoceptive perception (reduced capacity to understand one's own sensations and emotions, including visceral sensations of hunger and taste),
- fear of adulthood (reflects the desire to return to the safety of childhood and the fear of demands arising from adulthood).
- The new version of EDI 2 Test was supplemented by the author (Garner, 1991) with another scale focused on:
- self-renunciation (ascetism) (endeavor for self-discipline and excessive control, particularly of bodily needs),
- impulsive regulation (tendency to impulsivity, addictions, self-destructive and hostile behavior),
- social uncertainty (uncertain, tense and unsatisfactory social relationships) (Krch, 2005).

There also exists a computer version of the test.

We have performed tests of the relation to one's own body and somatoform dissociation (Uher et al., 2004) with the help of the BAT (Body Attitude Test) questionnaires and the SDQ-20 (Somatoform Dissociation Questionnaire) in validated Czech translation, which are used in research studies in the Specialized Centre for Eating Disorders of the Psychiatric Clinic in Prague. The scale of dissociation of one's own body (BAT II) appeared to be the best predictor of eating disorders. Somatoform dissociations were more frequent in both BN and AN. The body perception disturbances can be the manifestation of a more general mechanism, and it can be connected with non-sensitivity to pain, hunger and fatigue, as well as to other body signals. This may subsequently lead to the development of eating pathology or affect its course.

The EDE (Eating Disorder Examination) is the structured interview, which is considered the "golden standard" for diagnosis and assessment of eating disorder severity (Fairburn et al., 1993). A special training is required for its administration. The questionnaire version of this tool: the EDE-Q (Eating Disorder Examination-Questionnaire) has been translated into Czech and with the permission of its authors has been used in the research.

The basic battery of computerized or classical tests can be supplemented with special tasks to demonstrate cognitive deficit typical for anorexia and/or other diagnostic sub-groups. We have most often used verbal and non-verbal tasks, reliable even upon repeated testing (e.g., verbal tasks: Immediate and Delayed Recollection, Word Fluency and non-verbal tasks: attention flexibility—Brixton Task, spatial capacities—Mental Rotation Task, Complex Figure Recollection, arithmetic capacities—Number Sequence Test).

6. The Course of Cognitive Deficit

The course of AN and other eating disorders differs from fast remission to chronic disease. Despite the fact that neuronal changes in eating disorders are generally accepted, it is not clear which changes can be attributed to predisposition and which correlate with the course and prognosis of the disease. It is just cognitive changes that probably partake in the origin of eating disorders and severity of psychosocial impact of the disease. The symptoms of eating disorders usually exist for several months prior to the diagnosis specification (Lena et al., 2005). Cognitive dysfunctions probably precede the onset of the majority of psychiatric diagnoses. In children and adolescents, even a small cognitive dysfunction affects a number of personality and psychosocial characteristics. They apply mainly to the relationship to one's self and temperament features control. Particularly in adolescents, the psychosocial adaptation may be deteriorated as a consequence of cognitive impairment. It leads to deteriorated capacity to assess stressful situations and to solve problems and affects the process of physical and psychical maturation and control of interpersonal relationships. The authors describe hypersensitivity of bulimic girls to interpersonal interactions. The increased criticism and self-criticism can lead to overeating. The authors consider the manipulation with food as a "maladaptive mechanism" of individuals with worse social relationships.

Cooper et al. (2005) have even described a cognitive model of BN. It issues from current cognitive theories and follows up on the theories of Fairburn (1986) and Poliva, Herman (1985). Overeating episodes are triggered by negative self-assessment, negative assessment of one's own appearance, weight, body shapes and eating behavior, or other "degrading" events (criticism, argument at work, argument between partners). These are followed by negative automatic ideas that lead to the feeling of rejection by other people, depressions, anxieties and feelings of guilt. People suffering from eating disorders learn to disperse negative thoughts by increased concern and manipulation with food. This leads to physiological changes in cognitive functions, changed interoception (perception of hunger, satiety and emotions). Food is connected with the decreased arousal and overall intensity of emotional conditions. Individuals suffering from BN then have antagonistic ideas on positive effect of food (which helps control negative ideas) and its negative effects (fear of loss of control over food and body weight connected with negative self-assessment). They consider their eating behavior uncontrollable, which seemingly releases them from responsibility and leads to a vicious circle. It is made up of cognition, emotions, behavior and physiological effects of food. Negative self-assessment and dysfunction thoughts can be the result of negative or traumatic experience from childhood and can lead to ideas about dieting and compensation strategies: *When I do not eat, I will be slim and will be accepted by the others. When I eat, I am useless.* These predisposition factors can be triggered by various external stressors. Similar to other cognitive models, they activate long-term dysfunction schemes, which represent specific vulnerability and predict onset and course of the disease. Compared to the original theory, the recent model does not emphasize the previous restriction of food and caloric deficit. It works more with the anticipation of delight from eating, with inner and outer signals and the influence by learning. The advantage of this model consists of better testing, predicting and treatment of cognitive functions on the basis of cognitive and behavioral principles (work with verbal reconstructions, positive thoughts, dysfunction schemes and imaginative techniques).

The prospective studies have shown that after the treatment (weight increase and reduction of vomiting and overeating), some cognitive functions improved (Lauer et al., 2002), but functional damage of the right parietal association cortex in AN, impairment of visual and spatial orientation, nonverbal impairment (Neumarker et al., 2000) and reduced perception flexibility (Tchanturia et al., 2001) persist even after recovery. However, based on neuropsychological tests, the course of eating disorders has not yet been reliably predicted. They did not correlate with the extent of underweight, frequency of overeating and vomiting, EDI score or structural and functional changes (Uher, 2001).

In eating disorders, associations of cognitive dysfunctions with depressive symptoms have been excluded; however, they may result from long-term anxiety, perinatal damage and early traumas. Impairment of concentration, attention and psychomotor functions may be the effect of starvation and malnutrition, while the others (flexibility in decision-making, executive functions) may represent a predisposition feature (trait marker). The increased level of cortisol in acute phase of AN may cause disorders of vigilance and attention; Leasslie et al. (1992) pointed out the increased b-hydroxy butyric acid upon the metabolic adaptation to acute starving and its impact on the neurotransmitter system. The decreased levels of sex hormones, particularly estrogens, affect cognitive functions and are the subject of research in connection with hormonal substitution of women in menopause. As far as adolescents are concerned, the research has shown that the group with cognitive deficits differs from the group without such deficits in a number of personality and psychosocial characteristics, physical and emotional maturity, interpersonal relations, autonomy, healthy self-concept, self control and temperament (Huntigton a Bender, 1993). The problems in psychosocial development represent the risk, and the cognitive deficit increases the danger of onset of eating disorders.

7. Food Intake Control and the Results of Imaging Methods

The hypothalamus plays an important role in the complex control of appetite, hunger and body weight, and it is an integration centre for neuronal and humoral mechanisms of food intake control (Kalra et al., 1999). In the original dual model of the central food intake control, the principal role was played by ventromedial hypothalamic nucleus (VMH), whose damage led to overeating and significant weight gain. It was considered the centre of the sensation of satiety, while lateral hypothalamus (LH) was considered the centre of hunger. The current psychosomatic model of eating disorders corresponds to the concept of primary cortical dysfunction. Besides the hypothalamus, the prefrontal cortex, striatum, amygdala, midbrain and other brain areas also take part in the integration of signals from GIT and peripheral energy stores. In eating disorders, the food behavior is partially controlled also by the cortical and limbic neuronal circuits (orbitofrontal cortex, amygdala, insular cortex), while cognitive functions and motivation patterns are the responsibility of higher association areas of parietal and frontal cortex. The frontal cortex participates in motivation processes, narrowing attention to body scheme and nutrition. Perception of eating impulses is mediated by other structures: temporal cortex (integration of visual impulses), bulbus olphactorius and piriform cortex (flavors and fragrances), nc. tractus solitarius, thalamus, insula (taste). The damage of the hippocampus can be a part of pathology of eating disorders, particularly in connection with emotional stress and developmental trauma. The resulting maladaptive eating behavior then retrospectively affects functions of these neuronal circles e.g., by changes in gene expression (Papežová et al., 2002; Uher, 2004).

With the help of imaging methods, brain atrophy in AN can be detected already a few months after the onset of the disease. The structural measurement of brain tissue has proved that in acute AN, the grey and white brain mass is significantly reduced. Several studies focused on the combination of neuropsychological tests with the structural measurement by magnetic resonance (MRI) in order to find out whether there exists any relationship between structural changes (atrophy) and cognitive deficits. Neuropsychological damage (attention disturbances and visual and spatial orientation) together with signs of brain atrophy (extension of sulci and sulcal cavities) have been identified in the group of 46 patients with AN; however, correlations between structural and functional disorders were weak (Kingston et al., 1996). Neumarker et al. (2000) described the damage of numerical processes, which has disappeared after weight normalization. In patients with AN, some morphological pathological changes disappeared (extension of cavities), while the others (atrophy of mesencephalon) persisted (Neumarker et al., 2000). Out of the number of specific cognitive deficits described in AN, only some are reversible (or partially reversible) after recovery. Impaired attention, visuospatial and numeric processes, problem-solving and flexibility to change focus of attention have been sufficiently documented (see chapter 4.15 of the Annex, picture 4.1). While after successful realimentation the white brain mass returns to a premorbid level, the deficit of gray brain mass persists (Lambe et al., 1997 in: Uher, 2002). This may be explained partially by irreversible loss of neurons or glial cells, for example, by the increase of the level of cortisol. There may also an alternative explanation exist that the deficit is not the consequence but the cause of AN and that it reflects abnormal development of the nerve system. The atrophy particularly of the brain cortex was also detected in BN patients, but its development has not been investigated in such detail as in the event of AN.

Functional imaging methods (SPECT, PET and fMRI) provide relatively direct information on the functions of brain structures in eating disorders. The level of functioning of the brain and its parts can be roughly estimated according to blood flow (most often by the SPECT method), consumed glucose (by PET, consumption of radioactive fluorodeoxyglucose) or as waves of electric activity (with the EEG). Independent of the type of measurement in eating disorders, the brain functions less and economically: blood flow is lower (Krieg et al., 1989; Nozoe et al., 1995; Rastam et al., 2001), neurons consume less glucose (Delvenne et al., 1995; Delvenne et al., 1997) and electric response to standard impulses is slowed down (Bradley et al., 1997; Otagaki et al., 1998; Rothenberger et al., 1991). The brain most probably does not have sufficient energy. While in the rest condition, particularly, the prefrontal and parietal brain cortex in AN patients is less active (it metabolizes less glucose and has lower blood flow), in confrontation with food the medial frontal areas are activated (Delvenne, 1999; Nozoe, 1993; Ellison, 1998; Uher, 2001, 2002). Rest activity is more significantly reduced in frontal and parietal lobes, in association areas of brain cortex that are responsible for most complex tasks: integration of information from various resources, complicated logic thinking, imagination, creativity and planning. To a considerable extent, this also applies to patients with BN. Following the increase (normalization) of weight, parietal hypometabolism and hypermetabolism of lower frontal lobe persist, while the others (hypermetabolism in nc. caudatus and relative hypometabolism in frontal cortex) renormalize. This means that similar conclusions apply to functional abnormalities of the brain in eating disorders and to atrophy: they are mostly more significant in AN than in BN, and they are partially (but not completely) restored after the achievement of healthy body weight (Uher, 2001, 2002).

Activity of temporoinsular cortex (PET) changes with the exposition to and anticipation of food according to the accompanying emotions (desirable, disgusting), similarly as with sadness induced by memory, lactate-induced panic, anticipation anxiety, phobia, change in temperature, pain and visceral sensations (Gordon et al., 2000). Comparison of brain activity in eating disorders and in healthy individuals suggests that neutral brain circuits that normally provide food signals are replaced by pathological circuits like in obsessive-compulsive disorder, depression or addictions. They are created by connection of the originally neutral signal (in eating disorders it is food) with inadequate affective charge or compulsive behavior (Uher, 2002; Uher et al., 2003, 2004).

The authors studied reactions evoked by visual impulses connected with food and emotions with fMRI (functional magnetic resonance imaging) in nine long-term, recovered restrictive anorexic patients in comparison with eight chronic patients and nine healthy control individuals. In response to food signals, the activity of the medial prefrontal area and the anterior cingulum increased, and on the contrary, it decreased in lower parietal lobe compared to the group of healthy individuals and the group of recovered individuals. The recovered individuals manifested higher activity in the right lateral prefrontal cortex and apical prefrontal cortex and dorsal part of the anterior cingulum than chronic patients. Differences in brain activity between the groups were specific for food impulses, while the reactions to standard aversive emotional impulses did not differ. Here it is possible to differentiate "trait" and "state" characteristics of active disease and AN in remission. The medial prefrontal response to impulses specific for the disease is present in both, active disease as well as after remission. It can relate to genetic or development of vulnerability to the disease. During the food impulses' processing, lateral and apical prefrontal and dorsal parts of anterior cingulum are different in remission and in chronic disease and may be the sign of a good outcome of the disease (Uher, 2003, 2004).

8. Proposed Standardized Examination of Cognitive Functions

In the clinical examination, similarly to research projects that concentrate on individual tasks, it seems also inevitable to differentiate according to clinical purposes: for example, specification of the ability to change in the therapeutic program and prognostic factors particularly in long-term treatment, indications for specialized rehabilitation or forensic assessment of patient's capacity to evaluate severity of his/her own condition and to cooperate in adequate therapeutical program, and to give an informed consent to hospitalization (the issue of involuntary hospitalization) and disablement.

One of the cognitive functions that influence rehabilitation potentials damaged in AN patients is the so-called set-shifting. They have difficulties in using alternately various cognitive strategies, in perceiving various impulses and in doing several tasks at a time (multitasking). Set-shifting means the capacity to adjust one's one reactions to requirements of the environment. Tchanturia (2005) demonstrated that worse set-shifting capacity persists in patients even after long-term recovery. It seems that the reduced set-shifting capacity is not just the result of an acute state of the disease. Tchanturia has recently extended the battery of tests focused on set-shifting capacity in patients with AN. Some studies have shown the reduced set-shifting capacity in healthy sisters of AN patients. It seems that it represents an endophenotype of AN. As far as personality variables are concerned, the most connected with the reduced set-shifting capacity is the child's perfectionism.

So besides the above specified tests we can also use the following ones that are relatively easy for administration:

The Cat-Bat Test

The tested person is asked to fill in missing letters in a short story as quickly and accurately as possible. In the first part of the story, the letter c is always missing in the word *cat*. In the second part of the story (the part focused on *set-shifting*), the word "cat" does not at all fit the context of the story. It arises from the context that the letter to be filled in is b in the word *bat*. In the first part of the story, the tested person concentrates on filling the letter c in the word "*cat*", and in the second part of the test, he/she must adjust his/her cognitive focus to the change in context. Measured are perseverance errors and time that the tested person needs to complete the task.

The Trail Making Test

In the first part of the test, the tested person's task is to join on the screen the numbers from 1 to 26 placed on various places. In the second part of the test, numbers and letters are joined in the following order 1-A-2-B-3-C, etc. and the reaction time is measured..

The Brixton Test

The tested person is supposed to predict the movement of a blue ring whose position changes after each answer. From the current movement of the ring, the tested person must identify the rule according to which the ring moves in order to correctly predict its following position. However, in the course of the task, the rule changes,which means that the tested person must change his/her cognitive focus. Measured is the number of correct or incorrect answers.

The Haptic Illusion Test

This is the *set-shifting* perception task. During the test, three wooden balls are used: two of them of the same size (five cm in diameter) and one bigger ball (eight cm in diameter). The task of the tested person is to estimate, with his/her eyes closed, the relative sizes of two balls (always holding one ball in one hand). In the first part of the task, the tested person is always given a big ball to one hand and one of the small balls to the other hand. This procedure is repeated fifteen times (the tested person is always given the same ball to the same hand). Then follows the "critical stage" of the task, when the person is given two equal balls of five cm in diameter (always one ball to one hand). This procedure is repeated thirty times. The question is whether the balls are of the same size. The majority of healthy tested persons succumb to the illusion that the smaller ball is in the hand where they were previously holding the bigger ball. The number of repeating during which the illusion persists is the rate of perception rigidity.

The Wisconsin Card Sorting Test (WCST)

The tested person's task is to sort out the series of cards with various designs (one red triangle, two green stars, three yellow crosses, four blue rings) according to various rules they deduce from the testing person's feedback. Rules for cards classification to individual categories are defined by color, shape and number. Measured in this test are not just the capacity to generate and test various solutions, but also the flexibility to react upon changing conditions and the capacity to integrate new information into acquired knowledge in the manner so as to obtain the most effective reaction. The rate of *set-shifting* capacity is the number of perseverance errors (when the tested person classifies the card according to the previous rule and not according to the new one).

The Category Test from Halstead-Retain Battery

Commonly used technique to record capacities of the tested individual to flexibly use the feedback in order to find solution to the problem.

The Tower of London Test (Also Called the Tower of Hanoi Test)

The test consists of three wooden sticks and three balls (red, blue and green) attached to the sticks. The tested person's task is to reproduce the arrangement of balls according to the model of the testing person upon the observance of the following rules: Three balls can be concurrently attached to the first stick, two balls to the second stick, and one ball to the third stick. The tested person may at the same time always hold just one ball in his/her hand (this means that it is not possible to lift a ball and to move the one that is placed underneath). The test measures the capacity of planning. Measured is the number of moves necessary to obtain the correct answer and the number of correct answers upon the lowest number of moves in ten repeatings.

The Verbal Fluency Test

In the phonetic part of the test, the tested person is supposed to say as many words as possible starting with the same letter within the given time interval (the most often used letters in English are F and S). In the semantic part of the test, the tested person is instructed to specify as many words as possible falling within the given category (the most often used categories are animals and occupations).

9. Rehabilitation and Psychotherapy of Cognitive Deficit

The knowledge of cognitive dysfunctions in AN should contribute to our understanding of their influence upon everyday activities. In order to have a clinical impact, the testing should correspond to the maximum extent possible to realistic cognitive tasks and needs of the individuals. Despite the fact that the studies of neurobiology of the brain and brain cognitive functions are quite widespread, their significance from the viewpoint of treatment is yet small. Psychoeducation, including the presentation of atrophic brain, has a promotivation effect only on some patients with higher intellectual aspirations. A significant step in the rehabilitation of cognitive functions in eating disorders is cognitive remediation.

Cognitive Remediation Therapy (CRT)

Cognitive disturbances described in the literature reflect in patient's everyday life (reduced capacity to do various tasks at a time, reduced capacity to change strategies of problem solution in connection with changing requirements of the environment—in food as well as other areas of life, excessive focus on detail and insufficient regard to the whole). These characteristics are well known also from the clinical practice. Tchanturia (2007) has developed the therapeutic method known as *cognitive remediation therapy* (CRT), which is appropriate for work with seriouslyaffected patients in the acute stage of the disease. CRT is based on a number of tasks, in which the patients are provided feedback regarding their prevailing cognitive styles. They look for areas where this cognitive style is apparent in everyday life, and the possibilities to change it in common situations. In the centre of attention is not the content of thinking but its structure. CRT focuses on those areas of cognitive functions impairment that are particularly relevant for patients with eating disorders (*set-shifting*, focus on detail and neglect of the whole).

The tasks focused on *set-shifting* include:

1. The patient is asked to read the alphabet and come up alternately with female and male names starting with individual letters (it is the alternate focus of attention).
2. The following task is well known from Stroop's Test where words designating colors are written either in congruent or incongruent color (the word "green" is written in green or in blue color). The patient's task is either to read the words or to name colors. It again requires the patient to alternately focus attention according to feedback (instruction) of the testing person.
3. Token-Tower Task: The patient's task is to build a tower from tokens, while he/she has at his/her disposal tokens of various colors, sizes and shapes. Rules for token placing change during the course of the task (for example, at the beginning the patient places blue tokens disregarding their sizes and shapes, then tokens in the shape of a star disregarding their colors and sizes, then small tokens disregarding their shapes and colors). This is the training of capacity to adjust oneself to changing requirements of the environment.
4. Embedded-Word Task: The patient is submitted a list of words and his/her task is to underline words designating animals and circle words designating cities and towns.
5. Infinity-Sign Task: The patient's task is to draw the symbols for infinity with both his/her hands.
6. Number-Manipulation Task: The patient's task is to change the sequence of numbers in the row.

The tasks focused on global processing of information include:

1. The patient's task is to describe to the therapist a geometric figure in such manner so that the therapist is able to draw it according to such description. An excessive focus on detail and little regard to the whole contributes to the fact that the patient's description is incomprehensible and the therapist is thus unable to draw the figure.
2. The patient's task is to think up a title of an article or a short story. In this title, he/she must express a general message of the text without an excessive focus on details.

Tchanturia (2007) has developed the CRT model consisting of ten sessions twice a week.

The first part of CRT consists of individual tasks. In the second part, the patient with the help of a therapist tries to identify cognitive strategies he/she has used upon the solution of such tasks (e.g., an effort to precisely follow instructions, to alternately focus attention on various criteria, etc.). In the third part of the model, the patient, with the help of a therapist, tries to find situations in everyday life when he/she applies the same (unfavorable) strategies of information processing (e.g., inability to concurrently take care of a child and cook dinner as an example of little set-shifting ability, Tchanturia, 2007). The patient thus identifies the situations when his/her cognitive strategies are disadvantageous for him/her and tries to find alternative strategies. Two case reports (Davis and Tchanturia, 2005; Tchanturia et al., 2006), as well as the results of the pilot study (Baldock and Tchanturia, 2007; Whitney, Easter and Tchanturia, 2007) show that CRT may be an appropriate and effective intervention upon the improvement of cognitive strategies in patients with eating disorders and can facilitate subsequent psychological work.

4.10. Invalidity

Individuals with cognitive deficit use rigid compensation strategies that are little adaptive to relevant circumstances (Cohen, 1985). The disorder of an eating pattern can be considered a "coping" mechanism used particularly by adolescents with neuropsychological deficits to achieve the feeling of autonomy and internal control. Starving and overeating can modify by various mechanisms' dysphoric condition induced by stress. The combinations with a high score of perfectionism on the EDI scale contribute to rigid strategies for keeping control (Lena et al., 2004). The rigidity in problem-solving in stressful situations is often the cause of professional failure. Therefore, work capabilities and special treatment programs have been recently considered for physicians, medical students and healthcare employees with eating disorders (Australian Guidelines, 2004). The study compares possible negative affects on work capacities of healthcare professionals as a result of cognitive dysfunction, depressive symptomatics and somatic consequences, such as osteoporosis, hypotension and fatigue. According to the authors, insufficient judgment and rejection of change and treatment are considered the signs of a more serious disease. More often disabled becomethe girls with long-term, unfavorable somatic consequences and repeated study failures, i.e., the girls that have never worked. Inappropriate evaluation of disability can harm the patient and his/her further development and course of the treatment.

4.11. Conclusion

Despite the fact that the measurement of cognitive capacities in psychiatric disorders is well described, the long-term effect of rehabilitation programs focused on cognitive functions is still mostly the subject of the research.. As far as AN and other diagnostic subgroups of eating disorders are concerned, this area requires further long-term monitoring of better defined, larger groups. Measuring should be focused on the testing of specific clinical characteristics, at best together with neurophysiological factors (e.g., measurement of pain threshold). They may contribute to the creation of more effective psychoeducational and rehabilitation programs.

4.12. Summary

The neuropsychological tests originally detected deficits caused by brain injuries or neurological diseases. In the last decades, they have also been used in individuals with psychiatric disorders (Keefe, 1995; Heinrichs, 1998) to measure specific cognitive functions. The aim is to find out cognitive factors, manner of information perception, learning, remembering and processing (Sternberg, 2002), that take part in etiopathogenesis of the disease and therapeutically effective neuropsychological interventions. The data in eating disorders were inconsistent for quite a long period of time; original studies used broad batteries of tests on small and clinically heterogeneous groups and did not allow the detection of soft neuropsychological changes. Current researchers use hypotheses issued from the clinical practice that enable them to study selected functions in more depth and to detect problems specific for eating disorders with more specific tests relevant for the etiopathogenesis and the treatment. Examples are the studies focused on cognitive flexibility and on central coherence in AN, summarized by Tchanturia et al., in 2001–2007. Other studies are focused on interconnection of cognitive functions and specific psychopathological manifestations in eating disorders: changed body perception, pain and somatoform dissociation (Yamamotová and Papežová, 2001; Uher et al., 2004). Despite the fact that in AN, the overall IQ is usually not reduced, and on the contrary, there exist studies mentioning higher intelligence of girls with AN (Gordon et al., 1984; Rovet et al., 1988), there has been recently more proof regarding the impairment of specific cognitive functions. Some of them are considered secondary phenomenon caused by starving, while the other abnormalities precede the onset of the disease and persist even after recovery. These factors probably play their part in the development and in the course of the disease. In recent years, the new research findings in cognitive dysfunction in eating disorders has led to the development of specific rehabilitation approaches.

4.13. Key Words

Eating Disorders

Pathological eating behavior, biopsychologically conditioned; the most significant units are anorexia nervosa and bulimia nervosa; also included are atypical forms, psychogenic and night overeating, often related to obesity.

Disturbed Body Perception

A symptom represents an important diagnostical criterion. Its relation with other cognitive functions is the subject of the research.

Cognitive Impairment

Cognitive deficit is manifested first of all by deterioration of flexibility of thinking. However, the question remains as to what extent it precedes the disease and how the disease is affected by malnutrition and reduced hormonal levels.

Cognitive Deficit in Remission

The structural methods have identified the persisting deficit of the gray cerebral cortex, while the white cerebral cortex returns to the premorbid level after realimentation. The brain functional abnormalities also partly persist during remission, more significantly in anorexia. Attention is focused on the improvement of testing of specific dysfunctions and on the impact of rehabilitation (remediation).

4.15. Recommended and Used Literature

Australian guidelines for management of impaired doctors als mention Anorexia Nervosa. *Medical Journal of Australia*, 2004; 181, (Suppl. 7), 372–375.Beumont, P. J. V.: Neurobiology of eating behavior and weight control. In: Hoek, H. W.; Treasure, J. L.; Katzman, M. A., eds.: Neurobiology in the treatment of eating disorders. John Wiley and Sons, 1998, 431–455.

Baldock, E.; Tchanturia, K.: Translating laboratory research into practice: foundations, functions and future of cognitive remediation therapy for anorexia nervosa. *Future medicine,* 4 (3), 2007, 285-292.

Boleloucký Z.: O léčení dávkovaným hladověním (About dosing starvation used in the therapy) . Čas lék čes 1971, 110, 49.

Braun, C. M.; Chouinard, M. J.: Is anorexia nervosa a neuropsychological disease? *Neuropsychology Review*, 1992, 3, 2, 171–212.

Bishop, D.V.: Forty years on: Uta Frith's contribution to research on autism and dyslexia 1966-2006. *Quarterly Journal of Experimental Psychology*, 2008, 61 (1), 16-26.

Bulik, C. M.; Tozzi, F.; Anderson, C.; Mazzeo, S. E.; Aggen, S.; Sullivan, P. F.: The relation between eating disorders and components of perfectionism. *American Journal of Psychiatry*, 2003, 160, 2, 366–368.

Bulik, C. M.; Sullivan, P. F.; Wade, T. D.; Kendler, K. S.: Twin studies of eating disorders; a review. *J. Eat Disord.*, 2000, 27, 1–20.

Cavedini, P.; Riboldi, G.; D'Annucci, A.; Belotti, P.; Cisima, M.; Bellodi, L.: Decision-making heterogeneity in obsessive-compulsive disorder: ventromedial prefrontal cortex function predicts different treatment outcomes. *Neuropsychologia,* 2002, 40, 205–211.

Cassin, S. E.; von Ranson, K. M.: Word Lists for Testing Cognitive Biases in Eating Disorders. *Eur. Eat Disorders Review,* 2005, 13, 3, 216–221.

Cnattingius, S.; Hultman, C. M.; Dahl, M.; Sparen, P.: Very preterm birth, birth trauma, and the risk of anorexia nervosa among girls, Archives of General Psychiatry,1999, 56, 7, 634–638.

Connan, F.; Treasure, J.: Stress, eating and neurobiology. In: Hoek, H. W., Treasure, J. L., Katzman, M. A., eds.: Neurobiology in the treatment of eating disorders. John Wiley and Sons, 1998, 211–236.

Cummings, D. E.; Purnell, J. Q.; F Reyo, R. S.; Schmidova, K.; Wisse, B. E.; Weigle, D. S.: A preprandial rise in plasma ghrelin levels suggests a role in meal initiation. In: *Humans Diabetes*, 2001, 50, 1714–1719.

Damasio, A.: The feeling of what happens. Vintage, 1999.

Davies H.; Tchanturia K..: Cognitive Remediation Therapy as an intervention for acute Anorexia Nervosa: A Case Report. *Eur. Eat. Disorders Rev.*,2005, 13,311-316.

Delvenne, V.; Goldman, S., De Maertelaer V.; Lotstra, F.: Brain glucose metabolism in eating disorders assessed by positron emission tomography. *Int. J. Eat Disord.,* 1999, 25, (Suppl. 1), 29–37.

Dobson, K. S.; Dozois, D. J.: Attentional biases in eating disorders: A meta-analytic review of Stroop performance. *Clinical Psychology Review*, 2004, 23, 8, 1001–1022.

Duff, S. J.; Hampson, E.: A beneficial effect of estrogen on working memory in postmenopausal women taking hormone replacement therapy. *Horm. Behav*. 2000, 38, 262–276.

Ellison, Z.; Foong, J.; Howard, R.; Bullmore, E.; Williams, S.; Treasure, J.: Functional anatomy of calory fear in anorexia nervosa. *Lancet,* 1998, 352, (9135), s. 1192.

Fairburn, C. G.; Welch, S. L.; Doll, H. A.; Davies, B. A.; O´Connor, M. E.: Risk factors for bulimia nervosa—A community-based case-control study. *Arch. Gen. Psychiatry*, 1997, 54, 509–517.

Fairburn, C. G.; Harrison, P. J.: Eating disorders. *Lancet,* 2003, 361, 407–416.

Fox, C. F.: Neuropsychological correlations of anorexia nervosa. *Int. J. Psychiatry Med.* 1981, 11, s. 285–290.

Gillberg, C.; Gillberg, C.; Rastam, M.; Johansson, M.: The Cognitive Profile of Anorexia Nervosa: A Comparative Study Including a Community Based Sample, *Comprehensive Psychiatry,* 1996, 37, 1, 23–30.

Gordon, C. M.; Dougherty, D. D.; Rauch, S. L.; Emans, S. J.; Grace, E.; Lamm, R.; Alpert, N. M.; Majzoub, J. A.; Fischman, A. J.: Neuroanatomy of human appetitive function: A position emission tomography investigation. *Int. J. Eat Disord* .2000, 27, 167–171.

Green, M. W.; Elliman, N. A.; Wakeling, A.; Rogers, P. J.: Cognitive functioning, weight change and therapy in anorexia nervosa. *Journal of Psychiatric Research* 1996, 30, 401–410.

Green, M. W.; Rogers, P. J.: Impaired cognitive functioning during spontaneous dieting. *Psychol. Med.* 1995, 25, 1003–1010.

Grunwald, M.; Ettrich, C.; Assmann, B.; Dahne, A.; Krause, W.; Busse, F.; Gertz, H. J.: Deficits in haptic perception and right parietal theta power changes in patients with anorexia nervosa before and after weight gain. *International Journal of Eating Disorders*, 2001a, 29, 4, 417–428.

Grunwald, M.; Ettrich, C.; Krause, W.; Assmann, B.; Dahne, A.; Weiss, T.; Gertz, H. J.: Haptic perception in anorexia nervosa before and after weight gain, *Journal of Clinical and Experimental Neuropsychology*, 2001b, 23, 4, 520–529.

Hajek T.: Poškození hipokampu—klíčový patogenetický faktor v psychiatrii? (Damage of hippocampus - is it a key inpathogenesis in psychiatry ?*Psychiatrie,* 2001, 1, 20–26.

Hageman, I.; Andersen, H. S.; Jorgensen, M. B.: Post-traumatic stress disorder: A review of psychobiology and pharmacotherapy. *Acta Psychiatr. Scand*, 2001, 104, 412–422.

Hampson, E.: Spatial cognition in humans: possible modulation by androgens and estrogens. *J. Psychiatry Neurosci.*, 1995, 20, 397–404.

Hamsher, K. S.; Halmi, K. A.; Benton, A. L.: Prediction of outcome in anorexia nervosa from neuropsychological status. *Psychiatry Research*, 1981, 79–88.

Heim, C.; Nemeroff, C. B.: The impact of early adverse experiences on brain systems involved in the pathophysiology of anxiety and affective disorders. *Biol. Psychiatry*, 1999, 46, 1509–1522.

Heinrichs, R. W.; Zakzanis, K. K.: Neurocognitive deficit in schizophrenia: a quantitative review of the evidence. *Neuropsychology*, 1998, 12, 3, 426–445.

Holliday, J.; Tchanturia, K.; Landau, S.; Caspi, A.; Collier, D.; Treasure, J.: Neuropsychological Underpinnings of Personality in Anorexia Nervosa? submitted, 2004a.

Holliday, J.; Tchanturia, K.; Landau, S.; Collier, D.; Treasure, J.: Is impaired Set-Shifting an Endophenotype of Anorexia Nervosa. submitted, 2004b.

Jimerson, D. C.: Eating disorders and stress. Encyclopedia of Stress, 2000, 2, 4–8.

Johansson, L.; Ghaderi, A.; Andersson, G.: Stroop-interference for food- and body-related words: a meta-analysis. *Eating Behaviors*, 2005, 6, 271-281.

Jones, B. P.; Duncan, C. C.; Brouwers, P.; Mirsky, A. F.: Cognition in eating disorders. *J. Clin. Exp. Neuropsychol.*, 1991; 13, 711–728.

Kalra, S. P.; Dube, M. G.; Pu, S.; Xu, B.; Horvath, T. L.; Kalra, P. S.: Interacting appetite-regulating pathways in the hypothalamic regulation of body weight. Endocrine Reviews, 1999, 20, 1, 68–100.

Katzman, D. K.; Christensen, B.; Young, A. R.; Zipursky, R. B.: Starving the brain: Structural abnormalities and cognitive impairment in adolescents with anorexia nervosa. *Seminars in Clinical Neuropsychiatry*, 2001, 6, 2, 146–152.

Kaye W.: The new biology of AN and BN. *Eur. Eat Disorders Rev.*, 1999, 7.

Kaye, W. H.; Klump, K. L.; Frank, G. K.; Strober, M.: Anorexia and bulimia nervosa, *Annu. Rev. Med.*, 2000, 51, 299–313.

Kaye, W.: Neurobiology of anorexia and bulimia nervosa. Physiology and Behavior, 2007, doi. 10.1016/j.physbeh.2007.11.037

Keefe, R. S.: The contribution of neuropsychology to psychiatry, *American Journal of Psychiatry*, 1995, 152, 1, 6–15.

Kendler, K. S.; Walters, E. E.; Neale, M. C.; Kessler, R. C.; Heath, A. C.; Eaves, L. J.: The structure of the genetic and environmental risk factors for six major psychiatric disorders in women. *Arch. Gen. Psychiatry*, 1995, 52, 374–383.

Kingston, K.; Szmukler, G.; Andrewers, B.; Tress, B.; Desmond, P.: Neuropsychological and structural brain changes in anorexia nervosa before and after refeeding. *Psychological Medicine*, 1996, 26, 15–28.

Krch, F. a kolektiv: Poruchy příjmu potravy. (Eating Disorders). Praha, Grada 2005, 238.

Kuelz, A. K.; Hohagen, F.; Voderholzer, U.: Neuropsychological performance in obsessive-compulsive disorder: a critical review, *Biological Psychology*, 2004, 65, 3, 185–236.

Lilenfeld, L. R.; Kaye, W. H.; Greeno, C. G.; Merikangas, K. R. Plotnoicov, K., Pollice, C., Rao, R., Strober, M., Bulik, C. M., Nagy, L. A.: Controlled family study of anorexia nervosa and bulimia nervosa: psychiatric disorders in first-degree relatives and effects of proband comorbidity. *Arch. Gen. Psychiatry*, 1998, 55, s. 602–610.

Lauer, C. J., Gorzewski, B., Gerlinghof, F M., Backmund, H., Zihl, J.: Neuropsychological assessments before and after treatment in patients with anorexia nervosa and bulimia nervosa. *J.. Psychiatr. Res.* 1999, 33, 2, 129–138.

Lauer C.J.: Neuropsychological findings in eating disorders. InD'haenen H, den Boer J.A., Westenberg H., et al. (eds):

Biological psychiatry, Swansey, UK: Wiley, 2002. str. 1167

Lauer, C.: Neuropsychological Findings in Eating Disorders. In: D'Haenen, H., den Boer, J. A., Willner, P., eds.: Biological Psychiatry. Chichester, UK, John Wiley and Sons, 2002, 1167–1172.

Laessle, R. G.; Fischer, M.; Fichter, M. M.; Pirke, K. M.; Krieg, J. C.: Cortisol levels and vigilance in eating disorder patients. *Psychoneuroendocrinology*, 1992, 17, 465–484.

Maxwell, J. K.; Tucker, D. M.; Townes, B. D.: Asymmetric cognitive function in anorexia nervosa. *Int. J. Neurosci.* 1984, 24, 37–44.

Mazzeo, S. E.; Aggen, S.; Sullivan, P. F.: The relation between eating disorders and components of perfectionism, *American Journal of Psychiatry*, 2003, 160, 2, 366–368.

Miller, K. K.; Deckersbach, T.; Rauch, S. L.; Fischman, A. J.; Grieco, K. A.; Herzog, D. B.; Klibanski, A.: Testosterone administration attenuates regional brain hypometabolism in women with anorexia nervosa. *Psychiatry Research: Neuroimaging*, 2004, 132, 197–207.

Lezak, M.; Howieson, D.; Loring, D.: Neuropsychological Assessment, 4th ed., Oxford University Press, New York, 2004

Lopez, C.; Tchanturia, K.; Stahl, D.; Booth, R.; Holliday, J.; Treasure, J.: An Examination of Concept of Central Coherence in Women with Anorexia Nervosa. *International Journal of Eating Disorders*, 41, 2008, 143-152.

Monk, D.; Brodaty, H.: Use of estrogens for the prevention and treatment of Alzheimer's disease. Dement. Geriatr. *Cogn. Disord.*, 2000, 11, 1–10.

Murphy, R.; Nutzinger, D. O.; Paul, T.; Leplow, B.: Dissociated conditional-associative learning in anorexia nervosa. *J. Clin. Exp. Neuropsychol.*, 2002, 24, 176–186.

Neumarker, K. J.; Bzufka, W. M.; Dudeck, U.; Hein, J.; Neumarker, U.: Are there specific disabilities of number processing in adolescent patients with Anorexia nervosa? Evidence from clinical and neuropsychological data when compared to morphometric measures from magnetic resonance imaging. *Eur. Child Adolesc. Psychiatry*, 2000, 9, Suppl 2, II 111–II 121.

Nozoe, S.; Naruo, T.; Nakabeppu, Y.; Soejima, Y.; Nakajo, M.; Tanaka, H.: Changes in regional cerebral blood flow in patients with anorexia nervosa detected through single photon emission tomography imaging. *Biol. Psychiatry*. 1993, 34, 8, 578–580.

Papežová, H.: Poruchy příjmu potravy. In: Hoschl, C.; Libiger, J.; Švestka, J. eds.: Psychiatrie. Tigis, 2002, 599–605.

Papežová, H.: Poruchy příjmu potravy. (Eating Disorders).In: Houdek, L. eds.: Doporučené postupy v psychiatrii. (Therapeutic Guidelines in Psychiatry).Galén, 1999, 149–151.

Papežová, H.: Poruchy příjmu potravy. (Eating Disorders. In: Seifertová, D.; Praško, J.; Höschl, C.: Postupy v léčbě psychických poruch. (Therapeutic Approaches in Psychiatric Disorders).Medical Tribune Group. Praha 2004, 335–350.

Papežová, H.; Yamamotová, A.; Uher, R.: Elevated pain threshold in eating disorders. Physiological and psychological mechanisms. *Journal of Psych Research* 2005, 34, 431–438.Papežová, H.; Yamamotová, A., Uher, R.: Neurobiologie poruch příjmu potravy. Psychiatrie (Prague), 2002;6(4):268–275.

Pretorius, N.; Tschanturia, K.: Anorexia nervosa: How people think and how we address it in cognitive remediation therapy. *Therapy* 2007, 4, 423-431.

Rey, A.; Osterrieth, P.A.: Rey-Osterriethova komplexní figura, TKF, Příručka, Psychodiagnostika s.r.o., Brno 1997, 8.

Rovet, J.; Bradley, E.; Goldberg, E.; Wachsmuth, R.: Hemispheric lateralisation in anorexia nervosa. J. Clin. Exp. Neuropsychol., 1988, 10, 24.Schmidt, U. H.; Tiller, J. M.; Andrews, B.; Blanchard, M.; Treasure, J.: Is there a specific trauma precipitating the onset of anorexia nervosa? *Psychol. Med.*, 1997, 27, 523–530.

Smeets, M. A.; Kosslyn, S. M.: Hemispheric differences in body image in anorexia nervosa. *Int. J. Eat. Disord.*, 2001, 29, 409–416.

Szmukler, G. I.; Andrewes, D.; Kingston, K.; Chen, L.; Stargatt, R.; Stanley, R.: Neuropsychological impairment in anorexia nervosa: before and after refeeding. *J. Clin. Exp. Neuropsychol.*, 1992, 14, 347–352.

Southgate, L.; Tchanturia, K.; Treasure, J.: Neuropsychological performance in anorexia nervosa: A systematic review of Frontal Lobe functions. In progress.

Sternberg, R. J.: Kognitivní psychologie. Praha, Portál 2002, 636.

Strupp, B. J.; Weingartner, H.; Kaye, W.; Gwirtsman, H.: Cognitive processing in anorexia nervosa: A disturbance in automatic information processing. *Neuropsychology* 1986, 15, 89–94.

Swanda, R.M.; Haaland, K.Y.: Clinical Neuropsychology and Intellectual Assessment, in: Sadock, B.J., Sadock, V.A. (Eds.): Kaplan´s and Sadock´s Comprehensive Textbook of Psychiatry, I, Lipponcott Williams Wilins, Philadelphia, 2005, 2054.

Tchanturia, K.; Serpell, L.; Troop, N.; Treasure, J.: Perceptual illusions in eating disorders: rigid and fluctuating styles. *J. Behav. Ther. Exp. Psychiatry*, 2001, 32, 107–115.

Tchanturia, K.; Brecelj Anderluh, M.; Morris, R.; Rabe-Hesketh, S.; Collier, D.; Sanchez, P.; Treasure, J.: Cognitive Flexibility in anorexia nervosa and bulimia nervosa. *Journal of International Neuropsychological Society,* 2004a, 10, 1–8.

Tchanturia, K.; Davies, H.; Campbell, I.C.: Cognitive remediation therapy for patients with anorexia nervosa: preliminary findings. *Annals of General Psychiatry* 2007, 6:14 doi:10.1186/1744-859X-6-14

Tchanturia, K.; Whitney, J.; Treasure, J.: Can cognitive exercise help to treat anorexia nervosa?, A case report. *Weight. Eat. Disord.*, 2006, 11, 112-117.

Tchanturia, K.; Campbell, I.C.; Morris, R.; Treasure, J.: Neuropsychological Studies in Anorexia Nervosa. *International Journal of Eating Disorders,* 37, 2005,. 72-76

Tchanturia, K.; Morris, R.; Brecelj Anderluh, M.; Nikolaou, V.; Treasure, J.: Set Shifting in anorexia nervosa: An examination before and after weight gain, in full recovery and the relationship to childhood and adult OCPD traits. *Journal of Psychiatric Research*, 2004b, In: Press (available online).

Tchanturia, K.; Morris, R. G.; Surguladze, S.; Treasure, J.: An examination of perceptual and cognitive set shifting tasks in acute anorexia nervosa and following recovery, *Eating and Weight Disorders*, 2002, 7, 4, 312–315.

Tchanturia, K.; Morris, R. G.; Surguladze, S.; Treasure, J.: Evidence of mental rigidity in anorexia nervosa: set shifting paradigms. *Eating and Weight Disorders*. 2002, 7(4), 312-316.

Tomkins, S. S.; Miner J. B.: The Tomkins-Horn Picture Arrangement Test, Springer, New York, 1957

Uher, R., Papežová, H.: Strukturální a funkční abnormality mozku u osob trpících poruchami příjmu potravy. (Structural and Functional Abnormalities in Eating Disorders Sufferers)Čes. a slov. Psychiatrie, 2001, 97, 1, 27–30.

Uher, R.; Pavlová, B.; Probst, M.; Yamamotová, A.; Papežová, H.: Vztah k vlastnímu tělu a somatoformní disociace u poruch příjmu potravy. Čes. Psychologie, 2004, 48, 5, 385–396.

Uher, R.; Murphy, T.; Ng, V.; Phillips, M.; Dalgleish, T.; Treasure, J.: Perception of food and emotional stimuli in anorexia nervosa. *Neuroimage*, 2001, 13, 1022.

Uher, R.; Treasurem J.; Campbellm I. C.: Neurochemical Bases of Eating Disorders. In: D'Haenen, H., den Boer, J. A., Willner, P. eds.: *Biological Psychiatry*, John Wiley and Sons, Ltd, Chichester, UK, 2002, 1173–1179.

Uher, R.; Brammer, M. J.; Murphy, T.; Campbell, I. C.; Ng, V. W.; Williams, S. C. R.; Treasure, J.: Recovery and Chronicity in Anorexia Nervosa: Brain Activity Associated with Differential Outcomes. *Biol. Psychiatry,* 2003, 54, 634–642.

Uher, R.; Murphy, T.; Brammer, M. J.; Dalgleish, T.; Phillips, M. L.; Ng, V. W.; Andrew, C. M.; Williams, S. C.; Campbell, I. C.; Treasure, J.: Medial prefrontal cortex activity associated with symptom provocation in eating disorders. *American Journal of Psychiatry*, 2004a, 161, 1238–1246.

Uher, R.; Murphy, T.; Friederich, H. C.; Dalgleish, T.; Brammer, M. J.; Giampietro, V.; Phillips, M. L.; Andrew, C. M.; Ng, V. W.; Williams, S. C. R.; Campbell, I. C.; Treasure, J.: Functional neuroanatomy of body shape perception in healthy and eating disordered women. *Biological Psychiatry*, in press.

Uher, R.; Treasure, J.: Brain lesions and eating disorders. *J. of Neurology, Neurosurgery and Psychiatry*, 76, 852–857.

Whitney, J.; Easter, A.; Tschanturia, K.: Service users' feedback on cognitive training in the treatment of anorexia nervosa: a qualitative study, *International Journal of Eating Disorders*, 2007.

Yamamotová, A.; Papežová, H.: Změny prahu bolesti u mentální anorexie a bulimie v průběhu onemocnění.(Pain threshold changes during the course of anorexia and bulimia nervosa). Psychiatrie, 2001; 5, (Suppl. 2), 147–148.

Yamamotová, A.; Papežová, H.; Vurmová, I.: Vliv hormonální substituční terapie na nocicepci u pacientek s mentální anorexií.(Hormonal substitution therapy influence on nociception in patients with anorexia nervosa.*Psychiatrie,* 2005, 2, (Suppl. 2), 123–125.

In: Cognitive Deficit in Mental and Neurological Disorders ISBN: 978-1-60741-957-0
Editors: H. Kucerova, M. Preiss

Chapter III

Schizophrenia

Hana Prikrylova Kucerova, Radovan Prikryl, Zuzana Rihova, Petra Navratilova, and Eva Ceskova

Abstract

Schizophrenia is often associated with cognitive deficits, particularly within the domains of attention, memory, executive functions, and language skills. Specific cognitive deficits have recently been linked to psychotic phenomena, including verbal hallucinations and disorganized speech. Impairments of working and semantic memory are primarily due to dysfunction of the frontal cortex, temporal cortex, and hippocampus.

Examination of cognitive functions in patients with schizophrenia is complicated for many reasons. So far neither a unified examination battery nor a terminological consensus exists, which causes problems in the acquisition and interpretation of data (proposal of MATRICS initiative).

Cognitive skills in schizophrenia predict social functioning and may serve as outcome measures in the development of effective treatment strategies. There are extensive possibilities to therapeutically influence cognitive dysfunction; however, so far, their effects have not been investigated in detail. An integrated approach, including pharmacotherapy, social skills training and cognitive training, seems to be the optimal solution.

Keywords: *Cognitive function—epistemic function (memory, attention, executive functions).Cognitive disorder—according to ICD-10, impairment of thought processes, memory, reduced ability to learn, and reduced concentration and attention. Contextual reasoning—ability to maintain awareness of the source, quality, and location of input, and the ability to link those pieces of information. Disorders of contextual reasoning may cause failure on memory tests in patients with schizophrenia. Deficit—decrease, from the point of behaviorism, demonstrations that do not occur with adequate intensity or do not occur at all, and the absence of which is disruptive or undesirable. Dysfunction—disorder having a natural course of organic/psychic function; reaction that does not adequately correspond to its objective; disorder in the function of an organ/system. Executive functions—comprise* *cognitive processes influencing target oriented behavior—they provide for planning, ability of cognitive reconstruction and flexibility, and distribution of attention. It is a multi-component system that plays a significant role in every mental operation. Dysexecutive syndrome is most frequently connected with damage to the prefrontal cortex. Psychic deficit—permanent deviation, especially behavioral, from the psychic standard. Psychic function—psychic processes, the most important being cognitive processes, emotions, and will; humans predominantly interact with the outside world through psychic functions; these functions can last from a split second for sensomotor reactions to tens of seconds or hours while thinking; their course changes with developmental changes, condition of the organism, and environmental influences .Response inhibition—ability to suppress an automatic response; it is especially manifested in the interference Stroop test or WCST. In patients with schizophrenia, this ability is usually disrupted. Schizophrenia—generally a concept used for a whole group of psychoses characterized by loss of sense for the real world, plunging patients into fantasy, hallucinations, or possibly delusions, which are incomprehensible to others. Verbal fluency—ability to produce as many words, in a certain category, as possible during a timed interval; phonematic verbal fluency (category of words beginning with a certain letter) and categorical verbal fluency (animals, plants, means of transport) are distinguished. It is a sensitive indicator of the function of the frontal-temporal cerebral area. Working memory—provides for simultaneous registration of inputs and mental manipulation of these inputs, such inputs being only temporarily relevant. The basic characteristic of the working memory is the fact that inputs are carriers of new information that is not immediately transferred into long-term memory. It provides for continuity between past experiences and the present and is comprised of active selection, repetition and handling of information. Based on the Baddeley concept (1992), it consists of three systems: visuospatial sketchpad, phonological loop and a controlling system, providing for distribution of attention, selection of information and control of information operations (central executive). The phonological loop maintains acoustic and verbal inputs for one to two seconds, cooperates with the articulation control system, which is an analogy of internal speech and influences certain forms of acoustic projection, which does not depend on articulation. The visuospatial sketchpad consists of a passive component providing for maintenance of information about objects and scenes and an active component based on an internal spatial description and repetition of information and is responsible for planning and movement control. Baddeley A. Working Memory. Science 1992:556-559.*

1. Introduction

Schizophrenia is a severe mental disorder characterized by a variety of signs and symptoms. Since its earliest conception as "dementia praecox" (i.e., early onset dementia), impaired cognitive function has also been considered a core feature. Research into cognition and schizophrenia over the past years has recently been growing. Cognitive deficit is a virtually omni-present component of schizophrenic psychopathology, independent of other aspects of schizophrenia. It underlays other symptoms of schizophrenia and affects the success of therapy, ability of social adaptation and patient's quality of life.

The Concept of Cognitive Functioning in Schizophrenia in a Historic Perspective

Our understanding of the nature and causes of cognitive deficit in schizophrenia has a history of its own. The discussion was concerned with whether cognitive deficit is a primary or secondary symptom of the illness. Should cognitive impairment be a major part of the illness, its incidence would have to be associated with some etiological factors of the illness, specifically structural change in the CNS (Sharma and Harvey, 2000).

Cognitive deficit in schizophrenia was first observed by Kraepelin as early as a hundred years ago. He recorded a drop in the intellectual ability of his patients and regarded his finding as a characteristic important to such an extent that he proposed to use Morel's term *dementia praecox* to refer to the illness. Czech psychiatric literature of the end of the 19th century uses the term juvenile dementia (dementia juvenilis). Kufner (1897) explains in a textbook of psychiatry that "the nature of the illness consists in a relatively speedy and persisting weakening of the psychic ability. The degree of dementia differs with the individual" (quoted in Tuma, 1999).

Bleuler (1911) believed that cognitive deficit in schizophrenia has to do with a deficit of elementary cognitive processes. The intelligence quotient in schizophrenic patients was found diminished when compared with healthy subjects. Myslivecek (1959) writes in his textbook of *Special Psychiatry* that schizophrenic patients do not suffer from a real intellectual languor (dementia), but that "the patient does not use his intellectual ability adequately and does not control it efficiently" (Tuma, 1999).

The prevailing belief in the first half of the 20th century was that cognitive deficit in schizophrenia is not a primary symptom of the illness. It was regarded as a secondary phenomenon associated with the diminished motivation of the patients regarding testing, with positive symptoms, patients' long-term psychiatric hospitalization and, in the second half of the 20th century, with an undesirable inhibitory effect of typical antipsychotics (Tuma, 1999). Use of classic antipsychotics, the effect of long-term hospitalization and diminished motivation then play the role of secondary factors deepening the primary core deficit of cognitive functions (Rund, 1998).

Another shift in opinions about the nature of cognitive deficit came about with the development of new research methods. Imaging methods have confirmed and contributed further details about the incidence of specific structural and functional change in the brains of schizophrenic patients. Schizophrenia started to be regarded as an illness associated with impairment of certain brain areas (Tuma, 1999; Keefe et al., 2000; Gold et al., 1999; Green et al., 2000).

2. Prevalence

Clinically significant cognitive deficit is observed in 40 to 60% of patients. Only in about 15% of patients in good schizophrenic remission, the level of cognitive performance is comparable with that of healthy subjects (Palmer et al., 1997).

The level of cognitive deficit varies individually significantly. Harvey (1997) distinguishes between mild, medium and heavy cognitive deficit. Mild deficit represents a decrease by 0.5 to 1.0 of the standard deviation (SD) from the mean observed in healthy subjects. It is characterized by deficit of perception ability, memory deficit and attention deficit. Medium cognitive deficit is defined by the level of -1.1 to -2.0 of standard deviation. It is associated with attention deficit, delayed recall, working memory deficit and deficit of visuomotor skills. Heavy cognitive deficit is defined as -2.1 to -5.0 standard deviations. It involves learning deficit, deficit of executive functions, diminished psychomotor speed, speech fluency deficit, and vast memory deficits.

3. Areas of Cognitive Deficit in Schizophrenia

Schizophrenic patients show deficits in a variety of cognitive domains including executive function, attention, and memory. There is increasing evidence that such deficits are not global and generalized, but rather they are specific and selective, manifest by distinct patterns of association and dissociation of performance across different cognitive tasks (Kuperberg et al., 2000; Rossell and David, 1997; Gold et al., 1992; Saykin et al., 1991). Other symptoms may include motor skills deficit, some speech and language deficits and visual perception deficits (Calev, 1999). General intellectual performance decreases in some patients, too. Cognitive deficit may also be regarded as a result of bad coordination of individual component cognitive functions (Sharma and Harvey, 2000). Expressive vocabulary, general knowledge, and detail-abstraction skills remain relatively unimpaired (Tuma, 1999).

Attention

Schizophrenic patients often exhibit attention deficit, which has a negative impact on their overall cognitive performance (Neuchterlein, 1991; Cornblatt et al., 1994; Chen and Faraone, 2000; in Liu, Chiu, Chang, Hwang et al., 2002). The attention deficit is of a complex nature. Patients find focusing attention hard and are easily distracted by minor and banal external stimuli. In experimental settings of neuropsychological examinations, their attention seems to be constantly distracted by events other than those that are part of neuropsychological testing.

Schizophrenic patients can neither shift attention fast not sustain it. The Continuous Performance Test (CPT) is designed in such a way that patients are required to respond to targeted, previously set, and known stimuli. They are part of a series of other stimuli, which play the role of distracters, distracting attention. Schizophrenic patients have a significantly higher error rate in the test. They fail both due to neglecting the target stimuli and due to responding to non-target stimuli. Patients score significantly slower reaction times, being unable to divide attention between several simultaneous stimuli. Their ability to keep attention concentrated for a longer period of time is impaired. A sensitive measure of vigilance in schizophrenic patients is the Trail Making Test (TMT), especially its part B, which requires fast attention shifting between stimuli of different categories (letters and numbers). Both attention tenacity and vigilance are impaired; patients are unable to concentrate for a longer period of time and find shifting attention to different stimuli very hard.

Schizophrenic patients are, compared with healthy subjects, less apt at differentiating target objects against the background of unimportant stimuli (Oltmans et al., 1979). These patients respond to visual and auditory stimuli more slowly and often inadequately (Shakow, 1979; Libiger, 2002). Abnormal responses on the part of schizophrenic patients have been observed in reading evoked potentials during psychophysiological testing, too (Bratr et al., 1991).

In a number of patients, attention deficit is not associated with any other deficits of other parameters of cognitive functioning. In some patients, however, attention deficit has a negative effect on the working memory—especially during testing when patients sometimes make mistakes due to not being able to store the test instruction in their short-term memories.

Memory

Schizophrenic patients exhibit a wide range of memory deficits, showing deficient performance regarding almost all types of memory except for procedural (non-declarative) memory. The question, however, remains in which stage the impairment of the memory process occurs. Declarative memory may be divided by the type of information (e.g., visual, auditory, semantic, and episodic) and by the time for which information is retained (working, short-term, long-term memory).

A meta-analysis of 70 studies undertaken by Aleman et al. (1999; also Regland et al., 1996) shows that schizophrenic patients are characterized by diminished performance in terms of declarative memory compared with healthy subjects. Cirillo and Seidman (2003) analyzed 100 studies focusing on verbal declarative memory. Paulsen et al. (1995) found that schizophrenic patients perform by up to two standard deviations poorer when recalling words in California Verbal Learning Test (CVLT). On standardized Wechsler Memory Scale III (WMS-III; Psychological Corporation, 1997), the mean index of immediate auditory memory was one standard deviation lower than that of healthy subjects. The number of recalled items gets higher when patients are provided so-called key clues, and this improvement is higher in recognition than in free recall. Despite all this, the level of recall in all three modes (free recall, recognition and recall with code key) is poorer than in healthy subjects. The disproportion between performance on free recall and recognition supports the hypothesis that memory processes are affected in the recall stage rather than in the fixation or retention stage and that coordination of stimuli is less efficient than in healthy individuals.

The deficit of stimuli coding and consolidation is held to be associated with an impairment of the hippocampus and other structures of the temporal lobe (Squire, 1992; Hijman, 1996).

Verbal declarative memory depends on quality of information coding, storage and recall. It may be the case that the failure in memory tests that has been attributed to recall deficit is primarily due to a deficit in information coding. It is likely that this kind of deficit has to do with a deficit of spontaneous organization of material being stored in memory—i.e., rather with frontal brain area activity. This hypothesis was tested e.g., by Maher et al. (1995). They presented patients with a list of words whose repeated reading could highlight certain semantic relations and help patients arrange the words in a sentence. Most patients with schizophrenia and schizoaffective disorders were not capable of a contextual approach (coding the words based on arranging them in a sentence). Maher et al. (1995) were, therefore, basically exploring associational and contextual reasoning in patients. Contextual memory and information linkage ability is what the study by Waters et al. (2004) concentrated on, too. These researchers acted on the assumption that the awareness of context and memory item content are functionally independent components related to two anatomically distinct areas. Besides storing the relevant characteristic, retaining a certain event in memory requires the ability of contextual linkage, too. Contextual memory includes ability of information source identification, arranging the information in time, setting it and localizing it in space. Waters et al. (2004) examined 43 schizophrenic patients using a special method based on source identification, localization, and temporal arrangement of information (i.e., contextual reasoning). They found that patients performed poorer compared with healthy subjects both on free recall and on stimuli recognition. Patients found generating a clear contextual representation of the event heard (they failed in retaining some context characteristics).

Impaired recall ability is sometimes explained by a memory consolidation deficit (Goldberg et al., 1989; Gold et al., 1992), use of an inadequate strategy in free recall (Goldberg et al., 1989) and fast forgetting (McKenna et al., 1990). Another possible explanation for memory deficit in schizophrenia is the presence of a primary dysfunction of the executive component, namely inhibition deficit. Schizophrenic patients experience problems when they are to select relevant information in everyday situations. They find ignoring insignificant stimuli and inhibiting inadequate answers hard. The ability to suppress undesirable coding and information recall is examined using the directed forgetting (DF) paradigm. Müller et al. (2004) proved that schizophrenic patients are better at recognizing stimuli they were instructed to retain than stimuli they were instructed to forget. Up to this point, the results of patients and healthy subjects are the same. Schizophrenic patients in the study were, nevertheless, unable to adhere to the instruction regarding directed forgetting with the same success as healthy controls. The directed forgetting deficit was linked to the duration of the illness but not severity of symptoms. It may, therefore, be the case that the drop in items retained in memory is due to an inability to “filter out” irrelevant stimuli, causing a certain “contamination” to the patient’s memory capacity.

There has been evidence that episodic (autobiographical) memory is impaired in schizophrenic patients, too. Feinstein et al. (1998) found that compared with healthy subjects who remember their childhood, early adulthood and recent past just as well, the memory profile of schizophrenic patients forms a U-curve typical of schizophrenia. This means that they remember events from childhood and recent past relatively well, but are worse at recalling events from early maturity compared with healthy individuals.

One specific area of cognitive dysfunction in schizophrenic patients is working memory. Working memory mediates a temporary storage of information and mental manipulation of contents. Working memory deficit in schizophrenic patients is regarded as an irrefutable fact nowadays. At the same time, psychiatric literature keeps searching for evidence to support one of the following hypotheses: whether working memory deficit is one of the core neuropsychological deficits, causing patient failure in other cognitive areas, or whether it is a secondary deficit. For example Javitt et al. (1999) explain working memory deficit by an impairment of the ability of information coding. Tek at al. (2002) in their study consider the possible influence of perception recognition of object characteristics and space characteristics on working memory. Their schizophrenic patients performed poorer in recognition of object characteristics (e.g., color, shape, etc.) compared with healthy volunteers. Patients performed poorer in tests demanding in terms of spatial working memory. The authors conclude that schizophrenic patients suffer from dysfunction of posterior brain areas, which mediate visual information processing, and of the prefrontal area affecting information retention during short interference. The systems mediating operation of working memory for object and spatial characteristics seem to be distinct. The question whether working memory deficit is rather due to perception deficit however remains unanswered. E.g., Wexler et al. (1998) and Stevens et al. (2000) confirmed an auditory working memory deficit in schizophrenic patients, disproving impairment of the ability to discern between sounds.

Silver et al. (2003) argue in favor of the hypothesis that working memory deficit is one of the core cognitive symptoms of schizophrenia and therefore a primary deficit. They compared performance of a group of patients with a group of healthy controls, focusing on quality of verbal working memory and spatial working memory. They searched for correlations of the areas under examination with other cognitive functions (for their findings see Table 1).

Table 1. Adopted from Silver et al. (2003)

Verbal working memory	Spatial working memory
Visual retention	Visual retention
Visual orientation	Visual orientation
Motor functions	Object retention
Visuomotor coordination	Face retention
Executive functions	Motor functions

Silver et al. (2003) found working memory performance in schizophrenic patients to correlate with other cognitive functions, whereas no significant correlations were found in healthy subjects. Moreover, each type of working memory was found to correlate with a different group of cognitive functions. Compared with healthy individuals, patients had worse verbal working memory, but their performance in tasks testing spatial working memory was not impaired. Neither of the working memory domains tested correlated with attention, which the authors regard as an argument in support of the hypothesis that attention deficit is not at the core of working memory deficit in schizophrenic patients.

The way in which the operation of individual working memory types is organized varies (Tek, 2002). Dorsal prefrontal areas are reciprocally linked to inferior and posterior parietal areas, mediating thus spatial information processing (localization of information providing answers to "Where?" questions). Ventral prefrontal areas are linked to the inferior temporal visual area, mediating object information processing (i.e., information on "What" we see—e.g., color, shape, face, etc.).

Executive (Information-Management) Functions

Working memory deficit is held to be associated with the dorsolateral prefrontal cortex. Its dysfunction gets manifested, among other things, by the syndrome of executive (information-management) functions' deficit, i.e., the so-called "dysexecutive syndrome."

Prefrontal cortex is regarded as an area where internalized schemata for immediate further action, i.e., schemata into which multi-sensor information from dorsally situated association brain areas mingle and get formed. The linked limbic system signals information context based on long-term memory (the hippocampus) and emotional meaning (the amygdala). Schizophrenic patients, similar to patients with traumatic lesions of the prefrontal cortex, under-perform in a number of tests requiring the ability to retain information in memory for a short period of time and use it and its new combinations flexibly in further tasks. Working memory serves as a basis for activities typical of the humankind: understanding, planning and behavior algorithmization. Metaphorically speaking, it plays the role of a "writing pad" or a running plan of behavior. If this kind of information cannot be read from this "mental notepad," our behavior is devoid of management stimuli and our thoughts lack fluency and adequate context. If we forget to remove something from our "notepad," it comes back stereotypically. Working memory breakdown is manifested not by amnesia, but an inability to recall from memory and use a behavior- and action-organizing context (Libiger, 2002; in Höschl et al., 2002).

Deficit of executive functions in schizophrenia is manifested by hardships experienced by patients performing certain kinds of tasks. They are hardships in plan-making and implementation and difficulties at task solution (especially when new combinations of existing information are to be used), together with the consequence of a working memory deficit (Sharma and Harvey, 2000). Deficit of executive functions is, therefore, associated with patients experiencing difficulties in planning, cognitive reconstruction, flexibility and abstraction ability (Tuma and Lenderova, 2001).

In many schizophrenic patients, the core of functional deficit consists in the fact that behavior-management functions are impaired. They rely on:

- conation;
- attention regulation;
- the planning ability;
- the ability of purposeful behavior and goal attaining (Tuma, 1999).

According to Lezak (2004), the executive process involves several stages: decision, planning, purposeful action, and efficient performance. All individual components of the executive process are necessary to guarantee adequate, socially responsible, and self-caring behavior. Velligan et al. (1999) extend and specify the definition: executive functions include abstraction, activity initiation, planning and sequencing, self-monitoring, inhibition of behavior preventing goal attainment, and ability to organize and direct memory and attention. Other authors, e.g., Rossi et al. (1996) and Bustini et al. (1998), extend the definition of executive functions to include the ability of concept forming and mental flexibility.

Dysexecutive syndrome has been found in schizophrenic patients repeatedly and is currently regarded as one of the main cognitive deficits (Morice and Delahunty, 1996;

Goldsamt, 1993; Goldman, 1992 and others). In the Wisconsin Card Sorting Test (WCST), schizophrenic patients show a lower level of conceptualization and cognitive flexibility taking the form of an increased number of persevering mistakes and a small number of categories completed when compared with patients with affective disorders (Morice, 1996; Goldsamt, 1993). Considering that Goldman et al. (1992) found that schizophrenic patients are able to profit from key cues (i.e., administrator's instructions during the testing) in the test, this patients' failure is to be attributed to impaired concept-forming ability rather than failure in concept application. Goldberg et al. (1990), Schmand et al., (1992), Andreasen et al. (1992) and others have repeatedly confirmed that schizophrenic patients fail in Tower of Hanoi test. Patients are slower in the test than healthy individuals, using more steps to finish the task and exhibiting lower frontal activity. Probably due to the complexity of the executive functions construct, there is relatively little agreement about how the findings of individual studies should be interpreted. According to Morice and Delahunty (1996), failure in executive tests is underlain by a decreased level of analytical and anticipatory thinking. Other authors (Müller et al., 2004; Frith et al., 1991) believe the cause to be planning deficit and reduced rather than a deficit regarding inhibition of undesirable (automatic) responses or inability to remember the context (Bustini et al., 1998).

Executive deficit is one of the most important predictors of social skills, work efficiency, and life quality in schizophrenic patients.

Language and Speech Skills

Attention deficit, memory deficit and deficit of executive functions in schizophrenic patients are accompanied by an evident impairment of the speech ability.

As Timothy Crow has said, "schizophrenia is the price the humankind pays for speech development." Neologisms, paralogues, broken syntax, association disorders, and other disorders ranked with formal thinking disorders are the symptoms characteristic of impaired speech of schizophrenic patients. Verbal fluency (ability to recall as many words within a time interval as possible, word generation ability) is a function of the frontal lobes. As far as speech is concerned, their impairment is manifested by diminished spontaneity of verbal expression (Tuma, 1999).

Verbal fluency (VF) deficits have been observed in schizophrenic patients repeatedly. When VF is tested, two fundamental processes are activated: recall and vocabulary. The deficit may be due to an impairment of either or both processes. Chen et al. (2000) in their study tested the share of the individual processes on quality of verbal fluency in schizophrenic patients. They found not only decreased verbal production within a time limit, but also a restricted lexicon available to the patients. They found no connection between verbal fluency and the clinical profile (i.e., negative symptoms), education, age and duration of illness. Robert et al. (1997) considered in their research the possibility of decreasing verbal fluency by generation of the so-called semantic clusters (clusters of associations). They found patients had not only generally lower verbal fluency, but also produced lower numbers of clusters of associations compared with healthy subjects. (The term "clusters of associations" is used to refer to the approach to verbal fluency testing when the patients name e.g., cat, dog, cow, goat—domestic animals, mammals—within the "animals" category and then e.g., duck, goose, hen—poultry, etc.) On the other hand, Beilen et al. (2004) found based on their research that patients form just as many clusters as healthy individuals and switch from one cluster of associations to another just as often as healthy subjects but produce fewer words per cluster. Joyce et al. (1996) attempted to determine quality of recollection using keyword prompts (such as "farm animals" "domestic animals" "jungle animals", etc.). They found that patients were able to profit from the prompts—their performance improved significantly. Healthy individuals profited from the prompts just as well. The same conclusions were arrived at by Feinstein et al. (1998), who conclude that verbal fluency deficit is not due to impaired recollection. Moreover, they found that although healthy individuals produce more words in semantic (category) tests of verbal fluency and phonological category definition is more difficult for them, the situation is reverse in schizophrenic patients. Therefore, it seems that it is performance rather than recollection quality that influences the type of information solicited (semantic vs. phonological categories).

Freer associations and fragmentation of thinking are often manifested by irrelevant material included in the answer, which thus loses coherence and causes to be an adequate response to the question asked.

In heavy forms of schizophrenia, abstraction becomes less available; patients tend to provide concrete answers; the subjects are not able to abstract metaphorical meaning (Libiger, 2002).

In tests of semantic memory, patients respond increasingly to clues or priming (in the form of pairs of related concepts). Patients are to distinguish words from non-words on a computer screen and respond to them. If the word presented is proceeded by a related term (meadow—grass), the word is usually recognized faster by the person. If the words are not related, the decision about their meaning takes more time. According to some studies, patients with schizophrenia and formal thinking deficit need less time than healthy individuals to decide about the meaning of words. They are able to grasp the relation faster than healthy individuals. Patients' delay in some tests of semantic memory, evidencing harder access to concepts, can be regarded in the light of these findings as a kind of protective compensatory slow-down. It prevents them from generating excessively free associations, wiping away of differences between categories and over-inclusive thinking. Increased noise in the hyperplastic semantic network serves to reduce the ability to find more connections than useful (Libiger, 2002).

Motor Skills

The basic dysfunctions in schizophrenia include the inability of patients to perform some motor-skills-based tasks. They perform motor tasks inefficiently, slower; the movement is broken-down, and patients have an impaired ability to learn from their mistakes and correct them (Malenka et al., 1986). Their motor performance is characterized by perseveration patterns, their ability of behavior change is reduced and sometimes even an inability to finish an action started may be observed (Binder and Goldberg, 1987). Some authors regard tracking eye movement deficits as a marker of vulnerability to schizophrenia (Neuchterlein, 1991). If abnormal tracking eye movements are present, the finding is stable during the course of the illness (irrespective of the stage) and cannot be influenced by classic antipsychotics administration very much. Some studies demonstrated a connection between abnormal tracking eye movements and underperformance in neuropsychological tests of frontal functions (Levy et al., 1993).

Intellectual Skills

Intelligence quotient (IQ) may be regarded as a global output characterizing the quality of cognitive functions. IQ scores are less affected by schizophrenia as they depend on skills learned before the onset of the illness (Harvey, 1997).

Experts have recently been returning to the question whether schizophrenia is a dementia in the sense of a progressing intellectual decline or not. Poorer performance on IQ tests during the illness is explained by the effect of specific cognitive function deficits (Sharma and Harvey, 2000); as many as 51% of patients show a decline in premorbid IQ of over 10 points. This drop is due to memory deficit, attention deficit and executive functions deficit. Twenty-three percent of patients have mediocre IQ scores, showing no deterioration. In their case, memory, attention and executive functions deficits are joined by a speech deficit and a perception process deficit. Twenty-nine percent of patients have stationary, average IQ scores—they suffer from attention deficit and executive functions deficit (Weickert et al., 2000).

The study by Weickert et al. (2000) has also shown that intellectual and cognitive functions deficit need not be present in all patients before the onset of the psychosis. The finding supports the fact that in many, but not all, patients, a clinically manifested onset of the illness is followed by a cognitive decline.

The degree to which cognitive processes are influenced by IQ score has been unclear. Sharma found a connection between failure at school and retarded motor development, speech disorders and development of schizophrenia (Tuma and Lenderova, 2001).

Cognitive Deficit in Schizophrenia—Neuropsychological Studies

It is not the goal of the following chapter to provide a survey of all basic studies concerning cognitive deficit in schizophrenic patients. They are innumerable, and our understanding of the area has been developing constantly. Instead, our goal is rather to point out the stumbling blocks of research in cognitive functions—whether interpretational or terminological.

For the sake of completeness, we will mention several studies focusing on different aspects of cognitive deficit in schizophrenic patients. They will be described briefly, and some specifics to be paid increased attention will be pointed out.

Cuesta, Peralta and Zarzulela (1998) undertook research focused on the connection between duration of schizophrenia and depth of cognitive deficit. The study included 69 patients. Patients were evaluated on the SAPS and SANS scales (Scale for the Assessment of Positive Symptoms, Scale for the Assessment of Negative Symptoms) to determine positive and negative symptoms. Cognitive deficit was tested using an extensive battery including four WAIS subtests (Wechsler Adult Intelligence Scale; Information, Vocabulary, Cubes, Symbols) and WCST (Wisconsin Card Sorting Test). They also used a Spanish neuropsychological battery including a verbal fluency test (animals in one min, words beginning with P in three min), a test of visual and verbal memory (immediate and delayed recall of geometric shapes and text), and a discrimination test of attention (making out overlapping shapes). Patients were tested after the end of the acute stage of illness. Testing was done in two sessions as a maximum and lasted for not more than two hours. The findings of the study demonstrated a significant connection between duration of the illness and quality of the visuomotor process (TMT A, B, and Symbols) and delayed visual memory (accuracy of recollection of Rey-Osterrieth's complex figure). The longer the duration of the illness, the worse patients performed in these two areas.

Evans et al. (2004) observed cognitive and clinical predictors of success at work among schizophrenic patients. The study included 112 patients, who undertook a neuropsychiatric examination after being enrolled in one or another work scheme. The neuropsychological examination tested the level of learning and memory, attention, information-processing speed and executive functions. The neuropsychological battery included the following tests: California Verbal Learning Test (CVLT—learning a list of words in five attempts, recollection after interference and after delay), The Wisconsin Card Sorting Test (WCST), the Numeric Series subtest from WAIS-III, Symbols from WAIS-III and TMT—parts A and B. Clinical symptoms were assessed on PANSS (Positive and Negative Symptoms Scale). Success at work was monitored at four months after the basic examination, including tests of work success (earnings) and efficiency at work (measured by the Work Behavior Inventory questionnaire, WBI). Negative symptoms, learning and memory and cognitive disorganization correlated with duration of employment and wages. It was verbal learning and memory, together with cognitive disorganization, that proved to be significant predictors of work behavior.

Nathaniel-James et al. (1996) explored the relation between memory deficit and executive functions. They compared a group of 25 schizophrenic patients with 25 healthy subjects. Patients were examined using the following tests: Recognition Memory Test for Words, California Verbal Learning Test (CVLT), Verbal Fluency Test (phonematic version), Wisconsin Card Sorting Test (WCST), and Hayling Sentence Completion Test. Patients showed a significant drop in performance concerning immediate memory and a relatively unchanged recollection after delay. As far as verbal memory and re-identification were concerned, patients performed just as well as the control group. Memory deficit was present disregarding the coding strategy and had no connection to the duration of the illness. Patients also failed in executive functions tests, but a deeper deficit was observed in tests requiring initiation/inhibition of response. The authors conclude their study by saying that specific areas of executive functions (initiation and inhibition of response) seem to contribute to memory deficit.

Weickert et al. (2000) explored the connection between the level of cognitive functions and intellect. They examined 117 patients and 27 healthy controls. The actual level of IQ score was determined using four WAIS-R subtests (Counting, Symbols, Puzzles, and Details); premorbid intellect was assessed using the Reading subtest from WRAT (The Wide Range Achievement Test). The subtest is regarded as a sensitive method for premorbid IQ determination as it is believed that reading skills are something a person acquires prior to the onset of the illness. The neuropsychological battery contained subtests Logical Memory and Visual Memory from WMS-R (Wechsler Memory Scale Revisited), CVLT, Boston Naming Test, Verbal Fluency Test, CPT, WCST, The Benton Line Orientation Test, TMT (A, B) and The Finger Tapping Test.

In 60 patients (51%) who showed an IQ drop of 10 points or more, a deficit of executive functions, memory and attention was recorded. Twenty-eight patients (23%) with both premorbid and current IQ scores below average showed no drop in IQ scores. Patients from this group, however, failed in language and visual information processing, executive functions, memory and attention. Twenty-nine patients (25%) had average IQ scores; they showed no drop in intellectual skills, and their cognitive functions profile was comparable with that of healthy subjects except for the executive area. The authors of the study conclude from their findings that an IQ drop is not a universal characteristic of the illness and that deterioration of executive functions and attention are likely to be core symptoms of schizophrenia, regardless IQ change.

Table 2.

	Cuesta, Peralta and Zarzulela (1998)	Evans et al. (2004)	Nathaniel-James et al. (1995)	Ceskova (1999)	MATRICS (Kern et al., 2004)	Weickert et al. (2000)
CVLT—first attempts	learning		memory			declarative memory
CVLT— recall after interference and delayed recall	secondary verbal memory		memory			
WCST—perseverance errors	executive functioning	executive functioning	executive functioning	test of "frontal functions" insufficiently specific, measures rather generalized deficit		executive functioning and switching
WCST—number of categories completed	executive functioning	executive functioning	executive functioning			
TMT A	information processing speed and psychomotor speed	visuomotor functioning		visuomotor skills		psychomotor speed
TMT B	executive functioning	visuomotor functioning				
Numeric series (WAIS-III)	short-term memory					
Symbols (WAIS-III)	information processing speed and psychomotor speed					
Rey-Osterrieth's comprehensive figure		Memory				
Verbal fluency			executive functioning	speech functions	Information processing speed	recall and lexical integrity
Letter-Number Span Test				working memory	working memory	
CPT				attention	attention/ vigilance	attention

Since most neuropsychological tests measure several components simultaneously, approaches to interpreting their results differ, too; individual authors stress different parameters of the functions under analysis. Table 2 presents a review of methods used in the above research studies, including methods the authors use to interpret their findings.

Table 3. Tests of cognitive functioning

Test Cogn. function	Logical memory	Verbal pair associations	Verbal fluency	R-O figure	TMT A)	Numeric square	Tower of Hanoi	Stroop test (revised version)	WCST
Memory	++ 1)	++ 2)	++ 3)	+4)		++5)	++3)	+3)	++3)
PM			++	+	++	++	++	++	
Speech (verbal fluency, dysarthria, aphasia)	+	+	++					+	
Construction practice				++					
Visuomotor coordination				++	++	++			
Management functions (executive f.)				+			++	+	++
Attention	++	++	++	++	++	++	++	++	++
Resistance to stress	+	+	+	+	+	+	+	++	+

1) learning, short-term logical memory for auditory stimuli, 2) associative learning, 3) working memory, 4) memory for visual stimuli, 5) learning, memory for visual stimuli, spatial arrangement and movement.

Interpretation of test results is an extremely complicated issue, as most tasks require activating several cognitive areas. Quantitative data processing, moreover, misses information concerning patients and their performance that may otherwise be obtained only through observation and qualitative analysis.

Table 3 provides a list of some diagnostic methods in general use. It shows to what extent the individual methods are sensitive to areas of cognitive deficit (Tuma and Lenderova, 2001).

Although the study of cognitive deficit encompasses much research, there is little consistency among individual findings. We tend to ascribe the fact to the small number of comparative and double-blind studies. Small patient groups are tested, too. The period of monitoring (e.g., of influencing the deficit pharmacotherapeutically or rehabilitatively, its development in time, etc.) is usually relatively short. The study of development of the illness with respect to cognitive deficit is dominated by cross-sectional studies, although research would profit from a higher number of longitudinal ones. Control groups are based on sex, age and achieved education of the subjects as the main criteria, while balancing groups in terms of age, sex and IQ scores seems more useful. Moreover, no universal test battery has been available, as a consequence of which different studies use different examination methods and nonintegrated terminology. Distinguishing between long-term inpatients and outpatients is given little emphasis, too.

It is, therefore, a challenge for neurocognitive testing to develop an integrated neuropsychological battery and a unified terminology for future use.

Connections between Cognitive Deficit and Factors of the Illness (Age, Symptoms, Social Integration, Course, etc.)

Cognitive deficit is an important dimension of schizophrenia allowing us to observe certain principles of development over time. It is necessary to further study factors related to the degree of cognitive deficit—such as symptoms of the illness, demographic data, quality of social integration and also the course of the illness itself.

The study of the connection between parameters of cognitive deficit and clinical factors of schizophrenia (especially symptoms) has had unequivocal results, despite the fact that some studies in this area attempt to predict future development of clinical factors from the level of cognitive deficit at the onset of illness or the degree of its change over time.

Not all research did confirm a connection between change of symptomatology of the illness and cognitive deficit (Hoff et al., 2005; Heaton et al., 2001; Sweeney et al., 1991). These studies thus allow us to regard neuropsychological deficit as independent of the characteristics and change of the clinical status, regarding cognitive deficit as a "trait factor" of the illness.

A connection between cognition and symptoms was, conversely, suggested by other studies. Gold et al. (1999) found a connection between negative symptoms of schizophrenia and cognitive performance. Change of negative symptoms over time correlated with change of overall and verbal IQ scores. Performance IQ was in no relation to the symptoms. An improvement of verbal cognition was observed in cases when negative symptoms improved. Neither psychotic nor disorganized symptoms correlated with IQ. The study supports the view that negative symptoms are associated with a more serious course of development of cognitive performance, being linked to the primary cognitive deficit in schizophrenia. Nopoulos et al. (1994), too, found a correlation between the degree of improvement in some neuropsychological indicators and change of clinical symptoms. This concerned namely concentration of attention and inhibition of attention. Since these functions fluctuate over time, imitating clinical symptoms, referring to them as "state factors," seems useful.

Verdoux (Verdoux et al., 2002) attempted to determine whether an initial memory and executive deficit identified after two years predict worse social integration and clinical development in patients first treated with psychosis (irrespective of the diagnostic category). A worse memory performance proved to represent a greater risk of psychotic symptoms and rehospitalization. All in all, cognitive performance was a better predictor of clinical development than of social integration.

Chen et al. (2005) set out to identify cognitive predictors of a schizophrenic relapse. They found a significant difference between the relapse rate of patients with good compliance to therapy and patients without good compliance. Regression analysis used in checking the degree of compliance subsequently showed that the rate of perseverance errors in Wisconsin Card Sorting Test was a significant predictor of relapse (ratio 2:4). Cognitive flexibility and its impairment, therefore, can be an indicator of a tendency towards relapse. Carlsson et al.

(2006), too, used patients' cognitive performance to predict future development of schizophrenic symptomatology. They found that lower total IQ scores predict negative symptoms within one year.

The relation between response to therapy and cognitive performance was the subject of the study undertaken by Goldstein et al. (2002). They assumed that neurocognitive deficit may predict response to therapy in patients with first-episode schizophrenia. They namely explored the effect of cognition on adjustment of formal thinking deficit. Depending on change in this category, they divided the group into responders and non-responders and compared the subgroups. Compared with the nonresponders, the group of responders proved to be younger at the time of the testing, had a higher verbal IQ scores, higher scores in arithmetic WAIS-R subtests and lower rates of perseverance answers in Wisconsin Card Sorting Test. Responders had higher volumes of the frontal lobe, too. Semantically charged tasks had no connection to the number of responses. The study demonstrated a connection between improvement of formal thinking deficit and executive functions, which supports the hypothesis that the frontal system may play a role in response to therapy aimed at positive psychotic symptoms.

These results open the possibility of predicting different aspects of functional development of schizophrenia based on neurocognitive performance.

Visualization Methods for Schizophrenia

The greatest progress in research of cognitive functions is represented by functional visualization methods (functional nuclear magnetic resonance imaging—fMRI, single photon emission computer tomography—SPECT, positron emission tomography—PET, and magnetic resonance spectroscopy—MRS).

Structural magnetic resonance shows, thanks to its higher discrimination, the morphological finding of extended ventricles in schizophrenic patients, which were confirmed using computer tomography (CT) at the end of the 1980s. Nearly 200 MR studies (Hajek, 2002, in Höschl et al., 2002) monitoring cerebral changes in schizophrenic individuals are available. Of this set, 77% of the studies have confirmed an extension of the lateral ventricles, and 67% have confirmed an extension of the third chamber. Most structural abnormalities are locally concentrated in the area of the temporal lobe. Reduction of temporal lobe volume has been found in 62% of 37 studies. Most of the studies, which examined the temporal cortex, found a reduction in the volume of the gyrus temporalis superior, hippocampus, amygdala and gyrus parahippocampalis. Findings in the frontal lobe are somewhat less consistent—some reduction was found in 55% of focused studies. About two-thirds of the work focused on the subcortical structures found variations in the thalamus, corpus callosum, and basal ganglia areas. MRI studies have frequently shown a reduction in gray matter in the brain of schizophrenic patients. The reduction is more extensive in the temporal and prefrontal cortex than in other parts of the brain. MRI also revealed that, although the extension of the cerebral chambers and reduction of the gray matter is present in patients of childhood age and is largely static, in some patients, at least, a progression of the atrophic changes can still occur.

The atrophic changes are not accompanied by gliosis (hypertrophy of supportive cerebral cells that impair the cerebral activity and thus cognitive functions), as might be expected in cases of degenerative changes taking place during aging. The absence of the glial reaction is, therefore, indirect evidence supporting the theory of early development, in schizophrenia, of pathomorphological changes in the CNS. Structural changes in the brain of schizophrenics have been extensively reviewed by Koukolik (1992). A contrasting approach is offered by psychopathological findings related to schizophrenia in various anatomically localized brain injuries (Table 4) (Tuma and Lenderova, 2001).

Studies involving functional neuroimaging during several different cognitive tasks suggest that schizophrenia is associated with a widespread dysfunction within a network of brain areas involving the frontal and temporal cortex, the hippocampus, and subcortical regions.

Impaired dorsolateral prefrontal cortex (DLPFC) function has been linked with impaired working memory (WM)—the internal representation, maintenance and updating of sensory information—in schizophrenia (Goldman-Rakic et al., 1999). Several recent studies have given new insights into the precise relationships between DLPFC dysfunction and WM performance. DLPFC function may be dependent upon task "difficulty::" during tasks with a low WM load, DLPFC function lies within the normal range and only becomes abnormal when WM load increases and performance becomes less accurate (Carter et al., 1998; Fletcher et al., 1998; Manoach et al., 1999). Although this finding reconciles the divergent results of some previous studies, discrepancies still remain: both decreased (Carter et al., 1998) and increased (Manoach et al., 1999) recruitment of DLPFC have been described during high-load WM tasks, and both right (Carter et al., 1998) and left (Manoach et al., 1999) DLPFC dysfunctions have been documented.

Table 4. Organic brain injury and the psychopathology relation to schizophrenia (Tuma and Lenderova, 2001)

Anatomic localization of the lesion	Psychopathology	Reference
frontal lobe- medial part	Catatonic and hebephrenic symptoms; loss of initiative, volitional and intellectual activities, thinking arrests, mutism	Hilbom, 1951 Joseph, 1996
frontal lobe—lateral part (disruption of the frontal-thalamic-neocortical circuits)	information processing disorders, overloading with sensory inputs, confusion, working memory disorders, poverty of speech	Joseph, 1996 Lewis, 1995
nucleus caudatus (disruption of basal ganglia circuits—frontal cortex)	sensory disorders, agitation, hyperactivity or apathy, emotional flattening, catatonic conditions	Joseph, 1996 Spiegel a Szekeley, 1961
temporal lobe	inadequate emotional reactivity, aggressivity, aphasia, paranoia, hallucinations, memory disorders, magical/religious thinking	Crowe a Kuttner, 1991 Trimble a Perez, 1982
amygdala, hippocampus	complex hallucinations, speech/thinking disorders, memory/learning disorders, social-emotional agnosia	Dauphinais et al., 1990 Joseph, 1996

Moreover, deficits on different WM tasks are associated with distinct patterns of dysfunction: for example, WM deficit for words but not tones (Danion et al., 1999) is associated with an impaired recruitment of left inferior frontal cortex (Stevens et al., 1998).

Frontal dysfunction in schizophrenia may be associated with increases responses in distant yet highly connected areas such as the parietal cortex (Fletcher et al., 1998; Curits et al., 1999) and the superior temporal gyrus (Fletcher et al., 1998). Moreover, a recent PET study revealed abnormally high levels of hippocampal blood flow in schizophrenia: patients failed to show a normal modulation of hippocampal activity during word retrieval (Heckers et al., 1998).

There is increasing evidence that three brain regions that make strong connections with the frontal lobe—the thalamus, the striatum, and the cerebellum—are also abnormal in schizophrenia. First, thalamic glucose metabolism during verbal learning is reduced in schizophrenic subjects, primarily in the region of the mediodorsal nucleus (Hazlett et al., 1999). Second, both treated and untreated patient groups show decreased striatal metabolic rates during a verbal learning task (Shihabuddin et al., 1998). Third, studies of verbal learning and story recollection suggest that the cerebellum, via connections with both the DLPFC and the thalamus, is also part of the abnormal circuitry in schizophrenia (Crespo-Facorro et al., 1999; Andreasen et al., 1999).

Recent studies of eye-tracking dysfunction in schizophrenia provide further evidence for the involvement of both frontal and temporal regions (Chen et al., 1999, 1999, 1999; Maruff et al., 1998; Sweeney et al., 1998; Thaker et al., 1998). First, the observed pattern of impaired pursuit eye movements and intact catch-up saccades implicates the frontal eye fields or their efferent or afferent pathways (Sweeney et al., 1998). Second, a series of recent studies has described a motion perception deficit with impaired velocity discrimination, suggesting the involvement of the motion processing area MT (medial temporal area) in the temporal lobe (Chen et al., 1999, 1999, 1999).

In summary, perturbations of brain activity in schizophrenia are not localized to one brain region but to neural networks, primarily involving the frontal and temporal lobes as well as subcortical regions. It has been proposed that the functional connections between these regions may be abnormal in schizophrenia. This hypothesis has been tested using novel statistical approaches. For example, structural equation modeling (path analysis) of a semantic processing study using PET showed differences between schizophrenia and control groups in the neural interactions amongst frontal regions, and between the frontal and temporal regions, and between the frontal lobe and anterior cingulate cortex (Jennings et al., 1998). When PET data from a memory study were analyzed for the effects of one neuronal system over another (so-called effective connectivity analysis), the normal anterior cingulate modulation of frontal-temporal interaction was found to be disrupted in schizophrenia (Fletcher et al., 1999).

An imbalance along the frontal lobe-cerebellum-thalamus axis is interpreted by Andreasen (2000, in Crespo et al., 2000) as a neuronal base for permanent, non-progressing foundation of schizophrenia. The clinical correlate is a failure of the executive (controlling) functions linked with the activity of the prefrontal cortex; and an increase in thalamus/cerebellum activity is compensatory. To describe this proposed basic cognitive disorder in schizophrenia, Andreasen uses the term "cognitive dysmetria" (Hajek, 2002, in Höschl et al., 2002).

Interesting results have been revealed through MRS (magnetic resonance spectroscopy) in schizophrenic patients; this technique allows measurements of phospholipid metabolite concentrations. These metabolites influence the formation and degradation of phospholipid membranes, growth of dendritic spikes and synaptic dentition, among others, which are key processes in brain maturation. In vivo, MRS studies find lower concentrations of phosphomonoesters (PME) in the frontal lobes. In early phases of the disease, a concomitant increase in the concentration of phosphodiesters (PDE), i.e., products of their catabolism, were also found in addition to decreased concentrations of phospholipid membranes (PME) building stones. It seems that in the early stage of schizophrenia, MRS reflects a metabolic disorder of membrane phospholipids in the active phase, which later this process may be burned out. Such findings might be explained by differing maturation of CNS in schizophrenic individuals due to excessive synaptic elimination in the respective area. Some works have also described higher concentrations of PDE in the temporal lobe of schizophrenic patients. The most frequent replicated finding of proton spectroscopy in schizophrenia consists of a decrease in NAA (N-acetylaspartate) in temporal lobes, especially the hippocampus, and most frequently, bilaterally. A decrease in the NAA signal was also described for the frontal lobes. Generally, those findings have been most frequently interpreted as a result of neuronal dysgenesis or degeneration of those areas. In the coming years, there will probably be a trend to incorporate MRS findings into the broader context of neuronal dysfunction in schizophrenia. It appears that, for instance, a reduction of NAA concentration, revealed by SPECT, in the dorsolateral prefrontal cortex is correlated with lower resting dopaminergic activity in the striatum. Additionally, a correlation between NAA reduction in the prefrontal area and negative symptomatology in schizophrenic individuals has been found (Keshavan et al., 2000).

The PET/SPECT examinations of schizophrenia describe a decrease in sagittal, cortical-subcortical, and transversal gradient. Only 50% of the quiet studies (without stressing the patient with a neuropsychological paradigm) have confirmed a reduction in frontal cortex metabolism (hypofrontality). However, nearly all studies have confirmed activation hypofrontality. Frontal hypoactivity is most frequently connected with negative symptoms and psychomotor depletion syndrome. Hallucinations and delusions have been most frequently connected with abnormalities in temporal areas. The disorganized form of schizophrenia, characterized by formal thinking disorders and emotional inadequacy, is primarily connected with increased perfusion of the anterior cingulum (Liddle, 1996). Receptor studies have shown increased density of dopamine D2 receptors in schizophrenia. However, the presynaptic dopaminergic activity has also been found to be increased, e.g., increased uptake of F-DOPA or increased dopamine release after stimulation with amphetamine. The latest finding is, however, typical only for the exacerbation period; during dwell time, patients do not differ from healthy controls (Laruelle et al., 1999).

In the pathophysiology of cognitive disorders associated with schizophrenia, dysfunction of neurotransmitter systems (e.g., serotonin, excitation amino-acids, GABA, cholinergic system, neuropeptides) also plays a role (Libiger, 1990).

Some genetic studies have also provided evidence that the cognitive deficit seen in schizophrenia is part of the disease. An examination of monozygotic twins, who were discordant for schizophrenia, found that the schizophrenic twin showed significantly poorer cognitive performance (Goldberg, 1990, 1993a; Preiss, 1992). Bermann et al. (1992) found disruption of regional cerebral perfusion in the prefrontal area, in affected monozygotic twins, during test tasks requiring activity in this part of the cortex. No reduction in perfusion was observed in healthy siblings.

Egan et al. (2001) found that the polymorphism of the gene for enzyme catechol-O-methyl-transferase (COMT) is related to dopaminergic activity in the area of the prefrontal cortex and its functions, especially working memory. The COMT val allele is found more frequently in schizophrenic patients and is linked to a reduction in dopaminergic activity in the prefrontal cortex, especially in COMT val homozygotes. The reduced dopaminergic activity correlates with impaired performance.

4. Measurement of Cognitive Function

Recent proposals for inclusion of cognitive deficit in diagnostic indications of schizophrenia have occurred; e.g., Lewis (2004) suggested including a decrease in cognitive performance to the diagnostic B-criterion, which includes a reference to a reduction of efficiency in the areas of work, interpersonal relations, and patient self-care. Specifically, he suggests that cognitive dysfunction be defined as a deficit in at least two of the three cognitive areas: attention or vigilance (maintained attention), memory and executive functions.

Test Methods

Quality of attention may be assessed by a series of cognitive tests—the effect of attention on cognitive performance can, strictly speaking, never be isolated. Tests with greater sensitivity to attention disorders include: CPT (Continuous Performance Test), N-back test, Bourdon test, and the subtest Symbols from WAIS-R.

Examination methods are used to determine the quality of working memory, represented by the Verbal Fluency Test (FAS; phonematic and semantic version) and the Design Fluency Test, in which perseverance within a single category is considered to be an indicator of a working memory disorder. Other working memory tests include repetition of numbers in reverse order (Digit Span test of WMS or WAIS-R), Wisconsin Card Sorting Test—a disorder of the working memory is primarily manifested as a failure to complete the task—various alternatives to the "tower tasks" include the Tower of London, Tower of Hanoi, Trail Making Test B and N-back Test.

Examination of the short-term memory is mostly aimed at determination of capacity and quality in several modalities. We concentrated on variability of performance, based on the method of recall—we monitored free recall, cued recall and recognition, paid attention to the influence of input type (verbal or non-verbal, auditory or visual) and the effect of length of retention (immediate or remote recall). Standard, short-term memory examinations, e.g., subtests of the Wechsler Memory Scale, California Verbal Learning Test (CVLT), Rey-Osterrieth Complex Figure, and others, were used. The non-verbal tests of auditory memory included the Seashore Tonal Memory Test (Seashore et al., 1960). In this test, the patient should distinguish between tones that mark off two compared melodies (three to five tones) in a total of 30 paired melodies.

Methods used to examine executive functions included the Wisconsin Card Sorting Test (WCST), Tower of Hanoi, London, and Stroop test—an alternative of interference of a word and a color (Stroop Color Word Interference Test)—Test of Verbal Fluency ("FAS") and (Trail Making Test B). Each of the executive functions tests is aimed at a specific aspect of the neuropsychological area. WCST primarily measures concept-making, sensible flexible changes of strategy depending on feedback, ability of inhibition, abstraction and working memory. The more specific "tower tests" engage motor abilities, planning, fragmentation of long-term goals into individual steps and inhibition. The Stroop test, especially interference of a word and a color, requires a strong ability to inhibit automatic responses. The Trail Making Test B, on the other hand, puts a high demand on the ability to switch between attention and working memory.

Interpretation of the performance in tests of verbal fluency is a bit questionable. Generally, the test is considered a so-called prefrontal test, i.e., a tool that is sensitive to the function of the prefrontal brain area. We used either the phonematic or categorical version. However, patient performance is influenced by several factors, by the size of their vocabulary (i.e., also long-term memory) and the ability to search for proper words from their lexical reserve, and also recall ability and recall strategy. The test also places a demand on working memory; the patient must momentarily keep the words they have already listed in working memory in order to avoid repetition. However, this means they must suppress the answers that suggest themselves but that have already been used. Therefore, the test employs long-term memory, working memory, verbal fluency and executive functions (selection of strategy and inhibition). It turns out that while selecting words from the lexical reserve, the prefrontal lobe is activated, while recall from the lexical reserve tends to be limited to the temporal parts of the brain.

The difficulties in examination of cognitive functions in schizophrenic patients are not related to a lack of testing methods, but instead to questionable and often reductionist interpretations of patient performance. The communication between individual psychologists and sites is also complicated by inconsistent terminology used in the description of cognitive profiles. Another problem is associated with the wide spectrum of tests used and an unwillingness to accept the need for retesting using the same diagnostic tools. Also, in order to achieve a meaningful examination, it is important to determine the level of anxiety present in the patient prior to testing. Excessive anxiety may decrease the validity of the examination. Last but not least, we recommend focusing on the practical deficit-related impacts on the patient's everyday life.

5. Temporal Development of Cognitive Deficit

The study of the development of cognitive deficit over the period of duration of schizophrenia has been an important research area. Researchers are trying to find an answer to the question whether cognitive deficit in schizophrenic patients deteriorates, improves or remains stable in the course of the illness.

Change in cognitive deficit over time has been studied since Kraepelin, who regarded schizophrenia as a degenerative illness accompanied by a necessary decline of cognitive functions. On the other hand, Bleuler demonstrated on a big group of schizophrenic patients that the level of deterioration was only very mild in most of them, and the patients were able to engage in work activity (Kurtz et al., 2005). These two views have persisted until the present day. Schizophrenia is, on the one hand, being regarded as a degenerative neuropsychiatric illness characterized by a long, progressing, symptomatic, neurocognitive and psychosocial decline. The opposing view, however, presents schizophrenia as an illness characterized by neurocognitive deficit manifested at the beginning of its development and remaining more or less stable and without progression. So-called static encephalopathy is being referred to (Kurtz et al., 2005).

Both these views are reflected in research. Recent findings generally seem to support the hypothesis of static encephalopathy.

Cognitive deficit is present during the first schizophrenic episode already, remaining more or less stable later on, and persisting as long as the illness lasts (Gold et al., 1999; Ceskova et al., 1999). According to less recent studies, cognitive deficit deepens in states of acute exacerbation; cognitive functions are, however, largely not restored to a premorbid level in clinical remission (Sharma and Harvey, 2000). The persistent character of cognitive deficit after clinical symptoms of the illness abating was manifested by Goldberg et al. (1993). The authors observed a group of schizophrenic patients treated with clozapine. Their schizophrenic symptoms were reduced after 15 months, but cognitive functions did not improve. This persisting cognitive functions deficit was in the background of patients' inability of adequate social adaptation despite the fact that clinical symptoms were already gone.

Hyde et al. (1994) demonstrated in their cross-sectional study that intellectual functions do not show any marked drop in schizophrenic patients during their illness. A longitudinal study by Heaton (Heaton et al., 2001), also confirmed the stability of neuropsychological functions in schizophrenic outpatients over a period of three years. The group of patients with schizophrenia had a test-retest reliability and neuropsychological stability comparable to the control group both during short-term (1.6 year on average) and long-term (five years on average) observation. Sweeney (Sweeney et al., 1991) demonstrated by his research that in schizophrenic patients, along with stability in time of the neuropsychological deficit, an improvement of certain neuropsychological functions can be observed, too. In many patients, this improvement resulted in a test performance within the norm.

Rund's analysis (Rund et al., 1998) of longitudinal studies lasting for at least one year and mapping development of neurocognitive deficit in schizophrenic patients clearly demonstrated that cognitive deficit is relatively stable for a long period of time, and no cognitive functions' decline occurs in the course of the illness.

In contrast to that, Kurtz et al. (2005) found in their analysis of longitudinal studies dealing with temporal development of neurocognitive deficit in schizophrenic patients that the development of cognitive deficit may involve two different trajectories and that stability of cognitive deficit is not a general phenomenon. One of the two trends was typical of patients with a more favorable course of development of the illness (community-dwelling outpatients). In these patients, the level of cognitive functions remained the same throughout the illness. A potential amount of deterioration was consistent with deterioration of cognitive functions during normal aging. In some parameters (such as IQ), patients even improved—sometimes even after a period of 5 years. The findings were comparable for groups of patients experiencing their first episode of schizophrenia and chronic patients. The other, opposing trend was found in research focusing on middle-aged patients and elderly patients in institutional treatment. Their parameters of cognitive performance clearly indicated deterioration over the period of observation. The identification of these two differing trends in development of cognitive functions may, according to the author, suggest that different pathophysiological mechanisms may be manifested in different stages of schizophrenia. The study also showed that the hypothesis of static encephalopathy is not fully valid for development of cognitive deficit in schizophrenia and that other factors of this heterogeneous illness must be taken into account.

In a comparison of findings of studies dealing with the development of cognitive deficit solely in patients with first-episode schizophrenia (or those who were ill for a short time only), the findings were more consistent and confirmed that cognitive deficit is stabilized in time.

Hoff and his team (Hoff et al., 1999) demonstrated in their longitudinal research of patients with first-episode schizophrenia a relative stability of neuropsychological functions after four to five years from the onset of the illness. The degree of improvement was, however, smaller compared with the group of controls. The same observation was carried out after a period of 10 years (Hoff et al., 2005). No difference between the patients and the control group as to change of cognitive functions during the interval was detected either. In none of the tests did patients deteriorate more significantly than the group of controls.

Similar results and, moreover, an improvement over time were identified in other studies of patients with first-episode schizophrenia. Gold (Gold et al., 1999) found that the cognitive performance of a group of young patients treated with neuroleptics did not deteriorate and was even capable of improving. Nopoulos (Nopoulos et al., 1994), too, demonstrated that cognitive functions remained stable in most domains. A significant improvement was observed in tests of overall attention and response inhibition. Addington et al. (2005) identified several significant improvements of cognitive functions over the period of two years comparable with improvement in the control group.

These findings entitle us to expect cognitive performance to be stable or mildly improve in first-episode schizophrenia.

6. Proposal of Examination

The neuropsychological assessment of cognitive functions in schizophrenic patients is complex for several reasons. No diagnostic method that could separately evaluate single cognitive or intellectual functions is available. Each examination also involves a relationship between the patient and the investigator and the level of anxiety connected with the testing situation; quality of attention, as well as other variables, also actively intervenes. For instance, it is difficult to isolate the memory level, quality of attention and executive functions using memory tests. Because of this, most interpretations of test results are necessarily reductionist in nature. The most frequent questions we ask ourselves while examining schizophrenic patients include:

- Is there a neuropsychological deficit present? What is its character and extent?
- Which cognitive domains have been maintained?
- What effect has psychopharmacotherapy had on cognitive functions?

- Is the cognitive deficit developing progressively or is it stationary?
- To what extent and in which ways is the cognitive deficit influencing the social skills and quality of life of the patient?
- Which type of rehabilitation would be beneficial for the patient?

The clinical examination offers a scale of diagnostic opportunities. If we want to determine the individual cognitive profile of the patient in detail, his "weak," and "strong" points, it is useful to flexibly adapt the examination to relevant needs and intentions. This is especially true when our objective is to establish an individual plan of rehabilitation. There are many diagnostic methods suitable for examination of cognitive functions. A relatively comprehensive survey of the neuropsychological methods is given by Lezak (1995) in her book *Neuropsychological Assessment*. However, for research purposes, it is desirable to form a unified protocol for psychological examinations. MATRICS—Measurement and Treatment Research to Improve Cognition in Schizophrenia, an initiative of leading scientists dealing with cognitive affection in schizophrenic patients and its treatment, gives seven cognitive areas that are specific for schizophrenia (Kern et al., 2004): a) attention / vigilance, b) speed of information processing, c) working memory, d) verbal learning and memory, e) visual learning and memory, f) logical thinking and problem solving, and g) social cognition. The contemporary trend is towards creation of a neuropsychological battery of tests that could allow for a unified, adequately timed, exacting (lasting minimally 60 and maximally 120 minutes) examination aimed specifically at sensitive areas of the neurocognitive affection and fulfilling basic criteria for standardization. Such a battery should comply with requirements for test-retest reliability—offer an alternative form of examination and fulfill criteria of functional output prediction (i.e., influence of the cognitive deficit on "routine" functioning of the patient). It is still being considered whether computerized versions of the tests, or tests of the "pencil-paper" variety should be preferred. Computerized tests are easier for the psychologists—most of programs offer data processing as well, and thus their use is less time-consuming. However, for some patients, any contact with computers is too demanding and may negatively influence their test performance. In addition, computerized examinations lack direct contact between the test administrator and patient, which precludes any qualitative assessment of the patient's performance. MATRICS suggests the creation of a test battery that can also be administered by psychiatrists and nurses and recommends, in such cases, a two-day administrators' internship.

The MATRICS group has prepared a proposal for a battery for clinical purposes (www.matrics.ucla.edu, adapted according to Preiss, 2005)—see Table 5:

Table 5. Proposal of the MATRICS initiative, we enumerate methods which were best assessed by experts for respective area

Area of cognitive functions	Recommended tool (test)
Working memory	Letter Number Span (verbal) Spatial memory (from WMSIII)
Attention/vigilance	CPT-IP (Continuous Performance Test-Identical Pairs)
Verbal learning and memory	Hopkins Verbal Learning Test
Visual learning and memory	BVMT—Brief Visuospatial Memory Test
Reasoning and problem solving	Neuropsychological Assessment Battery—Mazes
Rate of information processing	Verbal fluency—category (Category Fluency)

7. Rehabilitation and Psychotherapy

The care for schizophrenic patients should integrate biological and psychological approaches. Although one therapeutic method for cognitive deficits involves treatment with modern antipsychotic drugs, the number of studies demonstrating their effectiveness is still insufficient. In the rehabilitation care of the schizophrenic patients, emphasis is put on the area of information processing, attention, memory, and the executive component. Although it has been found again and again that the rate of disruption of cognitive functions is reflected in the quality of social functioning of patients, therefore, treatment shouldn't be directed solely toward a remedy of the cognitive deficit. It appears that an appreciable part of stigmatization of schizophrenic patients is caused by persistent negative symptoms. When families of schizophrenic patients were questioned regarding what they considered to be the most troubling aspects of the patient's diseases, more than 85% of respondents cited loss of friends, hobbies, and lack of interest in what was happening around them (Runions and Prudo, 1983). Other negative symptoms include: poverty of speech, apathy, lack of motivation, emotional flattening and attention disorders (Andreasen and Olsen, 1982); a connection between negative symptoms and cognitive deficits has been found in some studies (Aleman et al., 1999, Braff et al., 1991, Buchanon et al. 1994). Neurocognitive deficits influence the successfulness of rehabilitation procedures (Green, 1996)—e.g., it was found that it was not the nature of the symptoms, but, more precisely, the seriousness of the cognitive affection that was the determining element for practicing of social skills—specifically, the executive functions, verbal memory and attention (McKee, 1997).

Smith et al. (1999) examined efficiency of two therapeutic approaches: training of skills and supportive psychotherapy. A total 32 patients with chronic psychotic disease, randomized in two groups, took part in the study. The first group was trained in skills; the training primarily utilized behavioral techniques, aimed at the ability to identify the risk factors, identify symptoms and effects of drugs and plan activities. The training consisted of 16 meetings carried out five times weekly for 60 minutes. The control group of the patients also came daily and took part in supportive group therapy, which involved discussions about problems the patients' faced during their daily routine. Both prior to the therapy and after it, the patients were examined with a battery of tests, covering both positive/negative symptoms, and a questionnaire that identified the rate of reintegration (social skills) of the patients and tests of attention, executive functions, and verbal memory. All three measured cognitive areas (most significantly verbal memory) correlated with the rate of therapeutic efficiency. The patients who were involved in the training program, showed a marked improvement in their social skills in comparison to patients under supportive therapy.

For now, combined treatment comprising pharmacotherapy, psycho-education, training of social skills and cognitive training seems to be effective. In this sense, H. D. Brenner's Integrated Psychotherapeutical Program (IPT) is the most elaborate program and, from the point of view of its effect, the most efficient one. It is concentrated on cognitive training, improvement of social perception and competence, increasing verbal communication abilities and solving interpersonal situations. In the area of cognitive rehabilitation, training is primarily focused on attention quality (targeted, selective attention and its switching), capability to develop and, depending on changing conditions, reevaluate strategic concepts leading to certain objectives and the ability to recall the concept (thus it is a development of abstract reasoning). In other IPT programs, patients are encouraged to improve skills in analyzing information (to be able to distinguish between relevant and irrelevant inputs), learn to view social situations from various angles, improve their conversation abilities, try to define behavioral objectives and choose successive steps to reach them. The efficiency of such an approach has been confirmed by many studies (Brenner et al., 1996). However, there remains a question regarding the success of the training effect over time. The longest period, during which the positive effects of IPT were monitored, has been 18 months (Brenner, 1996).

In contrast to the quite encouraging IPT results, the Goldberg (1987) plan to rehabilitate cognitive functions through training at solving the Wisconsin Card Sorting Test seems to be at an impasse. Studies (e.g., Delahunty et al., 1993) have shown that only through clear structuring of the task and specific instructions to the patient, was it possible to improve the patient's performance on the WCST.

Recently. computer programs have attracted the interest of therapists dealing with cognitive rehabilitation. The advantage of such a therapeutic approach is related to the complexity of the administered tasks, quality, and precise immediate feedback, often higher motivation of patients regarding their performance, flexibility of reaction to the performance and mistakes and the ability to store and process data (Rodriguez et al., 2002). Computerized rehabilitation may be carried out both in groups and individually, with a focus on specific or global deficits. Examples of these types of programs include Cognitive Enhancement Therapy (CET; Hogarty a Flesher, 1999), a technique combining interactive software and social training in groups, Cognitive Remediation Program (Vauth et al., 2000) and the Bracy PSS CogReHab program (Bracy, 1986). Despite the attractiveness of the computer programs, their efficacy is still debatable. Actually, one question remains regarding the effectiveness of isolating and rehabilitating a single cognitive domain; can the patient utilized the acquired skill in common daily activities, and to what extent does the therapeutic effect persist without additional training and revision. Although some programs are interactive (i.e., they offer feedback and motivational support to the patient), they are no substitute normal interpersonal contact. Despite these issues, it is an approach that may prove to be effective as we gain more experience with it.

Suslow et al. (2001) carried out a meta-analysis of nine studies monitoring efficacy of cognitive functions rehabilitation in schizophrenic patients. Of the nine studies, five studies were based on computerized rehabilitation and four studies included training using a pencil-paper method. Despite inconsistencies in rehabilitation procedures, it was shown that in 15 of 35 observed variables, which served as an index of efficacy, significant improvement occurred.

Although the results of research monitoring the efficacy of computerized rehabilitation are quite inconsistent, it seems that a certain rate of efficiency is now conclusive (review, Wykes, 2000). They are also two case reports demonstrating that rehabilitation of cognitive functions in schizophrenic patients may improve brain perfusion (Wykes, 1998).

So far, rehabilitation of cognitive functions has attracted relatively low attention. In addition, results from available studies are inconsistent, especially taking into account the view regarding the character of effective training. The question of duration of the therapeutic effect and its influence on common daily activates of patients has also not yet been answered. An ideal way to remedy the neuropsychological deficit seems to consist of a combination of pharmacotherapy, education, cognitive functions training, and social skills training.

Computerized training programs represent a relatively young, and so far unexplored, area of cognitive rehabilitation.

Conclusion

Cognitive deficit is considered one of the primary symptoms of schizophrenia; it affects approximately 40 to 60% of patients. The most disrupted cognitive processes include information processing, attention, memory, and executive functions. Again and again disorders of all memory types have been found; with the exception of procedural memory. However, so far the mechanism for memory deficits is not clear. It is speculated to be related to the influence of a reduced ability to select important inputs from among unimportant ones, the effect of attention and contextual reasoning disorders and problems in creating strategies which can provide recall of stored material. The dysexecutive syndrome is primarily manifested by disrupted ability to plan and change strategies based on changes in surrounding conditions. Both focused and divided and intermittent attention is usually disrupted.

Cognitive performance usually decreases after the first episode of disease; the deficit of cognitive functions are stable over time and are relatively independent of clinical symptoms associated with the disease.

The development of the imaging methods allows research into the neuro-anatomical correlates of cognitive deficits. Structural changes in the area of frontal and temporal lobe and extension of the ventricular system have been repeatedly found.

Examination of cognitive functions is complicated for many reasons. It is difficult to isolate individual cognitive domains; in addition, there is no unified test battery and terminological consensus that could facilitate interpretation of examination results and communication between clinics.

Therapy for schizophrenic patients should integrate pharmacological intervention, education, training of social skills and cognitive training. Also, computerized rehabilitation is available, although its efficiency has not been clearly proven yet.

Cognitive dysfunction significantly influences social competence of patients, their labor performance, and quality of life.

Future progress in research into the neuropsychological consequences of schizophrenia may help to prevent and diagnose the disease and find new efficient therapeutic treatments for schizophrenia.

References

Addington J, Addington D, Maticka-Tyndale E. Cognitive functioning and positive and negative symptoms in schizophrenia. *Schizophrenia Res.* 1991;5:123–134.

Alleman A, Hijman R, de Haan EHF, Kahn S. Memory Impairment in Schizophrenia: A Meta-Analysis. *Am. J. Psychiatry* 1999;156: 1358-1366.

Andreasen NC, Olsen S. Negative and positive schizophrenia: definition and validation. *Arch. Gen. Psychiatry* 1982;39:789-794.

Andreasen NC, Rezai K, Allinger R, Swayze HVW, Flaum M, Kirchner P, Cohen G, O´Leary D. Hypofrontality in neuroleptic-naive patients and in patients with chronic schizophrenia. *Archives of General Psychiatry* 1992;49:943-958.

Asarnow RF. Neurocognitive impairments in schizophrenia: a piece of the epigenetic puzzle. *Eur. Child Adolesc. Psychiatry* 1999;8(Suppl 1):15-18.

Aylward E, Walker E, Bettes B. Intelligence in schizophrenia: meta analysis of the research. *Schizophr. Bull.* 1984;10:430-459.

Bedwell JS, Keller B, Smith AK, Hamburger S, Kumra S, Rapoport JL. Why does postpsychotic IQ decline in childhood-onset schizophrenia? *Am. J. Psychiatry* 1999;156:1996-1997.

Berman KF, Torrey EF, Daniel DG, Weinberger DR. Regional cerebral blood flow in monozygotic twins discordant and concordant for schizophrenia. *Arch. Gen. Psychiatry* 1992;49:927–934.

Bleuler E. Dementia Preacox oder Gruppe der Schizophrenien. Franz Deuticke,Wien,1911: 420.

Borison RL. The role of cognition in the risk-benefit and safety analysis of antipsychotic medication. *Acta Psychiatry Scand* 1996;94:5-11.

Bracy OL. Cognitive rehabilitation: a process approach. *Cogn Rehabilit* 1986;4:10-17. In: Rodriguez M, Mohr P, Preiss M. Program počítačové rehabilitace kognitivních funkcí u schizofrenie. *Psychiatrie* 2002;6(Suppl.4):42-45.

Braff DL, Heaton R, Kuck J et al. The generalized pattern of neuropsychological deficits in outpatients with chronic schizophrenia with heterogeneous Wisconsin Card Sorting Test results. *Arch. Gen. Psychiatry* 1991;48:891-898.

Brenner HD, Hirsbrunner A, Heimberg A. Integrated Psychological Therapy Program: Training in Cognitive and Social Skills for Schizophrenic Patients. In: Corrigan PW and Yudofsky SC. Cognitive Rehabilitation for Neuropsychiatric Disorders. American Psychiatric Press 1996,459.

Buchanon RW, Strauss ME, Kirkpatrick B et al. Neuropsychological impairments in deficit vs. nondeficit forms of schizophrenia. *Arch. Gen. Psychiatry* 1994;51:804-811.

Bustini M, Stratta P, Daneluzzo E, Pollice R, Prosperini P, Rossi A. Tower of Hanoi and WCST performance in schizophrenia: problem-solving capacity and clinical correlates. *Journal of Psychiatric Research* 1999; 33: 285-290.

Calev A. Neuropsychological functions in psychiatric disorders. *American Psychiatric Press* 1999;2:33-66.

Cannon M, Caspi A, Moffitt TE, Harrington H, Taylor A, Murray RM, Poulton R. Evidence for early-childhood, pan-developmental impairment specific to schizophreniform disorder: results from a longitudinal birth cohort. *Arch Gen Psychiatry* 2002;59:449-456.

Cirillo MA, Seidman LJ. Verbal declarative memory dysfunction in schizophrenia: from clinical assessment to genetics and brain mechanisms. *Neuropsychology Review* 2003; 13: 43-77.

Cohen MR. Nejčastější psychické poruchy v klinické praxi. Portál, Praha,2002.

Cornblatt BA, Keilp JG. Impaired attention, genetics, and the pathophysiology of schizophrenia. *Schizophrenia Bull.* 1994;20:31–46.

Cornblatt B, Obuchowski M, Roberts S, Pollack S, Erlenmeyer-Kimling L. Cognitive and behavioral precursors of schizophrenia. *Dev. Psychopatol.* 1999; 11: 487-508.

Crespo-Facorro B, Kim JJ, Andreasen NC, O'Leary DS, Magnotta V. Regional frontal abnormalities in schizophrenia: A quantitative grey matter volume and cortical surface size study. *Biological Psychiatry* 2000;48:110-119.

Crow TJ, Done DJ, Sacker A. Childhood precursors of psychosis as clues to its evolutionary origins. *Eur. Arvh. Psychiatry Clin. Neurosci.* 1995;245:61-69.

Cuesta MJ, Peralta V, Zarzuela A. Illness duration and neuropsychological impairments in schizophrenia. *Schizophr. Res.* 1998;33:141-150.

Češková E. Kognitivní dysfunkce u schizofrenie. Č.S. Psychiat 1995;5:278-287.

Češková E, Drybčák P, Hrobař P, Lorenc M, Sedláková H, Špaček J. Význam biologických markerů v diagnostice a predikci výsledků akutní léčby. Čes Slov Psychiatrie 1998;94:245–251.

Češková E, Špaček J, Šindelářová M. Kognitivní dysfunkce a efekt léčby u schizofrenní poruchy. *Československá Psychologie* 1999;43:527–535.

Dauphinais ID, DeLisi LE, Crow TJ, Alexandropoulus K, Colter N, Tuma I, Gershon ES. Reduction in temporal lobe size in siblings with schizophrenia: a magnetic resonance imaging study. *Psychiat. Res* .1990;35:137–147.

Docherty NM, Hawkins KA, Hoffmen RE, Quinlin DM, Rakfeldt J, Sledge WH. Working memory, attention a*nd communication disturbances in schizophrenia. Journal of Abnormal Psychology* 1996;105:212-219.

Delahunty A, Morice R, Frost B. Specific cognitive flexibility rehabilitation in schizophrenia. *Psychol. Med.* 1993;23:221-227.

Dudek SZ, Kolivakis T. Stability of intellect and personality in schizophrenia. *Can. J. Psychiatry* 1983;28:2-7.

Feinstein A, Goldberg TE, Nowlin B, Winberger DR. Types characteristics of remote memory impairment in schizophrenia. *Schizophrenia Research* 1998;30:155-163.

Friedman JI, Harvey PD, Coleman T, Moriarty PJ, Bowie Ch, Parella M, White L, Adler D, Davis KL. Six-year follow-up study of cognitive and functional status across the lifespan in schizophrenia: A comparison with Alzheimer´s disease and normal aging. *Am. J. Psychiatry* 2001;158:1441-1448.

Egan MF, Goldberg TE, Kolachana BS, Callicot JH, Mazzanti CHM, Straub RE, Goldman D, Weinberger DR. Effect of COMT Val108/158Met genotype on frontal lobe function and risk fro schizophrenia. *Proc. Natl. Acad. Sci.* 2001;98:6917–6922.

Evans JD, Bond GR, Meyer PS, Won Kim H, Lysaker PH, Gibson PJ, Tunis S. Cognitive and clinical predictors of success in vocational rehabilitation in schizophrenia. *Schizophr. Res.* 2004;70:331-342.

Frith CD, Leary J, Cahill C, Johnstone EC. Performance on psychological tests: demographic and clinical correlates of the results of these tests. In: Johnstone EC (ed) Disabilities and circumstances of schizophrenic patients: A follow-up study. *Br. J. Psychiatry* 1991;159(Suppl 13):26-29.

Fucetola R, Seidman LJ, Kremen WS, Faraone SV, Goldstein JM, Tsuang MT. Age and neuropsychological function in schizophrenia: A decline in executive abilities beyond that observed in healthy volunteers. *Biol. Psychiatry* 2000;48:137-146.

Gold S, Arndt S, Nopoulos P, O´Leary DS, Andreasen NC. Longitudinal study of cognitive function in first-episode and recent-onset schizophrenia. *American Journal of Psychiatry* 1999;156:1342-1348.

Gold JM, Randolph C, Carpenter CJ. The performance of patients with schizophrenia on the Wechsler Memory Scale—Revised. *Clinical Neuropsychologist* 1992;6: 367-230.

Gold JM, Randolph, C, Carpenter CJ, Goldberg TE, Weinberger DR. Forms of memory failure in schizophrenia. *Journal of Abnormal Psychology* 1992;101:487-494.

Gold J.M. Cognitive deficits as treatment targets in schizophrenia. *Schizophrenia Research* 2004; 72: 21-28.

Goldberg TE, Gold JM. Neurocognitive deficits in schizophrenia. In: Hirsch SR, Weinberger DR. Schizophrenia. Blackwell Science Ltd 1995,146-162.

Goldberg TE, Torrey EF, Gold JM, Ragland JD, Bigelow LB, Weinberger DR. Learning and memory in monozygotic twins discordant for schizophrenia. *Psychological Medicine* 1993a;23:71–85.

Goldberg TE, Ragland JD, Torrey EF. Neuropsychological assessment of monozygotic twins discordant for schizophrenia. *Archive of Genetic Psychiatry* 1990;47:1066-1072.

Goldberg TE, Gold JM, Greenberg J, Griffin S, Schultz SC, Pickar D. Contrasts between patients with affective disorders and patients with schizophrenia on a neuropsychological test battery. *American Journal of Psychiatry* 1993b;150:1355-1362.

Goldberg TE, Winberger DR, Berman KF, Pliskin NH, Podd MH. Further evidence for dementia of the prefrontal type in schizophrenia? Arch Gen Psychiatry 1987;44:1008-1014. In: Rodriguez M, Mohr P, Preiss M. Program počítačové rehabilitace kognitivních funkcí u schizofrenie. *Psychiatrie* 2002;6(Suppl.4): 42-45.

Goldberg TE, Saint-Cyr JA, Weinberger DR. Assessment of procedural learning and problem-solving in schizophrenic patients by Tower of Hanoi tasks. *Journal of Neuropsychiatry and Clinical Neuroscience* 1990;2:165-173.

Goldman RS, Axelrod BN, Tompkins LM. Effect of instructional cues on schizophrenic patient´s performance on Wisconsin Card Sorting Test. *Am. J. Psychiatry.* 1992; 149: 1718-1722.

Goldsamt LA, Barros J, Schwartz BJ et al. Neuropsychological correlates of schizophrenia. *Psychiatr. Ann.* 1993; 23: 151-157.

Goldstein G, Shemansky WJ. Influences on cognitive heterogeneity in schizophrenia. *Schizophr. Res.* 1995;18:59-69.

Green MF. What are the functional consequences of neurocognitive deficits in schizophrenia? *Am. J. Psychiatry* 1996;153:321-330.

Green MF, Kern RS, Braff DL, Mintz J. Neurocognitive deficits and functional outcome in schizophrenia: are we measuring the "right stuff"? *Schizophr. Bull.* 2000;26:119-136.

Hájek T, Španiel F. Protonová rezonanční spektroskopie v psychiatrii. *Psychiatrie* 2000;4: 116-119.

Hanuš H, et al. Speciání psychiatrie. Karolinum,Praha, 2000.

Hartl P, Hartlová H. Psychologický slovník. Portál,Praha,2000.

Harvey P. Cognitive Function in patients with schizophrenia. Report from a roundtable meeting of experts in cognitive dysfunction in schizophrenia, Budapest, Hungary, September 1997.

Heaton RK, Gladsjo JA, Palmer BW, Kuck J, Marcotte TD, Jeste DV. Stability and course of neuropsychological deficit in schizophrenia. *Arch. Gen. Psychiatry* 2001;58: 24-32.

Heaton R, Paulsen JS, McAdams LA, Kuck J, Zisook S, Braff D et al. Neuropsychological deficits in individuals with schizophrenia: Relation to age, chronicity, and dementia. *Arch. Gen. Psychiatry* 1994;51:469-476.

Hijman R. Memory processes and memory systems: fractionation of human memory. *Neurosci. Res. Commun.* 1996; 19: 189-196.

Hilbom E. Schizophrenia-like psychoses after brain trauma. *Acta Psych* 1951;60:36–47.

Hogarty GE, Flesher S. Practice principles of cognitive enhancement therapy for schizophrenia. *Schizophr. Bull* 1999;25:693–708.

Horan WP, Goldstein G. A retrospective study of premorbid ability aging differences in cognitive clusters of schizophrenia. *Psychiatry Res.* 2003;118:209-221.

Höschl C, Libiger J, Švestka J. (Eds.).Psychiatrie. Tigis,Praha,2002.

Huag JO. Pneumoencephalographic studies in mental disease. *Acta Psychiatr Scand* 1962;38(suppl):1–114.

Huron C, Danion JM, Giacomony F, Grange D, Robert P, Rizzo L. Impairment of recognition memory with, but not without conscious recollection in schizophrenia. *American Journal of Psychiatry* 1995;152:1737-1742.

Chen RYL, Chen EYH, Chan ChKY, Lam LCW, Felice LM. Verbal fluency in schizophrenia: reduction in semantic store. *Australian and New Zealand Journal of Psychiatry* 2000; 34: 43-48.

Jacobi W, Winkler H. Encephalographische studien an chronisch schizophrenen. *Arch. Psychiatr Nerven*kr 1927;81:299–332.

Javitt DC, Liederman E, Cienfuegos A, Shelley AM. Panmodal processing imprecision as a basis for dysfunction of transient memory storage systems in schizophrenia. *Schizophr Bull.* 1999; 25: 763-775.

Jeste DV, Twamley EW, Eyler Zorrilla LT, Golshan S, Patterson TL, Palmer BW. Aging and outcome in schizophrenia. *Acta Psychiatr Scand* 2003;107:336-343.

Johnstone EC, Crow TJ, Frith CD, Stevens J, Kreel L. Cerebral ventricular size and cognitive impairment in chronic schizophrenia. *Lancet* 1976;2:924-926.

Jones P, Rodgers B, Murray M. Child developmental risk factors for adult schizophrenia in the British 1946 birth cohort. *Lancet* 1994;344:1398-1402.

Joseph R. Neuopsychiatry, neuropsychology, and clinical neuroscience. Emotion, evolution, cognition, language, memory, brain damage, and abnormal behavior. Williams and Wilkinson, 1996: 864.

Joyce EM, Collinson SL, Crichton P. Verbal fluency in schizophrenia: relationship with executive function, semantic memory and clinical alogia. *Psychological Medicine* 1996; 26: 39-49.

Keefe RS. Working memory dysfunction and its relevance to schizophrenia. In: Sharma T, Harvey P, (Eds) Cognition in schizophrenia. Oxford University Press, Oxford 2000: 16–50.

Kern RS, Green MF, Nuechterlein KH, Deng Bi-Hong. NIMH-MATRICS survey on assessment of neurocognition in schizophrenia. *Schizophrenia Research* 2004; 72: 11-19.

Keshavan MS, Stanley YA, Pettegrew, JW. Magnetic resonance spectroscopy in schizophrenia: methodological issues and findings-part II. *Biol. Psychiatry* 2000;48;369-380.

Koukolík F. Strukturální změny mozku při schizofrenii a afektivních psychózách. Čs *Psychiatrie* 1992;88:307–315.

Kuffner K. Psychiatrie pro studium i praktickou potřebu lékaře. Bursík a Kohout, Praha, 1897:274–279.

Kulišťák P. Neuropsychologie. Portál,Praha, 2003.

Laruelle M, Abi-Dargam A. Dopamine as the wind of the psychotic fire: new evidence from brain imaging studies. *J. Psychopharmacol.* 1999;13:358-371.

Lewis DA. Neural circuitry of the prefrontal cortex in schizophrenia. *Arch. Gen. Psychiatry* 1995;52:269–272.

Lezak MD. Neuropsychological Assessment. Oxford University Press, Oxford, 1995.

Lezak MD. Neuropsychological Assessment (4th ed.). Oxford University Press, New York, 2004.

Libiger J. Schizofrenní poruchy. In Höschl et al. (Eds) Psychiatrie.Tigis,Praha,2002.

Libiger J. Schizofrenie. Psychiatrické centrum Praha,Praha,1990.

Libiger J. Vyšetření regionální mozkové perfuze pomocí jednofotonové emisní tomografie (SPECT) v psychiatrii. *Psychiatrie* 1997;1:3–9.

Liddle PF. Functional brain imaging in schizophrenia. In: Lewis S, Higgins, N. *Brain Imaging in Psychiatry.* Blackwell Science, Oxford,1996.

Liu SK, Chiu ChH, Chang ChJ, Hwang TJ. Hwu HG, Chen WJ. Deficits in sustained attention in schizophrenia and affective disorders: stable versus state-dependent markers. *American Journal of Psychiatry* 2002;159:975-982.

Lysaker P, Bell M,Beam-Goulet J. Insight and cognitive impairment in schizophrenia. Performance on repeated administrations of the Wisconsin Card Sorting Test. *Journal of Nervous and Mental Disease* 1995;182:656-660.

Maher BA, Manschreck TC, Woods BT, Yurgelun-Todd DA,Tsuang MT. Frontal brain volume and context effects in short-term recall in schizophrenia. *Biol Psychiatry* 1995; 37: 144- 150. In: Cirillo MA, Seidman LJ. Verbal declarative memory dysfunction in schizophrenia: from clinical assessment to genetics and brain mechanisms. *Neuropsychology Review* 2003;13:43-77.

Malenka RC, Angel RW, Thiemann S. Central error correcting behavior in schizophrenia and depression. *Biological Psychiatry* 1986;21:263-273.

MATRICS (www.matrics .ucla.edu).

McGlashan TH, Hoffman RE. Schizophrenia as a disorder of developmentally reduced synaptic connectivity. *Arch. Gen. Psychiatry* 2000;57:637–648.

McKee M, Hull JW, Smith TE. Cognitive and symptom correlates of participation in social skills training groups. *Schizophr. Res. 1*997;23:223-229.

McKenna PJ, Tamlyn D, Lund CE, Mortimer AM, Hammond S, Baddeley AD. Amnestic syndrome in schizophrenia. *Psychological Medicine* 1990;20: 967-972 In: Hirsch SR, Weinberger DR. *Schizophrenia.* Blackwell Science Ltd, 1995:146-162.

Mockler D, Riordan J, Sharma T. Memory and intellectual deficits do not decline with age in schizophrenia. *Schizophr. Res.* 1997;26:1-7.

Mohr P. Deficitní syndrom ve schizofrenii: přehled. *Psychiatrie* 1998;2:94–102.

Morice R, Delahunty A. Frontal/executive impairments in schizophrenia. *Schizophr. Bull.* 1996;22:125-137.

Müller U, Ullsperger M, Hammerstein E, Sachweh S, Becker T. Directed forgetting in schizophrenia. Prefrontal memory and inhibition deficits. *Eur. Arch. Psychiatry Clin. Neurosci.* Published online 22November 2004.

Mysliveček Z. Speciální psychiatrie. Státní zdravotnické nakladatelství, Praha, 1959:154.

Nathaniel-James DA, Brown R, Ron MA. Memory impairment in schizophrenia: its relationship to executive function. *Schizophr. Res.* 1996;21:85-96.

Neuchterlein KH. Development processes in schizophrenia disorders: longitudinal studies of vulnerability and stress. *Schizophrenia Bulletin* 1991;18:387-425.

Niendam TA, Bearden CE, Rosso IM, Sanchez LE, Hadley T, Neuchterlein KH, Cannon TD. A prospective study of childhood neurocognitive functioning in schizophrenic patients and their siblings. *Am. J. Psychiatry* 2003;160:2060-2062.

Nelson HE, Pantelis C, Carruthers K, Speller J, Baxendale S, Barnes TR. Cognitive function and symptomatology in chronic schizophrenia. *Psychol. Med.* 1990;20:357-365.

Ober BA, Vinogradov S, Shenaut GK. Semantic priming of category relations in schizophrenia. *Neuropsychology* 1995;9:220-228.

Palmer BW, Heaton RK, Paulsen JS, Kuck J, Braff D, Harris MJ, Zisook S, Jeste DV. Is it possible to be schizophrenic yet neuropsychologically normal? *Neuropsychology* 1997;11:437-446.

Patterson TL, Moscona S, McKibbin ChL, Davidson K, Jeste DV. Social skills performance assessment among older patients with schizophrenia. *Schizophr. Res.* 2001;48:351-360.

Paulsen JH, Heaton RK, Sadek JR, Perry W, Delis DC, Braff D et al. The nature of learning and memory impairments in schizophrenia. *J Int Neuropsychol Soc* 1995;1:88-99. In: Cirillo MA, Seidman LJ. Verbal declarative memory dysfunction in schizophrenia: From clinical assessment to genetics and brain mechanisms. *Neuropsychology Review* 2003;13:43-77.

Preiss J, Dvořáková M, Zvárová J, Hynek K. Neuropsychologické testy u dvojčat a vliv schizofrenie. Čs. *Psychologie* 1992;36:257-266.

Preiss M. Klinická neuropsychologie. Grada, Praha,1998.

Preiss M, Laing H, Rodriguez M. Neuropsychologická baterie Psychiatrického centra Praha. Psychiatrické centrum Praha, Zprávy č. 154/2002.

Raboch J, Zvolský P.. Psychiatrie. Galén,Praha,2001.

Rapoport JL, Giedd JN, Blumethal J, Hamburger S, Jeffries N, Fernandez T, Nicolson R, Bedwell J, Lenane M, Zijdenbos A, Paus T, Evans A. Progressive cortical change during adolescence in childhood-onset schizophrenia: a longitudinal magnetic resonance imaging study. *Arch. Gen. Psychiatry* 1999;56:649–654.

Robert PH, Migneco V, Marmod D. Verbal fluency in schizophrenia: the role of semantic clustering in category instance generation. *European Psychiatry* 1997;12:124-129.

Roder V. Evaluation einer kognitiven Schizophrenietherapie. In: Kühne GE, Brenner HD, Huber G. Kognitive Therapie bei Schizophrenen. Fischer, Jena,1990.

Rodriguez M, Mohr P, Preiss M. Program počítačové rehabilitace kognitivních funkcí u schizofrenie. *Psychiatrie* 2002;6(Suppl.4):42-45.

Rossell SL, David AS. The neuropsychology of schizophrenia: recent trends. *Current Opinion in Psychiatry* 1997;10:26-29.

Rossi A, Daneluzzo E, Mattei P, Bustini M, Casacchia M, Stratta P. Wisconsin card sorting test and Stroop test performance in schizophrenia: a shared construct. *Neuroscience Letters* 1997;226:87-90.

Rund BR. A review of longitudinal studies of cognitive functions in schizophrenia patients. *Schizophrenia Bulletin* 1998;24:425-435.

Runions J, Prudo R. Problem behaviors encountered by families living with a schizophrenic member. *Can. J. Psychiatry* 1983;28:382-386.

Saykin AJ, Gur RC, Gur RE, Mozley PD, Mozley LH, Resnick SM, Kester DB, Stafiniak P. Neuropsychological function in schizophrenia: selective impairment in memory and learning. *Archive of Genetic Psychiatry* 1991;48:618–624.

Seashore CE, Lewis D and Saetveit DL. Seashore measures of musical talents (rev. ed.) The Psychological Corporation, New York, 1960.

Sedláková M, Hoskovec J, Nakonečný M. Psychologie XX. století. Karolinum,Praha,2002.

Sharma T, Harvey P. (Eds.) Cognition in Schizophrenia. Oxford University Press, Oxford, 2000.

Schmand B, Brand N, Kuipers T. Procedural learning of cognitive and motor skills in psychotic patients. *Schizophrenia Research* 1992;8:157-170.

Silver H, Feldman P, Bilker W, Ruben CG. Working memory deficit as a core neuropsychological dysfunction in schizophrenia. *Am J Psychiatry* 2003;160: 1809-1816.

Siris SG. Is life a Wisconsin card sorting test? *American Journal of Psychiatry* 1991;148:1413-1414.

Smith TE, Hull JW, Romaneli S, Fertuck E, Weiss KA. Symptoms and neurocognition as rate limiters in skills training for psychotic patients. *Am. J. Psychiatry* 1999;156:1817-1818.

Sternberg R. Kognitivní psychologie. Portál, Praha, 2002.

Stevens AA, Donegan NH, Anderson M, Goldman-Rakic PS, Wexler BE. Verbal processing deficits in schizophrenia. *J. Abnorm. Psychol.* 2000;109:461-471.

Squire LR. Memory and the hippocampus: a synthesis from findings with rats, monkeys and humans. Psychol Rev 1992;99:192-231.

Suslow T, Schonauer K, Arolt V. Attention training in the cognitive rehabilitation of schizophrenic patients: a review of efficacy studies. *Acta Psychiatr. Scand.* 2001;103:15-23.

Syřišťová E. Imaginární svět. Mladá fronta,Praha,1997.

Škoda C. Psychotický proces a postpsychotický defekt. SAV, Bratislava, 1963.

Tek C, Gold J, Blaxton T, Wilk Ch, McMahon RP, Buchanan R. Visual perceptual and working memory impairments in schizophrenia. *Arch Gen Psychiatry* 2002;59:156-153.

The Psychological Corporation. Wechsler Memory Scale- Third Edition. Technical Manual. In: Cirillo MA, Seidman LJ: Verbal declarative memory dysfunction in schizophrenia: From clinical assessment to genetics and brain mechanisms. *Neuropsychology Review* 2003; 13: 43-77.

Tsuang MT, Stone WS, Faraone SV. Toward reformulating the diagnosis of schizophrenia. *American Journal of Psychiatry* 2000;157:1041-1050.

Thagard P. Úvod do kognitivní vědy. Portál, Praha, 2001.

Trimble MR, Perez MM. The phenomenology of the chronic psychoses of epilepsy. *Adv. Biol. Psychiatry* 1982;8:98–105.

Tůma I. Schizofrenie a kognitivní funkce. Psychiatrické centrum Praha, Praha, 1999.

Tůma I, Lenderová Z. Schizofrenie a kognitivní funkce. *Psychiatrie* 2001;4:275-284.

Van Beilen M, Pijnenborg M, van Zomeren EH, Bosch RJ, Withaar FK, Bouma A. What is measured by verbal fluency tests in schizophrenia? *Schizophr. Res.* 2004;69: 267-76.

Vauth R, Dietl M, Stieglitz RD, Olbrich HM. Kognitive remediation. Eine neue chance in der rehabilitation schizophrener storungen? *Nervenarzt* 2000;71:19–29.

Velligan DI, Bow-Thomas CCh. Executive functions in schizophrenia. *Seminars in Clinical Neuropsychiatry*1999;1:24-33.

Walker EF. Neurodevelopmental precursors of schizophrenia. In: David AS, Cutting JC (Eds): The Neuropsychology of Schizophrenia. Lawrence Erlbaum Associates Ltd., 1994: 119-129.

Watters FAV, Maybery MT, Badcock JC, Michie PT. Context memory and binding in schizophrenia. *Schizophrenia Research* 2004;68:119-125.

Weickert TW, Goldberg TE, Gold JM, Bigelow LB, Egan MF, Weinberger DR. Cognitive impairments in patients with schizophrenia displaying preserved and compromised intellect. *Arch. Gen. Psychiatry* 2000;57:907-913.

Wexler BE, Stevens AA, Bowers AA, Sernyak MJ, Goldman-Rakic P. Word and tone working memory deficits in schizophrenia. *Arch. Gen. Psychiatry* 1998; 55:1093-1096.

Wykes T. What are we changing with neurocognitive rehabilitation? Illustrations from two single cases of changes in neuropsychological performance and brain systems as measured by SPECT. *Schizophr. Res.* 1998;34:77-86.

Wykes T. Cognitive rehabilitation and remediation in schizophrenia. In: Cognition in Schizophrenia. Eds.: Sharma T, Harvey P. New York: Oxford University Press, 2000:332-351.

Zapletálek M, Tůma I, Kudrnová K, Hubert J, Černoch Z. Atrofie mozku u schizofreniků. Klinická a skanografická studie. Čs *Psychiat* 1983;79:158–163.

This work was supported by the Ministry of Education Czech Republic (Project No. CEZ J07/18/141100001).

In: Cognitive Deficit in Mental and Neurological Disorders ISBN: 978-1-60741-957-0
Editors: H. Kucerova, M. Preiss

Chapter IV

Substance Use Disorder

Lenka Miovska, Michal Miovsky, Danica Klempova, Pavel Kubu, Karel Nespor, and Tomas Palenicek

Abstract

The chapter is divided into groups by different types of addictive substances with particular respect to specific features pertaining to the potential risks of the development of cognitive deficits associated with the use thereof. Considerably greater attention is paid to some of the substances, as the users of such substances and the consequences of using them are encountered more frequently in practice. For example, this emphasis was applied for cannabis and MDMA ("ecstasy"), as these are substances that have become very popular among adolescents and young adults, and there are no signs of any major reversal of this tendency. Significant attention was also paid to the group of stimulants whose risk in terms of cognitive deficits is unfortunately often underestimated in practice, as opposed to the risk associated with opioid use, which, conversely, is overestimated. A separate area of concern involves volatile substances whose significant risks, including those to cognitive functions, are well known—the professional community has been pointing this issue out—but these facts are not adequately reflected in writings published in professional journals, nor in other messages. Finally, the concluding section of the chapter deals with assessment methods and recommended procedures for the identification and proposal of treatment and rehabilitation interventions aimed at addressing cognitive deficits caused by addictive substance use.

1. Introduction

Evidence shows that when used over a long period of time, most addictive substances are associated with a negative impact on cognitive functions. However, as far as this impact is concerned, dramatic differences in their risk potential have been reported for individual substances. In order to make a correct assessment of the etiology of a cognitive deficit after it has been diagnosed, it is essential to know the broader context, as far as both the drug history and, naturally, other domains of the patient's life are concerned. It is not always the substance being used that is directly responsible for the development of a cognitive deficit. In some cases, patterns of use themselves may have a much stronger influence. In others, it may be the combination with other substances or that the user's overall lifestyle is associated with a virtually destructive way of living or other hazardous activities. In modern addictology, these factors are strictly distinguished, as such a distinction is of practical significance in terms of the therapy itself, as well as in terms of objective accuracy supported by the relevant evidence produced by research and clinical observations.

Given the economic cost and the broader social impacts of treatment and the consequences of cognitive deficits, addictive substances pose a major challenge for present-day society. The overall scope of illicit substances being used has reached a level that is far from negligible (Annual Report, 2007). A similar situation has been observed in the use of legal substances. The popularity of both alcohol and tobacco has grown significantly among young people in particular (Hibell et al., 2004). It should be stressed that alcohol, given the number of regular users and their patterns of use and consumption, may truly be considered the most pressing problem in terms of cognitive deficits.

2. Key Domains of Cognitive Functions Being Measured

If we are to summarise the basic requirements for the assessment of any cognitive deficits in a substance user, we can define several areas that need to be taken into consideration:

a) length and course of drug history;
b) type of substance used (or the combination of substances in the case of polydrug users);
c) use (including patterns of use and sources from which a substance is obtained);
d) occurrence of psychiatric disorders and illnesses in the past (addiction professionals generally report high rates of comorbid patients);
e) co-occurrence of another psychiatric disorder or illness; and
f) the patient's way of living and lifestyle.

Assessment of cognitive functions cannot be conducted under all circumstances. For some addictive substances (such as opioids and stimulants), it holds true that assessment should not be carried out until approximately eight to ten days into abstinence (after the substance was last used). This interval is longer for other substances. In the case of cannabis, for example, assessment should not be made until 30 days into abstinence. Still, it is imperative that any effects of acute intoxication or various residues are eliminated, as these may have an impact on the result of the assessment. It is also a matter of fact to assess for interaction with any pharmacotherapeutical treatment and eliminate (or control for, should they appear) other distorting factors, such as the occurrence of dual diagnoses. The differential diagnosis and etiological factors may be ranked among the most complex and, at the same time, crucial issues in the context of the assessment of cognitive deficits associated with addictive substance use. Other important elements are: the strict separation of the effects and impacts of the substance itself, in its pure form; the consequences related to the occurrence of contaminants and adulterants; the consequences related to the combination of various substances (and varying amounts of such substances and their possible interaction); the consequences related to patterns of use and the user's lifestyle (way of living, etc.). In terms of cognitive deficits, each of these aspects may play a role that has significant implications for treatment and rehabilitation options.

3. Measurement

One of the distinctive features of diagnosing cognitive deficits in substance users is the circumstances under which they are referred for assessment, as this very often happens in connection with conditions other than cognitive deficits. In practice, this may mean, for example, that patients who enter detoxification programmes or are admitted to structured treatment programmes undergo initial psychological and psychiatric assessment that identifies a suspected cognitive deficit that is to be confirmed or refuted by further examination. In addition, it needs to be taken into account that numerous substance users do not want to and refuse to associate their problems (including problems ensuing from cognitive deficits) with substance use. Moreover, some of them suffer from other serious psychiatric ailments that complicate the diagnostic process, as well as treatment intervention, if any. Certainly, the length of abstinence itself and general compliance with the treatment regimen are also of crucial significance for diagnostic assessment, as well as for a prognostic estimate of the potential therapeutic effect on possible cognitive deficits. Furthermore, these deficits may have a strong impact on the individual's quality of life (Goldstein et al., 2004). In some cases, the patient may experience rather serious ailments that require adequate assessment and intervention. As the data produced by common counselling sessions appear to be unreliable for detecting such problems, neuropsychodiagnostic methods need to be used for this purpose (Fals-Stewart, 1997). All this makes the diagnosis of such disorders in substance-using individuals a very specific process. Therefore, we have attempted to draw up a summary of methods that are used in practice as far as this area is concerned (Table 1).

Table 1. Description of neuropsychological tests with the highest frequency of use

Domain	Test	Description	Sources
Attention	Digit Symbol Substitution Test (DSST)	Numbers are matched with corresponding symbols according to a key.	Wechsler, 1955, 1981, 1997
	Digit Span (DS)	Participants hear a long succession of single digits and are asked to repeat them in the same/reverse order.	Wechsler, 1955, 1981, 1997
Vigilance	Continuous Performance Test (CPT)	Participants hear auditory signals through headphones and respond by pressing a button. Reaction times to stimuli are recorded.	Conners, 1995

Table 1. (Continued)

Domain	Test	Description	Sources
Working memory	Stroop Test (ST)	Participants are asked to read items in a table naming the meanings of words and then the colours in which the words are printed.	Trennery, Crosson, DeBoe, Leber, 1989
	Paced Auditory Serial Addition Test (PASAT)	Participants add pairs of sequential randomised digits presented verbally at varying speeds.	Gronwall, 1977
	Trail Making Test (TMT)	Participants rapidly track letters and numbers. Time to complete and errors are recorded.	Reitan, 1985
Verbal memory	Wechsler Memory Scale (WMS)—Logical memory	Participants listen to a short narrative story. They are asked to recall the story immediately and after a 30-minute delay. The number of items of information recalled is recorded.	Wechsler, 1987
	Hopkins Verbal Learning Test (HVLT)	Participants hear a list of words and are asked to recall them immediately.	Brandt, 1991; Shapiro, Benedict, Schretlen, Brandt, 1999
	Rey Auditory Verbal Learning Test (RAVLT)	Participants hear a list of words and are asked to recall them immediately.	Mitrushina, Satz, Chervinsky, D´Elia, 1991; Randall, Georgemiller, 1986
Problem-solving/logical reasoning	Logical Reasoning Test (LRT)	Participants are shown a list of verbal statements and must decide if they are true or false.	Baddeley, 1968
Fine motor coordination	Finger Tapping Test (FTT)	Participants rapidly press a button. The number of times it is pressed during a specific period of time is recorded.	Reitan, Wolfson, 1986; Spreen, Strauss, 1991
Pupillary reaction	Maddox-Wing Test (MWT)	Participants look through a device that measures relative position of the eyes—divergence.	Hannington-Kiff, 1970

Domain	Test	Description	Sources
Estimate of intelligence quotient	New Adult Reading Test (NART)	Participants read a list of words of increasing complexity. The number of correctly pronounced words is recorded.	Griffin, Rivera, Mindt, Rankin, Ritchie, Scott, 2002
Test batteries	Cognitive Drug Research (CDR)—reaction time, vigilance, memory, etc.		Wesnes, 1985

Naturally, apart from conventional assessment methods and approaches, modern imaging methods and computerised cognitive test batteries have been increasingly applied recently (e.g., Aharonovich, 2003; Chang et al., 2002).

4. Course of Cognitive Deficit

4.1. Cognitive Deficits Caused by Alcohol Use

4.1.1. Alcohol-Induced Short-Term Disorders of Cognitive Functions

Undoubtedly, acute intoxication with alcohol dramatically impairs cognitive functions. Evidence of this includes the very definition of acute alcohol intoxication presented in the International Classification of Diseases (ICD-10), which also refers to cognitive functions. The definition of acute intoxication as a result of the use of alcohol according to ICD-10 states the following:

- The general criteria for acute intoxication (F1*x*.0) must be met.
- There must be dysfunctional behaviour, as evidenced by at least one of the following: disinhibition, argumentativeness, aggression, lability of mood, impaired attention, impaired judgment, interference with personal functioning.
- At least one of the following signs must be present: unsteady gait, difficulty in standing, slurred speech, nystagmus, decreased level of consciousness (e.g., stupor, coma), flushed face, conjunctival injection.

The dangerousness of alcohol intoxication is aggravated by the intoxicated person not realising the impairment of his/her cognitive functions but, on the contrary, overestimating his/her abilities. For example, this significantly increases the risk of traffic accidents, injuries, violent acts, and other incidents.

Typical symptoms of an alcohol hangover include headache, diarrhoea, dysorexia, tremor, fatigue and nausea. Research purposes require at least two of the above symptoms to be present in such a serious form that normal daily activities and responsibilities are affected. It is noteworthy that, according to American estimates, alcohol hangovers cost the U.S. economy 148 billion dollars a year (Wiese et al., 2000). Other estimates refer to 3.3 billion pounds' worth of loss because of hangovers for the UK, 1.4 billion dollars for Canada, and 3.8 billion for Australia (*The Morning After the Night Before,* 2000).

An alcohol "blackout" is a period of alcohol-induced loss of memory (amnesia) of events in which an individual was actively participating. Alcohol "blackouts" are divided into two types: en bloc (continuous amnesia) and fragmentary (gaps in memory). En bloc "blackouts" are approximately three times less frequent and are perceived more negatively by the person experiencing them. Most frequently, alcohol "blackouts" occur after drinking a large quantity of alcohol within a short period of time or when drinking alcohol on an empty stomach. An alcohol "blackout" may be a sign of developing dependence, but it may also be observed in people who are not dependent. The occurrence of "blackouts" is considered a sign of higher brain vulnerability. People experiencing alcohol "blackouts" are assumed to be at greater risk of the development of more severe disorders, such as alcohol dementia and/or Korsakov's psychosis (White, 2003; Johnson et al., 2003). Alcohol strongly impairs hippocampal functioning. In particular, it affects the glutamate neurotransmitter function in this area (Oscar-Berman and Marinkovic, 2003). Both the alcohol exposure-related reduction in metabolism in the frontal lobe and clinical observations show that alcohol also has a significant impact on the frontal lobe, i.e., the part of the brain that is important in terms of planning, decision-making, and self-control. However, it is still unclear to what extent the frontal lobe is responsible for the occurrence of alcohol "blackouts" (White, 2003). If adequately processed, negative experience of alcohol "blackouts" may motivate the dependent person to treatment and abstinence. In our sample of 67 alcohol-dependent men, the average duration of an alcohol "blackout" was almost eight hours (Nešpor, 2004).

Craving has attracted increased attention in recent years, and now medications are also available that help alleviate craving. Craving is practically always present in the withdrawal state. However, craving may also occur in individuals who have been abstaining from alcohol for a long time, typically when confronted with a trigger (such as alcoholic drink, a setting that the dependent person has associated with drinking alcohol and alcohol advertisements). A craving for alcohol involves physical changes, including increased salivation and changes in skin galvanic reactions. There is also evidence of higher oxygen consumption in certain brain areas, such as the limbic system (e.g., Tapert et al., 2003). There are good reasons to assume a deterioration of cognitive functions during a craving for alcohol, as the dependent person experiencing such a state is often unable to foresee the consequences of his/her actions and fails to use his/her previous experience.

The temporary negative effect that the alcohol withdrawal state has on cognitive functions was confirmed by Seifert et al. (2003). The fact that repeated withdrawals may lead to a long-term impairment of cognitive functions has even greater clinical significance (Duka et al., 2003).

4.1.2. Alcohol-Induced Long-Term Disorders of Cognitive Functions

Alcohol worsens communication between brain cells. Initially, this happens at the receptor level. Then changes to the structure of neuron connections on both sides of synapses also occur. State-of-the-art imaging methods have proved that alcohol mainly causes damage to white brain matter, i.e., myelinated connections between brain cells (neurons). But the grey matter neurons also suffer damage. Cerebral tissue loss occurs especially in the frontal lobe, but the cerebellum and limbic system are affected, too. It is reported that approximately half of the Americans dependent on alcohol show alcohol-induced neurological and psychological impairments ranging from moderate to severe (Oscar-Berman and Marinkovic, 2003).

In particular, alcohol involves high risks for children and adolescents (*Underage Drinking*, 2003). New neuron networks are developed in the brain during adolescence (Spear, 2002). Even slight damage to cognitive functions due to alcohol use results in worse academic and, subsequently, occupational performance. Brown et al. (2000) found that alcohol-dependent adolescents of 15 to 16 years of age showed lower ability to remember words and geometrical patterns. These findings have also been confirmed by other studies (Tapert et al., 1999). Memory disorders are especially frequent in those adolescents who underwent withdrawal from alcohol, which is a sign of drinking high doses (Brown et al., 2000). Memory impairment as a result of alcohol use in adolescence may even persist until later on when the alcohol consumption decreases, as demonstrated by experiments on animals (Spear, 2002). Modern imaging methods identified the fact that 17-year-old adolescents whose alcohol use caused them problems had smaller hippocampi than their peers (De Bellis et al., 2000). The hippocampus is the brain area that is specifically important in terms of learning and memory.

Alcohol-induced impairment of cognitive functions may even occur in adults who are not dependent on alcohol. The dose of alcohol seems to matter in this respect. Parsons and Nixon (1998) report that individuals who drink a daily dose of 60 to 72 g of alcohol over a long period of time show some signs of the deterioration of cognitive functions, and those with a daily use of 84 to 108 g over a long period of time have a moderate cognitive deficit, while those drinking 120 g of alcohol and more suffer from impairments of medium severity (60 g of alcohol is equivalent to about two litres of beer, three two-decilitre glasses of wine, or 180 ml of liquor).

4.1.3. Foetal Alcohol Syndrome and Alcohol-Related Neurodevelopmental Disorder (ARND)

In the developing countries, foetal alcohol syndrome is one of the most common causes of congenital defects. The foetus is endangered by foetal alcohol syndrome if a woman drinks alcohol during pregnancy (throughout the entire pregnancy, although the foetus is at greatest risk in the first trimester, i.e., often before the woman knows she is pregnant). The signs of this disorder include congenital craniofacial abnormalities, lower birth weight, and brain damage manifested by behavioural disorders and lower intellect. Alcohol-induced impairments of the foetal brain without the expression of any other signs of foetal alcohol syndrome are sometimes referred to as “ARND” (alcohol-related neurodevelopmental disorder). However, alcohol-induced damage to the foetus is not limited to the above conditions and may be multifaceted—for a summary see, for example, American Academy of Pediatrics (2000). According to American sources, foetal alcohol syndrome accounts only for a quarter of all the foetal alcohol spectrum disorders.

4.2. Cognitive Deficits Caused By Nicotine Use

It is not easy to assess the risk potential of nicotine use in terms of cognitive disorders, particularly as far as patterns of use are concerned. While assessment of the impacts of pure nicotine appears to be a great deal more positive than one would expect, negative results have been achieved when considering the most frequent pattern of use (smoke inhalation) with respect to the length and intensity of use.

4.2.1. Nicotine to Compensate Cognitive Deficits of Various Etiologies

Positive associations between some psychiatric illnesses and smoking have been demonstrated by both retrospective and prospective clinical trials (Araki, Suemaru and Gomita, 2002). The prevalence of smokers among psychiatric patients tends to be two to three times higher than in the normal population. Studies conducted among various populations of psychiatric patients (Attention Deficit Hyperactivity Disorder—ADHD, formerly "minimal brain dysfunction," Alzheimer's disease, schizophrenia, Parkinson's disease, Tourette's syndrome, affective disorders) conclude in agreement that nicotine may be effective in remedying cognitive deficits associated with these illnesses and thus provide a framework for understanding these patients' specific vulnerability to the onset and continuation of smoking (Sacco, Bannon, George, 2004). Additionally, smoking is becoming more prevalent among individuals with co-factors such as depression, anxiety disorders, and bulimia (Pomerleau, 1997). For example, adolescents suffering from ADHD become cigarette smokers twice as often as their peers without this attention disorder, and this difference continues until adulthood (Potter, Newhouse, 2004). Abnormal cognitive inhibition, one of the main symptoms of ADHD, is the cause of impulsive behaviour in individuals with this disorder. The nicotine contained in cigarette smoke results in better attention, vigilance, and short-term memory on the part of these patients (Potter, Newhouse, 2004; Salin-Pascual, Alcocer-Castillejos, Alejo-Galarza, 2003).

Nicotine receptors in the central nervous system (CNS) are situated on the presynaptic membrane, which allows them to have an impact on the release of several neurotransmitters, including acetylcholine, dopamine, serotonin, and noradrenaline. In particular, the functional significance of nicotine receptor stimulation is apparent in the regulation of the sleep-vigilance cycle. Stimulation promotes waking time and reduces both the total time spent sleeping and the amount of REM sleep (Salin-Pascual, Alcocer-Castillejos, Alejo-Galarza, 2003). Working memory is influenced by alpha7 and alpha4beta2 nicotine receptors present in the hippocampus and amygdala brain areas. Lower numbers of alpha7 nicotine receptors are observed in schizophrenia patients. Stimulation of both types of nicotine receptors in the hippocampus is responsible for the improvement of cognitive functions in patients suffering from Alzheimer's disease, schizophrenia, and ADHD (Araki, Suemaru, Gomita, 2002). Cognitive functions are further influenced by the nicotine system interacting with the dopaminergic and glutamate neurotransmission systems (Levin, Detvani, 2002).

Some studies report that treatment with transdermally administered nicotine significantly improves attention in individuals suffering from Alzheimer's disease, schizophrenia, and ADHD, as well as in normal non-smokers (Levin, Detvani, 2002; Levin, Detvani, 2002). However, other research studies question the positive effect of nicotine on healthy non-smokers (Newhouse, Potter, Singh, 2004). Attention disorder symptoms can be influenced by nicotine treatment, as it produces minor but reliable changes in important cognitive and behavioural functions. Besides, the symptomatology of the above disorders may be unmasked or be exacerbated in the event of nicotine abstinence exceeding the usual time until the development of the first withdrawal symptoms compensated by the next cigarette. For example, a study carried out on military pilots in withdrawal from nicotine identified a deterioration in their performance and thus pointed out the safety risks of this state in activities requiring a high level of attention (Giannakoulas et al., 2003). The fact that nicotine is effective in compensating for cognitive deficits explains why individuals with psychiatric disorders accompanied by the deficit of cognitive functions find smoking so attractive and difficult to quit without having to undergo nicotine substitution (Pomerleau, 1997).

4.2.2. Effects of Prenatal Exposure to Smoking on Children's Cognitive Functions

A number of epidemiological studies describe the relationship between maternal smoking during pregnancy and adverse neurobehavioural effects on the child's later development. Prenatal tobacco exposure is reported as a factor increasing the risk of the development of ADHD (Laucht, Schmidt, 2004; Hellstrom-Lindahl, Nordberg, 2002), cognitive deficits (Hellstrom-Lindahl, Nordberg, 2002; Rauh et al., 2004), behavioural disorders, criminal activities in adulthood, and a predisposition to alcohol and tobacco abuse among offspring (Hellstrom-Lindahl, Nordberg, 2002). Nicotine easily penetrates the placenta. As a result, the foetus of a smoking mother is exposed to relatively higher concentrations of nicotine in serum than the mother herself. Thus, in foetal CNS, nicotine may activate nicotine receptors, which play an important role in brain development. The developing human brain may be directly affected by nicotine for most of the baby's prenatal life, as nicotine receptors are already present in the brain during the first trimester (Hellstrom-Lindahl, Nordberg, 2002).

4.3. Cognitive Deficits Caused by Stimulant Use

Addictive stimulants comprise a very rich group including both legal (such as caffeine and theine) and illegal addictive substances (such as amphetamine and methamphetamine). The risk potential of these substances is often strongly diversified and affects various areas of life. Different addictive stimulants bear varying degrees of risk in both somatic and psychological terms. Therefore, in drawing up the following section of the text, we mainly focused on those substances that are significant in terms of the current treatment intervention demand.

4.3.1. Acute Intoxication, Long-Term Stimulant Use, and the Related Cognitive Effect

Stimulating psychoactive substances have a range of impacts on the nervous system. The differences between patterns of damage caused by individual substances vary only slightly (Simon et al., 2002a). Neuropsychological deficits in stimulant users fall into two broad categories: mood disorders and cognitive disorders.

Despite its rapid development, stimulant neurotoxicology, like other areas of neuroscience, lacks many of the stones of its mosaic, especially those needed for the explanation of what we can observe using neuropsychodiagnostics and modern imaging methods. A limitation common to the majority of the existing studies, including those addressing changes at the brain level, is the "chicken-or-the-egg issue": there is a general lack of data on the level of premorbid capabilities/premorbid state of the CNS. Nevertheless, it is known that people who are inclined to seek psychostimulants (such as individuals with a sensation-seeking personality trait and people with ADHD in their history, to whom, paradoxically, these substances bring relief) show abnormalities on the neuro- and cognitive levels that are similar to those identified in stimulant users, including deficits in the dopaminergic system and attention disorders. Similar problems in the interpretation of impairments identified in psychostimulant users are caused by what has also been revealed in experiments on animals: animals with brain lesions similar to those identified in stimulant users were significantly more vulnerable to the self-administration of stimulants (Majewska, 1996). The identification of the extent to which stimulants damage the brain is further complicated by the fact that a large number of stimulant users also use other habit-forming substances. For example, strong intensification of the neurotoxic effect was identified in combination with alcohol use (Woods et al., 1996, Bolla et al., 2000).

4.3.2. Effects of Stimulants on the Brain

A number of studies suggest that the chronic use of stimulants may result in serious neuropathies—the most severe cases include seizures, optic neuropathy, brain infarctions, subarachnoidal and intracerebral bleeding, multifocal cerebral ischemia, cerebral atrophy, and myocardial infarction leading to global ischemia and cerebral oedema (Daras et al., 1991; Fredericks et al., 1991; Klonoff et al., 1989; Lathers et al., 1988; Lichtenfeld et al., 1984; Mody et al., 1988; Pascual-Leone et al., 1991).

In the past 15 years, a large number of studies using modern imaging methods have been carried out on long-term stimulant users, as well as after one-off use of a stimulating substance. Similarly, numerous studies have been conducted on animals in order to survey the impact of stimulants on the brain and, subsequently, its behavioural output.

In particular, modern diagnostic imaging methods suggest morphological, physiological, and neurochemical abnormalities in chronic users (Majewska, 1996; Bartzokis et al., 1996; Cascella et al., 1991; Pascual-Leone et al., 1991). The changes detected in the use of stimulants are summarised below.

- Vasoconstriction. Stimulant use induces vasoconstriction or even vasospasm of cerebral and other vessels (Vitullo et al., 1989; Flores, 1990; Gottschalk et al., 2001; Kaufman et al., 1998).
- Neurodegeneration. There is evidence of neurotoxity of the most common stimulants—methamphetamines, amphetamine, and cocaine; all these substances produce neurodegenerative changes. Various levels of cerebral atrophy and lesions, particularly in the frontal cortex and basal ganglia, have been demonstrated (Majewska, 1996). The neurotoxic effects of continuous stimulant use on the habenula are likely to create the basis for stimulant-induced psychosis (Ellison et al., 1996). Severe grey matter deficits in the cingulate, limbic, and paralimbic cortices have recently been discovered in chronic methamphetamine users. Compared to the control group, these users showed smaller hippocampal volumes and significant white matter hypertrophy. Hippocampal deficits were mapped and correlated with memory performance on a word-recall test. (Thompson et al., 2004).
- Cerebral blood flow. Chang et al. (2002) identified an increase and decrease in cerebral blood flow in the same areas. Chronic use results in a multiple focal decrease in cerebral blood flow (Volkow et. al, 1988; Strickland et al., 1998). Several research studies point out patchy cerebral blood flow deficits in the frontal,

periventricular, and temporal-parietal regions in cocaine users who also use other drugs (Holman et al. 1993; Strickland et al. 1993; Volkow et al. 1988). These circulation deficits are often acutely aggravated by cocaine. They may be a direct consequence of the vasoconstriction of cerebral vessels, as well as increased aggregation of thrombocytes and blood coagulability (Kosten et al., 1996; Rinder et al., 1994).

- Glucose metabolism abnormalities. Glucose metabolism abnormalities, a decrease in certain brain areas and an increase in others, were found after both acute and chronic stimulant use. For example, London et al. demonstrated that a reduction in glucose metabolism in the neocortex, basal ganglia, hippocampus, thalamus, and the mesencephalon in the intravenous administration of cocaine to volunteers correlated in time with euphoria. These changes correlated with the changes in neuropsychological performance, and both were controlled for with abstinence (Strickland et al. 1993; Holman et al., 1993; O'Malley, 1992).
- Bioenergetic balance deficits. The application of 31P spectrometry using magnetic resonance has also revealed that chronic stimulant users show deficits in bioenergetic balance (a significant reduction of ß-ATP/Pi ratio was demonstrated), similar to the deficits in patients suffering or recovering from cerebral hypoxia/ischemia, which may suggest that they have dysfunctional mitochondria in their brains, which could subsequently result in the disintegration of cell membranes and neuronal death (Majewska, 1996).
- Dopaminergic system deficits. Primarily, stimulants elicit euphoria by inhibiting the re-uptake of dopamine (as well as serotonin and noradrenaline) (Pettit et al., 1982; Roberts et al., 1989; Ritz et al., 1987). In chronic use, this mechanism probably results in a compensational regulation of dopaminergic systems—reduced dopamine production. A long-term decrease and increase in dopamine and prolactin blood levels, respectively, were identified among individuals dependent on stimulants (Wilson et al., 1992; Dackis and Gold, 1985; Mendelson et al., 1988). Moszczynska et al. (2004) found that some individuals using methamphetamines show a dopamine loss as great as 97% in certain brain regions. Hypodopaminergy, probably acting concurrently with impairments of the basal ganglia, seems to be responsible for extrapyramid symptoms found in chronic stimulant users, which are similar to those occurring in individuals suffering from Parkinson's disease (Bartzokis et al., 1996; Bauer, 1996; Daras, 1996).
- Changes in neuropeptidergic systems. Equally, there is evidence of persisting changes in neuropeptidergic systems among chronic stimulant users (reduction in enkephalinergic systems and rise in dynorphinergic systems). These are considered to be the mechanisms related to withdrawal from stimulant use.
- Changes in bioelectric brain activity. Applied to stimulant users, the EEG method revealed diffuse theta activity and a rise in both theta and delta activities, which increased as use continued (Pascual-Leone and Dhuna 1990; Newton et al., 2003).

Although it has been proved that the severity of such variations depends on the length and intensity of use, the pathophysiological mechanisms that cause them and their specific consequences for the brain are not clear yet. Even more effort is required to clarify the relationship between these variations and the neuropsychological functioning of the patient. Various authors have tried to link the results of imaging methods with neuropsychological testing results and the progress made in cognitive-behavioural therapy, suggesting certain associations between them (e.g., Paulus et al., 2002; Volkow et al., 2001a; Gottschalk et al., 2001). Majewska suggests that cognitive disorders in stimulant users are caused by the loss of neurons (1996). Another feasible hypothesis, referring rather to the possible influence of neuroadaptive mechanisms on cognition (such as the reduced production of neurotransmitters, especially dopamine, to set off the chronic impact of stimulants) could be derived from Simon (2004), for example, who found that, of three study groups of chronic methamphetamine users (abstaining for six months, after relapse, and continuing using respectively), those who continued using showed the highest performance in cognitive tests.

4.3.3. Cognitive Deficits in Stimulant Users

Following one-off administration of stimulants, study subjects show less fatigue and a rise in cognitive performance, without any increase in the tendency towards impulsive responses to stimuli (Wiegmann et al., 1996). Reaction time accelerates, too (Halliday, 1994). However, people with high working memory capacity prior to the administration may show deterioration in their subsequent cognitive performance (Mattay, 2000).

In the clinical picture of a chronic stimulant user, variations on the brain level manifest themselves in problems in motivational and behavioural areas, emotional instability, impulsiveness, aggression, depression, anhedonia, and persistent motor problems, as well as problems in the attention and cognition domains. These are closely interrelated. Current stimulant users were found to show deficits (Ardila et al., 1991; O'Malley et al., 1992; Weinrieb and O'Brien, 1993; Simon et al., 2000; Simon et al., 2002b) in performance in memory tests, including the recall of audio stimuli, in perception-motor pace, reaction time, inhibition and attention concentration, problem-solving, information processing, abstract thinking, and mental flexibility.

Studies indicate that former stimulant users who have abstained for periods of from five days to several years still show impaired performance in tests that require the ability to inhibit irrelevant information (Kalechstein et al., 2003; Salo et al., 2002) and concentration of one's attention (O'Malley et al., 1990, 1992; Herning et al., 1990), decision-making (Paulus et al., 2001), the use of memory functions (Chang et al., 2002; McKetin and Mattick, 1998; Cunha, 2004), especially short-term memory (O'Malley et al., 1990, 1992; Herning et al., 1990), the processing of spatial tasks and the organisation of information (Kalechstein et al., 2003; Ornstein et al., 2000), and learning ability (Simon et al., 2001). Other studies with these patients identified various deficits in motor tasks similar to Parkinsonian symptoms (Bauer, 1993; Roberts and Bauer, 1993) and deficits in verbal fluency (Cunha, 2004).

Both these groups (both current and abstaining stimulant users) show intact performance in other cognitive tests, including overall IQ and verbal IQ scores (Sim et al., 2002; Simon et al., 2000; Volkow et al., 2001b).

4.4. Cognitive Deficits Caused by MDMA Use

MDMA ("ecstasy") is a substance whose neurotoxic effect has been proved by a range of animal studies, as well as by studies conducted with ecstasy users. These works indicate that, in particular, MDMA has a selective impact on the CNS serotonergic system. The impairment mainly involves axons of serotonergic neurons that degenerate as a result of the action of a range of processes induced by the acute effect of MDMA (Fišerová, Páleníček, 2001; Páleníček, Šustková, 2003; Baggott et al., 2001). No specific borderline dose of MDMA neurotoxicity in humans has been determined yet. Nevertheless, on the basis of animal studies and comparative methods (such as the interspecies scaling method), a neurotoxic dose of MDMA in humans has been predicted to be 1.28 (1.4) mg/kg (20 mg/kg in rats, 5 mg/kg in primates). Recalculated to the mean weight of an adult person, i.e., 75 kg, the total dose amounts to 96 mg (105 mg). This dose basically corresponds to the amounts that are regularly used by recreational users (a typical single dose used is 75 to 125 mg MDMA), but in a number of cases, this dose is dramatically exceeded (during one night, an amount ten times higher may often be used) (Ricaurte et al., 2000). This implies that common recreational MDMA use may already lead to the development of neurotoxicity. The development and degree of the neurotoxic effects of MDMA also depends on a wide range of external factors. The factors that significantly increase MDMA's neurotoxic effects include hyperthermia and dehydration. MDMA itself may induce a hyperthermic reaction (Mills et al., 2003; Sprague et al., 2003; O'Loinsigh et al., 2001), which is strongly potentiated by a high ambient temperature (which is often the case in the party settings where MDMA is most frequently used) and increased physical activity (excessive dancing at parties), resulting in an increased metabolic demand on the part of the body and, accordingly, a rise in body temperature. Dehydration is an accompanying condition related to excessive perspiration elicited by the above mechanisms and insufficient intake of mineralised fluids during MDMA intoxication (Fišerová, Páleníček, 2001; Baggott et al., 2001; Burgess et al., 2000; Páleníček, Šustková, 2003).

The serotonergic system is involved in the regulation of a range of mental processes in the human brain. They include the control of affectivity, impulsiveness, and aggression, social behaviour, sleep, and cognitive functions. Therefore, it is apparent that any damage to the system may manifest itself in a disorder concerning these areas. Indeed, as far as MDMA users are concerned, all these areas are somehow affected. Compared to control subjects, MDMA users tend to be more depressive, anxious, impulsive, and aggressive, and have sleep disorders and, naturally, various deficits in cognitive functions (Burgess et al., 2000; Cole, Sumnall, 2003; Parrott, 2000; Montoya et al., 2002; Fišerová, Páleníček, 2001; Páleníček, Šustková, 2003; Baggott et al., 2001).

One of the main problems encountered in most of the projects studying the consequences of MDMA use is the issue of polydrug use (Csémy et al., 2000). The point is that the majority of MDMA users combine various drugs (polydrug users), whose effects are then difficult to rule out (Baggott et al., 2001; Parrott, 2000; Montoya et al., 2002). In this respect, perhaps the most discussed problem is the use of cannabis, which is the most frequent concomitant illicit drug among MDMA users. Therefore, a number of recent studies compare groups of MDMA users ranking among polydrug users with polydrug users who do not use MDMA, cannabis users who do not use other drugs and drug-naïve controls (Gouzoulis-Mayfrank et al., 2000; Milani et al., 2004; Fox et al., 2001; Morgan et al., 2002). Another major limitation of most of the works is the method used for the selection of the study population and the actual number of doses and amount of MDMA. Most projects apply a similar technique to recruit study subjects from among MDMA users, namely by means of the snowball sampling method (Hartnoll et al., 2003). However, considering the significant media coverage of MDMA's adverse effects, voluntary subjects may be joining the study so as to confirm their already existing concerns that their current problems are related to MDMA use (Cole, Sumnall, 2003; Turner, Parrott, 2000). It also needs to be pointed out that these studies are very often initiated among university students, which results in a higher representation of students or, generally, people with higher academic education in the study population as compared to the general population (Cole, Sumnall, 2003). The amounts of doses used by MDMA users very often vary dramatically. Therefore, users are frequently divided into light and heavy users. Nevertheless, the variation in the number of doses consumed (usually tablets) within each group is very wide. Moreover, the amount of the active ingredient in tablets varies within a range of 0 to 150 mg/tab. However, in most countries, the highest percentages of tablets that have been analysed contain 50 to 80 mg MDMA/tab. Another aspect that needs to be taken into account is that 10 to 30% of tablets contain no MDMA whatsoever and may contain scores of other substances (such as amphetamine, ketamine, and PMA) (Parrott, 2004). Finally, these individuals' premorbidity is a limiting factor. People using MDMA may be driven to it on the basis of certain pre-existing factors, which are very difficult to analyse *ex post*. Certain difficulties in childhood or personality traits such as antisocial behaviour or impulsiveness are risk factors in terms of future experimentation with drugs and the development of dependence. In addition, they are often associated with lower cognitive performance and an increased risk of the development of psychopathologies in adulthood. This would imply that certain individuals might be much more inclined to use MDMA (as well as other drugs) (Cole, Sumnall, 2003; Baggott et al., 2001). We are currently unable to rule out this premorbidity by any means. On the contrary, a great deal of evidence suggests that it is necessary to take it into account.

The cognitive deficit in chronic MDMA users, as evidenced by many studies, covers a wide range of cognitive functions, including disorders of short-term memory, medium-term memory, visual memory, working memory, episodic memory, and memory of new information; disorders of central executive functions, judgment, and reasoning, and semantic recognition. The general indicators of intelligence and psychomotor performance also show certain abnormalities (Montoya et al., 2002). The most commonly studied parameters include verbal memory and executive functions (Baggott et al., 2001) (see Tab. 1.1). The first work that suggested a possible cognitive deficit in the group of MDMA users was a 1992 study involving nine MDMA users (with a five-year use history), which discovered lower performance in memory tests for short-term and medium-term memory (Krystal et al., 1992). In a different research project in 1998, Parrott discovered a deficit in the immediate and deferred recall of words, where the users repeated significantly fewer words than did the control group (Parrott et al., 1998). Many studies that followed identified similar results covering a wide range of cognitive functions (Baggott et al., 2001). Numerous authors correlated their findings with measures attained by means of biochemical and imaging methods. Reneman et al. (2000) found that, in users abstaining for an average of 4.6 months, memory disorders correlated with an increased density of post-synaptic serotonin 5-HT2a receptors (Reneman et al., 2000). Studies using PET and SPECT revealed changes in metabolism, as well as in the density of serotonin transporter in the hippocampus, amygdala, and neocortex (especially the frontal areas) (Montoya et al., 2002), i.e., regions that are very important for cognitive functions, particularly memory and learning (Altman, Normile, 1988). Similar results were also observed when using fMRI. Most of the studies provided evidence of a significant correlation between the severity of the defect and the amount of the drug used.

A number of recent studies take into account the significance of polydrug use in terms of the possible development of a cognitive deficit. In general, these studies suggest that polydrug users who combine MDMA with other drugs have more severe cognitive deficits than individuals using MDMA only. Cannabis use combined with MDMA use, in particular, leads to more serious consequences. Morgan et al. (2001) allowed for polydrug use by evaluating groups of current MDMA users, MDMA ex-users, polydrug users who had never used MDMA, and naïve controls. They found that cognitive dysfunction is likely to correlate with previous experience with MDMA, while other psychopathologies rather correlate with cannabis use (Morgan et al., 2002). One of the factors that may complicate the interpretation of the deficits identified in MDMA users to a great degree is the lack of sleep. Most MDMA users have a highly irregular sleep regimen, and sleep deprivation is known to have a negative impact on cognitive abilities and emotiveness (Páleníček, Šustková, 2003). In conclusion, it should be noted that most of the differences identified, as compared to the normal population, are of a subclinical nature and can be detected using a battery of sensitive cognitive tests.

Although today we still do not have a clear picture of the role of 5-HT in cognition, we know that it is involved in a range of cognitive processes, including memory and information processing speed. Moreover, it is possible that cognitive deterioration in users may be caused by secondary regulatory mechanisms, including other neurotransmitter systems that are not directly impaired by the neurotoxic effect of a drug. Subjects themselves may not register a subclinical cognitive impairment for a long time. As a result, they continue using the drug and thus expose themselves to a risk of damage that may not take effect until years later. In theory, a cognitive impairment may not manifest itself until many years later, when the damage brought about by the neurotoxic mechanism is enhanced by common changes occurring as a result of aging.

4.5. Cognitive Deficits Caused by Cannabis Use

The issue of health and the psychosocial consequences of cannabis use has been dealt with by a large number of research studies (see, for example, the WHO reviews and the UK Royal Commission and Canadian reports); but generally speaking, the international literature in this field is rather inconsistent and much discussion and many research studies addressing this topic are constantly being initiated.

4.5.1. Effects on the Brain

The main active substance contained in the plant named *Cannabis sativa* is delta-9-tetrahydrocannabinol (Δ^9-THC). Delta-9-tetrahydrocannabinol is a primary cause of marijuana's psychoactive properties. The THC content in a marijuana plant usually ranges from 6 to 8%; however, as far as the currently widespread application of indoor cultivation technologies is concerned, in Holland and elsewhere in Europe we may encounter a THC content of 12 to 16% (EMCDDA, 2004). The neurochemical processes causing cognitive deficits in marijuana users are not known to a sufficient degree (Fišar et al., 2005). Given cannabinoids' lipophilic qualities, in the beginning it was assumed that their effect involves the disruption of the arrangement of cellular membranes. Although this mechanism cannot be completely ruled out, the receptor mechanism is the main candidate for the mediation of the central effects of cannabinoids. Delta-9-tetrahydrocannabinol is an agonist of CB_1 and CB_2

cannabinoid receptors. Endogenous ligands of these receptors (endocannabinoids) include anandamide (arachidonylethanolamide) and 2-arachidonyglycerol (Fišar et al., 2005). The CB1 and CB2 receptors are located in the central nervous system, as well as in its peripheries. They include the frontal and parietal regions of the cortex (higher cognitive functions), cerebellum (movement coordination), hippocampus (learning and memory), nucleus accumbens (reward and pleasure), basal ganglia (motor control), as well as, to a lesser extent, the hypothalamus (basic body functions—body temperature regulation, balance of salt and water in the body), amygdala (emotions, fear), spinal cord (peripheral perception, pain), and the brain stem (sleep, excitement, thermoregulation, motor control).

4.5.2. Effects of Acute Intoxication

Depending on dosage, intoxication with cannabis is associated with relaxation, euphoria, perceptual alterations, distorted perception of time, and intensification of ordinary sensory experiences. Short-term memory and attention, learning abilities, reaction time and coordination, and motor functions are also impaired during acute intoxication (Miovský, 2003).

Marijuana use affects cognitive and behavioural functions, which may have a negative influence on those driving a motor vehicle or operating a machine. These impairments depend on the amount of THC used, and the manifestation of the impairment increases as the task becomes more complex and demanding in terms of focus of attention (Hall, Solowij, 1998).

The effects of recreational marijuana use on driving have been examined with laboratory stimulators and in standardised driving courses. These studies identified that the effects are similar to those at a 0.07 to 0.1% blood alcohol content (Hall, Solowij, 1998). The reason why the studies conducted under more realistic conditions on roads show more moderate results is probably that, because of their superior self-reflection, marijuana users tend to be more careful and less inclined to take risks while driving than alcohol users (Robe, 1994; Smiley, 1998).

The results of epidemiological studies pertaining to traffic accidents are not unequivocal, as a number of drivers with cannabinoids in their blood also had high blood alcohol concentrations. Two studies were carried out with individuals who had used marijuana only, but these drivers were not found guilty of causing the accident (Hall, Solowij, 1998). These conclusions were also confirmed by the only Czech study into this area conducted using toxicological examination of bodies of all the drivers involved in fatal traffic accidents (Vorel, 2003). Of the 166 bodies of drivers subjected to the toxicological examination, only one had THC metabolites in their blood. On the other hand, blood samples taken from 72 dead drivers (37%) contained alcohol and eight (4.8%) had used medication with psychotropic effects. However, as far as THC is concerned, it is very difficult to determine the likely degree of guilt for the road accident, as this relies on the types of metabolites detected and many other circumstances (including whether the driver had been using cannabis regularly and for how long). Therefore, forensic assessment of these cases is a great deal more complex than in the case of alcohol and many other drugs.

4.5.3. Consequences of Short-Term and Long-Term Cannabis Use

Experimental studies with control groups of cannabis non-users support the notion of the existence of a short-term influence of cannabis use on attention, ability to perform psychomotor tasks, and short-term memory (Pope et al., 1995; Pope et al., 1996; Fletcher et al., 1996; Pope et al., 1997; NIDA, 2002b ad.). Short-term marijuana users show impairments that are not so severe as to have a negative impact on cognitive functioning in daily life. Evidence has suggested that the length of marijuana use is the key factor in the development of the impairment of cognitive functions (Solowij et al., 2002). Another assumption is that marijuana may cause potential irreversible neurotoxic effects in individuals who begin using it at an early age (prior to the fifteenth year of their life) (Pope et al., 2002).

No irreversible impact of long-term cannabis use on cognitive functions has been proved yet and experts have not reached a consensus on this point (Lyketsos et al., 1999; Martin, 2000; Jentsch et al., 2002). Bolla et al. (2002) state that heavy cannabis users show a persistent reversible decrease in cognitive functions for up to 28 days into abstinence. Other studies report that negative effects may persist for as long as several weeks after use (NIDA, 2002b). Hall and Solowij (1998) indicate a deterioration of attention and memory that persists during use and may, but may not, be reversible after lengthy abstinence. Another study (Solowij et al., 2002) confirms the deterioration of cognitive functions, particularly memory and attention, in long-term cannabis users. This deficit became most evident in the abilities to learn and retain and recall information. As for the speed of comprehension, marijuana users did not differ from the non-user control group in terms of speed, but made more mistakes. Another study (Fletcher et al., 1996) dealing with cognitive functions in long-term marijuana users concluded that the impairments are most apparent in attention-demanding tasks that are performed quickly under time pressure. All these functions worsen as the length and frequency of use increase. On the other hand, heavy long-term marijuana use does not produce such a severe deterioration of memory, attention, and other cognitive functions as is found in chronic alcohol users, for example. It rather produces less severe memory impairments, particularly in the domain of attention and the organisation and integration of comprehensive information. As regards these impairments, it still remains unclear to what extent they influence daily life and what options and limits in terms of compensation mechanisms they involve (Hall, Solowij, 1998; Pope, Yurgelum-Todd, 1996; Solowij et al., 1995).

According to a number of studies, long-term marijuana use affects short-term memory. Some studies also indicate that long-term use in adolescents may result in the impairment of long-term memory. Some evidence suggests that people with learning disorders may be more susceptible to these memory deficits. However, all the studies show that marijuana use has no impact on the recall of material that has already been acquired or learned (Martin, 2000; Schwartz, 1993). Another factor that may have a significant influence on cognitive functions is the frequency of cannabis use. Having compared the memory performance of light and heavy cannabis users, Pope et al. (1996) did not find any significant differences between these two groups in tasks involving the immediate recall of text passages, word pairs, or pictures and figures. Only the deferred recall of pictures and numbers was significantly worse in heavy cannabis users.

Among long-term marijuana users, cognitive deficits were mainly identified in the following domains: attention concentration, selectivity, and oscillation; short-term memory, verbal memory, and working memory; registration, organisation, and use of new information (work with information); perceptive-motor pace and reaction time, and ability to learn.

4.6. Cognitive Deficits Caused by Opioid Use

Opioids, substances structurally derived from morphine, elicit feelings of euphoria. This term is a summary name for natural vegetable alkaloids and their semisynthetic derivatives, synthetically prepared drugs derived from the morphine structure (opiates), as well as animal peptides found in some parts of the brain. Opioid peptides occur in the limbic system regions (hippocampus and archistriate), in the reticular formation monoaminergic system, particularly in the basal ganglia neostriate, where there is a great concentration of neuroactive substances such as dopamine, acetylcholine, enkephalines and neuropeptides. The opioid action mechanism takes effect by means of opioid receptors (Blahoutová et al., 2003).

Morphine has been identified as the active ingredient of opium. Other opium components include codeine, papaverine, thebaine, and narcotine. A range of other opiates, including semisynthetic opioids, such as heroin (diacetylmorphine) and hydromorphone, and synthetically manufactured opiates, such as pethidine (meperidine), methadone, and buprenorphine, are derived from morphine. Opioids play a crucial role in the management of pain (both acute and long term), particularly in patients with tumours in advanced stages of the disease. Pain affects one-third of patients suffering from malign tumours and 60 to 90% of those with advanced malign tumours. Heroin prevails among the opioids used illegally.

4.6.1. Effects on the Central Nervous System

Opioids have a depressant effect on the central nervous system; they suppress the perceptive, localisation, and psychological elements of pain and elicit euphoria and tranquillisation or even drowsiness. They induce inhibition of the respiratory centre and reduce sensitivity to the stimulating effects of acidosis and CO_2. Respiratory arrest may even occur. Opioids suppress the cough centre, stimulate the chemoreceptor zone triggering vomiting, induce miosis, and are also responsible for an overall drop in body temperature (Kalina et al., 2003). Opioid dependence is primarily associated with changes in the frontal lobes, which are mainly manifested by deficits in executive functions (Lyvers, Yakimoff, 2002). However, when administered orally under medical supervision, opioids, even if used for a long time, do not produce any significant toxic side effects on the physiological system. In some individuals, prolonged exposure to opioids is likely to cause long-term adaptive changes that require the continuing administration of opioids in order to maintain a normal mood and normal responses to stress. In contrast with the moderate side effects caused by opioids administered orally under medical supervision, the toxic side effects associated with the illicit use of opioids, often contaminated, applied parenterally, are serious and very frequent. The wide range of these toxic effects includes acute and sometimes fatal cases of overdose, an array of infections associated with the sharing of injecting equipment, and neurological, muscular, pulmonary, and renal impairments (Lowinson et al., 1997; Preston, 1999).

4.6.2. Opioid Use in Pain Management

Opioids are widely used to treat acute and long-lasting pain, particularly in patients with advanced cancer. Patients in the less advanced stages of the disease suffer from slight impairments of their cognitive functions. In the terminal stages of a tumour disease and in elderly patients admitted to hospital for acute pain, cognitive dysfunctions in the form of delirium may occur (Bowen, Larson, 1993; Lawlor et al., 2000; Morrison et al., 2003; Schor et al., 1992). Cognitive deficits may interfere with everyday functioning, as well as the ability to drive. Management of these problems requires careful clinical assessment, the identification of risk factors, objective monitoring of cognitive functions, maintenance of adequate hydration, and even a reduction in the dose or change of a drug-opioid. Responsible decision-making about opioid use requires an understanding of the incidence, severity and picture of side-effects (Lawlor, 2002; Ersek, 2004).

Several studies investigated the acute and long-term effects of opioids in healthy volunteers. A number of these studies focused on investigating the dependence potential (Hill, Zacny, 2000; Walker, Zacny, 1999; Zacny, Conley, Galinkin, 1997), and the assessment of cognitive functions was one of the areas that this investigation addressed. These studies show that significant cognitive impairment is associated with parenterally administered opioids and that this deficit is associated with the amount used. The results of studies dealing with orally administered opioids vary. Nevertheless, some of them indicate moderate but significant impairment associated with the size of the dose (Ersek, 2004). The designs of these studies usually employed randomisation, control groups, and blinding. However, the results would be difficult to extrapolate to a clinical setting. It is also noteworthy that pain in itself may cause cognitive impairment, which is the reason why the control group should include individuals suffering from pain and not using opioids in order to ensure a better comparison (Lorenz, Beck, Bromm, 1997).

Other studies examined the cognitive functions of patients suffering from chronic pain caused by a tumour disease (Banning, Sjogren, 1990; Banning, Sjogren, Kaiser, 1992; Bruera et al., 1989). Bruera et al. (1989) compared the performance of 20 hospitalised cancer patients who were on stable doses of opioids with the performance of 20 hospitalised patients who were receiving increased doses of opioids. Although increased doses were associated with impaired memory, reasoning, and reaction time, stable doses had no negative impact on cognitive functioning. On the basis of these findings, the authors posited that tolerance to cognitive deficits occurs in time. Using the reaction time test, Banning and Sjogren (1990) compared the performance of 34 cancer patients who received stable oral doses of morphine with the performance of 32 healthy control subjects. A small but significant prolongation of average reaction time was found in the opioid-treated group. Clemons et al. (1996) administered a battery of neuropsychological tests to three groups: 16 healthy volunteers not receiving opioids, six advanced cancer patients not receiving opioids, and seven advanced cancer patients receiving stable, regular oral doses of opioids.

Significant differences were found in the tests for reaction time and attention between the cancer patients and the healthy control group, but not between the two groups of cancer patients. Thus, cancer patients using opioids show moderate cognitive impairments in comparison to the healthy controls. Naturally, pain, the opioids used, and the state of functioning need to be taken into account, as all these factors have a negative impact on cognitive functions (Ersek, 2004).

Research into the cognitive effects of opioids in patients with chronic non-malign pain produces conflicting results. The generalisation of results is limited by methodological shortcomings that include insufficient sample size (Lorenz et al., 1997), non-randomised selection of subjects (Haythornthwaite et al., 1998; Lorenz et al., 1997), limited neuropsychological testing (Rowbotham et al., 2003), and non-experimental study design (Haythornthwaite et al., 1998). The study with the most rigorous design (Raja et al., 2002) did not find any cognitive impairment associated with opioid use. The influence of opioid side-effects on the ability to drive a motor vehicle has been examined using several different methodologies. No study has provided evidence that opioid use impairs the ability to drive. It is not clear, however, whether these findings may be applied to patients suffering from pain and using opioids on a long-term basis. For the time being, it is not possible to give a distinct answer (because of a number of other factors) to the question about the degree to which it is possible, in this area, to compare the results obtained for substances officially used for analgesic purposes (registered preparations) and substances that are legally manufactured and distributed (Ersek, 2004).

The long-term use of opiods to relieve pain does not affect neuropsychological performance. Pain and functional impairment may have a more severe neuropsychological impact than opioids. Cognitive deficits induced by the controlled use of opioids under medical supervision are very moderate and include delayed recall, impaired coding and processing of verbal information, and lower velocity of pupillary responses, as well as deficits in concentration and swapping of attention, the recall of images, working memory, and fine motor coordination.

4.6.3. Cognitive Dysfunctions in Heroin Users

The long-term use of illegally obtained opiates such as heroin may lead to long-lasting brain dysfunctions. These negative side-effects complicate treatment and require additional rehabilitation focused particularly on the cognitive deficits that interfere with daily functioning. There are relatively few detailed studies examining the nature of possible neuropsychological changes related to long-term opiate use (Ornstein, 2000). Heavy long-term opiate users show neuropsychological impairments more frequently (Grant et al., 1978). Hill and Mikhael (1979) studied heroin users' cognitive functioning and found impairment of memory and spatial orientation. Chronic use may lead to changes in dopaminergic transmission in the nucleus accumbens, caudate-putamen, and frontal cortex, which results in impaired processing of cognitive and emotional information (Alexander et al., 1986). In addition, patients with lesions in the frontal lobe show deficits in cognitive and executive functioning, particularly as regards tests focusing on working memory, shifting of attention, and planning abilities (Owen et al., 1995, 1990, 1991; Milner, 1963). Similar to other groups of drugs, valid assessment is limited by the problem of polydrug use. It is very common for users of heroin (or other opioids) to consume other addictive substances, and often in large quantities (in terms of both dosage and frequency). Thus, there is also a problem here with the determination of etiological fraction with respect to the cognitive deficit identified. In general, cognitive deficits in heroin users are evident in concentration and planning ability, problem-solving, spatial memory, verbal fluency, spatial orientation, abstract reasoning, working memory, and psychomotor pace.

Studies examining the cognitive functioning of patients in methadone substitution therapy only found minimal impairments (Appel, Gordon, 1976). The results of the studies that provide evidence of cognitive impairment are limited for several reasons, including: no urine drug analysis being carried out prior to the commencement of testing; during the study, most users subjected to testing also using other drugs than opioids, including benzodiazepines, whose negative side-effects on cognitive functioning are well-documented; or the study lacking an adequately selected control group. Moderate impairments were found in psychomotor pace, verbal memory, memory for complex word pairs, short-term memory, attention, and problem-solving.

4.7. Cognitive Deficits Caused by Volatile Substance Use

Volatile substances are present in a wide range of household products that are used for different purposes. They include paints, glues, diluents, ether, detergents, nail varnish removers, deodorants, and lighter gas. Most of the products contain several dramatically different volatile substances, each with its unique toxicity. They are toluene, which is used most frequently, as well as ethyl acetate, methyl chloride, acetone, trichloroethylene, tetrachlorethylene, butane, propane, isopropane, fluorocarbon, ethyl chloride, nitrous oxide, and many other substances. Products containing these psychoactive substances are not expensive and are readily available, which is one of the reasons why they are used to such a great degree by children and young adults from a lower socioeconomic environment. Nevertheless, this problem is often underestimated not only by the public but also by parents, who may show proper interest in the issue of illicit drugs but very often ignore the risks associated with the use of readily available household products containing volatile substances. In addition, these substances are used in order to achieve quick intoxication without concern about serious health consequences. Intoxication only lasts a few minutes and so the users continue sniffing for up to several hours, which may result in dangerous loss of consciousness and even death (NIDA, 2004).

4.7.1. Effects on the Central Nervous System

The majority of volatile substances have a sedative affect on the central nervous system, which slows down neural processes. Before these relaxing effects occur, an excitation phase characterised by energy and loss of inhibitions may develop (Meadows, Verghese, 1996).

Volatile substances are highly lipophilic and tend to spread into organs rich in lipids, such as the brain, liver, and adrenal glands, on which they have a strong toxic effect. The impact of volatile substances on the brain and its functions is the most important and widely debated issue. The toxic effects of chronic volatile substance use cause widespread and long-lasting damage to the brain and other parts of the nervous system. Long–term toluene use, for example, damages the protective layer around certain nerve fibres in the brain and in the peripheral nervous system. In clinical terms, this extensive destruction of nerve fibres is similar to that found in neurological illnesses such as multiple sclerosis (Finch, Lobo, 2005; Lowinson et al., 2004; NIDA, 2004).

The toxic effects of prolonged use occur on many levels. Their manifestations include lower cognitive functioning, difficulties in movement coordination, and impairment of visual and auditory functions. These deficits may range from moderate impairment to severe dementia (Lowinson et al., 2004; NIDA, 2004). The features of these impairments are rarely specific enough to be visualised using computer tomography (CT) or magnetic resonance imaging (MRI) (Schaumburg, Spencer, 1987). The main reasons are that many neurotoxic effects are short-term and reversible and, also, some neurotoxic injuries of the brain may not be associated with brain damage sufficiently large enough to be detected by MRI. However, recent studies indicate that MRI may be the most sensitive and specific method to reliably detect brain impairments related to long-term exposure to high doses of volatile substances (Lowinson et al., 2004).

As far as reversibility is concerned, one-off exposure to both low and high doses of volatile substances is associated with full reversibility of cognitive functions. However, this finding cannot be used as the basis for an assumption that long-term exposure to low doses results in irreversible neurological impairments. The impairment caused by long-term exposure to high doses of volatile substances is slowly and incompletely reversible and does not usually have a progressive character after use has been discontinued. The length of use and the amount of the toxic substance used have a direct impact on the extent, degree, and reversibility of neurological impairment (Lowinson et al., 2004).

4.7.2. Acute Intoxication

Initially similar to those induced by alcohol, the effects of acute intoxication with volatile substances include excitation, euphoria, and agitation, followed by drowsiness, daze, and disinhibition. Increased intoxication elicits ataxia, dizziness, nausea and vomiting, disorientation, and lower movement coordination ability. The signs of extreme intoxication include sleeplessness, muscle weakness, dysarthria, and nystagmus, and occasionally, hallucinations and delusions, disruptive behaviour, slurred speech, unsteady gait, difficulty standing up, balance disorders, and lethargy; the qualitative disturbance of consciousness may also turn into a quantitative disturbance, a stupor or even coma in which heart arrest, respiratory arrest, or suffocating on vomit may occur. Cerebral anoxia associated with fatalities may be related to multiple factors including asphyxia, cerebral and pulmonary oedema, cardiac arrhythmia and arrest, unconsciousness that may lead into a coma, hyperpyrexia, and others. Several hours after intoxication, mostly followed by sleep, lethargy and mild to severe headaches are experienced (Al-Alousi, 1989; Kalina et al., 2003; Lowinson et al., 2004; Rosenberg, 2002; Smolík, 1996).

4.7.3. Effects of Short-Term and Long-Term Use

Major injuries caused by long-term volatile substance use include encephalopathy (non-specific acute encephalopathy as a result of high-level exposure, chronic encephalopathy as a result of repeated exposure to high doses over several years), cerebellar ataxia, peripheral neuropathy, cranial neuropathy (nerves V and VII), Parkinsonism, visual function disturbance (eye neuropathy), and auditory function disturbance (Filley et al., 1990; Lowinson et al., 2004). Long-term exposure to low doses of volatile substances may also result in an organic psychosyndrome (also referred to as the "painter's syndrome"), which includes delirium, dementia, hallucinosis, personality changes and marked deterioration of memory or recall rate concerning past experience, and difficulty in focusing attention (Lowinson et al., 2004; Smolík, 1996).

A large number of studies address neurological deficits in individuals who are exposed to volatile substances at work. Although this damage is minute, mild deficits do occur in learning, short-term memory, attention, spatial orientation, and psychomotor pace; tremor, ataxia, and impairments of fine motor functioning and eye and arm coordination are also present (Baker et al., 1985; Chouaniere et al., 2002; Ellingsen et al., 1997; Marrow et al., 2001; Ryan et al., 1988). Some well-controlled studies even report no evidence of any effect of volatile substances on this population after the cessation of exposure and their disappearance from the blood (Deschamps et al., 2001; Seeber et al., 2004) or no evidence of any relationship between the level of exposure (dose) and the presence of a psycho organic syndrome (Rosenberg, 1995).

Investigating the impact of volatile substances on individuals who work with them, many studies address the issue of colour discrimination, finding out that styrene, for example, impairs colour discrimination, especially blue and yellow, and sometimes also red and green

(Campagna et al., 1996; Lomax et al., 2004), while toluene has no direct impact on colour discrimination (Lomax et al., 2004; Schaper et al., 2004).

5. Proposed Standardized Cognitive Functioning Assessment

See Chapter 3 Measurement, Table 1.

6. Cognitive Deficit Rehabilitation and Psychotherapy

The effective treatment of substance use-related consequences is based on an interdisciplinary approach (Kalina et al., 2003). Therefore, the effective treatment of cognitive deficits caused by addictive substance use needs to involve a comprehensive approach to the patient, i.e., it needs to address different levels of the problems associated with addictive substances. The treatment of cognitive disorders cannot be expected to be successful if the patient's needs pertaining to the socio-psychological, social, and criminal justice areas are not dealt with adequately. It also needs to be noted that, from the etiological point of view, addictive substance use can be perceived, in most cases, as a consequence of a failure to cope with other predicaments. One significant group of such problems includes undiagnosed and mistreated depression, severe personality disorders, psychotic illnesses, family and partner difficulties, and unemployment (Lowinson et al., 2004). When disregarding or underestimating these factors, we may still achieve partial results in the treatment of cognitive deficits, but, sooner or later, the patients are likely to progress in their drug careers through recurring relapses until the pattern of use of the original drug, or a different drug, is restored. This, of course, hampers the results of cognitive disorder treatment and, if such a situation occurs, the treatment cannot be considered effective. Thus, a specific feature of the treatment of and rehabilitation from cognitive disorders associated with addictive substance use is the necessity to refer these patients to adequate treatment programmes. One of the key concepts involved in the result of the initial examination and assessment of the patient's condition is "matching," which, in this context, is understood as the allocation of the patient to a suitable programme that can address the patient's needs (Miovský, 2003; Rotgers, 1999). The programme must correspond to the nature of patients' problems and their specific needs, as well as addressing all the crucial domains. This implies, for example, that if the patient's possible retention in medium-term or long-term residential treatment is conditioned by their conflict with the law being solved, an adequate solution must be integrated into the programme. This may include social and legal counselling during criminal proceedings and arranging a possibility of alternative punishment or court-ordered treatment for the patient so that the patient can enter and duly complete the treatment programme.

One of the preconditions of successful treatment on the patient's part is his/her perspective on and motivation to treatment, which can only be successful if the patient is actively involved in the process and other addictive substance use-related problems are addressed at the same time. Addictive substance use in itself and the related behaviour are conditioned by multiple factors (Lowinson et al., 2004) and by no means can it be considered as being within the cause-effect category, i.e., the category that, in medical terms, would imply the application of conventional causal treatment.

A large number of cognitive deficits usually improve as early as in the initial stages of the treatment process. These deficits are compensated for or even remedied (in the case of reversible impairments) as the period of abstinence grows longer and a suitable combination of therapeutic procedures is applied. For example, most alcohol-induced brain impairments improve, at least in part, during the first year of abstinence, although recovery sometimes requires even more time (Oscar-Berman and Marinkovic, 2003). The greatest improvement in intellectual functioning seems to occur during the first month of abstinence. This is the reason why the dependent in residential treatment are subjected to psychological assessment of their cognitive functions not sooner than after one month into abstinence, if possible. The improvement in the condition is enhanced by the multiplication of connections between nerve cells, i.e., the reconstruction and reorganisation of the neural network. Recent evidence shows that neurogenesis, i.e., the creation of new neurons from stem cells, is also possible in the adult brain. Stem cells can divide without limit to give rise to various other cells. It has been proved that, even in a healthy adult brain, neurogenesis takes place in at least two regions. One of them is the above-mentioned hippocampus, i.e., the part of the brain that is important for memory. Cameron and McKay (2001) even state that new cells generated in the hippocampal gyrus dentatus during one month comprise up to 6% of the total population in that region. Alcohol slows down the proliferation of neural stem cells and thus the creation of new neurons (Crews, Nixon, 2003). The newly generated cells do not begin functioning until two to four weeks later, which implies that, for example, the influence of alcohol on neurogenesis becomes evident after longer latency.

Conclusion

Evidence shows that, when used over a long period of time, most addictive substances are associated with a negative impact on cognitive functions. However, as far as this impact is concerned, dramatic differences in their risk potentials have been reported for individual substances. In order to make a correct assessment of the etiology of a cognitive deficit after it has been diagnosed, it is essential to know the broader context, as far as both the patient's drug history and, naturally, other domains of his/her life are concerned. The substance used is not always directly responsible for the development of a cognitive deficit. In some cases, patterns of use themselves may have a much stronger influence. In others, it may be the combination with other substances or the user's overall lifestyle associated with a virtually destructive way of living or other hazardous activities. Modern addictology draws a strong distinction between these factors, as it has its practical significance in terms of the therapy itself, as well as in terms of objective accuracy supported by the relevant evidence produced by research and clinical observations. In the context of the assessment of cognitive deficits associated with addictive substance use, the differential diagnosis and etiological factors may be ranked among the most complex and, at the same time, crucial issues. An important element is the strict separation of the effects and impacts of the substance itself, in its pure form; the consequences related to the occurrence of contaminants and adulterants; the consequences related to the combination of various substances (and varying amounts of such substances), and the consequences related to patterns of use and the user's lifestyle (way of living, etc.). In terms of cognitive deficits, each of these aspects may play its role, which has significant implications for treatment and rehabilitation options. The effective treatment of substance use-related consequences is based on an interdisciplinary approach. Therefore, the effective treatment of cognitive deficits caused by addictive substance use needs to involve a comprehensive approach to the patient, i.e., it needs to address different levels of the problems associated with addictive substances. Thus, a specific feature of the treatment of and rehabilitation from cognitive disorders associated with addictive substance use is the necessity to refer these patients to adequate treatment programmes that must respect the multifaceted nature of substance-related problems and permit a comprehensive approach to patients and their specific needs.

References

Al-Alousi, L. M.: Pathology of volatile substance abuse: a case report and literature review. *Med Sci Law*, 29, 1989, 189–208.

Alexander, G. E.; DeLong, M. R. and Strick, P. L.: Parallel organization of functionally segregated circuits linking basal ganglia and cortex. *Rev. Neurosci.*, 9, 1986, 357–381.

Altman, H. J. & Normále, H. J.: What is the nature of the role of the serotonergic nervous system in learning and memory: prospects for development of an effective treatment strategy for senile dementia? *Neurobiol. Aging* 9, 1988, 627–638.

American Academy of Pediatrics (2000). Fetal Alcohol Syndrome and Alcohol-Related Neurodevelopmental Disorders. *Pediatrics,* 106(2), 358–361.

Annual report on the state of the drugs problem in Europe (2007). EMCDDA, Lisboa. Source: http://www.emcdda.europa.eu/html.cfm/index419EN.html (1.3.2008, 18:40).

Appel, P. W.; Gordon, N. B.: Digit-symbol performance in methadone-treated ex-heroin addicts. *Am. J. Psychiatr.* 133, 1976, 1337–1340.

Araki, H.; Suemaru, K. & Gomita, Y.: Neuronal nicotinic receptor and psychiatric disorders: functional and behavioral effects of nicotine. *Jpn. J. Pharmacol.*, Feb; 88 (2), 2002, 133–8.

Baggott, M.; Jerome, L. & Start, R.: 3,4-Methylenedioxymethamphetamine (MDMA): A Review of the English-Language Scientific and Medical Literature, www.maps.org., 2001.

Baker, E. L.; Jr., Smith, T. J. and Landrigan, P. J.: The neurotoxicity of industrial solvents: A review of the literature. *Am. J. Ind. Med.,* 8, 1985, 207–217.

Banning, A. and Sjogren, P.: Cerebral effects of long-term oral opioids in cancer patients measured by continuous reaction time. *Clinical Journal of Pain*, 6, 1990, 91–95.

Banning, A.; Sjogren, P. and Kaiser, F.: Reaction time in cancer patients receiving peripherally acting analgesics alone or in combination with opioids. Acta Anaesthesiologica Scandinavica, 36, 1992, 480–482.

Bartzokis, G.; Beckson, M. and Ling, W.: Clinical and MRI Evaluation of Psychostimulant Neurotoxicity. In: Majewska MD, ed.: Neurotoxicity and Neuropathology Associated with Cocaine Abuse. NIDA Research Monograph 163, National Institute on Drug Abuse, Rockville, 1996.

Bauer, L. O.: Psychomotor and Electroencephalographic Sequelae of Cocaine Dependence. In: Majewska, M.D. ed. (1996). Neurotoxicity and Neuropathology Associated with Cocaine Abuse. NIDA Research Monograph 163, National Institute on Drug Abuse, Rockville, 1996.

Blahoutová, V.; Zajícová, A.; Wilczek, H. and Holáň, V.: Opiáty a jejich imunomodulační vlastnosti [Opiates and Their Immunomodulation Properties]. Časopis lékařů českých, 142, 4, 2003, 244–47.

Bolla, K. I.; Brown, K. and Eldreth, D.: Dose-related neurocognitive effects of marijuana use. *Neurology,* 59, 2002, 1337–1343.

Bolla, K. I.; Funderburk, F. R. and Cadet, J. L.: Differential effects of cocaine and cocaine alcohol on neurocognitive performance. *Neurology* 54 (12), 2000, 2285–92.

Bowen, J. D. and Larson, E. B.: Drug-induced cognitive impairment. Defining the problem and finding solutions. *Drug and Aging*, 3, 1993, 349–357.

Bruera, E.; Macmillan, K.; Hanson, J. and MacDonald, R. N.: The cognitive effects of the administration of narcotic analgesics in patients with cancer pain. *Pain*, 39, 1989, 13–16.

Burgess, C.; O'Donohoe, A. & Gill, M.: Agony and ecstasy: a review of MDMA effects and toxicity. *Eur. Psychiatry,* 15, 2000, 287–294.

Buschke, H.: Retention in immediate memory estimated without retrieval. *Science,* 140, 1963, 56-67.

Buschke, H.: Selective reminding for analysis of memory and learning. *Journal of Verbal Learning and Verbal Behavior* 12, 1973, 543–550.

Campagna, D.; Gobba, F.; Mergler, D. et al.: Color vision loss among styrene-exposed workers neurotoxicological threshold assessment. *Neurotoxicology*, 17(2), 1996, 367–73.

Cascella, N. G.; Perrlson, G.; Wong, D. F.; Broussole, E.; Nagoshi, C.; Margolin, R. A. and London, E. D.: Effects of substance abuse on ventricular and sulcal measures assessed by computerized tomography. *Br. J. Psychiatry* 159, 1991, 217–221.

Clemons, M.; Regnard, C. and Appleton, T.: Alertness, cognition and morphine in patients with advanced cancer. *Cancer Treatment Reviews*, 22, 1996, 451–468.

Cole, J. C. & Sumnall, H. R.: Altered states: the clinical effects of Ecstasy. *Pharmacol. Ther.,* 98, 2003, 35–58.

Csémy, L.; Sadílek, P.; Sovinová, H. & Lejčková, P.: ESPAD 03. Přehled hlavních výsledků z let 1995, 1999 a 2003 [Summary of Main Results from 1995, 1999 and 2003]. Press release. Praha, Úřad vlády ČR, 2003.

Csémy, L.; Sovinová, H. & Komárek, J.: Drogy na taneční scéně [Drugs and the Dance Scene]. Praha, Státní zdravotní ústav 2000.

Cunha, P. J.; Nicastri, S.; Gomes, L. P.; Moino, R. M. and Peluso, M. A.: Neuropsychological impairments in crack cocaine-dependent inpatients: preliminary findings. *Rev. Bras. Psiquiatr.* 26 (2), 2004, 103–6.

Dackis, C. A. and Gold, M. S.: New concepts in cocaine addiction: The dopamine depletion hypothesis. *Neurosci. Biobehav. Rev.* 9, 1985, 469–477.

Daneman, M. and Carpenter, P. A.: Individual differences in working memory and reading. *Journal of Verbal Learning and Verbal Behavior*, 19, 1980, 450–466.

Daras, M.; Tauchman, A. J. and Marks, S.: Central nervous system infarction related to cocaine abuse. *Stroke*, 22, 1991, 1320–1326.

Daras, M.: Neurologic Complications of Cocaine. In: Majewska MD, ed.: Neurotoxicity and Neuropathology Associated with Cocaine Abuse. NIDA Research Monograph 163, National Institute on Drug Abuse, Rockville, 1996.

Delis, D. C.; Squire, L. R.; Bihrle, A. and Massman, P.: Componential analysis of problem-solving ability: Performance of patients with frontal lobe damage and amnestic patients on a new sorting test. *Neuropsychol.,* 30: 1992, 683–697.

Deschamps, D.; Geraud, C. and Dally, S.: Cognitive functions in workers exposed to toluene: evaluation at least 48 hours after removal from exposure. *Int. Arch. Occup. Environ. Health*, 74(4), 2001, 285–8.

Ellingsen, D. G.; Lorentzen, P. and Langard, S.: A Neuropsychological study of patients exposed to organic solvents. *Int. J. Occup. Environ. Health*, 3(3), 1997, 177–183.

Ellison, G.; Irwin, S.; Keys, S.; Noguchi, K. and Sulur, G.: The Neurotoxic Effects of Continuous Cocaine and Amphetamine in Habenula: Implications for the Substrates of Psychosis. In: Majewska MD, ed.: Neurotoxicity and Neuropathology Associated with Cocaine Abuse. NIDA Research Monograph 163, National Institute on Drug Abuse, Rockville, 1966.

EMCDDA. An overview of cannabis potency in Europe. Lisbon, EMCDDA, 2004.

EMCDDA. Komorbidita: užívání drog a duševní poruchy [Comorbidity—Drug Use and Mental Disorders]. *Drugs in Focus*, 14, Lisbon, EMCDDA. 2004.

Ersek, M.; Cherrier, M.; Overman, S. S. and Irving, G. A.: The Cognitive effects of opioids. *Pain Management Nursing,* Vol. 5, No 2, 2004, 75–93.

Fals-Stewart, W.: Ability of counselors to detect cognitive impairment among substance-abusing patients: An examination of diagnostic efficiency. *Experimental and Clinical Psychopharmacology*, Vol. 5 (1), 1997, 39–50.

Filley, C. M.; Heaton, R. K. and Rosenberg, N. L.: White matter dementia in chronic toluene abuse. *Neurology,* 40, 1990, 532–534.

Fišar, Z.; Velenovská, M. and Hanuš, Z.: In vitro vliv kanabinoidů na vlastnosti buněčných membrán [In vitro Effect of Cannabinoids on Characteristics of Cell Membranes]. Poster session presented at the 47th Czech-Slovak Psychopharmacological Conference, 5-9 January 2005, Lázně Jeseník, 2005.

Finch, C. K. and Lobo, B. L.: Acute inhalant-induced neurotoxicity with delayed recovery. *Ann. Pharmacother.*, 39 (1), 2005, 169–72.

Fišerová, M. & Páleníček, T.: MDMA (3,4-methylendioxymetamfetamin)—"Extáze" [MDMA (3,4-methylendioxymethamphetamine)—"Ecstasy"]. *Adiktologie*, 2, 2001, 48–59.

Fletcher, J. M.; Page, J. B.; Francis D. J. et al.: Cognitive Correlates of Long-term Cannabis Use in Costa Rican Men. *Arch. Gen. Psychiatry*, 53(1), 1996, 1051–1057.

Flores, E. D.; Lange, R. A.; Cigarroa, R. G. and Hilus, L. D.: Effect of cocaine on coronary artery dimensions in atherosclerotic coronary artery disease: enhanced vasoconstriction at sites of significant stenoses. *J. Am. Coll Cardiol.* 16, 1990, 74–79.

Fox, H. C.; Parrott, A. C. & Turner, J. J.: Ecstasy use: cognitive deficits related to dosage rather than self-reported problematic use of the drug. *J. Psychopharmacol.*, 15, 2001, 273–281.

Fredericks, R. K.; Lefkovitz, D. S.; Challa, V. R. and Troost, B. T.: Cerebral vasculitis associated with cocaine abuse. *Stroke.* 22, 1991, 1437–1439.

Giannakoulas, G.; Katramados, A.; Melas, N.; Diamantopoulos, I. and Chimonas, E.: Acute effects of nicotine withdrawal syndrome in pilots during flight. *Aviat. Space Environ. Med.*, 74, 3, 2003, 247–251.

Goldstein, R. Z.; Leskovjan, A. C.; Hoff, A. L.; Hitzemann, R.; Bashan, F.; Khalsa, S. S. ; Wang, G. J.; Fowler, J. S. and Volkow, N. D.: Severity of neuropsychological impairment in cocaine and alcohol addiction: association with metabolism in the prefrontal cortex. *Neuropsychologia* 42 (11), 2004, 1447–58.

Gottschalk, Ch.; Beauvais, J.; Hart, R. and Kosten, T.: Cognitive Function and Cerebral Perfusion During Cocaine Abstinence. *Am. J. Psychiatry*, 158, 2001, 4.

Gouzoulis-Mayfrank, E.; Daumann, J.; Tuchtenhagen, F.; Pelz, S.; Becker, S.; Kuvert, H. J.; Fimm, B. & Sass, H.: Impaired cognitive performance in drug free users of recreational ecstasy (MDMA). *J. Neurol. Neurosurg. Psychiatry*, 68, 2000, 719–725.

Grant, I.; Adams, K. M.; Carlin, A. S.; Rennick, P. M.; Judd, L. L. and Schooff, K.: Collaborative neuropsychological study of polydrug users. *Arch. Gen. Psychiatry*, 35, 1978, 1063–74.

Hall, W. and Solowij, N.: Adverse effects of cannabis. *The Lancet,* 352, 1998, 1611–1616.

Halliday, R.; Naylor, H.; Brandejs, D.; Callaway, E.; Yano, L. and Herzig, K.: The effect of D-amphetamine, clonidine, and yohimbine on human information processing. *Psychophysiology* 31 (4), 1994, 331–337.

Hartnoll, R. et al.: Příručka k provádění výběru metodou sněhové koule (Snowball Sampling) [Handbook on Snowball Sampling]. Praha, Úřad vlády ČR 2003.

Haythornthwaite, J. A.; Menefee, L. A.; Quatrano-Piacentini, A. L. and Pappagallo, M.: Outcome of chronic opioid therapy for non-cancer pain. *Journal of Pain and Symptom Management*, 15, 1998, 185–194.

Hellstrom-Lindahl, E. & Nordberg, A.: Smoking during pregnancy: a way to transfer the addiction to the next generation? *Respiration.*, 69 (4), 2002, 289–293.

Hibell, B. et al.: The ESPAD Report 2003. Alcohol and other drug use among students in 35 European countries. Stockholm, CAN 2004.

Hill, S. Y. and Mikhael, M. A.: Computerised transaxial tomographic and neuropsychological evaluations in chronic alcoholics and heroin abusers. *Am. Psychiatry*, 136, 1979, 598–602.

Hill, J. L. and Zacny, J. P.: Comparing the subjective, psychomotor, and physiological effects of intravenous hydromorphone and morphine in healthy volunteers. *Psychopharmacology* (Berl), 152, 2000, 31–39.

Holman, B. L.; Mendelson, J.; Garada, B.; Teoh, S. K.; Hallgring, E.; Johnson, K. A. and Mello, N. K. Regional cerebral blood flow improves with treatment in chronic cocaine polydrug users. *J. Nucl. Med.* 34, 1993, 723–727.

Chany, L.; Ernst, T.; Speck, O.; Patel, H.; DeSilva, M.; Leonido-Yee, M. and Miller, E. N.: Perfusion MRI and computerized cognitive test abnormalities in abstinent methamphetamine users. *Psychiatry Res.* 114 (2), 65–79.

Chouaniere, D.; Wild, P.; Fontana, J. M. et al.: Neurobehavioral disturbances arising from occupational toluene exposure. *Am. J. Ind. Med.*, 41 (2), 2002, 77–88.

Jacobsen, L. K.; Krystal, J. H.; Mencl, W. E.; Westerveld, M.; Frost, S. J. and Pugh, K. R.: Effects of smoking and smoking abstinence on cognition in adolescent tobacco smokers. *Biol. Psychiatry,* 57, 1, 2005, 56–66.

Jentsch, J. D.; Roth, R.; Taylor, J. and Verrico, C.: Cannabinoid effects on neurocognition: implications for psychosis. 2002.

Kalechstein, A. D.; Newton, T. F. and Green, M.: Methamphetamine dependence is associated with neurocognitive impairment in the initial phases of abstinence. *Neuropsychiatry Clinical Neuroscience* 15, 2003, 215–220.

Kalina, K. et al.: Drogy a drogové závislosti 1, 2. Mezioborový přístup [Drugs and Drug Addiction 1, 2. An Interdisciplinary Approach]. Praha, Úřad vlády ČR 2003.

Kampman, K.; Majewska, M. D.; Tourian, K.; Dackis, C.; Cornish, J.; Poole, S. and O'Brien, C.: A pilot trial of piracetam and ginkgo biloba for the treatment of cocaine dependence. *Addict. Behav.* 28 (3), 2003, 437–48.

Kaufman, M. J.; Levin, J. M.; Ross, M. H.; Lange, N.; Rose, S. L.; Kukes, T. J.; Mendelson, J. H.; Lukas, S. E.; Cohen, B. M. and Renshaw, P. F.: Cocaine-induced cerebral vasoconstriction detected in humans with magnetic resonance angiography. *JAMA* 279, 1998, 376–380.

Klonoff, D. C.; Andrews, M. D. and Obana, W. G.: Stroke associated with cocaine use. *Arch. Neurology* 46, 1989, 989–993.

Kosten, T. R., Malison, R. and Wallace, E.: Neuropsychological Abnormalities in Cocaine Abusers: Possible Correlates in SPECT Neuroimaging. In: Majewska, M. D., ed. (1996). Neurotoxicity and Neuropathology Associated with Cocaine Abuse. NIDA Research Monograph 163, National Institute on Drug Abuse, Rockville, 1996.

Krystal, J. H.; Price, L. H.; Opsahl, C.; Ricaurte, G. A. & Heninger, G. R.: Chronic 3,4-methylenedioxymethamphetamine (MDMA) use: effects on mood and neuropsychological function? *Am. J. Drug Alcohol Abus*e, 18, 1992, 331–341.

Lathers, C. M.; Tyau, L. S.; Spino, M. M. and Agarawal, I.: Cocaine induced seizures, arrhythmias and sudden death. *J. Clin. Pharmacol.* 28, 1988, 584–593.

Laucht, M. & Schmidt, M. H.: Maternal smoking during pregnancy: risk factor for ADHD in the offspring? In: Kinder Jugendpsychiatr Psychother. Jul; 32(3), German, 2004, 177015085.

Lawlor, P. G.; Gagnon, B.; Mancini, I. L.; Pereira, J. L.; Hanson, J.; Suarez-Almazor, M. E. and Bruera, E.: Occurance, causes, and outcome of delirium in patients with advanced cancer: A prospective study. Archives of Internal Medicine, 160, 2000, 786–794.

Lawlor, P. G.: The panorama of opioid-related cognitive dysfunction in patients with cancer: A critical literature appraisal. *Cancer,* 94, 2002, 1836–1853.

Levin, E. D. & Detvani, A. H.: Nicotinic treatment for cognitive dysfunction. Curr Drug Targets CNS Neurol Disord., Aug; 1 (4), 2002, 423–31.

Levin, E. D. & Detvani, A. H.: Development of nicotinic drug therapy for cognitive disorders. *Eur. J. Pharmacol.*, Mar 30, 393(1-3), 2000,141–6.

Lichtenfeld, P.; Rubin, D. B. and Feldman, R. S.: Subarachnoid hemorrhage precipitated by cocaine scoring. *Arch Neurology* 41, 1984, 223–224.

Lomax, R. B.; Ridgway, P. and Meldrum, M.: Does occupational exposure to organic solvents affect colour discrimination? *Toxicol. Rev.*, 23 (2), 2004, 91–121.

Lorenz, J.; Beck, H. and Bromm, B.: Cognitive performance, mood and experimental pain before and during morphine-induced analgesia in patients with chronic non-malignant pain. *Pain,* 73, 1997, 369–375.

Lowinson, J. H.; Ruiz, P.; Millman, R. B. and Langrod, J. G. (Eds.): Substance abuse. A comprehensive textbook. Philadelphia: Lippincott Williams and Wilkins 2004.

Lyketsos, C. G.; Chen, L. S. & Anthony, J. C.: Cognitive decline in adulthood: an 11.5-year follow-up of the Baltimore epidemiologic catchment area study. *Am. J. Psychiatry*, 1999, 156 (58), 58–65.

Lyvers, M. and Yakimoff, M.: Neuropsychological correlates of opioid dependence and withdrawal. *Addictive Behaviors*, 2002, 28, 605–611.

Majewska, M. D.: Cocaine Addiction as a Neurological Disorder: Implications for Treatment. In: Majewska MD, ed.: Neurotoxicity and Neuropathology Associated with Cocaine Abuse. NIDA Research Monograph 163, National Institute on Drug Abuse, Rockville, 1996.

Marrow, L. A.; Stein, L.; Bagovich, G. R.; Condray, R. and Scott, A.: Neuropsychological assessment, depression, and past exposure to organic solvents. *Appl. Neuropsychol.*, 8(2), 2001, 65–73.

Martin, B. R.: Marijuana. http://www.acnp.org/g4/GN401000170/Default.htm., 2000.

Matysy, V. S.; Callicott, J. H.; Bertolino, A.; Newton, I.; Frank, J. A.; Coppola, R.; Berman, K. F.; Goldberg, T. E. and Weinberger, D. R.: Effects of dextroamphetamine on cognitive performance and cortical activation. *Neuroimage* 12 (3), 2000, 268–75.

McKetin, R. and Mattick, R. P.: Attention and memory in illicit amphetamine users: comparison with non- drug-using controls. *Drug and Alcohol Dependence.* 1998, 50: 181–184.

Meadows, R. and Verghese, A.: Medical complications of glue sniffing. *South Med. J.*, 1996, 89, 455–62.

Mendelson, J. H.; Teoh, S.; Lange, U.; Mello, N. K.; Weiss, R.; Skupny, A. and Ellingboe, J.: Anterior pituitary, adrenal, and gonadal hormones during cocaine withdrawal. *Am. J. Psychiatry*, 1988, 145: 1094–1098.

Milani, R. M.; Parrott, A. C.; Turner, J. J. & Fox, H. C.: Gender differences in self-reported anxiety, depression, and somatization among ecstasy/MDMA polydrug users, alcohol/tobacco users, and nondrug users. *Addict. Behav.*, 2004, 29, 965–971.

Mills, E. M.; Banks, M. L.; Sprague, J. E. & Finkel, T: Pharmacology: uncoupling the agony from ecstasy. *Nature,* 2003, 426, 403–404.

Milner, B.: Effects of different brain lesions on card sorting. *Arch. Neurol.*, 1963, 9, 90–100.

Miovský, M.: Konopné drogy [Cannabis]. In: Kalina, K. et al.: Drogy a drogové závislosti 1, 2. Mezioborový přístup [Drugs and Drug Addiction 1, 2. An Interdisciplinary Approach]. Praha, Úřad vlády ČR. 2003, 174–179.

Miovský, M.: Problémy meziborového přístupu k léčbě závislostí [Issues of the Interdisciplinary Approach to Addiction Treatment]. In: Kalina, K. et al. Drogy a drogové závislosti 2. Mezioborový přístup [Drugs and Drug Addiction 2. An Interdisciplinary Approach]. Praha, Úřad vlády ČR 2003, 14–15.

Miovský, M.; Šťastná, L. & Řehan, V.: Aktuální přehled stavu užívání konopných drog v České republice z perspektivy školních a celopopulačních studií [Summary of the Recent Cannabis Use Situation in the Czech Republic from the Perspective of School and General Population Surveys]. Psychiatrie, 3, 2004, 196–201.

Miovský, M.; Šťastná, L. & Řehan, V.: Indikátory rizikového chování v kontextu užívání konopných drog [Risk Behaviour Indicators in the Context of Cannabis Use]. Psychiatrie, 2004, 4, ročník 8, 200–205.

Mody, C. K.; Killer, B. L.; McIntyre, H. B. and Goldberg, M. A.: Neurologic complications of cocaine abuse. *Neurology*, 1988, 38: 1189–1193.

Montoya, A. G.; Sorrentino, R.; Lukáš, S. E. & Price, B. H.: Long-term neuropsychiatric consequences of "ecstasy" (MDMA): a review. *Harv. Rev. Psychiatry,* 2002, 10, 212–220.

Morgan, M. J.; Mafie, L.; Fleetwood, H. & Robinson, J. A.: Ecstasy (MDMA): are the psychological problems associated with its use reversed by prolonged abstinence? Psychopharmacology (Berl), 2002, 159, 294–303.

Morrison, R. S.; Magaziner, J.; Gilbert, M. et al.: Relationship between pain and opioid analgesics on the development of delirium following hip fracture. *Journals of Gerontology Series A-Biological Sciences and Medical Sciences,* 2003, 58, M76-M81.

Moszczynska, A.; Fitzmaurice, P.; Ang, L.; Kalasinsky, K. S.; Schmunk, G. A.; Peretti, F. J.; Suken, S. S.; Wickham, D. J. and Kish, S. J.: Why is parkinsonism not a feature of human methamphetamine users? *Brain.*, 2003, 127 (2): 363–70.

Newhouse, P. A.; Potter, A. & Singh, A.: Effects of nicotinic stimulation on cognitive performance. *Curr. Opin. Pharmacol.*, Feb, 2004, 4 (1), 36–46.

Newton, T. F.; Cook, I. A.; Kalechstein, A. D.; Duran, S.; Monroy, F.; Ling, W. and Leuchter, A. F.: Quantitative EEG abnormalities in recently abstinent methamphetamine dependent individuals. *Clin. Neurophysiol.* 114, 2003, (3): 410–5.

NIDA (2002b). Marijuana abuse. Research Report. NIDA.

NIDA (2004). Inhalant abuse. Research Report Series. www.drugabuse.gov.

O'Loinsigh, E. D.; Boland, G.; Kelly, J. P. and O'Boyle, K. M.: Behavioural, hyperthermic and neurotoxic effects of 3,4-methylenedioxymethamphetamine analogues in the Wistar rat. Prog. Neuropsychopharmacol. *Biol. Psychiatry*, 2001, 25, 621–638.

O'Malley, S.; Adamse, M.; Newton, R. K. and Gawin, F. H.: Neuropsychological impairment in chronic cocaine abusers. *Am. J. Drug Alcohol Abuse*, 1992, 18: 131–144.

Ornstein, T. J.; Iddon, J. L.; Baldacchino, A. M. et al.: *Neuropsychopharmacology*, Vol. 23, No. 2, 2000, 113–126.

Owen, A. M.; Downes, J. J.; Sahakian, B. J. et al.: Planning and spatial working memory following frontal lobe lesions in man. *Neuropsychologia*, 1990, 28 (10), 1021–1034.

Owen, A. M.; Roberts, A. C.; Polkey, C. E. et al.: Extra-dimensional versus intra-dimensional set shifting performance following frontal lobe ixcisions, temporal lobe excisions or amygdala-hippocampectomy in man. *Neuropsychologiea,* 1991, 29 (10), 993–1006.

Owen, A. M.; Sahakian, B. J.; Hodges, J. R. et al.: Dopamine-dependent frontostriatal planning deficits in early Parkinson's disease. *Neuropsychology*, 1995, 9 (1), 126–140.

Páleníček, T. & Šustková, M.: "Ecstasy"—A Mysterious Dance. *Psychiatrie*, 2003, 7 (2), 101–109.

Pascual-Leone, A.; Dhuna, A. and Anderson, D. C.: Long-term neurological complications of chronic, habitual cocaine abuse. *Neurotoxicology*, 1991, 12: 393–400.

Parrott, A. C.: Human research on MDMA (3,4-methylene-dioxymethamphetamine) neurotoxicity: cognitive and behavioural indices of change. *Neuropsychobiology*, 2000, 42, 17–24.

Parrott, A. CIs ecstasy MDMA? A review of the proportion of ecstasy tablets containing MDMA, their dosage levels, and the changing perceptions of purity. *Psychopharmacology* (Berl), 2004, 173, 234–241.

Parrott, A. C.; Lees, A.; Garnham, N. J.; Jones, M. & Nesnes, K.: Cognitive performance in recreational users of MDMA of "ecstasy": evidence for memory deficits. *J. Psychopharmacol.*, 1998, 12, 79–83.

Paulu, M. P.; Hozack, N. E.; Zauscher, B. E.; Frank, L.; Brown, G. G.; Bratr, D. L. and Schuckit, M. A.: Behavioral and functional neuroimaging evidence for prefrontal dysfunction in methamphetamine-dependent subjects. *Neuropsychopharmacology*, 2002, 26 (1): 53–63.

Pettit, H. O.; Ettenberg, A.; Bloom, F. E. and Koob, G. F.: Destruction of dopamine in the nucleus accumbens selectively attenuates cocaine but not heroin self-administration in rats. *Psychopharmacology*, 1982, 84: 167–173.

Pomerleau, C. S.: Co-factors for smoking and evolutionary psychobiology. Addiction. Review, Apr; 1997, 92 (4): 397–408.

Pope, H. G. Jr.; Gruber, A. J. & Yurgelum-Todd, D.: The residual neuropsychological effects of cannabis: the current status of research. *Drug Alcohol Depend*, 1995, 38, 25–34.

Pope, H. G. Jr. & Yurgelum-Todd, D.: The residual cognitive effects of heavy marijuana use in college students. *The Journal of the American Medical Association*, 1996, 275(7), 521–527.

Pope, H. G. Jr.; Jacobs A. & Mialet J. P. et al.: Evidence for a sex-specific residual effect of cannabis on visuospatial memory. *Psychother. Psychosom.*, 1997, 66, 179–184.

Pope, H. G. Jr.; Gruber, A. J.; Hudson, J. I.; Cohane, G.; Huestis, M. A. & Yurgelum-Todd, D.: Early-onset cannabis use and cognitive deficits: what is the nature of the association? *Drug and Alcohol Dependence*, 2002, 69, 303–310.

Preston, A.: Drogy na předpis II. Vše o metadonu. Olomouc, Votobia 1999.

Psychiatrické centrum Praha GENACIS (Gender and alcohol comparative international study) 2003. Unpublished results of research conducted in 2002.

Raja, S. N.; Haythornthwaite, J. A.; Pappagallo, M. et al.: Opioids versus antidepressants in postherpetic neuralgia: A randomized, placebo-controlled trial. *Neurology*, 2002, 59, 1015llaceb

Rauh, V. A.; Whyatt, R. M.; Garfinkel, R.; Andrews, H.; Hoepner, L.; Reyes, A.; Diaz, D.; Camann, D. & Perera, F. P.: Developmental effects of exposure to environmental tobacco smoke and material hardship among inner-city children. *Neurotoxicol Teratol.*, May-Jun, 2004, 26 (3), 373–85.

Reneman, L.; Booij, J.; Schmand, B.; van den Brink; W. & Gunning, B.: Memory disturbances in "Ecstasy" users are correlated with an altered brain serotonin neurotransmission. *Psychopharmacology* (Berl), 2000, 148: 322–324.

Ricaurte, G. A.; Juan, J. & McCann, U. D.: (+/-)3,4-Methylenedioxymethamphetamine ('Ecstasy')-induced serotonin neurotoxicity: studies in animals. *Neuropsychobiology*, 2000, 42, 5–10.

Rinder, H. M.; Ault, K. A.; Jatlow, P. I.; Kosten, T. R. and Smith, B. R.: Platelet alpha-granule release in cocaine users. *Circulation.*, 1994, 90: 1162–1167.

Ritz, M. C.; Lamb, R. J.; Goldberg, S. R. and Kuhar, M. J.: Cocaine receptors on dopamine transporters are related to self-administration of cocaine. Science, 1987, 237: 1219–1223.

Robe, H. W. J.: Influence of marijuana on driving. Maastricht, University of Limberg: *Institute for Human Psychopharmacology,* 1994.

Roberts, D. C.; Koob, F.; Klonoff, P. and Fibiger, H. C.: Extinction and recovery of cocaine-self administration following 6-hydroxydopamine lesions of the nucleus accumbens. *Pharm. Biochem. Behav.*, 1989, 12: 781–787.

Rotgers, F. et al.: Léčba drogových závislostí [Treating Substance Abuse]. Praha, Grada Publishing 1999.

Rowbotham, M. C.; Twilling, L.; Davies, P. S. et al.: Oral opioid therapy for chronic peripheral and central neuropathic pain. *New England Journal of Medicine*, 2003, 348, 1223–1232.

Ryan, C. M.; Morrow, L. A. and Hodgson, M.: Cacosmia and neurobehavioral dysfunction associated with occupational exposure to mixtures of organic solvents. *Am. J. Psychiatry*, 1988, 145, 1442–1445.

Rosenberg, N. L.: Neurotoxicity of organic solvents. In Occupational and Environmental Neurology; Rosenberg, N. L., Ed., Butterworth/Heinemann Publishers: Stoneham, MA 1995, 71–114.

Rosenberg: Neuropsychologic Impairment and MRI abnormalities associated with chronic solvent abuse. *Clinical Toxicology*, 2002, 40 (1), 21–34.

RVKPP: Standardy odborné způsobilosti služeb pro uživatele omamných a psychotropních látek [Professional Qualification Standards for Drug Treatment Services]. Praha, RVKPP 2003.

Sacco, K. A.; Bannon, K. L. & George, T. P.: Nicotinic receptor mechanisms and cognition in normal states and neuropsychiatric disorders. *J. Psychopharmacol. Dec*, 2004, 18 (4): 457 Dec

Salin-Pascual, R. J.; Alcocer-Castillejos, N. V. & Alejo-Galarza, G.: Nicotine dependence and psychiatric disorders. *Rev. Invest. Clin. Nov-Dec*, 2003, 55 (6), 677–93.

Salo, R.; Nordahl, T. E.; Posaun, K.; Leamon, M.; Gibbon, D. R.; Galloway, G. P.; Flynn, N. M.; Henik, A.; Pfefferbaum, A. and Sullivan, E. V.: Preliminary evidence of reduced cognitive inhibition in methamphetamine-dependent individuals. *Psychiatric Research.,* 2002, 111: 65–74.

Seeber, A.; Schaper, M.; Zupanic, M. et al.: Toluene exposure below 50 ppm and cognitive function: a follow-up study with four repeated measurements in rotogravure printing plants. *Int. Arch. Occup. Environ. Health*, 2004, 77 (1), 1–9.

Schaper, M.; Demes, P.; Kiesswetter, E. et al.: Colour vision and occupational toluene exposure: results of repeated examinations. *Toxicol. Lett.*, 2004, 151 (1), 193–202.

Schaumbur, H. H. and Spencer, P. S.: Recognizing neurotoxic disease. *Neurology*, 1987, 37, 276–278.

Sim, T.; Simon, S. L.; Domier, C. P.; Richardson, K.; Rawson, R. A. and Ling, W.: Cognitive deficits among methamphetamine users with attention deficit hyperactivity disorder symptomatology. *J. Addict. Dis.*, 2002, 21 (1): 75–89.

Simon, S. L.; Domier, C.; Carnell, J.; Brethen, P.; Rawson, R. and Ling, W.: Cognitive impairment in individuals currently using methamphetamine. *Am. J. Addict.* 2000, 9 (3): 222–31.

Simon, S. L.; Dacey, J. M.; Glynn, S.; Rawson, R. A. and Ling, W.: Learning difficulties in abstinent methamphetamine abusers. Paper presented at the sixty/third annual meeting of the College on Problems of Drug Dependence, Scottsdale, AZ 2001.

Simon, S. L.; Domier, C. P.; Sim, T.; Richardson, K.; Rawson, R. A. and Ling, W.: Cognitive performance of current methamphetamine and cocaine abusers. *J. Addict. Dis.*, 2002a, 21 (1): 61–74.

Simon, S. L.; Dacey, J. M.; Glynn, S. and Rawson, R. A.: Treatment implications of cognitive deficits in methamphetamine abusers. Poster session presented at the annual meeting of the Western Psychological Association, Irvine, CA 2002b.

Simon, S. L.; Dacey, J.; Glynn, S.; Rawson, R. and Ling, W.: The effect of relapse on cognition in abstinent methamphetamine abusers. *Journal of Substance Abuse Treatment*, 2004, 27: 59–66.

Sprague, J. E.; Banks, M. L.; Cook, V. J. & Mills, E. M.: Hypothalamic-pituitary-thyroid axis and sympathetic nervous system involvement in hyperthermia induced by 3,4-methylenedioxymethamphetamine (Ecstasy). *J. Pharmacol. Exp. Ther.*, 2003, 305, 159–166.

Schor, J. D.; Levkoff, S. E.; Lipsitz, L. A. et al.: Risk factors for delirium in hospitalized elderly. *Journal of the American Medical Association*, 1992, 267, 827-831.

Schwartz, R. H.: Chronic marihuana smoking and short-term memory impairment. In: Nahas, G. G., Latour, C. (Eds.) Cannabis: Physiopathology, Epidemiology, Detection. Boca Raton, FL, CRC Press 1993, 61-71.

Smiley, A.: Marijuana: on road and driving simulator studies. In: Kalant, H., Corrigal, W., Hall, W., Smart, R., eds. The health effects of cannabis. Toronto, Addiction Research Foundation, 1998.

Smolík, P.: Duševní a behaviorální poruchy [Mental and Behavioural Disorders]. Praha, MAXDORF 1996.

Snodgrass, J. G. and Vanderwart, M.: A standardized set of 260 pictures: Norms for name agreement, image agreement, familiarity and visual complexity. Journal of Experimental Psychology: *Human Learning and Memory*, 1980, 6: 174–215.

Solowij, N.; Michie, P. & Fox, A.: Differential impairments of selective attention due to frequency and duration of cannabis use. *Biological Psychiatry*, 1995, 37, 731–739.

Solowij, N.; Stephens, R. S.; Roffman, A. R. And Babor, T. et al.: Cognitive functioning of long-term heavy cannabis users seeking treatment. *The Journal of the American Medical Association*, 2002, 287 (9), 1123–1131.

Srisurapanont, M.; Jarusuraisin, N. and Kittirattanapaiboon, P.: Treatment for amphetamine dependence and abuse (Cochrane Review). The Cochrane Library, Issue 1. Chichester, UK, John Wiley and Sons, Ltd. 2005.

Strickland, T. L.; Miller, B. L.; Kowell, A. and Stein, R.: Neurobiology of cocaine-induced organic brain impairment: contributions from functional neuroimaging. *Neuropsychol. Rev.*, 1998, 8: 1–9.

The Morning After the Night Before, The Globe, volume not indicated, 2000, 4–7 and 18–19.

Thompson, P. M.; Hayashi, K. M.; Simon, S. L.; Gesta, J. A.; Hong, M. S.; Sui, Y.; Lee, J. Y.; Toga, A. W.; Ling, W. and London, E. D.: Structural abnormalities in the brains of human subjects who use methamphetamine. *J. Neurosci.* 2004, 24 (26): 6028–36.

Turner, J. J. & Parrott, A. C.: "Is MDMA a human neurotoxin?": diverse views from the discussants. *Neuropsychobiology*, 2000, 42, 42–48.

ÚZIS: Psychiatrická péče 2002 [Psychiatric Care 2002]. Praha, ÚZIS 2003.

ÚZIS: Psychiatrická péče 2003 [Psychiatric Care 2003]. Praha, ÚZIS 2004.

Vitullo, J. C.; Karam, R.; Mekhail, N.; Wicker, P.; Engelmann, G. L. and Khairallah, P. A.: Cocaine-induced small vessel spasm in isolated rat hearts. *Am. J. Pathol.* 1989; 1998, 135: 85–91.

Volkow, N. D.; Mullani, N.; Gould, L.; Adler, S. and Krajewski, K.: Cerebral blood flow in chronic cocaine abusers: a study with positron emission tomography. *Br. J. Psychiatry* 1998, 152: 641–648.

Volkow, N. D.; Chany, L.; Wang, G. J.; Fowler, J. S.; Leonido-Yee, M.; Franceschi, D.; Sedler, M. J.; Gatley, S. J.; Hitzemann, R.; Ding, Y. S.; Logan, J.; Wong, C. and Miller, E. N.: Association of dopamine transporter reduction with psychomotor impairment in methamphetamine abusers. *Am. J. Psychiatry* 2001, 158 (3), 377–82.

Volkow, N. D.; Chang L.; Wang G. J.; Fowler J. S.; Franceschi D.; Sedler M. J.; Gatley S. J.; Hitzemann R.; Ding Y. S.; Wong C. and Logan J.: Higher cortical and lower subcortical metabolism in detoxified methamphetamine abusers. *American journal of Psychiatry.* 2001B, 158: 383–389.

Vorel F.: Mortalita řidičů 1998–2002 [Driver Mortality 1998-2002]. Praha, Sekretariát Rady vlády pro koordinaci protidrogové politiky. Pracovní skupina NMS "Drogová mortalita" 2003. IN: Mravčík V et al., 2003. Výroční zpráva o stavu ve věcech drog v České republice v roce 2002 [Annual Report on the 2002 Drug Situation in the Czech Republic]. Úřad vlády ČR.

Walker, D. J. and Zacny, J. P.: Subjective, psychomotor, and physiological effects of cumulative doses of opioid mu agonists in healthy volunteers. *Journal of Pharmacology and Experimental Therapeutics,* 1999, 289, 1454–1464.

Wiese, J. G.; Michael, G.; Shlipak M. G.; Browner, W. S.: The Alcohol Hangover. Ann *Intern Med.* 2000, 132, 897–902.

Wiegmann, D. A.; Stanny, R. R.; McKay, D. L.; Neri, D. F. and McCardie, A. H.: Methamphetamine effects on cognitive processing during extended wakefulness. *Int J Aviat Psychol.* 1996, 6 (4): 379–97.

Wilson, J. M.; Nobrega, J. N.; Corrigall, W.; Shannak, K.; Deck, J. H. N. and Kish, S. J.: Influence of chronic cocaine on monoamine neurotransmitters in human brain and animal model: Preliminary observations. *Ann. NY Acad Sci.* 1992, 654: 361–363.

Woodcock, R. W. and Johnson, M. B.: Woodcock-Johnson Psycho-Educational Battery. Allen TX: DLM Teaching Resources 1997.

Woods, S. W.; Cheeves, C.; Palubo, J.; Hoffer, P. B.; Price, L. H. and Kosten, T. R.: Regional cerebral blood flow during acute and chronic and combined cocaine-alcohol abuse abstinence. In: Kosten, T. R.; Malison, R., Wallace, E: Neuropsychological Abnormalities in Cocaine Abusers: Possible Correlates in SPECT Neuroimaging. In: Majewska, M. D., ed.: Neurotoxicity and Neuropathology Associated with Cocaine Abuse. NIDA Research Monograph 163, National Institute on Drug Abuse, Rockville, 1996.

Zacny, J. P.; Conley, K. and Galinkin, J.: Comparing the subjective, psychomotor and physiological effects of intravenous buprenorphine and morphine in healthy volunteers. *Journal of Pharmacology and Experimental Therapeutics*, 1997, 282, 1187–1197.

In: Cognitive Deficit in Mental and Neurological Disorders ISBN: 978-1-60741-957-0
Editors: H. Kucerova, M. Preiss

Chapter V

Antidepressants and Cognitive Function

Radovan Prikryl

Antidepressants globally belong to the most frequently prescribed medicinal products. This is supported by the fact that the depressive condition is one of the five most frequent diseases that significantly decrease working abilities of the patients, disable them or lead to their untimely death (Látalová et al., 2004).

It is generally known that antidepressants lead to the remission of depression and improve the general health including the patient's quality of life. However, many antidepressants may show undesirable impact on a series of the cognitive function domains (Amado-Boccaro et al., 1994). Only antidepressants with no negative effects on the cognitive functions should be considered optimal. The older tricyclic antidepressants (TCA) show very strong anticholinergic and antihistamine effects (Rudorfer et al., 1994). Histamine is a neurotransmitter that modulates the neuron path with its origin in the hypothalamus, projecting through telencephalon to the limbic structures (Schwartz, 1991). In the brain, histamine preferentially binds to its post-synaptic histamine H_1 receptors and, using this mechanism, it facilitates the neuron excitation. This is also an explanation of a well-known sedative effect of antihistamine drugs used for the treatment of allergies. The antihistamine agents penetrate into the brain, crossing the hematoencephalitic barrier, and block the postsynaptic histamine H_1 receptors. Within the therapeutical dose, the degree of a sedative effect of antihistamine drugs is low; however, it may already disrupt the cognitive performance or lead to psychomotor lapse. Similar to the histamine system, the cholinergic system also takes part in neuron excitation; in addition, it directly influences the so-called encoding, which is an active process helping to store new information into the short-term memory (Lane et al. 1999).

Antihistamine and anticholinergic effects of the TCA cause disruption of the psychomotor rate by decelerating the reception of sensomotor information that disrupts many common daily routines, especially the ability to drive. The anticholinergic activity then leads to a more specific disorder of cognitive functions because it disrupts the ability to immediately use information, working memory and, possibly, their transfer into the long-term memory including their later recall (Riedel and van Praag, 1995). It seems that tolerance to sedation or psychomotor lapse is probably developed during the course of a long-term TCA treatment, however, this does not apply to the memory disruption. A monthly treatment with amitriptyline, a principal representative of the TCA, dosed daily from 50 to 350 mg, led, besides the remission of depression, to gradual adjustment of the psychomotor rate while the memory functions remained disrupted (Spring et al., 1992).

The disruption of memory caused by the TCA is similar to the deterioration of memory functions, which is apparent after scopolamine administration. Scopolamine is a strong anticholinergic drug used in pharmacological experiments like memory disorder model in Alzheimer's-type dementias (Wesnes, Anand and Lorscheid, 1990). Molecules that enhance cholinergic neurotransmission, especially acetylcholine inhibitors (donepezil, rivastigmine, galantamine) are used in the clinical practice to treat dementias. The potentiation of the cerebral cholinergic system shows antidementia effects, while the anticholinergic activity is connected with memory functions disorder. An antidepressant called trazodone shows strong sedative effects, despite the minimum anticholinergic activity. The explanation consists in the relatively strong antagonism to adrenergic alfa$_1$-receptors from the trazodone side. It is a difference in comparison to amitriptyline, which, even though it shows sedative effects similar to trazadone, it also shows important anticholinergic activity. Although both antidepressants lead to various types of the psychomotor/cognitive disruption, amitriptyline has a stronger effect on the short-term memory (Sakulsripong et al., 1991; Branconnier and Cole, 1981). The memory disorder is, therefore, a key cognitive domain distinguishing antidepressants with or without anticholinergic activity.

Effect on Cognition after the Administration of a Single Dose to Healthy Volunteers

The measurement of antidepressive effect on cognitive functions may help objectively assess their impact on possible disruption of everyday activities, e.g., driving, remembering to purchase items, etc. The studies with healthy volunteers have shown diverse impact of individually tested antidepressants on the cognitive performance. Based on the neuropsychological data from many studies, an index of neurobehavioral toxicity of antidepressants in relation to the cognitive functions was constructed (Kerr et al., 1991). All studies had a very similar design. The healthy volunteers were neuropsychologically tested every hour for the period of six hours after the administration of a single dose of the tested antidepressant or placebo. After a week-long washout period, they were again tested using the same design with one exception: if they had been previously treated with the tested substance, they were taking a placebo and vice versa. Cognitive functions were tested by a standardized battery of neuropsychological tests containing critical flicker fusion (CFF) threshold, choice reaction time (CRT), compensatory tracking test (CTT) and subjective assessing scales. The TCA and other sedative antidepressants, e.g., mianserin or trazodone (antidepressants of the first and second generations), disrupted the cognitive performance and information processing to a significantly higher extent than the SSRI (selective serotonin re-uptake inhibitors, antidepressants of the third generation). The SSRI effect on the cognition was in principle neutral, very similar to placebo, with the exception of paroxetine and sertraline, which significantly increased the CFF threshold. In addition, sertraline improved the CRT.

A more complex view on the same data as Kerr (Kerr et al., 1991) was later offered by Sherwood (Sherwood et al., 1995). Sertraline (100 mg) a paroxetine (30 mg) significantly increased the CFF threshold. However, the CFF threshold increase may be caused by mydriasis rather than change in alertness or attention. Mydriasis may be induced by the anticholinergic effect of paroxetine. Mydriasis itself influences the CFF threshold and may lead to false-positive results (Freeman and O'Hanlon, 1995). Sertraline, which does not show any anticholinergic effect, did not improve the CRT, which means attention, information processing and sensomotor performance including reaction times. An improvement of the CRT may probably be ascribed to the sertraline effect on alertness because its impact on reaction times has not been proved. Despite the fact that paroxetine significantly improves the CFF threshold, it probably does not have any extensive impact on the CRT, although it improves reaction times that are a part of the CRT test (Robbe and O'Hanlon, 1995; Hindmarch and Harrison, 1988; Kerr et al., 1992).

The single administration of 40 mg citalopram increased the tapping rate (TAP) and the symbol coping rate; the reaction times were not influenced (Lader et al., 1986). The single administration of fluoxetine, paroxetine, a fluvoxamine, led to the disruption of psychomotor and cognitive performance in healthy volunteers. In healthy women, the administration of 30 mg paroxetine in combination with alcohol led to the impairment of the ability of driving and subjective feeling of fatigue for the period of four hours following the administration (Hindmarch and Harrison, 1988). In another study, fluoxetine was administered in the evening at bedtime, and the neuropsychological performance was then tested on the next day, immediately after awakening. It has been found out that even nine hours after the administration, fluoxetine significantly disrupts the number of substitution on the Digit Symbol Substitution Test (DSST) (Nicholson and Pascoe, 1988). The single administration of 100 mg fluvoxamine significantly disrupted the performance in divided visual attention task (Weinstein et al., 1996).

The studies using healthy volunteers are criticized because their results are often generalised for the population of patients with depressive disorders. However, this is questionable for two reasons. Any changes in the performance in neuropsychological tests should ideally reflect the abilities to perform common daily activities, especially when they reach clinical significance. It is always problematic to say that a certain product has actually no impact on a certain skill, only because it shows a negative result in the test testing the respective skill. The predictive value of neuropsychological tests has not yet been reliably proven (O'Hanlon and Freeman, 1995). Another significant reason consists in the difference between the population of healthy volunteers and that of the patients with depressive disorders. The patients with depression have real potential to utilize the therapeutical effect of antidepressants, while the healthy volunteers do not use their potential in any way, and may only be burdened by possible undesirable effects of the drugs. An exception may be the patients with depression who were tested either at the very beginning of the treatment when the effect of antidepressants had not yet been developed or, on the contrary, after the treatment in cases when satisfactory reaction to such treatment had not been reached and the original symptomatology persists. In patients reacting to the antidepressive treatment, the final result of the effect on the cognition will always be a balanced relation between the beneficial effect of the drug and concurrent undesirable effects.

The sedative, psychomotor and cognitively deteriorating impact of antidepressants, especially caused by the anticholinergic effects, is manifested within minutes or hours after the drug administration. However, this means that particularly in case of the TCA or antidepressants of the second generation, their adverse effect on cognition is manifested long before commencement of their own therapeutic effect, which starts approximately two to three weeks after the beginning of the therapy. This is important information, especially for those patients who depend on outpatient care. This problem may be, to a certain extent, attenuated by postponement of the administration of antidepressants to night hours or division of the total therapeutical dose to several partial doses. When amitriptyline dosed 75 mg in divided/night dose (Seppala et al., 1984; Lader et al., 1986; Allen et al., 1988; Robbe and O'Hanlon, 1995), clomipramine dosed 50 mg three times daily (Allen et al., 1991), or dothiepin dosed 150 mg at night (Ramaekers et al., 1995) were administered, the acute undesirable effects on cognitive performance were attenuated similarly to the increase of tolerance in healthy volunteers.

Several times, it was shown that the cognitive deficit in depression is improved with the remission of depressive symptomatology (Peselow et al., 1991). In patients who had responded to antidepressive treatments, the memory functions have been normalized to the level of healthy volunteers within a four-week interval after the remission (Peselow et al., 1991). On the other hand, the cognitive performance of non-responders remained even after the treatment beyond the level of both healthy volunteers and patients who benefited from the treatment. Since the depression itself is connected with cognitive deficit, it may seemingly be incomprehensible to treat depression with drugs whose acute administration may further deepen the cognitive deficit. This could be significant, especially in the event of antidepressants whose possible undesirable effect on the cognition in healthy volunteers, caused by a single administration, would persist even after repeated administration, and possibly after commencement of the antidepressive effect itself. Although it is well known that especially the sedative effect of the TCA shows a tendency to tolerance in the event of continuous administration, this may not apply to all domains of cognitive functions or to all sedative antidepressants (Curran et al., 1988).

The Effect on Cognition after Repeated Administration of an Antidepressant to Healthy Volunteers

A series of studies during which an antidepressant of the SSRI group was administered to healthy volunteers did not show any negative impact on the cognition. More specifically, the following antidepressants were tested: citalopram 40 mg daily (Lader et al., 1986), fluvoxamine 100 mg daily (Curran et al., 1986), paroxetine 20 mg daily and 30 mg daily (Deijen et al., 1989; Kerr et al., 1992) and sertraline 200 mg daily (Hindmarch et al., 1990). Unlike the SSRI, dothiepin dosed 75 mg daily significantly disrupted the concentration on visual inputs in comparison to placebo after 17 days of administration (Stille and Herberg, 1989). The same drug, administered at night, dosed 75 to 150 mg, impaired the CFF performance after 22 days of administration (Ramaekers, Muntjewereff and O'Hanlon, 1995). Also, clomipramine impaired the performance in the Digit Symbol Substitution Test (DSST) in comparison to a placebo after ten days of administration (Allen et al., 1991). Similar results, confirming the disruption of cognitive functions, were also reported for amitriptyline, imipramine, mianserin and trazodone, which belong to antidepressants of the first and second generations (Volz and Sturm, 1995; van Laar et al., 1995; Ramaekers et al., 1992; O'Hanlon et al., 1998). Although tolerance may, but also may not, solve the deteriorating effect on the cognition in case of a single administration of an antidepressant, the same mechanism may attenuate potential impacts on the cognition, even in case of a long-term administration of antidepressants to healthy volunteers. Therefore, the results shown on the generation of healthy volunteers may be generalised only with extreme caution to the population of patients suffering from the depressive disorder.

In addition to the development of tolerance, in the event of long-term administration of antidepressants, it remains unknown whether the possible undesirable effect of antidepressants on the cognition is manifested or highlighted after days or weeks of administration. This problem was solved in the study of van Laar (van Laar et al., 1995). One of the following substances was administered to twenty volunteers for the period of one week: nefazodone (100/200 mg daily), imipramine (50 mg daily) and placebo, dosed twice daily. The cognitive performance aimed at memory and psychomotor rate, including ability to drive, was assessed after the morning doses on the first and on the last (i.e., the seventh) day of the experiment. Imipramine disrupted the memory and abilities to drive as early as on the first day. On the seventh day, imipramine continued to impair the memory; however, the disruption of the ability to drive was alleviated and compared to the assessment on the first day, it did not reach the statistical significance. On the other hand, nefazodone disrupted the ability to drive both on the first and seventh day of the experiment. The nefazodone impact on cognitive functions was more important in both testing events than that of imipramine. In view of the fact that nefazodone does not show any sedative effect, there must be another reason explaining the deteriorating effect of nefazodone on the cognition. Nefazodone and its active metabolite interact both agonistically and antagonistically with a series of serotonin receptors; and nefazodone, in addition, slightly blocks the presynaptic serotonin carrier. Although there is no clear evidence that just the influence of the serotonin system by means of serotonin receptors is the reason why nefazodone significantly disrupts cognitive functions, this fact is considered very likely.

The repeated administration of fluoxetine to healthy volunteers has brought equivocal results in the area of influence of cognitive functions. Both acute and subchronic effect of dothiepin (75 to 100 mg daily) and fluoxetine (20 mg daily) on cognitive functions was compared with placebo in the double-blind, crossed study on 18 healthy volunteers (Ramaekers et al., 1995). The drugs were administered for the period of 22 days in the form of a night dose. The dothiepin effect on cognitive functions was as expected; the attention was disrupted on day one and the CFF threshold on day 22. The effect of fluoxetine was very similar to that of dothiepin. The administration of fluoxetine led to the disruption of attention and CFF threshold, and therefore statistically, this parameter differed significantly from that of placebo on day 22. Both monitored parameters of cognition have linearly impaired during the period of the fluoxetine administration. A similar result to that of fluoxetine was also seen in case of venlafaxine. In the double-blind, crossed study, venlafaxine, mianserin or a placebo was administered to healthy volunteers for the period of 15 days (O'Hanlon et al., 1998). Venlafaxine, similarly to fluoxetine and unlike mianserin, did not significantly disrupt the ability to drive. As far as the attention is concerned, venlafaxine, unlike mianserin, disrupted the attention only slightly after the initial dose; however, after two weeks of administration, the significant disruption of attention was proven. The effect of mianserin was an inverse one. The initial administration of mianserin led to the significant disruption of attention; however, in case of a long-term administration, the attention has slowly adjusted. The volunteers also subjectively assessed the influence of venlafaxine on their attention as worse than that of the placebo.

Sertraline dosed daily 100/200 mg administered to healthy volunteers for a period of nine days, did not lead to any disruption of cognitive functions or psychomotor rate (Hindmarch, 1990). On the other hand, it has turned out that the long-term administration of paroxetine leads to the disruption of the cognitive functions (Robbe and O'Hanlon, 1995). The impact of paroxetine (20 and 40 mg daily) and amitriptyline (75 mg daily) on cognitive functions was compared with placebo in the double-blind, crossed study. The neuropsychological examination was administered on the first and on the last day of an eight-day experiment. Amitriptyline led to sleepiness and disruption of practically all tested domains of cognition on the first day; however, this negative effect virtually disappeared during the experiment. Paroxetine in its daily dose of 20 mg did not disrupt cognitive functions in any way. Paroxetine dosed 40 mg daily significantly disrupted the performance in the CTT, Divided Attention reaction time and reaction time on the Sternberg Test. The disruption of cognition was not as significant as in the event of amitriptyline, but it persisted during the whole period of the study. In addition, no tolerance to subjective sleepiness has been described in the event of paroxetine (40 mg daily) after eight days of administration. For the ability of driving, particularly important is the ability of quick attention transfer. This cognitive domain is especially important in the event of increased demands on the driver, e.g., in dense urban traffic (Parasuraman and Nestor, 1993). The disruption of such abilities is, in case of paroxetine, dependant on the dose; in healthy volunteers, already the daily dose of 40 mg significantly disrupts this ability, and, in addition, it persists for the minimum period of one week.

Similarly, also the study with volunteers aged over 60 who were administered 20 mg daily dose of paroxetine for the period of 13 days has shown that paroxetine statistically significantly disrupts, in comparison to the placebo, the reaction times in the Sternberg Test of scanning and retrieval from short-term memory and also on reaction time to matched stimuli in the Stroop test (Kerr et al., 1992). In another study, the effect of a week-long administration of sertraline and paroxetine to healthy volunteers on their cognitive functions was compared (Schmitt et al., 1999). Paroxetine, but not sertraline, have more disrupted the unaltered attention compared to placebo. In addition, paroxetine extended the reaction times; on the other hand, sertraline reduced them, and, therefore, the resulting difference was statistically significant. The disruption of cognitive functions by paroxetine was of similar extent as in the event of fluoxetine or venlafaxine. In addition to the fact that it did not significantly disrupt cognitive functions, sertraline has also improved the parameters of strategic recall of information from the semantic memory, which are cognitive domains considered as frontal executive functions. The administration of 40 mg citalopram for a period of eight days caused the disruption in DSST and free recall of information from memory in healthy volunteers (Lader et al., 1986).

The Impact on Cognition upon the Long-Term Administration of an Antidepressants to Patients Suffering from Depressive Disorders

Cognitive deficit is the symptom of depression, and it recedes with mood clarification during the treatment with antidepressants. During the treatment with antidepressants, any possible impact of antidepressants on the cognition is concealed by cognitive deficit of depression itself. In the patient who sufficiently responds to the administered antidepressant, the resulting effect on the cognition will be given by mutual coincidence of depression, potential short-term or long-term negative effect of the antidepressant on the cognition, and last but not least, also by own therapeutic effect of such antidepressant. A seven-week study on 66 elderly patients suffering from depression, who were treated either with fluoxetine dosed 20 mg daily, administered in the morning, or amitriptyline dosed 75 mg, administered in the evening, may serve as an example (Fairweather et al., 1993). Although the therapeutical efficacy of the assessed antidepressants was similar, they differed from each other in the ability to affect cognitive functions, which were tested every week using the CFF and CRT. The average CFF threshold was statistically significantly improving during the course of the fluoxetine treatment; however, such effect was not observed in the event of amitriptyline. The fluoxetine/amitriptyline treatment led to the improvement of the CRT parameters, while in the fluoxetine arm, the improvement was more noticeable; at the end of monitoring, a significant difference was found in the CRT performance between fluoxetine and amitriptyline in favour of fluoxetine. Sabbe examined cognitive performance in 22 patients suffering from depression; six of them demonstrated the psychotic symptoms. The patients were treated with fluoxetine dosed 20 mg daily for a period of six weeks. The identified cognitive performance of the patients was subsequently compared with cognitive performance of 22 healthy volunteers of similar age and education. During the course of treatment, the determined cognitive deficit in patients with depression was reduced; however, it did not completely disappear. After the end of the treatment, statistically significant differences between the cognitive performance in healthy volunteers and patients with depressive disorder still persisted. The authors ascribe the persisting cognitive deficit after the end of the antidepressive treatment to insufficient clinical response to fluoxetine and recommend examining cognitive functions only after real remission/recovery is reached. They also believe that any adjustment to cognitive deficit falls behind the clinical remission, the delay being in the order of weeks or even months (Sabbe et al., 1997).

The occurrence of cognitive deficit in the sense of delirium and memory/attention disorders was described in connection with both acute and long-term fluoxetine treatment (Mirow, 1991; Nicholson and Pascoe, 1988; Ramaekers et al., 1995; Singh et al., 1995; Bangs et al., 1994; Hoehn-Saric et al., 1990; Bradley and Kulik, 1993; Hoehn-Saric et al., 1991). As an example of the above mentioned, can serve the case report of a 60-year-old woman treated for recurrent depression by fluoxetine in 20 mg daily dose. During the period of her nine-month treatment, she repeatedly complained of problems with memory, impaired ability to remember and learn new things, sedation, anticholinergic signs or sleeping disorders. Laboratory, neurological and neuroimaging examinations did not reveal any abnormality that could explain the above-mentioned symptoms. After discontinuation of the fluoxetine treatment, the patient subjectively relished the improvement of memory and attention. For prophylaxis of other possible depressive episodes, the patient started the treatment with nortriptyline. Roughly three weeks after discontinuation of her fluoxetine treatment, the patient underwent a complex neuropsychological examination that showed significant improvement of all parameters of cognition that had been defective during the fluoxetine treatment. The next neuropsychological examination after another three months did not reveal any deficit in cognitive functions. It is important to stress that upon the fluoxetine discontinuation, the patient was in a long-term remission; the improvement of cognitive functions may not be ascribed to the nortriptyline impact, but only to discontinuation of the fluoxetine administration (Mirow, 1991). A similar case was described in the event of a 60-year-old woman treated with fluvoxamine (300 mg daily) for obsessive-compulsive disorder (Tourjman and Fontaine, 1992).

Fluoxetine (20-60 mg daily) and paroxetine (20-40 mg daily) showed comparable efficacy and tolerance in a six-week, double-blind study on 106 patients with involutive depression (Shone and Ludwig, 1993). The cognitive functions were assessed by means of an 18-item Sandoz Clinical Assessment Geriatric Scale (SCAG), which is the scale generated for the assessment of cognitive performance of geriatric patients and allowing to distinguish between depression and dementia, using the test of Minimental State Examination (MMSE), which is the scale used for screening examination of dementia. Unfortunately, the selected scales are not optimal for the assessment of the cognitive deficit in depression. SCAG is not able to quantify the cognitive performance, and MMSE only covers the gross disruption of cognition, which is not present in the depression. This is the reason why the results of this study practically cannot be generalized and compared with other studies. Fluoxetine and paroxetine led to the improvement of cognitive functions, the improvement being more distinct in the paroxetine arm. This may be ascribed to a faster onset of paroxetine effect compared to fluoxetine. Nevertheless, at the end of the study, there was no statistically significant difference in the level of cognition between the patients treated with fluoxetine and those treated with paroxetine.

From the viewpoint of methodology, the two studies with sertraline, which compared it with fluoxetine and nortriptyline, were more genuine. As far as the clinical efficacy is concerned, there was no significant difference between the compared antidepressants. However, compared to fluoxetine and nortriptyline, sertraline significantly better influenced cognitive functions. Both studies were carefully prepared from the methodological point of view, no patients with significant cognitive deficit were included, and the cognitive deficit was assessed by validated neuropsychological tests (McEnttee et al., 1996).

Sertraline was also compared with nortriptyline in a 12-week, double-blind study including 210 elderly patients with involutive depression. The cognitive performance, measured by means of DSST, has statistically significantly improved during the sertraline treatment; on the contrary, in patients treated with nortriptyline, it was impaired. At the end of the study, cognitive deficit in patients treated with nortriptyline was statistically significantly worse than in patients treated with sertraline (McEntee et al., 1996). The fact that nortriptyline impairs cognitive deficit in older patients had already been described in another study, in which the nortriptyline treatment led to impairment of the short-term memory (Young et al., 1991).

The studies, which only use MMSE for the assessment of cognitive deficit in the depressive disorder, are controversial from the viewpoint of methodology. The MMSE is a screening scale developed for the detection of dementia, and therefore, it is not suitable for identification of small cognitive deficits that are characteristic of depression (Nadler et al., 1993). The study in which the MMSE was not able to distinguish between cognitive performances of two equally aged groups of geriatric patients with involutive depression with early or late onset may serve as an example. The detailed neuropsychological examination revealed that patients with the late-life-onset depression suffer from considerably worse memory, verbal fluency and executive functions (Salloway et al., 1996).

The studies have repeatedly shown that sertraline leads to the significant improvement of cognitive functions assessed by means of DSST (the Digit Symbol Substitution Test) scores. The improvement appears after two to four weeks of treatment and persists up to the end of monitoring. The DSST assesses a series of the cognitive processes, e.g., unaltered attention, short-tem memory or psychomotor rate. These cognitive domains are conditioned especially by neuronal activity of cortex, which is modulated by neuronal subcortical projections. There exists a hypothesis that sertraline does not affect directly cognitive functions but rather facilitates neuronal arousal from subcortex to cerebral cortex. It seems that this function is specific only for sertraline. Why it does not appear in connection with other SSRI remains a mystery. In the event of TCA, the explanation is simpler: these substances block the subcortical cholinergic system and thus inhibit neuronal paths from subcortex to cerebral cortex. The cholinergic system is the function of memory and this is the reason why TCA impairs the memory functions (McEntee et al., 1996). On the other hand, SSRI, specifically sertraline and fluoxetine, improve the memory both in animals and in men. Fluvoxamine has proved useful for attenuation of amnesic symptoms within the Korsak's syndrome in patients suffering from alcohol addiction. The explanation of a positive impact of SSRI on memory is seen in facilitation of the respective neuronal circuits, absence of the anticholinergic effects, and, last but not least, also in specific influence on serotonin receptors.

Out of new antidepressants, the most extensively studied was the affect of milnacipran (antidepressant of the fourth generation) on the level of cognitive functions in depression. It has been proved that a 100 mg daily dose does not affect the quality of cognitive functions in healthy volunteers. After the administration of milnacipran, an increased extracellular release of dopamine in prefrontal cortex was reported, which, according to many authors, may be a sign of potential positive impact on cognition in patients with depression. Milnacipran has proved to be effective in the reduction of cognitive dysfunction in patients with organic depression resulting from vascular cerebral event (Sato et al., 2006). Navrátilová has shown that both milnacipran and antidepressants of the SSRI group are effective in affecting cognitive deficit in the depressive disorder, however, only on condition they are also efficient in affecting the clinical symptomatology of depression. Attenuation of cognitive deficit occurred in responders, while in non-responders, it remained virtually unaltered. It was interesting that cognitive functions were adjusted with a certain delay following the clinical remission of depression. On the basis of her own results, the author assumes that for the reduction of cognitive deficit in the depressive disorder, the type of antidepressant is not so much important as is particularly its efficacy on core symptoms of depression (Navrátilová, 2007).

Similarly to milnacipran, bupropion has also improved cognitive deficit in patients with depression. The authors believe that positive pro-cognitive effect of bupropion is linked to the facilitation of the brain dopaminergic system (Gualtieri et al., 2007).

Summary

The cognitive deficit represents an important dimension of the depressive disorder. It is expected from new, modern antidepressants that in addition to a sufficient effect on the basic depressive symptoms, they will also show a positive impact on cognitive functions. Any impairment of cognitive deficit in the depressive disorder during the course of treatment is connected either with insufficient clinical efficacy or concomitant undesirable effects of the respective antidepressant. The undesirable effects are caused especially by antagonism to muscarine/histamine receptors. This applies primarily to older antidepressants, drugs of the TCA group. Newer antidepressants, drugs of the third and fourth generation, are already free of such undesirable effects, and therefore, they should also be free of the negative impact on cognitive functions. In some antidepressants, especially in drugs of the fourth generation, the positive effect on cognitive deficit has been manifested. This is probably due to their pharmacodynamic profile and particularly their impact on noradrenergic and dopaminergic neurotransmitter system of the brain. However, the drug's own efficacy on the basic depression symptoms seems to be a very important fact. It follows from a number of studies that if the antidepressive treatment leads to the sufficient therapeutic response, then the reduction of cognitive deficit occurs, although with a certain time interval after the clinical response. Therefore, the selection of such antidepressants seems to be desirable for the clinical practice, which will be free of undesirable effects on some receptors (muscarine/histamine ones) and which will be efficient enough for treatment of the depressive disorder.

Keywords: *antidepressants, cognition, deficit, performance, SSRI, TCA, milnacipran, bupropion.*

This chapter was supported by the research program of the Ministry of Education of the Czech Republic MSM0021622404.

References

Allen D, Lader M, Curran HV. A comparative study of the interactions of alcohol with amitriptyline, fluoxetine and placebo in normal subjects. *Prog. Neuropsychopahracol. Biol. Psychiatry* 1988;12:63-80.

Allen D, Lader M, Curran HV. The effects of repeated doses of clomipramine and alprazolam on physiological, performance and cognitive functions in normal subjects. *Eur. J. Clin. Pharmacol.* 1991;40:355-62.

Amado-Boccara I, Gougolis N, Poirier Littre MF, Galinowski A, Loo H. Effects of antidepressants on cognitive functions. Review of the literature. *Encéphale* 1994;20:65-77.

Bangs ME, Petti TA, janus M-D. Fluoxetine-induced memory impairment in an adolescent. *Journal of the American Academy of Child and Adolescent Psychiatry* 1994;33:1303-1306.

Bradley SJ, Kulik L. Fluoxetine and memory impairment. *Journal of the American Academy of Child and Adolescent Psychiatry* 1993;32:1078-1079.

Branconnier RJ, Cole JO. Effects of acute administration of trazodone and amitriptyline on cognition, cardiovascular function and salivation in the normal geriatric subjects. *J. Clin. Psychopharmacol.* 1981;1:82S-88S.

Curran HV, Lader M. The psychopharmacological effects of repeated doses of fluvoxamine, mianserin and placebo in healthy human subjects. *Eur. J. Clin. Pharmacol.* 1986;29:601-607.

Curran HV, Sakulsripong M, Lader, M. Antidepressants and human memory: an investigation of four drugs with different sedative and anticholinergic profiles. *Psychopharmacol.* 1988;95:520-7.

Deijen JB, Loriaux SM, Orlebeke JF, de Vrues J. Effects of paroxetine and maprotiline on mood, perceptual motor skills and eye movements in healthy volunteers. *J. Psychopharmacol.* 1989;3:149-55.

Fairweather DB, Kerr JS, Harrison DA, Moon CA, Hindmarch I. A double-blind comparison of the effects of fluoxetine and amitriptyline on cognitive function in elderly depressed patients. *Hum. Psychopharmacol.* 1993;8:41-7.

Freeman HL, O'Hanlon JF. Acute and sub-acute effects of antidepressants on performance. *J. Drug. Dev. Clin. Pract.* 1995;7:7-20.

Gualtieri CT, Johnson LG. Bupropion normalizes cognitive performance in patients with depression. *Med. Gen. Med.* 2007;9:1-22.

Hindmarch I, Harrison C. The effects of paroxetine and other antidepressants in combination with alcohol on psychomotor activity related to car driving. *Hum. Psychopharmacol.* 1988;3:13-20.

Hindmarch I, Barwell F, Alford C. Behavioural toxicity of antidepressants. In: Antidepressants: 30 years on 1990. CNS Publishers, London, 404-409.

Hoehn-Saric R, Lipsey JR, McLeod DR. Apathy and indifference in patients on fluvoxamine and fluoxetine. *J. Clin. Psychopharmacology* 1990;10:343-5.

Hoehn-Saric R, Harris GJ, Pearlson GD, Cox CS, Machlin SR, Camargo EE. A fluoxetine-induced frontal lobe syndrome in an obsessive-compulsive patient. *J. Clin. Psychiatry* 1991;52:131-133.

Kerr JS, Sherwood N, Hindmarch I. The comparative psychopharmacology of 5-HT reuptake inhibitors. Hum Psychopharmacology: *Clin. and Exper.* 1991;6:313-7.

Kerr JS, Fairweather DB, Mahendren R, Hindmarch I. The effects of paroxetine, alone and in combination with alcohol on psychomotor performance and cognitive function in the elderly. *Int .Clin. Psychopharmacol.* 1992;7:101-8.

Lader M, Melhuis A, Freka G, Fredricson Overo K, Christensen V. The effects of citaloprame in single and repeated doses and with alcohol on physiological and psychological measures in healthy subjects. *Eur .J. Clin. Pharmacol.* 1986;31:183-90.

Lane MR, O'Hanlon JF. Cognitive and psychomotor effects of antidepressants with emphasis on selective serotonin reuptake inhibitors and the depressed elderly patient. German *Journal of Psychiatry* 1999;2:1-28.

Látalová K, Pidrman V. Antidepresiva s duálním působením—účinnost a indikace. *Klin. Farmakol. Farm.* 2004;18:218-222.

McEntte W, Ko G, Richter E. Sertraline and nortriptyline: heart rate, cognitive improvement and quality of life in the depressed elderly. *Eur. Neuropsychopharmacol.* 1996;6:36.

Mirow S. Cognitive dysfunction associated with fluoxetine. *Am J Psychiatry* 1991;148:948-9.

Nadler JD, Richardson ED, Malloy PF. The ability of the dementia rating scale to predict everyday functioning. *Arch. Clin. Neuropsychol.* 1993;8:449-460.

Navrátilová P, Češková E, Přikryl R, Kučerová H. Profil a dynamika kognitivního výkonu při léčbě antidepresivy. *Čes a slov. Psychiatr* .2007;4:168-174.

Nicholson AN, Pascoe PA. Studies on the odulation of the sleep-wakefulness continuum in man by fluoxetine, a 5-HT uptake inhibitor. *Neuropharmacol.* 1988;27:597-602.

O'Hanlon JF, Freeman HL. Categorizing the behavioural toxicities of antidepressants. *Br. J. Psychiatry* 1995;166:421-3.

O'Hanlon JF, Robbe HWJ, Vermeeren A, van Leeuwen C, Danjou PE. Venlafaxine effects on healthy volunteers during 15-day fixed (75mg/day) and incremental (75-150mg/day) dosing regiments. *J. Clin. Psychopharmacol.* 1998;18:212-221.

Parasuraman R, Nestor P. Attention and driving assessment in elderly individuals with dementia. *Clin. Geriatr. Med.* 1993;9:377-87.

Peselow ED, Corwin J, Fieve RR et al. Disappearance of memory deficits in outpatient depressives responding to imipramine. *J. Aff. Disord* .1991;21:173-83.

Ramaekers JG, Swijgman HF, O'Hanlon JF. Effects of moclobemide and mianserin on highway driving, psychometric performance and subjective parameters, relative to placebo. *Psychopharmacol.* 1992;106:62-67.

Ramaekers JG, Muntjeweroff ND, O'Hanlon JF. A comparative study of acute and subchronic effects of dothiepin, fluoxetine and placebo on psychomotor and actual driving performance. *Br. J. Clin. Psychopharmacol.* 1995;39:397-404.

Riedel WJ, van Praag HM. Avoiding and managing anticholinergic effects of antidepressants. *Drugs* 1995;3:245-59.

Robbe HWJ, O'Hanlon JF. Acute and subchronic effects of paroxetine 20 and 40 mg on actual driving, psychomotor performance and subjective assessments in healthy volunteers. *Eur. Neuropsychopharmacol.* 1995;5:35-42.

Rudorfer MV, Manji HK, Potter WZ. Comparative tolerability profiles of the newer versus older antidepressants. *Drug. Safety* 1994;10:18-46.

Sabbe B, van Hoof J, Hulstijn W, Zitman F. Depressive retardation and treatment with fluoxetine: assessment of the motor component. *Journal of Affective Disorders* 1997;43:53-61.

Sato S, Yamakawa Y, Terashima Y, Ohta H, Asada T. Efficacy of milnacipran on cognitive dysfunction with post-stroke depression: Preliminary open-label study. *Psychiatry and Clinical Neurosciences* 2006;60:584-589.

Sakulsripong M, Curran HV, Lader M. Amitriptyline versus trazodone. *Eur. J. Pharmacol.* 1991;40:43-8.

Salloway S, Malloy P, Kohn R, Gillard E, Duffy J, Rogg J, Tung G, Richardson E, Thomas C, Westlake R. MRI and neuropsychological differences in early- and late-life onset geriatric depression. *Neurology* 1996;46:1567-1574.

Seppala T, Stromberg C, Bergman J. Effects of zimelidine, mianserine and amitriptyline on psychomotor skills and their interaction with ethanol: a placebo controlled cross-over study. *Eur. J. Pharmacol.* 1984;27:181-9.

Sherwood N. Comparative behaviour toxicity of the selective serotonin reuptake inhibitors. *Hum. Psychopharmacol.* 1995;10:159-162.

Shone W, Ludwig M. A double-blind study of paroxetine compared with fluoxetine in geriatric patients with major depression. *J. Clin. Psychopharmacol.* 1993;3:34-39.

Schmitt J, Kruizinga M, Teunisse S, Riedel WJ. SSRIs effects on vigilance and cognition: A placebo-controlled comparison of sertraline and paroxetine. Poster presented 39th Annual Meeting New Clinical Drug Evaluation Unit, Boca Raton, Florida, June 1-4, 1999.

Schwarz JC, Arrang JM, Gartburg M, Pollard H, Ruat M. Histaminergic transmission in the mammalian brain. *Physiological Reviews* 1991;71:2-51.

Singh RK, Gupta AK, Singh B. Acute organic brain syndrome after fluoxetine treatment. *Am. J. Psychiatry* 1995;152:295-6.

Spring B, Gelenberg AJ, Gardin R, Thompson S. Amitriptyline, fluvoxamine and cognitive function: a placebo-controlled comparison in depressed out-patients. *Psychopharmacology* 1992;108:327-332.

Tourjman S, Fontaine R. Fluvoxamine can induce confusion in the elderly. *J. Clin. Psychopharmacol.* 1992;12:203.

van Laar M, van Willigenburg APP, Volkerts ER. Acute and subchronic effects of nefazodone and imipramine on highway driving, cognitive functions and daytime sleepiness in healthy adult and elderly subjects. *J Clin Psychopharmacol* 1995;15:30-40.

Volz HP, Sturm Y. Antidepressant drugs and psychomotor performance. *Neuropsychobiology* 1995;31:146-55.

Weinstein A, Wilson S, Bailey J, Nutt D. Sedative antidepressants impair visual detection mechanism in humans. *Psychopharmacol.* 1996;10:141-145.

Wesnes K, Nand R, Lorscheid T. Potential of moclobemide to improve cerebral insufficiency identified using a scoppolamine model of aging and dementia. *Acta Psychiatr. Scand.* 1990:82:71-2.

Young RC, mattis S, Alexopoulos GS, Meyers BS, Shindledecer R, Dahr AK. Verbal memory and plasma drug concentrations in elderly depressives treated with nortriptyline. *Psychopharmacology Bulletin* 1991;27:291-294.

In: Cognitive Deficit in Mental and Neurological Disorders ISBN: 978-1-60741-957-0
Editors: H. Kucerova, M. Preiss

Chapter VI

Pharmacological Management of Cognitive Deficit in Schizophrenia

Pavel Mohr

1.1. Schizophrenia and Cognition

The subject of cognitive dysfunction in schizophrenia patients is discussed at large in other sections of the book; this chapter reviews both currently available and experimental options of pharmacological treatment. It has been postulated that a cognitive deficit represents the core impairment of schizophrenia with considerable negative impact on the course and functional outcome of the illness (Sharma a Harvey, 2000; Harvey et al., 2004). The deficit, presumably generalized, thus interferes with basic everyday functioning, including integration into the community, ability to cope with social problems, or acquisition of psychosocial skills. Effective remediation of a cognitive dysfunction is one of the unmet needs in the complex schizophrenia treatment. The schematic relationship between real (functional) outcome and various therapeutic interventions is depicted in the Figure 1.1 (adapted from Green and Nuechterlein, 1999). The scheme illustrates the fact that psychotic symptoms have little impact on outcome, which largely depends on cognitive performance and can be affected by pharmacotherapy mostly indirectly.

In addition to the rehabilitation and remediation strategies, much attention has been paid to procognitive effects of the drugs commonly used in treatment of schizophrenia (conventional and atypical antipsychotics), in primary cognitive disorders such as Alzheimer's Dementia (cognitive enhancers), or other agents modifying hypothesized etiopathogenetic mechanisms of cognitive impairment (reviews in: Harvey, 2009; Galletly, 2009). For example, an initiative of the U.S. National Institute of Mental Health, MATRICS (Measurement and Treatment Research to Improve Cognition in Schizophrenia; Marder and Fenton, 2004) represents a comprehensive program that supports development of pharmacological agents to improve cognitive deficit in schizophrenia.

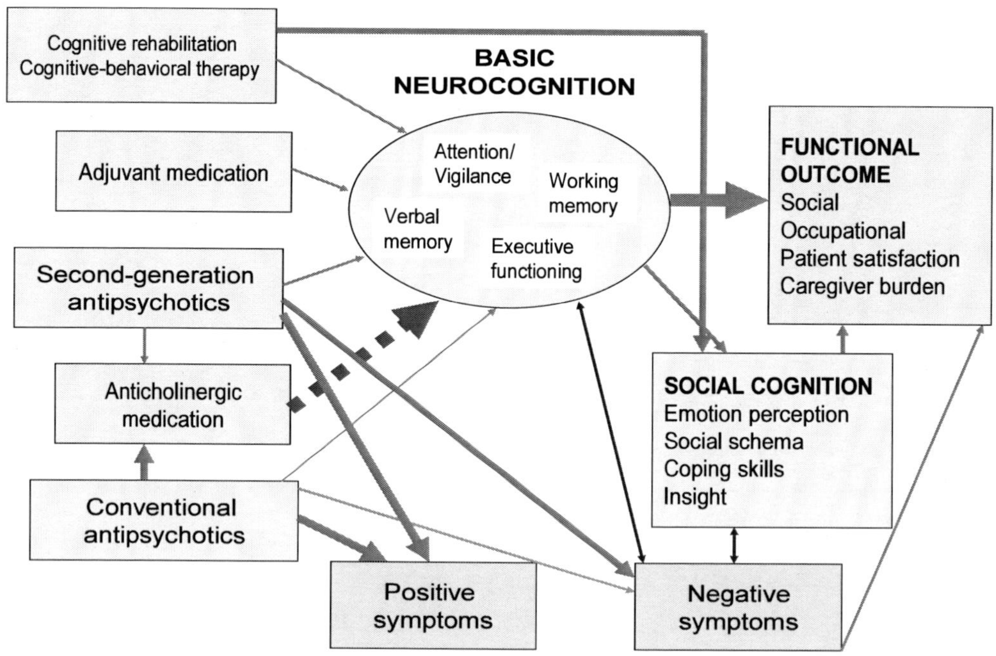

Figure 1.1. The relationship between treatment, symptoms, cognitive functions, and functional outcome (adapted from Green and Nuechterlein, 1999).

1.2. Antipsychotics

Introduction of antipsychotic drugs (synonymously labeled as neuroleptics) into the treatment of schizophrenia in the 1950s became a major therapeutic breakthrough. Antipsychotics effectively control symptoms of illness and are essential in relapse prevention. Furthermore, their administration results in shortening episodes of illness, reduces the number of hospital inpatients and improves overall the patient's quality of life.

1.2.1. Conventional (Typical) Antipsychotics

The group of first neuroleptics, now called conventional or typical antipsychotics (e.g., chlorpromazine, haloperidol, perphenazine, etc.) is characterized by nonselective blockade of dopamine D_2 receptors, reliable control of positive psychotic symptoms (delusions, hallucinations, behavioral disturbances, etc.) and a high incidence of side effects. The most troublesome are neurological and endocrine adverse events: extrapyramidal symptoms (EPS; parkinsonism), dystonia, dyskinesia, akathisia, hyperprolactinaemia and others. Conventional antipsychotics are typically considered to be less effective in the treatment of negative symptoms (emotional and social withdrawal, flat affect, etc.) and are associated with a high number of residual states and treatment resistance.

The generally held view has been that conventional antipsychotics are also somewhat less potent in alleviation from a cognitive deficit or that their effects are at least questionable

(Blyler and Gold, 2000). Additional cognitive impairment can be caused by adjuvant anticholinergic medication prescribed for control of antipsychotic-induced EPS. However, some earlier and more recent reports challenged this assumption and suggested that typical antipsychotics could display procognitive effects. Green and collaborators (2002), in a two-year, double-blind trial, compared cognitive functions of 62 schizophrenia patients treated with low dose of a typical antipsychotic haloperidol or an atypical antipsychotic risperidone. The results showed that both drugs improved cognitive functions to the same degree. No difference was detected in the score clusters or in the global score of neurocognitive test battery. Similarly, Keefe et al. (2004) found comparable effects of an atypical antipsychotic olanzapine and low-dose haloperidol given to 167 first-episode psychosis patients. Olanzapine and haloperidol reduced the cognitive deficit according to the composite score consisting of verbal fluency measures, motor functions, working memory, verbal memory, and vigilance. Olanzapine showed marginal superiority just in weighted composite score. Nonetheless, in the long-term follow-up of the study sample, the difference between the typical and atypical antipsychotic was completely lost; after two years, haloperidol was just as effective as olanzapine (Keefe et al., 2006a). Mishara and Goldberg (2004) published a meta-analysis of placebo-controlled studies comparing cognitive effects of typical antipsychotics with those of atypical drugs and/or a placebo in schizophrenia. The results confirmed mild-to-moderate gains in cognitive performance with conventional medications. The greatest improvement was achieved in automatic and perceptual processing, then attention, language, tests of general intellect, and memory. Only mild changes were observed in executive and oculomotor functions and, as expected, there was deterioration in motor functions. The authors failed to find a relationship between antipsychotic dose and cognitive change. The procognitive effect of haloperidol confirmed another meta-analysis by Woodward and collaborators (2007). Haloperidol improved cognition in both low- and high-dose regimes (below and above 10 mg, respectively). The deleterious effect on cognitive functions was observed only in extremely high doses, above 24 mg. The analysis showed that the improvement could not be attributed to the practice effect. Cognitive enhancement with low-dose haloperidol treatment, identical to that seen with risperidone or olanzapine, was found in other recent controlled trials, as well (Harvey et al., 2005; Keefe et al., 2006b). The latest piece of evidence represent the analyses of neurocognitive data from two large prospective randomized studies, CATIE (Clinical Antipsychotics Trials of Intervention Effectiveness) and EUFEST (The European First Episode Schizophrenia Trial). In CATIE, the improvement of cognition after 2 and 18 months treatment with a typical antipsychotic perphenazine was equivalent and in some respects even greater than the change after administration of olanzapine, risperidone, quetiapine, or ziprasidone (Keefe et al., 2007). Similar results yielded EUFEST; all drugs showed moderately positive effect on cognition in first episode-patients, with no difference between a typical comparator haloperidol and amisulpride, olanzapine, quetiapine, or ziprasidone (Davidson et al., 2009).

Despite the above-cited positive indications, the utilization of conventional antipsychotics in the clinical management of a cognitive deficit should be viewed with caution. The major impediments are the risk of serious adverse events plus the existence of a viable therapeutic alternative, atypical natipsychotics.

1.2.2. Second-Generation Antipsychotics (Atypical)

Novel, second-generation antipsychotics (e.g., clozapine, olanzapine, risperidone, quetiapine, ziprasidone, zotepine, amisulpride, aripiprazole) is a heterogeneous groups with respect to chemical structure or pharmacological profile. Their common denominator is a distinction from the typical antipsychotics: reliable efficacy not just on positive but also negative and affective symptoms and lower incidence of serious adverse events, especially EPS. Virtually all atypical antipsychotics have been also tested for their efficacy on cognitive functions in schizophrenia. Positive effects on cognition were first demonstrated in separate studies with every drug of this class and subsequently confirmed by meta-analyses and reviews (Keefe et al., 1999; Woodward et al., 2005). The hypothesized mechanism of action of antipsychotics on cognitive functions is an increased release of dopamine in the prefrontal cortex (PFC). The release may be stimulated directly or indirectly through blockade of the serotonin 5-HT_2 receptors in the ventral tegmental area that have inhibiting effects on the dopamine projection into the PFC. The blockade of serotonin inhibition may subsequently result in increased activity of the dopamine D_1 receptors.

Some of the authors speculated about selectively different effects of individual antipsychotics on specific cognitive functions, or superiority of one drug over the other. However, the current evidence does not support such assumptions, and the direct head-to-head drug comparisons suggest their comparable efficacy (Keefe et al., 2007; Davidson et al., 2009).

One of the most important factors affecting the assessment of drug effects on cognition are the methodological issues (Harvey and Keefe, 2001; Harvey, 2009). It is necessary to take into consideration lingering effects of previous drug treatments, including adjuvant medications (anticholinergic, anxiolytic, hypnotic), dosing schedules of the experimental and control substances. New treatment can be given in too-low doses and conversely, control drugs are often prescribed in disproportionate high doses that make any comparison unfair. Objective evaluation requires a controlled, randomized, double-blind study with parallel design and of sufficient duration in order to be able reliably differentiate early and late treatment effects. Selection of study subjects and sample size play also important role, as well as the careful choice of the neuropsychological test battery, its composition, features, number of tests, time to administer, interpretation of results, etc. Investigators have to take into account the practice effect in repeated testing, especially over shorter time intervals. For example, Goldberg with collaborators (2007) in a recent study showed that although a sixteen-week administration of either olanzapine or risperidone significantly improved cognitive performance, identical improvement as measured by effect size was observed in healthy, non-medicated volunteers. The results clearly indicate that practice effect considerably interferes with the interpretation of effects of cognitive training. Finally, true improvement of cognitive deficit should be separated from other cognitive changes, such as improvement of negative symptoms.

1.3. Pharmacological Interventions on Specific Neurotransmitter Systems

1.3.1. Dopamine

There is a general agreement that dopamine activity in the prefrontal cortex, mediated by D_1 receptors, plays a key role in cognition (Goldman-Rakic et al., 2004). In addition to the above described effects of atypical antipsychotics, cognitive performance in schizophrenia has been improved following administration of D_1 agonists and worsened with D_1 blocking agents. Catechol-O-methyltransferase (COMT) is an enzyme deactivating dopamine in the cortex and high activity of COMT has a deleterious effect on cognitive performance. COMT inhibitors, e.g., tolcapone, thus may be hypothetically used as cognitive enhancers (Harvey, 2009). Currently, there is only limited experimental experience with some indirect D_1 agonists (amphetamine, bromocriptine, pergolide, dihydrexidine, SKF-38393). The administration of full dopamine agonists, such as amphetamines, to schizophrenia patients is associated with a significant risk of exacerbation of psychosis. Moreover, first results indicate that stimulation of dopaminergic neurotransmission is dose-limited: low doses improve cognition while higher doses may on the contrary lead to cognitive impairments.

1.3.2. Serotonin

The interaction of serotonin (5-HT) receptors with the dopaminergic system mediating procognitive effects of atypical antipsychotics has been already discussed. Available cognitive research data suggest that the most promising pharmacological approach is to selectively target individual 5-HT receptor groups: 5-HT_{1a} partial agonism, 5-HT_{2a} antagonism, 5-HT_4 partial agonism, or 5-HT_6 antagonism (Roth et al., 2004). In a small controlled trial of 30 schizophrenia patients, adjuvant therapy with 5-$HT_{2a/2c}$ antagonist mianserin, an antidepressant, outperformed a placebo on memory/learning tests (Poyurovsky et al., 2003). Another antidepressant mirtazapine, an indirect 5-HT_{1a} agonist and 5-HT_2 and 5-HT_3 antagonist, also demonstrated procognitive effects in a placebo-controlled study of 37 patients treated with antipsychotics (Stenberg et al., 2009). Positive results of the 5-HT_{1a} receptor stimulation as add-on therapy in schizophrenia were confirmed in several clinical trials from Japan, where two selective 5-HT_{1a} agonists, buspirone and tandospiron, significantly improved attention and verbal memory and executive functions, respectively (Sumiyoshi et al., 2008).

1.3.3. Norepinephrine

Norepinephrine activity plays an important role in cognition, too (Arnsten, 2004). The main noradrenergic nucleus, locus coeruleus, projects into the prefrontal cortex and is simultaneously activated by new stimuli. Locus coeruleus then subsequently attenuates distracting perceptions and enables the focus of attention on the activities necessary to complete the task. $Alpha_{2a}$ selective agonists (guanfacine, clonidine) improve cognitive performance (working memory), while $alpha_1$ agonists have deleterious effects. Complex memory modulation is also mediated via beta adrenergic receptors: their activation enhances consolidation of declarative memory, whereas beta blockers (propranolol) ameliorate cognitive flexibility, problem-solving, and executive functions. Promising procognitive effects were observed in selective norepinephrine reuptake inhibitors, such as atomoxetine, a stimulant that increases norepinephrine levels in the PFC.

1.3.4. Acetylcholine

The relationship between impaired cholinergic neurotransmission and cognitive dysfunction has been well documented in primary cognitive disorders, e.g., Alzheimer's Dementia. There is also evidence suggesting a role of acetylcholine in schizophrenia (Friedman, 2004). Therefore, acetylcholinesterase inhibitors (ACEI), drugs widely used for treatment of Alzheimer's Dementia, have been tested in remediation of cognitive deficit in schizophrenia. The most studied agent is donepezil as adjuvant therapy. However, the controlled trials unanimously failed to detect a significant amelioration of cognitive functions (Friedman et al., 2002; Tugal et al., 2004; Pérez et al., 2006; Keefe et al., 2008). Similarly, negative findings yielded studies with another ACEI, rivastigmine. On the other hand, mostly positive results were found in add-on studies with galantamine, e.g., better performance in attention tasks and verbal memory in small case series (Bora et al., 2005), or improvement of processing speed and verbal memory (Buchanan et al., 2008). Alternative treatment strategy is to target the nicotinic and muscarinic receptors directly. Although administration of nicotine indeed enhances some areas of cognitive functioning in schizophrenia patients, it carries serious health risks. A more viable approach thus may be a stimulation of the muscarinic receptors (Friedman, 2004), for example with M_1/M_4 agonist xanomeline.

1.3.5. Glutamate

Impaired glutamatergic neurotransmission in schizophrenia has been associated with negative and cognitive symptoms, in particular memory and learning deficits (Coyle and Tsai, 2004). This assumption has been supported by the results of several studies investigating effects of add-on therapy with N-methyl-D-aspartate (NMDA) receptor agonists, especially d-serine, cycloserine, and glycine on negative symptoms with subsequent improvement of a cognitive deficit. Another pharmacological technique is the enhancement of glutamate alpha-amino-3-hydroxy-5-methyl-4-isoxazolepropionic (AMPA) receptors involved in the modulation of long-term memory with the use of so called "ampakines," e.g., CX516 or farampator. Thus far, published clinical results are equivocal (Goff et al.,2008). Likewise adjuvant treatment with medications that regulate glutamatergic activity, such as lamotrigine, has so far produced inconclusive findings (Goff et al., 2007).

1.3.6. γ-aminobutyric acid (GABA)

$GABA_A$ receptors were identified as the regulators of cognitive and emotional processing. While $GABA_A$ agonists, e.g., benzodiazepines, have an adverse impact, more selective modulation of various receptor subtypes is expected to enhance cognitive performance cognition (Möhler, 2009). This assumption was supported by two small placebo-controlled studies of schizophrenia patients. $GABA_A$ antagonist flumazenil enhanced working memory, whereas agonist lorazepam impaired cognitive performance (Menzies et al., 2007). Furthermore, functional magnetic resonance imaging revealed corresponding changes in the brain activation. More nuanced and complex interplay between the GABA neurotransmission and cognition was suggested by the improvement of attention and working memory after 4-week administration of MK-0777, a selective agonist on the α2 and α3 $GABA_A$ receptor subunits (Lewis et al., 2008).

1.3.7. Other Pharmacological Interventions

Among other experimental strategies for cognitive remediation, administration of stimulants may be considered. Nevertheless, due to the risk of deterioration or exacerbation of primary psychotic symptoms, their utilization in the clinical practice is limited. In addition to the above-mentioned atomoxetine, another stimulant, modafinil, a drug that unlikely other stimulants do not affect catecholamine system, has been tested in the treatment of a cognitive deficit with mixed results. A critical review of the data available from six small trials, five controlled and one open-label study, stated that effects of modafinil on cognitive deficit in schizophrenia are still inconclusive (Saavedra-Velez et al., 2009). Improvement of short-term memory, attention, and the ability to shift mental sets was observed only in three studies. Modafinil was well tolerated, with a 6.0% risk of psychosis exacerbation (2.9% in the placebo groups).

Encouraging are the results from a controlled trial testing cognition in schizophrenia by modulation of immune reaction with adjuvant administration of celecoxib, cyclooxygenase 2 enzyme inhibitor (Müller et al., 2004). Though numerous studies suggested procognitive effects of non-saturated fatty acids in non-psychiatric population, the results of a single placebo-controlled trial of omega-3, ethyl eicosapentaenoic, acid, were disappointing (Fenton et al., 2001). Contradictory results yielded tests with other potential cognitive enhancers under investigation: neurosteroids, or selective phosphodiesterase inhibitors (Galletly, 2009).

1.4. Conclusion

An overview of the potential pharmacological interventions modulating specific neurotransmitter systems is summarized in the Table 1.1. Other experimental compounds modifying cognitive functions through alternative mechanism of action (e.g., modulation of immune response, gene expression, etc.) are in various phases of development and testing. The most widely accessible pharmacological option is the therapy with the second-generation antipsychotics. Atypical antipsychotics demonstrated improvement of cognitive functions in controlled trials and clinical practice. Their role in cognitive remediation is further stressed by the expert consensus (Harvey et al., 2004) or by the MATRICS' initiative. The utilization of conventional antipsychotics should be re-valuated and their positive effects with low-dose treatment acknowledged. Nevertheless, it must be said that, from a clinical perspective, the procognitive effects of the available drugs are not robust, so we have to keep looking for new therapeutic options or to combine pharmacological and non-pharmacological interventions.

1.5. Summary

Cognitive deficit represents the core impairment in schizophrenia that fundamentally affects course and functional outcome of illness. Thus far, generally held views claim that conventional antipsychotics are less effective in cognitive remediation; furthermore, cognition may be worsened by the adjuvant anticholinergic medication used to alleviate from side effects. However, several earlier and recent reports indicated that a low dosage of typical antipsychotics may possess procognitive properties. Unequivocally positive effects of virtually all second-generation antipsychotics in remediation of a cognitive deficit have been shown in both individual studies and meta-analyses. The key role in cognition is played by dopamine activity in the prefrontal cortex. Dopamine action is mediated through D_1 receptors, as evidenced by the improvement of cognitive performance following administration of D_1 agonists. Stimulation of dopamine neurotransmission is rate-limited: low doses enhance cognition whereas higher doses may cause cognitive impairments. Dopamine activity can be also modulated indirectly, via serotonin receptor system, either with 5-HT_{1a} agonists or 5-HT_2 antagonists.

Table 1.1. Potential therapeutic options in remediation of cognitive deficit with pharmacological interventions on specific neurotransmitter systems

Intervention goal	Effective drugs
Increase of dopamine in the prefrontal cortex	Second-generation antipsychotics D_1 receptor agonists 5-HT_{1a} receptor agonists 5-HT_2 receptor antagonists
Enhancement of noradrenergic neurotransmission in the prefrontal cortex	Selective alpha $_2$ receptor agonists Selective norepinephrine reuptake inhibitors Stimulants
Enhancement of cortical cholinergic activity	Muscarinic M_1/M_4 and nicotinic receptors agonists Acetylcholinesterase inhibitors?
Enhancement of glutamate neurotransmission	NMDA receptor agonists AMPA receptor agonists Glutamate activity regulators
Regulation of GABA-ergic activity	$GABA_A$ receptor modulators

1.6. Key Words (Glossary)

Antipsychotics

Drugs used to treat psychotic symptoms, their common mechanism of action is the blockade of dopamine D_2 receptors. They are classified into two groups: conventional (typical) and second-generation (atypical) antipsychotics.

Neurotransmitters

Chemicals that, through their affinity to the receptors at the binding sites, mediate transmission of neural signals between the neurons on synapses.

Dopamine

A neurotransmitter that is essential in the control of movement, motivation, and pleasure. Dopamine action in the prefrontal cortex plays a key role in cognitive functions. Dopamine hyperactivity evokes psychotic symptoms and its blockade during antipsychotic treatment may lead to movement and endocrine side effects.

Norepinephrine (Noradrenaline)

A neurotransmitter that plays a role in the regulation of attention, impulsiveness and partially of cognition and emotionality. In addition to the CNS, it acts in the sympathetic nervous system; it is one of the stress hormones.

Serotonin

A neurotransmitter, primarily involved in the regulation of emotionality, anxiety, and impulsivity.

Acetylcholine

An excitatory neurotransmitter that mostly regulates cognitive and motor functions. Besides the CNS, it acts in the parasympathetic nervous system.

Glutamate

The main excitatory neurotransmitter, it modulates cognitive functions, learning and memory. Glutamate deficit is associated with negative symptoms.

γ-aminobutyric acid (GABA)

The main inhibitory neurotransmitter in the CNS. GABA regulates neuronal excitability and is directly responsible for the regulation of muscle tone.

Agonist

A compound that enhances signal transmission through its affinity to the receptor.

Antagonist

A compound that attenuates or blocks signal transmission through its affinity to the receptor.

References

Arnsten, A. F.: Adrenergic targets for the treatment of cognitive deficits in schizophrenia. *Psychopharmacology* 2004; 174: 25–31.

Bilder, R. M.; Goldman, R. S.; Volavka, J.; Czobor, P.; Hoptman, M.; Sheitman, B.; Lindenmayer, J. P.; Citrome, L.; McEvoy, J.; Kunz, M.; Chakos, M.; Cooper, T. B.; Horowitz, T. L.; Lieberman, J. A.: Neurocognitive effects of clozapine, olanzapine, risperidone, and haloperidol in patients with chronic schizophrenia or schizoaffective disorder. *Am. J. Psychiatry* 2002, 159: 1018–1028.

Bora E., Veznedaroglu B., Kayahan B.: The effect of galantamine added to clozapine on cognition of five patients with schizophrenia. *Clin. Neuropharmacol.* 2005; 28:139-141.

Blyler, C. R.; Gold, J. M.: Cognitive effects of typical antipsychotic treatment: another look. In: Sharma, T.; Harvey, P. eds.: Cognition in Schizophrenia. New York, Oxford University Press 2000; 241–265.

Buchanan, R.W.; Conley, R.R.; Dickinson, D.; Ball, M.P.; Feldman, S.; Gold, J.M.; McMahon, R.P.: Galantamine for the treatment of cognitive impairments in people with schizophrenia. *Am. J. Psychiatry* 2008, 165: 82-89.

Coyle, J. T.; Tsai, G.: The NMDA receptor glycine modulatory site: a therapeutic target for improving cognition and reducing negative symptoms in schizophrenia. *Psychopharmacology* 2004, 174: 32–38.

Davidson, M.; Galderisi, S.; Weiser, M.; Werbeloff, N.; Fleischhacker, W.W.; Keefe, R.S.; Boter, H.; Keet, I.P.; Prelipceanu, D.; Rybakowski, J.K.; Libiger, J.; Hummer, M.; Dollfus, S.; López-Ibor, J.J.; Hranov, L.G.; Gaebel, W.; Peuskens, J.; Lindefors, N.; Riecher-Rössler, A.; Kahn, R.S.: Cognitive effects of antipsychotic drugs in first-episode schizophrenia and schizophreniform disorder: a randomized, open-label clinical trial (EUFEST). *Am. J. Psychiatry* 2009, 166: 675-682.

Fenton, W. S.; Dickerson, F.; Boronow, J.; Hibbeln, J. R.; Knable, M.: A placebo-controlled trial of omega-3 fatty acid (ethyl eicosapentaenoic acid) supplementation for residual symptoms and cognitive impairment in schizophrenia. *Am. J. Psychiatry* 2001, 158: 2071–2074.

Friedman, J. I.; Adler, D. N.; Howanitz, Harvey P. D.; Brenner, G.; Temporini, H.; White, L.; Parrella, Davis, K. L.: A double-blind placebo controlled trial of donepezil adjunctive treatment to risperidone for the cognitive impairment of schizophrenia. *Biol. Psychiatry* 2002, 51: 349–357.

Friedman, J. I.: Cholinergic targets for cognitive enhancement in: schizophrenia: focus on cholinesterase inhibitors and muscarinic agonists. *Psychopharmacology* 2004, 174: 45–53.

Galletly, C.: Recent advances in treating cognitive impairment in schizophrenia. *Psychopharmacology* 2009, 202: 259-273.

Goff, D.C.; Keefe, R.; Citrome, L.; Davy, K.; Krystal, J.H.; Large, C.; Thompson, T.R.; Volavka, J.; Webster, E.L.: Lamotrigine as add-on therapy in schizophrenia: results of 2 placebo-controlled trials. *J. Clin. Psychopharmacol.* 2007, 27: 582-589.

Goff, D.C.; Lamberti, J.S.; Leon, A.C.; Green, M.F.; Miller, A.L.; Patel, J.; Manschreck, T.; Freudenreich, O.; Johnson, S.A.: A placebo-controlled add-on trial of the Ampakine, CX516, for cognitive deficits in schizophrenia. *Neuropsychopharmacology* 2008, 33: 465-472.

Goldberg, T.E.; Goldman, R.S.; Burdick, K.E.; Malhotra, A.K.; Lencz, T.; Patel, R.C.; Woerner, M.G.; Schooler, N.R.; Kane, J.M.; Robinson, D.G.: Cognitive improvement after treatment with second-generation antipsychotic medications in first-episode schizophrenia: is it a practice effect? *Arch. Gen. Psychiatry* 2007, 64: 1115-1122.

Goldman-Rakic, P. S.; Castner, S. A.; Svensson, T. H.; Siever, L. J.; Williams, G. V.: Targeting the dopamine D1 receptor in schizophrenia: insights for cognitive dysfunction. *Psychopharmacology* 2004, 174: 3–16.

Green, M. F.; Nuechterlein, K. H.: Should schizophrenia be treated as a neurocognitive disorder? *Schizophr. Bull.* 1999, 25: 309–318.

Green, M. F.; Marder, S. R.; Glynn, S. M.; McGurk, S. R.; Wirshing, W. C.; Wirshing, D. A.; Liberman, R. P.; Mintz, J.: The neurocognitive effects of low-dose haloperidol: a two-year comparison with risperidone. *Biol. Psychiatry* 2002, 51: 972–978.

Harvey, P. D.; Keefe, R. S.: Studies of cognitive change in patients with schizophrenia following novel antipsychotic treatment. *Am. J. Psychiatry* 2001, 158: 176–184.

Harvey, P. D.; Green, M. F.; Keefe, R. S.; Velligan, D. I.: Cognitive functioning in schizophrenia: a consensus statement on its role in the definition and evaluation of effective treatments for the illness. *J. Clin. Psychiatry* 2004, 65: 361–372.

Harvey, P.D.; Rabinowitz, J.; Eerdekens, M.; Davidson, M.: Treatment of cognitive impairment in early psychosis: a comparison of risperidone and haloperidol in a large long-term trial. *Am. J. Psychiatry* 2005, 162: 1888-1895.

Harvey, P.D.: Pharmacological cognitive enhancement in schizophrenia. *Neuropsychol. Rev.* 2009, 19:324-335.

Keefe, R. S.; Silva, S. G.; Perkins, D. O.; Lieberman, J. A.: The effects of atypical antipsychotic drugs on neurocognitive impairment in schizophrenia: a review and meta-analysis. *Schizophr. Bull.* 1999, 25: 201–222.

Keefe, R. S. Seidman, L. J.; Christensen, B. K.; Hamer, R. M.; Sharma, T.; Sitskoorn, M. M.; Lewine, R. R.; Yurgelun-Todd, D. A.; Gur, R. C.; Tohen, M.; Tollefson, G. D.; Sanger, T. M.; Lieberman, J. A.: Comparative effect of atypical and conventional antipsychotic drugs on neurocognition in first-episode psychosis: a randomized, double-blind trial of olanzapine versus low doses of haloperidol. *Am. J. Psychiatry* 2004, 161: 985–995.

Keefe R.S.; Seidman L.J.; Christensen B.K.; Hamer R.M.; Sharma T.; Sitskoorn M.M.; Rock S.L.; Woolson S.; Tohen M.; Tollefson G.D.; Sanger T.M.; Lieberman J.A.; HGDH Research Group: Long-term neurocognitive effects of olanzapine or low-dose haloperidol in first-episode psychosis. *Biol. Psychiatry* 2006a, 59: 97-105.

Keefe, R.S.; Young, C.A.; Rock, S.L.; Purdon, S.E.; Gold, J.M.; Breier, A.; HGGN Study Group.: One-year double-blind study of the neurocognitive efficacy of olanzapine, risperidone, and haloperidol in schizophrenia. *Schizophr. Res.* 2006b, 81: 1-15.

Keefe, R.S.; Bilder, R.M.; Davis, S.M.; Harvey, P.D.; Palmer, B.W.; Gold, J.M.; Meltzer, H.Y.; Green, M.F.; Capuano, G.; Stroup, T.S.; McEvoy, J.P.; Swartz, M.S.; Rosenheck, R.A.; Perkins, D.O.; Davis, C.E.; Hsiao, J.K.; Lieberman, J.A.; CATIE Investigators; Neurocognitive Working Group.: Neurocognitive effects of antipsychotic medications in patients with chronic schizophrenia in the CATIE Trial. *Arch. Gen. Psychiatry* 2007, 64: 633-647.

Keefe, R.S.; Malhotra, A.K.; Meltzer, H.Y.; Kane, J.M.; Buchanan, R.W.; Murthy, A.; Sovel, M.; Li, C.; Goldman, R.: Efficacy and safety of donepezil in patients with schizophrenia or schizoaffective disorder: significant placebo/practice effects in a 12-week, randomized, double-blind, placebo-controlled trial. *Neuropsychopharmacology* 2008, 33: 1217-1228.

Lewis, D.A.; Cho, R.Y.; Carter, C.S.; Eklund, K.; Forster, S.; Kelly, M.A.; Montrose, D.: Subunit-selective modulation of GABA type A receptor neurotransmission and cognition in schizophrenia. *Am. J. Psychiatry.* 2008, 165: 1585-1593.

Marder, S. R.; Fenton, W.: Measurement and Treatment Research to Improve Cognition in Schizophrenia: NIMH MATRICS initiative to support the development of agents for improving cognition in schizophrenia. *Schizophr. Res.* 2004, 72: 5–9.

Menzies, L.; Ooi, C.; Kamath, S.; Suckling, J.; McKenna, P.; Fletcher, P.; Bullmore, E.; Stephenson, C.: Effects of gamma-aminobutyric acid-modulating drugs on working memory and brain function in patients with schizophrenia. *Arch. Gen. Psychiatry.* 2007, 64: 156-167.

Mishara, A. L.; Goldberg, T. E.: A meta-analysis and critical review of the effects of conventional neuroleptic treatment on cognition in schizophrenia: opening a closed book. *Biol. Psychiatry* 2004, 55: 1013–1022.

Möhler, H.: Role of $GABA_A$ receptors in cognition. *Biochem. Soc. Trans.* 2009, 37 (Pt 6): 1328-1333.

Müller, N.; Ulmschneider, M.; Scheppach, C.; Schwarz, M. J.; Ackenheil, M.; Moller, H. J.; Gruber, R.; Riedel, M.: COX-2 inhibition as a treatment approach in schizophrenia: immunological considerations and clinical effects of celecoxib add-on therapy. *Eur. Arch. Psychiatry Clin. Neurosci.* 2004, 254: 14–22.

Pérez, M.; Tuma, I; Pytela, O.; Kadlecova, E.; Zemanova, M.; Lenderova, Z.: Acetylcholinesterase inhibitor donepezil in the treatment of cognitive deficit in schizophrenia. Subanalysis of the active branch from Czech extended double-blind study. *Eur. Psychiatry* 2006, 21: 548-550.

Poyurovsky, M.; Koren, D.; Gonopolsky, I.; Schneidman, M.; Fuchs, C.; Weizman, A.; Weizman, R.: Effect of the 5-HT2 antagonist mianserin on cognitive dysfunction in chronic schizophrenia patients: an add-on, double-blind placebo-controlled study. *Eur. Neuropsychopharmacol.* 2003, 13: 123-128.

Roth, B. L.; Hanizavareh, S. M.; Blum, A. E.: Serotonin receptors represent highly favorable molecular targets for cognitive enhancement in schizophrenia and other disorders. *Psychopharmacology* 2004, 174: 17–24.

Saavedra-Velez, C.; Yusim, A.; Anbarasan, D.; Lindenmayer, J.P.: Modafinil as an adjunctive treatment of sedation, negative symptoms, and cognition in schizophrenia: a critical review. *J. Clin. Psychiatry.* 2009, 70: 104-112.

Sharma, T.; Harvey, P. eds.: Cognition in Schizophrenia. New York, Oxford University Press, 2000, 363.

Stenberg, J.H.; Terevnikov, V.; Joffe, M.; Tiihonen, J.; Tchoukhine, E.; Burkin, M.; Joffe, G.: Effects of add-on mirtazapine on neurocognition in schizophrenia: a double-blind, randomized, placebo-controlled study. *Int. J. Neuropsychopharmacol.* 2009, 27: 1-9.

Sumiyoshi, T.; Bubenikova-Valesova, V.; Horacek, J.; Bert, B.: Serotonin$_{1A}$ receptors in the pathophysiology of schizophrenia: development of novel cognition-enhancing therapeutics. *Adv. Ther.* 2008, 25: 1037-1056.

Tugal, O.; Yazici, K. M.; Yacolu, A. E.: A double-blind, placebo controlled, cross-over trial of adjunctive donepezil for cognitive impairment in schizophrenia. *Int. J. Neuropsychopharmacol.* 2004, 7: 117–123.

Woodward N.D., Purdon S.E., Meltzer H.Y., Zald D.H.: A meta-analysis of neuropsychological change to clozapine, olanzapine, quetiapine, and risperidone in schizophrenia. *Int. J. Neuropsychopharmacol.* 2005; 8:457-742.

Woodward N.D., Purdon S.E., Meltzer H.Y., Zald D.H.: A meta-analysis of cognitive change with haloperidol in clinical trials of atypical antipsychotics: dose effects and comparison to practice effects. *Schizophr. Res.* 2007, 89: 211-224.

Supported by the research project CNS 1M0517.

In: Cognitive Deficit in Mental and Neurological Disorders ISBN: 978-1-60741-957-0
Editors: H. Kucerova, M. Preiss

Chapter VII

Non-Psychopharmacological Cognitive Interventions for Neuropsychiatric Disorders

Mabel Rodriguez, Mirka Mirka Benešová and Radka Čermaková

I. Introduction

Training of cognitive functions has become so popular recently that the British newspaper *The Guardian* is offering aides for the improvement of basic cognitive abilities via their online interactive brain training games, including memory and processing speed (www.lumosity.com/guardian). As these and other training methods become more popular, the training of cognitive functions continues to be developed in both a scientific and professional framework.

Cognitive deficits related to neuropsychiatric disorders have been studied, accepted, described, and treated since early last century. One cannot claim that every neuropsychiatric patient suffers from a deficit of cognitive functions, but a considerable number of these patients do suffer deficits of varying degrees; a notable percentage of them are living with permanent disabilities. The social and financial impact, as they relate to severity and duration of such cognitive deficits, then becomes significant for both health and social care institutions throughout the world. People with neuropsychiatric disorders become isolated from their communities. This isolation, in turn, impacts patients and their families, cooperation with treatment, and the psychiatric state of the patient. Neuropsychiatric patients face stigmatization, not only in terms of society, but also a self-stigma with regard to the patient's perception of "self." Pharmacological treatment seems to influence cognition at least in part, and laboratories have shifted their attention to the development of new molecules that can improve cognition. Currently, however, there are no psychopharmacological treatments capable of restoring cognitive function to the patient's premorbid state, or even levels that can dramatically improve patient's cognition. Therefore, we are looking for non-psychopharmacological approaches to improve and enhance the effect of drugs on cognitive deficits.

Cognitive remediation[1] of neuropsychiatric disorders originated from the rehabilitation treatment of neurological disorders. It is difficult, however, to say exactly when cognitive rehabilitation as field began. One of the oldest documents related to brain dysfunctions treatmeant is the "Edwin Smith Papyrus" discovered in Luxor in 1862[2] (Helgason, 1987). More recently, there have been three key moments in the history of rehabilitation that should be mentioned. The first took place during the seventeenth century and involved Itard's work with the Averon child[3]. The second, considered to be the beginning of the modern era of rehabilitation, is connected with the following German, Russian, and British neurologists working with soldiers with brain damage during the first half of the twentieth century: Kurt Goldstein, Alexander Lurja, Richie Russell, Henry Head, and Henri Hecaen. Their work produced new knowledge of language disorders, perception, and memory, executive and social functions and introduced this knowledge to the field of rehabilitation. The aim of rehabilitation was not only helping the patient regain practical skills, i.e., walking, talking, reading, and writing, but also working with family and society in order to facilitate the patient's return to society and work. The third event, more related to neuropsychiatric remediation is the discovery that patients with schizophrenia could improve their cognitive performance during executive function testing, particularly through training with the Wisconsin card test (WCST). Patients with schizophrenia very often fail tests involving executive strategies because they often fail to develop adequate problem-solving strategies and are inflexible with regard to new solutions. Goldberg et al. (1987) reported that the training of patients with schizophrenia failed to improve their performance on the WCST. However, Delahunty et al. (1993) proved that these patients are able to improve their results after training on cognitive flexibility.

Since these three major events, there has been a substantial effort to develop new methods in the field of cognitive rehabilitation, remediation, and training (or however our esteemed colleagues choose to label their attempts to influence cognition) for neuropsychiatric disorders. Whether it's the simple training of functions, the search for compensatory strategies, paper-pencil or computer-training paradigms, or the more complex social training or training combined with some enhancer (e.g., repetitive transcranial magnetic stimulation rTMS), scientists and clinicians are searching their entire fields for non-psychopharmacological interventions in neuropsychiatry.

Remarkably, we are now able to measure improvement in remediation with clinically verified neuropsychological tests and functional brain imaging methods. Recently, however, a

---

[1] The term rehabilitation, in this text, refers to any process of therapy. The terms cognitive rehabilitation, remediation and cognitive training refer to specific interventions in order to improve cognition (not necessarily to restore functions back to normal).

[2] The surgical papyrus dated from the pyramid age 3,000-2500 BC was acquired by Edward Smith in 1862, and translated and published by James Henry Breasted in 1930. The document contains mention about the brain and meninges, functional localization in the brain and spine, and calvarial and cervical vertebral injuries in details of pathology, symptomatology, but also on treatment and prognosis and the medical ethic of its time (Helgason, 1987).

[3] In 1799, three French hikers found, in the forest, a boy around 11 years old. The boy was dirty, naked and with scars all over his body. The boy was transferred to Paris, where he was assessed as mentally retarded. Jean-Marc Gaspard Itard, a French physiologist who was delegated to take care of the boy, did not agree with the diagnosis. Itard claimed that the retardation was due the absence of interaction with people. In order to prove his hypothesis, Itard started to stimulate the boy using a holistic approach. The aim was to integrate the problems and needs of Victor, the name given to the boy. Itard summarized his objectives in five points: to wake up social interest, to improve stimulus processing, to expand the range of thought, to teach him how to speak and to teach him communication through symbols (images, words).

new issue has come up; ecological validity and the question of how to prove such training has had a positive impact on a patient's performance within the scope of their personal environment.

There are many additional questions being raised as well, e.g., when to start cognitive remediation; who benefits from these methods; how long do patients need to be trained, who is the best person to perform remediation, and what is the effect of "on-line" training?

It would seem that healthier patients could start training earlier. However, there are still unanswered questions regarding spontaneous improvement following a neuropsychiatric episode and the need to let the brain recover, at least in part, by itself. We are not yet sure which mechanisms are associated with improvement in these disorders. Additionally, with regard to the question "when to start," we need to establish which patients are best suited for which type of intervention. Based on extensive experience with cognitive enhancement therapy, it is clear that neuropsychiatric disorders require their own remediation approach.

This chapter considers previously mentioned and related topics in an effort to summarize ways to improve/enhance cognition with non-psychopharmacological interventions in four main categories of neuropsychiatric disorders: schizophrenia, depression, bipolar disorder, and obsessive-compulsive disorder (OCD). However, the bulk of this chapter relates primarily to schizophrenia, the neuropsychiatric disorder that has inspired a dramatic increase in the interest of cognitive disorders in the field of neuropsychiatry, and where the majority of cognitive rehabilitation efforts have been directed. A recently Meta-Analysis of cognitive remediation in schizophrenia showed improvement on cognitive performance, and when combined with psychiatric rehabilitation, also improves functional outcome (McGurk et al, 2007)

Hopefully, this chapter may bring more than just answers; it should also provoke new questions.

II. Rationale for Non-Psychopharmacological Cognitive Interventions

As a biopsychosocial entity, humans are permanently under the influence of three factors—biological, psychological, and social—the combination of which, both positively and negatively, influence human functioning, health, and quality of life. In people who suffer from neuropsychological diseases, these three factors collectively influence the start of their problems as well as the course of the illness and therapy. Therefore, when trying to affect cognitive deficits, we use this three-factor model and gradually present the biological, psychological, and social rationales.

II.1. Biological Rationales

The brain is a fascinating organ that undergoes both permanent and non-permanent changes. It is currently the most complex and dynamic structure known. It represents an almost perfect organ, finely tuned for the changes and evolutionary demands originating from the external and internal environment. The basis for this adaptation is "whole-life" neuronal plasticity which is the underlying principle for modern neuro-remediation. In addition to its use in molecular medicine, the development of neuroimaging methods, and the practical application in neuropsychiatry, has neuroplasticity played an important role in the theoretical principles of non-pharmacological interventions for cognitive deficit.

II.1.1. Neural Plasticity

Neural plasticity represents the specific ability of the nervous system to undergo regular development, to adapt to changes in both the internal and external environment with the aim of maintaining maximum functionality of the whole system. By means of learning, memory, perception, cognition and motor experience, the brain adapts to all varying conditions of the environment and, in the process, creates an incredible number of neural networks (Johansson, 2004). Due to neural plasticity, throughout its life, the brain is able to continually structurally and functionally adapt to new stimuli, reorganize neural pathways based on experience and also change in response to functional and organic damage (Wieloch, Nikolich, 2006). The potential of neuronal cells to build, reorganize, and repair cerebral tissue is fascinating. However, this ability is based especially on new learning experiences (Gage, 2002). A stimulus-rich environment and active mental activity plays a key role in this process. Gould et al. (1999) suggests that environmental complexity makes the process of learning easier and activates hippocampal functions. Tasks aimed at associative learning increase the hippocampal volume, support production of stem cells, survival of new neurons and their integration into existing circuits. A higher number of mutually related stimuli support cell and neural network reparation. However, active, long-term, intensive, and conscious activity is necessary to improve cognitive abilities (Johansson, 2004). Exposure to stimuli alone does not lead to desired results without practice of the specific cognitive functions and individual activity (Gage, 2002).

The neuroplastic process can run on various levels, and it can be seen over a broad time span, from milliseconds up to years (Trojan, Pokorný, 1999). Neuronal cells extend and amplify their sprouts, join together to form new synapses and are incorporated into existing systems. Previously formed neural circuits change their shape. Modern neuroscience confirms that new axons are generated from existing neurons and new synaptic connections formed, and it was more recently confirmed that new neurons are also produced. This is supported by multipotent neural stem cells and nerve growth factors that are preserved in the human brain, in lesser quantities, even into adulthood. They represent a potential source of new cells that can replace those cells that disappear because of injury or disease (Kulišťák, 2003; Johansson, 2004). Although the human brain has the greatest plasticity during youth, this ability has been found to remain preserved, to some degree, in adults and even the elderly. Learning, mental and physical activity, as well as a stimuli-rich environment, plays a key role in the success and extent of these processes (Huttenlocher, 2002; Kolb, Gibb, 1999; Nelson, 1999; Trojan, Pokorný, 1999). This knowledge creates rationales for modern cognitive rehabilitation that focuses on increasing the functional potential of the brain and cognitive functions.

I.1.2. Imaging Methods in Neuropsychiatry

A continual development of imaging methods that enable monitoring of the living brain in various stages and cognitive processes has helped the neurosciences to gradually and increasingly understand the complex relation between cognitive functions and neural structures of the brain. For example, the above-mentioned neural plasticity associated with learning and development is increasingly investigated using functional neuroimaging techniques such as positron emission tomography (PET) and functional magnetic resonance (fMR).

In recent years, diagnosis of brain injury has significantly improved due to the implementation of imaging and neurophysiological techniques. Currently, they represent an important part of clinical examination in neuropsychiatric disorders. Obsessive-compulsive disorder, depression, schizophrenia and other psychoses are currently considered to be neurodevelopmental diseases (Bradshaw, Sheppard, 2000; Angelucci et al., 2005; Singh et al., 2004). Imaging methods inform us about morphological changes in brain tissue and blood perfusion changes in various areas of the brain. They provide information regarding the location of possible deviations. Presently, there is an increasing trend to implement these methods as part of the verification process relative to the effect of rehabilitation of cognitive functions. For example, in an fMRI study, Wexler has confirmed an association between an improvement of working memory and the activation of frontal lobes in schizophrenia (Wexler et al., 2000); Penades et al. (2002) showed in an SPECT study, results of increased prefrontal blood flow after cognitive and social performance training.

I.2. Psychological Aspects

In the biopsychosocial model of neuropsychology, psychological aspects are those that can be measured and observed by behavior and that constitute a link between the biological and social aspects. Therefore, psychological aspects are those that we try to affect directly during remediation programs in order to have an impact on both—biological and social aspects. According to Lezak (1995), behavior and its disabilities can be divided into three functional systems: cognitive, emotional, and executive. The relationship among these systems and their respective components is so close that is difficult to differentiate the degree of influence of each one separately. However, we are, to some degree, able to measure, study, and influence components of these systems separately. Taking into account Lezak's division, and focused on the cognitive remediation for neuropsychiatric patients, we can also find rationales for each of the dimensions of behavior.

I.2.1. Cognition

The possibility to improve cognition is based on two fundamental assumptions: the theory of brain neuronal plasticity and the results of neuroimaging studies (mentioned previously). Therefore, we assume that effective stimulation may affect the ability to regain certain skills or influence compensation for lost abilities. It appears that not every component of cognitive function can be influenced identically. We distinguish these components of cognition by separating them into three main areas: receptive functions; memory and learning; thought and metacognition.

Receptive functions in neuropsychiatric disorders are often studied in the context of schizophrenic disorders. Schizophrenia is characterized by problems associated with information filtering. Deficits in receptive functions affect social functional outcomes (Cadenhead et al., 2000). Studies of prepulse inhibition (PPI) in humans show that schizophrenia patients, when compared with healthy subjects, activate different regions in the brain (Kumari et al., 2003). Despite the fact that animal studies using the PPI model have suggested that PPI deficits should be reversible through antipsychotic treatment as opposed to training (Geyer, Ellenbroek, 2003), these results do not apply to schizophrenia patients. While some improvement in PPI can be seen post-medication, improvement does not approach the level of normalization and is not present in all patients (Kumari, Ettinger, 2004). On the other hand, there are several cognitive rehabilitation procedures that offer evidence of improvement in neurological and neuropsychiatric disorders by using information processing as the basic model for rehabilitation (Bracy, 1986; Rodriguez et al., 2002)

It appears that *Learning and Memory* are affected in almost every neuropsychiatric disorder, although not always to the same extent or in the same way. There are three important aspects that play an important role in learning and especially in complex learning: first, the associative processes determined by repetition and enhancement; second, the processes of memory and thought; and third, the creation of cognitive maps. Additionally, the abilities of generalization, differentiation, and the creation of strategy are important factors in the process of learning (Atkinson et al., 1995). Therefore, Wykes and Reeder (2005) assert that various learning techniques must be combined in remedial therapy. Methods in which the patient is permitted to find suitable strategies in order to solve the problem seem to be effective in learning. By means of practicing within the patient's actual ability, we can provide help through tasks that are too difficult, while at the same time allowing the patient to use preserved abilities to solve the problem. In addition to gradual involvement, i.e., making tasks more difficult, Socratic dialogue can also be used to help facilitate problem-solving. Below, we also include the subject of metacognition, another area of significant importance in learning and relearning processes.

It appears as though, apart from attentional aspects, one of the main benefits of cognitive rehabilitation in patients with schizophrenia involves the domain of memory/learning. Patients with schizophrenia do not show the same pattern of deficit as those with brain injuries; therefore, remediation is able to provide more substantial benefits (Wykes, 2000). Also it seems that the pattern of training should work different. McGurk et al (2007) found that hours of training, use of drill and practice are related to improvements in verbal learning and memory. In our cognitive remediation computer program for patients with schizophrenia, we have found significant improvements in working memory (Rodriguez et al., 2004). These findings agree with other rehabilitation programs around the world (Hogarty et al., 2004). There is no evidence in the literature about the effect of targeted memory training on memory/learning functions in other neuropsychiatric disorders.

Thought and Metacognition—Metacognition is a person's general capacity to think about his or others' thinking. Recently, Lysaker et al. (2007) found a strong correlation between neurocognitive capacities such as working and visual memory, executive functions and metacognition in patients with schizophrenia. Moreover, metacognitive abilities have a great impact in social cognition (Hoekert et al., 2007). At the conference "Cognition and Schizophrenia: Improving real life function" held at the institute of psychiatry in London, Wykes pointed out that "improvements in cognition would only impact efficiency if the person uses metacognition to decide to use the improved cognitive functions" (Wykes 2006). Our Prague rehabilitation programs have also attempted to improve the efficacy of metacognition as one of the strategies for psychiatric rehabilitation (Rodriguez et al., 2004; Perglová, 2006; Benešová, 2007). Later in this chapter, we will evaluate metacognition as a method in cognitive rehabilitation.

I.2.2. Emotions

Deficits in processing of emotions may contribute to social isolation (Hoekert, 2007). People with both schizophrenia and depressive disorders have a tendency toward inappropriate processing of emotions, although in different ways. Patients with schizophrenia tend to produce emotions with reduced intensity in relation to unipolar depressive patients and normal controls. In contrast, patients with unipolar depressive disorders show more intensity than patients with schizophrenia and normal controls (Yecker et al., 1999). A meta-analytical study, by Hoekert et al. (2007), found a significant deficit in perception and expression of emotional prosody (emotional tone of voice—how something is said) in schizophrenia. Recent research has found that perception of facial emotions can be successfully trained in schizophrenia (Brenner et al., 1996; Wolwer et al., 2005; van der Gaag et al., 2002). Training of emotion processing must be a routine part of cognitive rehabilitation in neuropsychiatric disorders.

I.2.3. Executive Functions

Both emotions and executive functions have great influence on expression and treatment of cognitive deficits. Therefore, a severe impairment of executive functions will have an impact on functional outcomes (Palmer and Heaton, 2000). Moritz et al. (2002) found impaired executive control in patients with obsessive-compulsive disorder, unipolar depression, and schizophrenia, in comparison to normal health subjects. Improvement of performance on the Wisconsin card sorting test, in patients with schizophrenia who were provided with instructions on which strategy to choose for solving the test, was one of the milestones that caused a shift in interest from neurology to neuropsychiatry with regard to cognitive rehabilitation (Delahunty et al, 1993). Since then, several remediation programs for schizophrenic, and lastly for bipolar disorders have demonstrated improvements of both executive test measures after strategic-learning-based programs (Krabbendam and Aleman 2003; Rodriguez et al., 2004) and an improvement in functional outcomes (Wexler et al., 2005, Deckersbach et al., 2009).

We have given a brief overview of the psychological rationales of the three major areas of cognition, which deserve consideration for cognitive rehabilitation in neuropsychiatric disorders. Nevertheless, we need to keep in mind that these three major areas are also dependent to some degree on attention, consciousness, and motivation (Lezak, 2004). Educational literature stresses the importance of attention, consciousness, and motivation in learning; therefore, good cognitive remediation programs for neuropsychiatric disorders should also include these three aspects.

I.3. Social Rationales

With the progress of therapy in psychiatric diseases, and an improvement in the ability to affect symptoms of disease, greater attention to the patient's quality of life, his/her integration and independence have become important pillars. Rehabilitation that improves the quality of life of people with neuropsychiatric diseases becomes important once the acute psychotic or depressive condition is under control. Modern concepts of rehabilitation go beyond health-care and psychological treatment; it is included in the documentation and recommendations of international and national organizations (OSN, WHO, European Council, relative legislation of the Czech Republic). This issue involves the whole of society, with emphasis placed on the integration of handicapped persons, achievement of maximum independence, active participation in rehabilitation and availability of rehabilitation services as close as possible to the client's home (community-based rehabilitation; Švestková and Angerová, 2006).

Psychiatric disorders, residual symptoms and frequently associated cognitive deficits result in failure of the social aspects of patients' lives. Impairment of psychosocial function also persists in the remission phase. An association between single cognitive deficit domains and the level of social functions, e.g., the ability to solve interpersonal relationship problems, as well as the level of working assignment and self-functioning, has been repeatedly confirmed in patients with schizophrenia (Addington et al., 1998; Hofer et al., 2005; Laes and Sponheim, 2006). Problems with social functioning also appear in patients with other neuropsychiatric disorders. In a meta-analysis of studies that investigated long-term social functioning in patients following a depressive episode associated with bipolar disorder BAP, Kennedy et al. (2007) describe aspects of social impairment, including both residual symptoms and mild neurocognitive deficits. Neuropsychological development is a predictive marker of regaining social function in the same group of patients (Jaeger et al., 2007).

In psychiatric patients, we can observe failure in social relations both in close relations (marriage, parent-child, or friends) and in the broader social context (social isolation, meeting people outside the home). Patients also have difficulty meeting their socioeconomic needs.

The number of people in the Czech Republic on temporary disability due to a psychiatric indication is 0.8 to 1.6% (999 out of 100,000 insured people). The largest group of these is represented by people with neurotic disorders. However, patients with psychoses and affective disorders make up the group requiring the longest period of care. Psychiatric disease is a common reason patients are given invalid status. In 2001, 8.5% of all newly recognized disability pensions were due to psychiatric diseases, most often due to mental retardation and psychotic diseases. Only one out of seven people who receive a disability pension is able to return to daily work (Baudiš, 2006). In addition, mental disorders are the leading cause of disability in the U.S. and Canada in people aged 15 to 44. (http://www.nimh.nih.gov/health /publications/the-numbers-count-mental-disorders-in-America).

Young people with a psychotic disease must often interrupt their studies due to their illness. In addition to effective therapy for the underlying disease, they also require continual care, both in terms of cognitive rehabilitation and the training of educational and social skills needed to successfully finish their studies (e.g., The STUDENT program in the Czech Republic for young people following a psychotic onset; www.baobab.cz).

Other social aspects that particularly affect patients with psychotic diseases, as well as their relatives, include the development of independence and the handling of personal issues (care, hygiene, etc.).

It is clear from those studies that investigated the association among cognitive function, their possible deficits and the level of social functioning, that cognitive function, and especially executive function, generally appear to be good predictors. Employability, as well as the level of everyday functioning, i.e., money management, cooking, safety, compliance with medication, and social functioning, significantly correlate with cognitive functions in both the healthy population (Bell-McGinty et al., 2002) and in patients with neurodegenerative (Aronson and Vrooland, 1993; Nadler et al., 1993) and neuropsychiatric disease (McGurk and Meltzer, 2000).

People with psychosis are probably the most affected group among the psychiatric patient population. Patients trained for cognitive functions who are hospitalized with schizophrenia show improvement not only in single cognitive domains such as overall cognitive flexibility, verbal memory, verbal working memory (Rodriguez et al., 2004), but also, in social functioning, as has been recently shown (Wykes et al., 2007[a, b]). The question, regarding which cognitive dimensions are "responsible" for the individual aspects of social functioning, remains open.

During cognitive remediation, we assume that the change in cognitive deficits in psychiatric patients is possible, and we expect, at the same time, that these changes will be reflected in social behavior. One of the main assumptions of cognitive remediation is as follows: if we are able to facilitate a reduction in the cognitive deficit and its devastating effects on patients´ lives, we can improve social adaptation (i.e., more social contacts, work in protected workshops, education, higher quality of life, etc.).

II. Targets and Evidences

A summary of the main cognitive deficit domains in four selected neuropsychiatric diseases are presented in this part of the chapter (Tab. I). Additionally, we present a summary of the most common forms of therapy and possibilities for affecting cognitive deficit by means of cognitive remediation (Tab. II).

Clinical experience indicates that certain dynamics (see further) are generally typical for neuropsychiatric diseases, and it is similar with regard to cognitive deficits, which are related to these types of diseases. Frith (1995) found an association between the symptoms of a disease and the type of cognitive deficit. For example, positive symptoms (delusions, hallucinations) in schizophrenia are considered to be associated with predominant attention and self-monitoring disorders. On the other hand, predominant negative symptoms (volitional deficit, emotional flattening) are more often linked with increased rigidity and perseverations. Findings that support the idea that neurocognitive remediation may, to some extent, affect the symptoms of a disease were published. Bark et al. (2003) presented findings indicating that even short cognitive remediation in people who suffer from schizophrenia had some positive, though non-significant, influence on the patients´ psychopathology. On the other hand, as the first results with cognitive training in people with recurrent depressive disorder show, there was no affect on the extent of their depression while trying to improve cognitive functions. However, it significantly affected the quality of their cognitive performance (Elgamal et al., 2007). The above-stated findings support the hypothesis that there is only a partial dependence between cognitive deficit and actual psychopathology and provide further arguments for gradual extension of cognitive remediation in people with psychiatric diseases.

In acute phases, there is a tendency toward worsening cognitive performance, which is dependent on the symptoms of a disease (see episode of psychosis, mania, and decompensation of OCD).

Table I. The major domains of cognitive deficit

	Attention/ Processing speed	Memory	Visuospatial	Executive functions	Reasoning
Schizophrenia (Heinrichs, 2001)	X	X		X	X
Bipolar Disorder (Torres et al., 2007)	X	X		X	
Unipolar Depression Preiss, in press)	X			X	X
Obsessive-compulsive Disorder (Aouizerate et al, 2004)			X	X	

Table II—The most commonly used types of therapy and cognitive rehabilitation/remediation

	Therapy	Cognitive training/ Rehabilitation
Schizophrenia	Psychoeducation, occupational therapy, social skills training	Cognitive remediation (computer/ pencil-paper/combined; Penadés et al., 2006; Rodriguez et al., 2004; 2009; Wykes et al., 2007) Training of social skills (Cohen et al., 2005)
Bipolar Disorder	Cognitive-behavioral therapy, interpersonal therapy, psychoeducation, psychosocial therapy	Cognitive Rehabilitation for Bipolar Disorder: Deckersbach T, Nierenberg AA, Kessler R, Lund HG, Ametrano RM, Sachs G, Rauch SL, Dougherty D.: 2009
Unipolar Depression	Cognitive-behavioral therapy, interpersonal therapy	Computer-assisted cognitive remediation—early trials (Elgamal et al., 2007)
Obsessive-compulsive Disorder	Cognitive-behavioral therapy	Cognitive training aimed at organization strategies—experimental (Park et al., 2006; Buhlmann et al., 2006)

Nevertheless, cognitive deficits often persist after the acute symptoms disappear. Studies have shown that it especially concerns psychotic diseases. Moreover, cognitive deficit is considered to be a core symptom of schizophrenia (Heinrichs and Zakzanis, 1998). However, even in remission, cognitive deficits can be observed in patients who suffer from unipolar depression. A controlled study performed by Preiss et al. (2008) revealed the occurrence of cognitive deficits during remission of depressive symptoms. A persistent deficit of attention and executive was found.

Instability is typical for cognitive functioning in neuropsychiatric diseases. In contrast to cognitive deficits following brain injuries, which represent an area where cognitive rehabilitation is extensively used, psychiatry works with conditions in which the effects of pathological processes are still actively present and may continue to affect the possible results of remediation activities. This basic premise must be considered during attempts to affect cognitive deficit.

The following section of the chapter will focus on the questions that arise from our collective years of experience in training of cognitive functions in patients with schizophrenia and that are topical in the scientific literature as well. Due to the fact that most research studies have been performed in the schizophrenia population, answers to questions must necessarily be based on the available literature. Nevertheless, we can see that similar questions has started to appear with gradual development of cognitive remediation in other groups of psychiatric diseases.

How long will the effects of cognitive rehabilitation last? Studies show improvement of cognitive variables after both short (e.g., 10 sessions; Bark et al., 2003) and long (one year; Greig et al., 2007) periods of cognitive training. Fiszdon et al. (2004) compared performance of patients in a paradigm of work therapy and cognitive remediation versus performance of people undergoing work therapy alone. Patients who also underwent cognitive training showed more improvement, which was comparable to other studies (Rodriguez et al., 2004; Wykes et al. 2007). These patients had still maintained their progress, based on neuropsychological tests (e.g., digit span), six months after the rehabilitation program had concluded. Based on this, the authors reasoned that the effects of rehabilitation would persist even though they emphasized that these findings do not apply to all cognitive areas (Fiszdon et al., 2004). Other authors suggest that rehabilitation effects may last one year, whereas the main variable for the maintenance of this effect is considered to be an immediate improvement in the speed of processing and other attention/vigilance determinants during training (Hogarty et al., 2006). A limited amount of studies on the impact of amount of cognitive remediation on the maintenance of treatment effects point the need for further research.

What are the predictors of successful cognitive rehabilitation? Not all patients should benefit from training of cognitive functions. The level of premorbid intelligence and the extent of its deterioration at the beginning of training probably affect the ability to profit from training of cognitive functions, i.e., the ability to transfer learned skills to untrained tasks. Patients with the greatest degree of deterioration of intellectual abilities are those who, based on researchers, have the greatest problems using what they learned during neurocognitive remediation (Fiszdon et al., 2006). In addition to cognitive variables, such as good attention functions or short-term memory, motivation factors and good co-operation play an important role in successful remediation (see low scores of hostility in the PANSS scale in patients with normalized cognitive performance). On the other hand, variables related to the chronic nature of the disease, such as disease duration, number of hospitalizations, etc., appears to be insignificant (Fiszdon et al., 2005). Motivation, as an important factor for training benefit, has been confirmed by other authors in an extensive study aimed at possible predicative factors for cognitive remediation benefits. Motivation is measured from the regular attendance, and it appears that people with normalization of cognitive performance had more regular appointments compared to people who had no improvement. These authors also found that people with delayed onset of disease profited more often from remediation. It also appears that some training variables, such as intensity of training, are important in later effectiveness of the program. Training at higher intensities or with greater frequencies, usually results in the desired effect. The authors mention the role of the therapist or training assistant. The best improvement occurred in patients who were trained by therapists with postgraduate education (PhD level clinician; Medalia et al., 2005). Lastly meta-analysis found that in general, the number of hours of the program did not correlated with the improvement on coginition domains. Hours of training, as well as use of drill and practice were related just to improvement in verbal learning memory. (Mc Gurk et al. 2007)

Who, which patients, when, and at which phase of the disease, should rehabilitation start? Most of the studies that have investigated neurocognitive remediation include patients who had previously received long-term treatment for a psychotic disease, e.g., in one of the first studies performed, (Wykes et al., 2002) disease duration was more than 10 years in two-thirds of patients. This could suggest that remediation programs in clinical settings are mainly concentrating on patients with a chronic form of disease. There are new studies in which cognitive functions are successfully remediated in patients at the beginning of their disease as well (Wykes et al, 2007). Related to age, younger people benefit more than older in some cognitive domains, but in memory training both younger and older inidividuals benefit from training. Regarding symptomatology, it seems that cognitive remediation does not have effect in older people with negative predominant symptomatology (Wykes, 2009). The questions that remain open are as follows: to what extent do we perform remediation, and to which degree do we help the self-curative process at the onset of disease?

The topic for research and clinical practice is to determine which patients are suitable for cognitive remediation. In recent years, as with schizophrenia, remediation is expanding to other neuropsychiatric diseases, such as OCD, bipolar affective disorder, and unipolar depression. These first attempts will be discussed further.

Literature data shows that training of organizational strategies has a positive effect on performance, on the Rey figure test, in people with anxiety disorders, obsessive-compulsive disorder (OCD) in particular (Buhlmann et al., 2006). In another study, a longer, five-day training of planning and organizational activities affected both neurocognitive performance and disease symptoms (Park et al., 2006). These patients are generally motivated with regard to therapy, but we consider their primary anxiety, and low tolerance for frustration, to be a potentially disturbing variable for success of long-term programs, such as cognitive training.

Cognitive remediation is a very young procedure in patients with bipolar disorder; literature provides just few information of studies investigating remediation of cognitive deficits in people with bipolar affective disorder (Deckersbach et al. 2009). However, cognitive training is a suitable alternative to affect cognitive deficits associated with the disease (Burdick et al., 2007).

Cognitive remediation in patients with unipolar depression is also just beginning. The first successful study was presented by Elgamal et al. last year (2007). Twelve patients in the stabilized phase of major depression underwent a 10-day training of cognitive functions. After the training, patients showed improvement in a series of neuropsychological tests that measured attention, verbal learning, and memory, processing speed, and executive functions.

IV. Training Methods and Measurement of their Efficacy[4]

Cognitive remediation of neuropsychiatric diseases currently offers a relatively broad spectrum of interventions ranging from narrow-focused trainings to complex programs. They aim to improve cognitive functions or compensate for their deficits. Complex programs aspire toward improvement of social competence, support of adaptive functions, and influencing the environment itself. These basic programs, except for trainings such as "pencil and paper" exercises, which have been successfully used for decades, currently also include computer-based training software. This software usually contains various modules focused on the training of a single cognitive function or a combination and is a good aid for cognitive therapists.

At the beginning, it must be noted that the presented methods are used, and some of them designed mainly for patients with schizophrenia, and most of the studies were performed on these patients. Remediation of cognitive functions and effect of cognitive deficits in other neuropsychiatric diseases represent new challenges and await an opportunity.

IV.1. Cognitive Training—Differences in Approaches: Pencil-Paper versus Computer Software

The classical “pencil and paper” procedures, which may include various riddles, brain-teasers, cross-words puzzles, etc., may cover a broad spectrum from single to more complex tasks and can also be used during the training of cognitive functions in patients with neuropsychiatric diseases. Training can be focused on various areas of cognition, e.g., visual searching and scanning, memory and learning, numerical abilities, verbal comprehension and skills, judgment and logical problem-solving, and social skills (recognition of emotions from the pictures of human faces). The pencil-paper approach enables an accurate and flexible selection of tools, focus on the training of specific areas of cognition and intensive contact between therapist and patient. Various manipulation techniques, such as brain-teasers, visuospatial memory training tools, ranking of sequences of picture stories, jugglers, etc., are other possible tools (Benešová, 2007). In addition to these classical procedures for training cognitive functions using pencil-paper techniques, manipulation tasks and group games, computer software is an increasingly popular aid used in the remediation of cognitive functions (Rodriguez et al., 2002, 2004). Software, such as the American PSS CogReHab or

[4] During measurement of efficacy of intervention, the authors recommend performing the first measurement several weeks prior to the beginning of remediation (the number of previous weeks should correspond to duration of the training program), the second measurement before remediation and another measurement after termination of the program and the final several weeks after the end of rehabilitation (again dependant on duration of the program). This should ensure monitoring of the cognitive dynamics of the brain.

German neurorehabilitation and diagnostic program NEUROP-2, are commonly used in the Czech Republic. The PSS CogReHab (Bracy, 2007) is based on the theory of information processing and has been developed over the past 25 years. They contain eight modules with modified parameters and are comprised of a total of 64 tasks. Training gradually escalates from focusing attention, to visuospatial and memory tasks, to executive skills and situation solving. The advantages of Bracy's software are ease of use, comprehensibility, individual settings, laterality and flexibility training for each task and emphasis on client independence (results are displayed for each individual task; Kulišťák, 2002; Rodriguez et al., 2002). However, the disadvantages of this software are its exceptionally high price, as some organizations cannot afford it, and the limited possibility to adapt verbal tasks in languages other than English.[5] The software NEUROP-2 was developed by the Slovak psychologist Ladislav Gaál (2002), who works in Germany. It involves a diagnostic-rehabilitation program that is often used in neurologically affected patients. This software tool contains over forty modules with an inexhaustible amount of freely programmable trainings focused on various cognitive functions and their combinations. Each module is equipped with an ancillary file containing a description of the program, instructions for use and examples of how to create your own exercise for a given module. It enables creative and enjoyable multimedia training with or without a therapist. Its indisputable advantage compared to other globally recognized tools is its relatively low price and the potential to be used at home by the patient. There is also the ability to exchange homework between patient and therapist by e-mail. The disadvantage of this program is the occasional instability of the software itself. The program also needs to be more extensively (scientifically) tested in patients with neuropsychiatric disorders. A very challenge program seems to be the Computerised Interactive Remediation of Cognition – Training for Schizophrenia (CIRCUITS), developed inside the team of Till Wykes (Reeder, Wykes, 2008). The aim of the program is to goal a transfer of acquiered skills from abstract context through more real-life situations. Task are more ecologically valid, using as background a villague where the patient needs to carry out with every daylife activities (e.g. planning a meal, remembering a shopping list, etc.).

Working with the computer programs is possible as a separate method or in combination with the pencil-paper technique, manipulation techniques (brain-teasers, puzzles, etc.) and training of social skills. Computer neurorehabilitation software offers a wide range of possibilities that enable specific or general training of impaired functions (Bracy, 2007; Brieff, 1994). Their advantage lies in complexity, flexibility in setting the level of difficulty of training, the ability to provide exact and rapid feedback, the ability to archive and statistically process data (including comparison of single results and trends over time), game characteristics, flexibility and variability (Brieff, 1994; Kulišťák, 2003). Patients typically tolerate and adjust to these software programs well. Last, but not least, computers facilitate the work of the therapist and save time (Preiss, 1998). The disadvantages of software programs lies in the use of mechanical drills, which involve practicing singular tasks, which may or may not be done correctly and offer a low level of generalization to more difficult everyday tasks (Kulišťák, 2003; Preiss, 1998; Rodriguez, 2006). Problems may occur if a therapist incorrectly interprets the patient's results or does not correctly match the level of

[5] Rodriguez also draws attention to worsening of the symptomatology in patients who underwent computer program (three times a week for 90 minutes) and had other activities at the same time. Because of this, he proposes to include only those patients who will have no other load activities during the program (eight weeks).

difficulty with the actual condition of the patient. Moreover, unassisted computer remediation, can lead to a reduction of benefits in the individualized approach (training of metacognition strategies, solution planning, and single-step procedure, targeted feedback, etc.) due to a weakened therapeutic relationship. A purely computer-based form of training should, rather, be one part of a more complex cognitive function remediation. Increased generalization and transfer of “clinical” effects of computer cognitive training into real life situations can be partially solved by using virtual reality within the software. It offers the potential to create an environment that enables practicing from the simplest motor activities to the most complex cognitive functions, removes “drill,” is able to approximate real environments, and, due to this fact it, can partially solve the problem of skill transfer and generalization (Kulišťák, 2002, 2003). However, interdisciplinary dialogue and connection of psychological, neuropsychological and information technologies to produce quality programs are needed.

The question, whether training performed using "pencil-paper" methods is more effective than specialized software dedicated to neurorehabilitation, is still open. Comparisons of both strategies are still taking place. Twamley’s summary study investigating cognitive function training in patients with schizophrenia (Twamley et al., 2003) comprised sixteen studies. Seven of these studies were performed by means of “pencil-paper” methods and nine used computers. In view of the relative success of these training approaches, it was found that the approach did not play an important role. Six out of seven "pencil-paper" studies were successful and six out of nine computer studies were also successful. The results of this research also show that the training approach and its strategy (e.g., orientation to the process of solution versus repeated practicing of skills) may be much more important and has been documented by other authors (e.g., Medalia, Richardson, 2005).

IV.2. EEG Biofeedback

Another globally known, non-pharmacological method is EEG biofeedback. This method is based on the basic clinically verified assumption that patients are capable of learning to regulate their own brain activity. Training is performed under the principle of operative conditioning and EEGs are recorded on the patient. The EEG signal is transmitted to a computer and displayed on screen. The display provides the patient with positive or negative feedback relative to positive or negative results in the computer game. This method has been implemented in work with epileptics and in pediatric psychiatry where it is used during attention deficit disorder therapy (ADD/ADHD; Kopřivová et al., 2007). The scientific literature does not mention this method for use as a targeted method with cognitive deficits in neuropsychiatric diseases. However, there are human studies following traumatic brain injuries (Thatcher, 2000). It has also been used as a method for improving cognitive deficits in healthy individuals (Vernon, 2005). We assume that, due some similarities in cognitive patterns, EEG biofeedback, which is still underused, has potential in neuropsychiatry. The rationale for using neurofeedback therapeutically is that it corrects deficits in brain cerebral regulatory function related to arousal, attention, vigilance and affect.

IV.3. Repetitive Transcranial Magnetic Stimulation (rTMS)

The use of noninvasive Transcranial Magnetic Stimulation (TMS) had been well documented in clinical neurophysiologic studies. During the last century, the power of this method was studied in the cognitive neurosciences in correlation with perception, attention, learning, plasticity, language and awareness and in the field of neuropsychiatric disorders in correlation with depression, anxiety disorders, and schizophrenia. Repetitive Transcranial Magnetic Stimulation (rTMS) a variation of TMS, is also noninvasive and uses repetitive short magnetic pulses to the cortex, through the scalp, in order to influence specific neural circuits. rTMS can directly affect cortical excitability and metabolism and subsequently affect cognition. Several trials, including our study, showed rehabilitation efficacy after cognitive training (Rodriguez et al. 2004; Mohr et al. 2007). The aim is to enhance the improvement of cognitive functions with a direct modification of cortical excitability with repetitive transcranial magnetic stimulation (rTMS). Effect of rTMS on cognitive functions was shown in healthy, elderly, volunteers with memory dysfunction and in schizophrenia patients (Fitzpatrick and Rothman, 2000; Solé-Padullés et al., 2006; Rollnik et al., 2000; Huber et al., 2003; Mohr et al., 2006[6]; Rodriguez et al. 2007). However, the final benefits and protocol for use, of rTMS with regard to remediation of cognitive functions in neuropsychiatric disorders, is still basically an unanswered question. Combinations of rTMS stimulation with neuroimaging methods may provide new information with regard to modulation of cortical regions, trans-synaptic effects and the effects on other, more remote, brain areas.

IV.4. Combined Methods

A complex and extensively used rehabilitation approach is the Integrated Psychotherapeutic Program (IPT) that was developed during the latter half of the 1970s, in Switzerland. It was introduced to the scientific community in 1990 by physicians Hans Brenner and Volker Roder. IPT is a structured therapeutic program for people suffering from schizophrenia. The program combines rehabilitation of cognitive functions and social cognition training through both group and individual activities. It is used in small groups and proceeds through single sub-programs from (i) training of cognitive differentiation, (ii) social perception and communication, (iii) social skills, and finally to (iv) interpersonal problem-solving. The complexity and difficulty of the tasks are gradually increased. The first sub-program includes cognitive training focused on concentration, vigilance, ability to abstract, and creation of a solution plan. Another is concentrated on social perception and understanding social situations. The third is focused on verbal communication; the fourth on social skills; and the fifth on interpersonal situations and problems. The tasks proceed (in the spirit of metacognition) from (i) identification of the problem, (ii) the solution proposal, (iii) critical review of the solution and possible solution modification, and (iv) solution application

[6] We studied in a group of 34 patients with schizophrenia, treated with second-generation antipsychotics, except for clozapine, the effect of augmentation of computer-assisted cognitive remediation in schizophrenia with rTMS. The results showed an after training significant improvement in severity of cognitive deficit in schizophrenia in many domains, especially executive functions: attention shift–flexibility, attention control, and working memory. The output was faster, more precise, and more reliable. Results also showed some trend of augmentation effect due rTMS.

and evaluation of feedback. The work includes cards, slides, interviews, and role-playing (Roder et al., 1993). Efficacy of the program has been verified by Spanish researchers (Penadés et al., 2003), and their data correspond with the results provided by Brenner and Roder. Accordingly, patients who participated in this program achieved improvement on neuropsychological tests (in vigilance, memory, and executive functions) together with higher levels of autonomy and social skills.

In the 1970s, Robert Paul Liberman developed a complex rehabilitation program called Social Skills Training for patients with schizophrenia who are in remission and live at home. During the program, patients learn how to increase social competence, i.e., their ability to communicate with other people and solve interpersonal problems (Liberman et al., 1998). The program includes systematic training of communication and complex social skills; its level of difficulty can be gradually increased to meet the needs of each patient. It is usually set in small groups, and it uses instructions, role-playing, modeling of interpersonal situations, training of social sensitivity, and communication. Patients are provided permanent and targeted feedback. They rehearse skills such as perception of social situations, nonverbal communication, active listening, empathy, appreciation, appraisal, compliment, introduction, maintenance, and discontinuation of short interviews, demonstration of negative emotions in appropriate ways, self-enforcement, compromising skills, and problem-solving training. They also learn how to regularly take medication and how to cope with the symptoms of their disease. Throughout the program, therapists use techniques as schematic aids, learning through stimulation, contextual hints, corrective feedback, and reinforcement of the effective behavior (Liberman et al., 1998). Patients do their homework in-between sessions, which consist of practical applications of what they have learned.

Efficacy of this program has been verified by several studies. Benton and Schroeder compared four comparative studies from 1990, in a meta-analytic study and described a non-significant therapeutical effect of practicing of social skills on reduction of psychopathology (Benton and Schroeder, 1990). However, meta-analytical studies have shown that the effect of generalization of learned behavioral patterns in practical life is mild (Benton and Schroeder, 1990) or moderate (Corrigan, 1991). Patients were able to use learned social skills mainly in situations that were similar to the practiced situations. Simple skills (e.g., motor) were better generalized into the practical life than complex behavioral patterns (Wallace et al., 1992).

Another example of a comprehensive complex program is Cognitive Enhancement Therapy (CET) developed by Hogarty and Flesher (1999) that initially uses computer training and in later phases provides group tasks focused on development of cognitive abilities and social skills. CET stems from methods used in the rehabilitation of patients following brain injury. The program consists of assisted computer rehabilitation, training groups for social perception and social skills, support groups and psychoeducational meetings for better disease control (Hogarty, Flesher, 1999; Wykes and Reeder, 2005). Verifying studies (Hogarty et al., 2004; Hogarty et al., 2006) have confirmed acceleration of information processing, improvement of verbal memory and problem-solving skills.

IV.5. Social Cognition within Cognitive Function Rehabilitation

Social cognition (or self-cognition) can be described as the ability to correctly evaluate the meaning of social situations (social scheme), reading of emotionally colored contexts, interpretation of verbal and nonverbal demonstrations of a communication partner, differentiation of changes of mental states within the communication and social interactions with other people as well as perception and disease-coping mechanisms (Green and Nuechterlein, 1999). It also includes the schemes of persons, roles, events, self-schemes and procedural social schemes (Burns, 2006). Healthy people often have a so-called social appearance; they are able, for example, to deduce significant communication information from the expression of the other person. People with cognitive deficits due to neuropsychiatric diseases often lack this ability (Lewis and Mitchell, 1994). Some people experience this problem during an episode of their disease or due to a deficit in cognitive function. Other people stopped using these skills as a result of social isolation and eventually lost the skills altogether (Motlová and Koukolík, 2004). A lack of social skills can lead to repeated social failures and a reduction in, or loss of, self-confidence, people and communication fears (social phobia), as well as an increase in stress, which can threaten their mental condition and trigger a relapse of the disease. While direct training of social cognition is not a common facet of cognitive training, it can be found in the combined training of social skills and social perception (see IPT, Liberman's program, and CET).

For instance, social cognition was included as one of the basic elements of cognitive impairment in schizophrenia (MATRICS—NIMH Measurement and Treatment Research to Improve Cognition in Schizophrenia—American National Institute of Mental Health); it was added after the revision of results from extensive meta-analyses (Nuechterline et al., 2004). It was found to repeatedly impact the quality of interpersonal relations, final functional conditions and was important in evaluating the efficacy of cognitive rehabilitation programs. Interest in this problem is growing, and it is often investigated in relation to the theory of mind. This theory studies social cognition with regard to understanding the behavior of other people and the ability to assign various mental conditions to ourselves and others that can then be used to describe, understand, and predict behavior (Premack and Woodruff, 1978; Brüne, 2005).

Patients with schizophrenia can have problems recognizing emotion in the faces of people in videotapes or photographs (Bellack et al., 1999; Brüne, 2005). However, the number of relevant studies in this area is limited, and diagnostic tools are rare. Some studies (e.g., Bellack et al., 1999) used the Social Problem-solving Assessment Battery, in which the probands act out a series of three-minute, imaginary interviews with a relative (brother, parent, friend). The role of the relative is played by a member of the staff. Interactions are recorded on videotape and then evaluated in accordance with various nonverbal and verbal criteria.

Frommann et al., (2003) focused on affect recognition problems among rehabilitation patients. They developed a special training program called Training of Affect Recognition (TAR), which focused on the recognition of faces and emotions from the expressions on other peoples' faces. Training takes place in small groups with the support of computers. The authors verified its efficacy in relation to the computer training called Cognitive Remediation Therapy (CRT) as well as with a control group. The study included a total of 77 stabilized patients who were randomly divided into groups and assessed both at the beginning and the end of training. The results of the study showed significant improvement in the recognition of emotions (scores of patients at the end of the study were near to the results of healthy people). Results showed that it could be necessary to use specifically focused social skills programs (a group undergoing CRT and a control group did not achieve corresponding results) (Wölwer et al., 2005). During the training of social skills, patients learn specific skills to improve their competency in interpersonal relations and increase levels of personal satisfaction. They practice and learn how to correctly perceive and understand verbal and nonverbal communication, how to cope with social situations, and how to maintain sufficient eye contact with the corresponding strength of voice (Glynn, 2003; Häfner, 1996). Group trainings and role-playing are often used in rehabilitation with positive results (e.g., Cohen et al., 2005; Green, 2000). These trainings involve instructional techniques such as modeling of situations, providing feedback, and strengthening of effective behavior (Kopelowicz et al., 2003; Roder et al., 1993). We have previously mentioned related programs such as Liberman's and Wallace's complex training program for social skills or the Integrated Psychotherapeutic Therapy (IPT) of Roder and Brenner.

One of the research programs that relates to the association between cognitive functions as measured by neurocognitive tests, is the so called "role-play" test for functioning in everyday life, provided by A. Cohen et al. in 2005. Based on his results, it is clear that "Role-play" tests, and the related capacity regarding social skills and the ability to cope with everyday life, only modestly correlates with functioning in everyday life. The characteristics of cognitive deficits seem to be a more significant factor (whether specific or generalized). Therefore, it is important to measure the capacity of social skills; the results that follow can then be considered to be in the upper range of success of the subject (Cohen et al., 2005).

Evaluation of the level of social cognition brings purely clinical evaluations closer to the everyday life of a patient and could, therefore, be a bridge between neuropsychological diagnostics and the evaluation of functions in everyday life (Nuechterlein et al., 2004). Tůma and Lenderová (2001) state that impairments of social abilities occur in relation to insufficiently received and decoded information, its processing, decision-making, and transmission of socially adequate responses. This causes reduced sensitivity to interpersonal signals, insufficient cognitive flexibility, and expression. MATRICS, in its battery for measurement of social cognition, proposes to use the Mayer-Salovey-Caruso Emotional Intelligence Test-Managing Emotions tools (Green, 2007). Bellack et al. (1999) assume that social cognition, recognition of emotions from facial expressions and correct evaluation of social situations should be the main goals of cognitive remediation.

IV.6. Strategies of Cognitive Remediation

IV.6.1. Should We Restore or Compensate?

In our approach to remediation of cognitive functions, we can differentiate between restorative and compensatory strategies. The *restorative* approach is based on the assumption that a particular deficit of cognitive function can be improved. It uses direct and repetitive practice. The restorative approach has dominated the field of cognitive function training for many years. The approach emphasizes the volume of training and an adequate load in attenuated areas. The strengthening of an impaired function should be achieved by means of repeated and regular practice and gradually increasing levels of difficulty. Over-learned or gained skill can also become automated by gradual training that can then facilitate, for example, working memory (Bellack et al., 1999; Rodriguez, 2006; Wykes, 2000). This model applies more to training utilizing computer software.

The *compensatory* strategy is based on the assumption that the impaired function cannot be significantly affected but can be bypassed through various surrogate strategies and aids such as changes in working procedures (various cognitive heuristics), self-instruction, reduction of impulsivity or the substitution of other preserved cognitive functions, etc. (Twamley et al. 2003; Wexler and Bell, 2005). This strategy stresses individual feedback and supports the effective use of cognitive functions (see the metacognition concept). The purpose of compensation is to minimize the limitations resulting from the impairment of cognitive function (Bellack et al., 1999). Therefore, it does not focus, for instance, only on the improvement of verbal memory and attention in order to achieve higher functioning in social relations, but also stresses a reduction in environmental (day-to-day) demands.

Based on the principle of "bridging" the cognitive deficits by compensatory strategies, Velligan et al. founded (2000) the Cognitive Adaptation Training for patients with schizophrenia. Later, the effect of this method was verified in a study that included experimental and control groups and concluded that the compensatory strategy had an unambiguous positive impact on patients. Wexler and Bell (2005) also concluded that clients who underwent this type of training had lower rates of positive and negative symptoms, higher motivation, and functioned better under general conditions.

Should we arrange Individual or group settings?

Another question that therapists must consider is whether an individual or group setting is more suitable for the training of cognitive functions in patients with neuropsychiatric disorders, especially those with Schizophrenia. The *individual setting* is more flexible when responding to specific needs, the picture of cognitive deficit and suits the individual personalities of patients. Another advantage is feedback; it can be immediate and targeted. Various metacognition techniques, in conjunction with error-free learning or the analysis of working procedures during task-solving, (i.e., focus on executive functions and metacognition) can be used as well. Therefore, some authors (e.g., Bellack, 1999; Koren et al. 2006; Wykes et al., 1999) recommend the individual approach. However, the *group design of training* cognitive function has advantages as well; meeting with clients in a group improves the client's social skills, develops feelings of belonging, communication, cooperation, and mutual support. The client receives constructive correction and helpful feedback from more people, particularly when the training of social cognition is included in the program. In addition, it is less demanding on time and cost (Wykes et al., 2003).

IV.6.2. Rewards, Feedback

We usually stress immediate feedback during cognitive training. This strategy is based on commonly observed problems in neuropsychiatric patients with self-appreciation or over-appreciation of their own behaviors (Wykes, 2000, Rodriguez 2004) and on the basic theoretical principles of learning (see above). Targeted and precise feedback from a therapist fills this void and helps the client correct his/her own behavior and modify his/her problem-solving strategies. Effective feedback provides the patient with the experience of success, positively affects his/her motivation and self-confidence and helps him/her develop cognitive skills at the same time (Brown et al., 1993). Therefore, several principles must be kept in mind: to recognize and reflect even the smallest success of the patient; to provide concrete, precise, consistent, and immediate (during task-solving) feedback; and to remain flexible, empathic, and cooperative. Positive performance feedback (e.g., average time or standard deviation in attention tasks) can also be provided by computer training software, which can show current performance, a comparison with past results, performance trends, etc. (Perglová, 2006). However, the fundamental training aid is personal, immediate, and targeted feedback provided by a therapist to the patient. It enables the correction of non-specific procedures, the development of metacognitive skills and error-free learning, as well as the maintenance of motivation, initiative, and endurance. By virtue of this feedback, the patient learns to accurately evaluate his own performance and behavior (Koren et al., 2006). Some studies also had positive results when using remuneration as a form of the feedback (e.g., Woonings et al., 2002).

IV.6.3. Metacognition

Efficacy of cognitive functions can be improved by various metacognitive techniques and mental aids. The aim is to have patients learn to plan and monitor their actual performance and evaluate conceptualized procedures and strategies with realized outcomes and to use these comparisons as part of recognition and modification of their behaviors (Koren et al., 2006; Sternberg, 2002; Wykes and Reeder, 2005). Metacognition theory assumes that an individual can comply with environmental requirements even with decreased levels of cognitive functions, if he learns how to reflect his mental processes, is aware of key moments susceptible to errors, and makes associations between the activity and results (Koren et al., 2006).

The metacognitive strategies are not geared directly toward a result, but more toward a process that leads to this result. They emphasize motivation and patient's disposition for self-development. They support active efforts to explore, ask questions, respond, sort, categorize, and re-process tasks and procedures for solving. The therapist should deliberately interfere with the process of cognition in order to regulate these activities and redirect them toward higher reflection of the patient, improved self-cognition, reflection of strategies and procedures of learning. Optimally, this regimentation is gradually changed based on the patient's auto-regulation, ability to perform self-monitoring, self-evaluation, and self-instruction (Wykes, 2000). For example, at the beginning of training, tasks based on executive functions, patients are focused on recognition of the basic steps associated with reliable performance, supported in estimation of the difficulty of the task, finding a strategy for effective solution, self-instruction, estimation of time needed to solve the task, and estimated success. During this type of training, feedback is provided at each level with regard to the selected strategies or mistakes, and therapists assist clients in their search for a broader range of possible approaches from which they can select that which is most suitable. Later, the therapist gives the client initiative and, if necessary, warns them of possible limits of the chosen procedure.

IV.6.4. Error-Free Learning

Error-free learning is a training method based on the strengthening of correct and effective procedures for acquiring skills. It starts with a simple visual discrimination task with a high probability of success and proceeds to those requiring complex solutions (e.g., tasks that are similar to the Hanoi or London tower test), while minimizing the test-error strategy (Green et al. 1999; Sachs, 2000). It is also focused on avoiding repetition of erroneous strategies and the strengthening of new, more effective procedures for task resolution and behavior. One of the techniques used in the method of error-free learning involves a gradual increase in the task's degree of difficulty, which encourages the patient to seek and strive for the correct solution, provided the tasks stay within the patient's level of competence[7] (this strategy is also called scaffolding) (Koren et al., 2006; Wykes, 2002). For example, after managing the tasks focused on vigilance and concentration, the patient moves on to memory tasks, decision-making tasks and solution planning. The therapist increases the load gradually, makes an effort to help the patient adequately learn how to communicate difficulties, avoids acting impulsively and tries to eliminate non-productive solutions.

IV.7. Ecological Validity and Transfer into Everyday Life

The aim of the assessment of cognitive functions is mainly that of helping to reveal and understand the nature of cognitive deficits, to explain whether and how deficits affect the patient's behavior and which problems in the patient's everyday life are related to the deficit. However, most psycho diagnostic tools often fail to meet this prerequisite and are often based on tasks that are far removed from everyday situations. The relationship between the test and assessment results and their relation to ecological validity in everyday situations is more and more discussed in recent years. Ecological validity expresses a level in which the tool is able to predict functionality or behavior in everyday conditions and situations (Lezak, 1995; Preiss et al., 2006). It is an external, criterion-based form of validity where the measure reflects certain aspect of the patient's functionality in everyday life. e.g., if the patient is able to drive a car, take care of him/herself, or work. Ecological validity helps to better estimate the quality of life of a patient or the ability to live independently. The results of neuropsychological tests are usually unable to provide this information alone. Psychologists often must rely on clinical impressions and information received from the patient or his/her relatives. In addition, clinical assessment may not reflect various compensatory mechanisms that help people cope with similar tasks in everyday life (Preiss et al., 2006).

Prouteau et al. (2004) compared the results of neuropsychological tests and subjectively conveyed problems directly from patients. Based on the results, they recommend using subjective and objective measures of cognitive deficits to develop a more complex view. However, they recommend being careful with regard to interpretations of statistical results due to possible discrepancies between subjective complaints and objective measures, which are apparent during clinical analysis. In recent years, there has been a growing emphasis on improving the ecological validity of diagnostic procedures as well as a call for ecologically valid tools. For example, Koren et al. (2006) proposes several procedures for increasing the ecological validity of research into cognitive deficits in schizophrenia. They mention the need to find out what is actually being measured by particular neuropsychological tests, to produce new ecologically valid tools that would be more similar to real-life situations and implementation of theoretical constructions that are able to better reflect the complexity of real life. However, they are scarce. Additionally, more frequent use of imaging techniques

[7] The author of the theoretical rationale is Lev Vygotsky, who talks about a "zone of the closest development" and describes it as a range of potential between the observable level of realized abilities and the latent capacity of a person (Sternberg, 2002).

during neuropsychological assessment could markedly extend the spectrum of information on the nature and symptoms of cognitive deficits and possibilities for neuronal plasticity in neuropsychiatric diseases as well (Preiss, 1998; Wykes, 2002).

Although a number of studies focused on remediation interventions have confirmed better function and good results (e.g., Barton, 1999; Glynn, 2003; Maj and Sartorius, 2002; Kopelowicz et al., 2003, etc.), it is apparent that benefits of using psychosocial interventions and trainings of skills are inhibited by problems associated with the transfer of learned skills to everyday life. In some cases, the failure of this transfer is related to neurocognitive damage resulting from neuropsychiatric diseases. Sometimes, it is a lack of social opportunity in the natural environment and the low level of stimulation coming from the environment (Glynn, 2003). The more difficult the skill, the lower the level of generalization in everyday conditions. The potential for transfer arises from: sufficient training or practice and its intensity; the ability of said training to be incorporated into real life situations of the patient; an increase in environmental support; and the possibility of repeated testing of the learned skills in everyday situations (Häfner, 1996; Kopelowicz et al., 2003). Other effective possibilities include “life” practicing, role-playing, and homework that prolongs the effects of training in everyday life. The development of techniques with higher degrees of generalization is currently the biggest challenge and another important step in strengthening of efficacy of cognitive remediation in neuropsychiatric diseases (Glynn, 2003).

V. Conclusion

Taking into consideration the evidence provided in this chapter, it is clear that both a good theoretical background (rationales) and additional studies aimed at understanding what we are targeting during cognitive remediation are key topics in need of further research. We must also find better means of marrying neurological cognitive remediation experience with neuropsychiatric needs. In the field of neurology, there are a variety of complex cognitive rehabilitation programs that have strengths in areas that are not fundamental to our neuropsychiatric patients. With this in mind, we have written about very simple training methods, as well as important theories of learning (including the neuronal plasticity of brain), that could constitute great inspiration and provide the solid theoretical background needed for further exploration in the field of cognitive remediation of the neuropsychiatric population.

Social and cognitive remediation of cognition in neuropsychiatric patients makes, without discussion, sense. Our work arises from both theories of learning and information processing, and deals with both paper-pencil and computer-training methods. Patients could be treated individually or in groups, in accordance with patients’ needs. Currently, however, the main clinical and scientific questions regard (i) which approaches of cognitive remediation programs and their lengths are the most effective, (ii) what can be considered as a brain self-recovery process and when to start cognitive remediation with the patient, and (iii) how to obtain maximum benefits from cognitive rehabilitation relative to the patient’s everyday activities?

Despite these and other questions, there is an excellent theoretical background, as well as both recent and older studies, that support and rationalize the importance of cognitive rehabilitation for people in our community suffering from neuropsychiatric disorders.

Supported by the research project CNS 1M0517

VI. Keywords

Rehabilitation

Rehabilitation is the minimum grade of support for people with disabilities. The aim of rehabilitation is to achieve the maximum level of independence, providing high levels of continuous supervision.

Neuropsychological Rehabilitation

A component of the whole rehabilitation field focused on the improvement of cognitive functions. Neuropsychological rehabilitation involves the treatment of emotional, personality, and physical deficits resulting from illness.

Cognitive Rehabilitation-Remediation

A field of neuropsychology that combines several methods of rehabilitation based on both neuropsychological and cognitive theories to correct an underlying cognitive impairment, developing new skills that replace or compensate for lost ones and facilitating a naturally occurring recovery process.

Cognitive Training

Cognitive training is a neuropsychological method of cognitive rehabilitation—remediation, which uses both systematic and repeated training and re-training of cognitive functions.

Appendix 1—CASE VIGNETTE

Hannah is a 28-year-old single female, living with her parents. She is a college drop-out, living on a disability pension and concurrently has a supported job in a cafeteria. Seven years ago, she was diagnosed with Paranoid Schizophrenia and so far had three hospitalizations. During remissions, she took several work trials (in a graphic studio, as a cleaning woman). Hannah is on a stable dose of second-generation antipsychotics plus supplemental vitamins. Perceived side effects are morning fatigue, sluggishness, and problems with concentration. She gets along with her parents fairly, they spend vacations together, share various activities in their leisure time. However, despite the Hannah's illness, the parents still have high expectations, and it is hard for them to put up with the situation. Hannah often goes for walks, likes to converse, is comfortable working with other people. She reads a lot, practices her German language skills and has started study English.

She is optimistic about her future, plans to take a one-year English language course or to get a job as a receptionist. Hannah also participated in a retraining course for librarians, which she could not complete due to her attention problems. She was slow at school but otherwise performed well, had some difficulties with writing and petty manual labor. However, her parents wanted her to excel.

She entered the program of cognitive training with aims "to be able to calculate change money from memory, swiftly type in data into a computer and to improve my concentration so I could do better at work and deal well with other people." Hannah also complained that "I have often hard time to find something on a list and can't remember it by heart." Training goals were later on broadened mainly to include an estimate what Hannah could do by herself and where she needed assistance. The additional focus was on impulse control and planning ahead. At the same time, Hannah attended a social skills training where she developed the ability to express and recognize emotions and worked on a more effective way to communicate with customers.

The baseline diagnostic examination of cognitive functions revealed that Hannah's strongest part was verbal abstraction, with average to above-average performance. Hannah worked well with language, understood verbal relations, and had a large vocabulary. She was primarily focused on performance. Due to the absence of depressive symptoms, she had a positive attitude towards the diagnostic examination and training itself.

She took badly any failure. The support of visual detection, attention, and enhancement of verbal and visual memory proved to be very helpful. She practiced change of work style, how to reduce error rate, which was one of Hannah's problems: distortions and a high number of omissions. She worked on the improvement of planning, vocal self-instructions, and self-awareness of ongoing actions. Training of impulse control was needed to prevent her from the tendency to pick recklessly the first option without consideration other alternatives. She was aware of her slower pace and attempted to compensate with initiative, but with a negative impact on the performance quality. If Hannah controlled her impulsiveness, then the execution was more accurate. She gradually learned to work with time estimates and to assess output. Hannah also trained in calculus and to recognize what she would be able to calculate in her head and what needs to be counted with pen and paper or a calculator.

In the course of training, Hannah was enthusiastic and active, looking forward to the sessions and highly cooperative. She was always on time and motivated; she never missed a class. Hannah by herself conceived various home exercises and tested the training methods in a cafeteria, utilizing various mnemonics. In total, she completed 23 sessions. After the completion of cognitive training, Hannah was looking for a job and found an English course where she enrolled. There was no change in the medication and her mental status was stable; she was in a good and optimistic mood.

The endpoint examination showed, compared to the baseline testing, the following results (abbreviated): inconsistent processing speed, while in some tasks was low (TMT), in the D2 test significantly increased with a higher error rate. Moreover, her performance in the first part of the Numeric Square Test improved dramatically. However, there was increasing time in the repeated trials. The results in all attention tests significantly improved; however, there was a higher error rate in the D2 test. The execution curve was getting more balanced without signs of weariness. The memory and learning tests showed improvement of visual learning (the most remarkably, in the first part of the Numeric Square Test) and on the delayed recall of the Rey-Osterrieth Figure. A significant increase of the short-term memory was found in the verbal learning, with a higher number of distortions and repetitions. The similar trend for higher error rate could be observed in every test. It was very likely caused by the subjectively perceived pressure on the performance that interfered with the behavior control under testing conditions. No change was detected in working memory. In the executive functions, there was a mild improvement in the distribution of attention and procedure planning. All questionnaires evaluating impact of cognitive deficit indicated positive changes in self-reported measures (significantly) and objective reports by a caregiver.

The recommendations made at the conclusion of the training were to repeat actions regularly during the learning process, to learn short parts and add new items gradually. Hannah was advised to practice acquisition of unusual situations, to pace their solutions and executions stepwise, to work on a realistic estimate of performance, to make a stop at every little progress and compliment herself. She should learn to accept her limitations and to take them easy—to remind herself that quality should prevail over quantity and to insist on accuracy. Hannah was told to follow time-undemanding activities, where she could verbally express herself. In all activities, including conversation, Hannah should practice self-reflective awareness of her thought processes, learn to take a break, plan the task solution, design potential strategies, keep in mind accuracy, and have time for insight into the situation.

Table III. Hannah—the baseline and endpoint test scores

TEST PARAMETERS	BEFORE*	AFTER*	DIFFERENCE
AVLT			
Trials I-V	38	52	14
Trial B	5	7	2
Trial VI	9	10	1
Reproduction after 30 min.	11	11	0
Repetition	2	8	6
Confabulation	1	2	1
REY FIGURE			
Copy	22	28	6
Reproduction after 3 min.	14	13	-1
Reproduction after 30 min.	9.5	22	12.5
D2			
Total number	292	342	50
Errors 1 (omissions)	13	17	4
Errors 2 (commissions)	1	4	3
% of errors	4.79	6.14	1.35
Overall performance	278	321	43
Fluctuation range	15	12	-3
Concentration	106	112	6
Curve	Relatively OK	Fluctuating	
VERBAL FLUENCY			
Word count	51	52	1
STROOP TEST			
Words W (time)	70	71	1
Colors C (time)	110	115	5
Word Color WC (time)	155	150	-5
Interference Factor WC-C (time)	45	35	-10

TEST PARAMETERS	BEFORE*	AFTER*	DIFFERENCE
Errors	2	4	2
TMT			
Part A time	58	57	-1
Part B time	120	115	-5
NUMERIC SQUARE			
Mean of trials 1-5 (time)	53.9	34.4	-19.5
Mean of trials 6-10 (time)	25.4	29.8	4.4
Mean of 1-5/mean of 6-10 (time)	2.12	1.15	-0.97
Mean of 1-10 (time)	39.7	32.1	-7.55
Curve	Fluctuating	More stable	
DIGIT SPAN			
Forward	8	8	0
Backward	3	4	1
Total	11	12	1
QUESTIONNAIRES			
DEX	44	35	-9
CFQ	54	48	-6
EMQ	78	66	-12
DEX-SO	17	14	-3
CFQ-SO	32	30	-2

* values are in raw scores; time in seconds.

References

Addington J, McCleary L, Munroe-Blum H. Relationship between cognitive and social dysfunction in schizophrenia. *Schizophrenia Research* 1998;34(1-2):59-66.

Angelucci F, Brené S, Mathé AA. BDNF in schizophrenia, depression and corresponding animal models. *Molecular Psychiatry* 2005;10(4):345-352.

Aouizerate B, Guehl D, Cuny E, Rougier A, Bioulac B, Tignol J, Brbaud P. Pathophysiology of obsessive–compulsive disorder. A necessary link between phenomenology, neuropsychology, imagery and physiology. *Progress in Neurobiology* 2004;72:195–221.

Aronson J a Vroonland JP. The Residual Cognitive Competence of Elderly Females. *J. Clin. Psychol.* 1993;49(5):724-31.

Atkinson R.L, Atkinson RC, Smith EE, Bem DJ. Psychologie; 1995. Victoria Publishing Praha.

Bark N, Revheim N, Huq F, Khalderov V, Ganz ZW, Medalia A. The impact of cognitive remediation on psychiatric symptoms of schizophrenia. *Schizophrenia Research* 2003;63(3):229-35.

Barton R. Psychosocial Rehabilitation Services in Community Support Systems: A Review of Outcomes and Policy Recommendations. Psychiatric Services; 1999; 50(4):525-534.

Baudiš P. Psychiatry in Numbers—Psychiatrie v číslech; 2006, *Prague Psychiatric Center*,

Bellack A, Gold JM, Buchanan RW. Cognitive Rehabilitation for Schizophrenia: Problems, Prospects, and Strategies. *Schizophrenia Bulletin* 1999; 25(2):257-274.

Bellack AS. Rehabilitative treatment of schizophrenia. In Liberman JA, Murray RM, eds. Comprehensive Care of Schizophrenia: A Textbook of Clinical Management. 2001, Martin Dunitz, London, UK.

Bell-McGinty S, Podell K, Franzen M, Baird AD a Williams MJ. Standard Measures of Executive Functioning in Predicting Instrumental Activities of Daily Living in Older Adults. *Int. J. Geriatr. Psyc.* 2002;17:828-834.

Benešová M. Rehabilitace pacientů se schizofrenním onemocněním—trénink kognitivních funkcí; 2007, Filozofická fakulta Karlova Univerzita, Praha.

Benton MK, Schroeder TJ. Social skills training with schizophrenics: a meta-analytic evaluation. *J. Consult. Clin. Psychol.* 1990; 58:741–747.

Bracy OL. Cognitive rehabilitation: a process approach. Cogn Rehabilit 1986, 4: 10-17.

Bracy O. Cognitive Functioning and Rehabilitation. Psychological Software Services [online]. 2007 [cit. 2007-06-03]. From: <http://www.neuroscience.cnter.com /pss/article_cognitive_functioni.html>.

Bradshaw JL, Sheppard DM. The Neurodevelopmental Frontostriatal Disorders: Evolutionary Adaptiveness and Anomalous Lateralization. *Brain and Language* 2000; 73(2):297-320.

Brenner HD, Hirsbrunner A, Heimber A.: Integrated Psychological Therapy Program: Training in Cognitive and Social Skills for Schizophrenic Patients. In: Corrigan PW and Yudolfsky SC.: Cognitive Rehabilitation for Neuropsychiatric Disorders. *American Psychiatric Press* 1996.

Brieff R. HCP MAR94: Personal computers in Psychiatric Rehabilitation: A New Approach to Skills Training. *American Psychiatric Press* 1994; 45(3):257-260.

Brown C, Hartwood, K., Hays, C., Heckman, J. and Short, J. Effectiveness of Cognitive Rehabilitation for Improving Attention in Patients With Schizophrenia. *Spring.* 1993, vol. 13, no. 2, s. 71-86.

Brüne M. "Theory of Mind" in Schizophrenia: A Review of the Literature, *Schizophrenia Bulletin* 2005; 31:21–42.

Buhlmann U, Deckersbach T, Engelhard I, Cook LM, Rauch SL, Kathmann N, Wilhelm S, Savage CR. Cognitive retraining for organizational impairment in obsessive-compulsive disorder. *Psychiatry Res.* 2006;144(2-3):109-16.

Burdick KE, Braga RJ, Goldberg JF, Malhotra AK. Cognitive dysfunction in bipolar disorder: future place of pharmacotherapy. : *CNS Drugs* 2007;21(12):971-81.

Burns J. The social brain hypothesis of schizophrenia. *World Psychiatry* 2006; 5(2): 77–81.

Cadenhead KS., Swerdlow NR, Shafer KM, Diaz M, Braff DL. Modulation of the startle response and startle laterality in relatives of schizophrenic patients and in subjects with schizotypal personality disorder: evidence of inhibitory deficits. *AM. J. Psychiatry* 2000; 157 (10): 1660-1668.

Cohen AS, Forbes CB, Mann MC, Blanchard JJ. Specific cognitive deficits and differential domains of social functioning impairment in schizophrenia. *Schizophrenia Research* 2005; 81:227-238.

Corrigan PW. Social skills training in adult psychiatric populations: A meta-analysis. *J. Nebav. Ther. Exp. Psychiatry* 1991; 22:203–210.

Corrigan PW, Yudofsky MD. Cognitive Rehabilitation for Neuropsychiatric Disorders. 1996, *American Psychiatric Press*, Inc. NY.

Deckersbach T, Nierenberg AA, Kessler R, Lund HG, Ametrano RM, Sachs G, Rauch SL, Dougherty D. Cognitive Rehabilitation for Bipolar Disorder: An Open Trial for Employed Patients with Residual Depressive Symptoms. CNS Neurosci Ther. 2009 Nov 6

Delahunty, A., Morice, R., Frost, B.: Specific cognitive flexibility rehabilitation in schizophrenia. *Psychol. Med* 1993; 23: 221-227.

Elgamal S, McKinnon MC, Ramakrishnan K, Joffe RT, MacQueen G. Successful computer-assisted cognitive remediation therapy in patients with unipolar depression: a proof of principle study. *Psychol. Med.* 2007;37(9):1229-38.

Fiszdon JM, Bryson GJ, Wexler BE, Bell MD. Durability of cognitive remediation training in schizophrenia: performance on two memory tasks at 6-month and 12-month follow-up. *Psychiatry Res.* 2004;125(1):1-7.

Fiszdon JM, Cardenas AS, Bryson GJ, Bell MD. Predictors of remediation success on a trained memory task. *J. Nerv. Ment. Dis.* 2005;193(9):602-8.

Fiszdon JM, Choi J, Brusin GJ, Bell MD. Impact of intellectual status on response to cognitive task training in patients with schizophrenia. *Schizophr. Res.* 2006;87:261–269.

Fitzpatrick SM., Rothman DL. Meeting report: transcranial magnetic stimulation and studies of human cognition. *J. Cognitive Neurosci.* 2000; 12:704-709.

Frith CD. The cognitive abnormalities underlying the symptomatology and the disability of patients with schizophrenia. *Int. Clin. Psychopharmacol.* 1995;10 (Suppl 3) :87-98.

Fromann N, Streit M, Wölwer W. Remediation of facial affect recognition impairments in patients with schizophrenia: a new training program. *Psychiatry Research* 2003; 117(3):281-284.

Gaál, L. Neurop-2: Užívatelská príručka. 2002; Bratislava.

Gage F. Neurogenesis in the Adult Brain. *Journal of Neuroscience* 2002; 22(3):612-613.

Geyer MA, Ellenbroek B. Animal behavior models of the mechanisms underlying antipsychotic atypicality. Prog Neuropsychopharmacacol. *Biol. Pyschiatry* 2003; 27 (7): 1071-1079.

Glynn SM. Psychiatric rehabilitation in schizophrenia: advances and challenges. *Clinical Neuroscience Research* 2003; 3:23-33.

Goldberg TE, Weiberger DR, Berman KF, Pliskin MH, Podd MH. Further evidence for dementia of the prefrontal type in schizophrenia a controlled study of teaching the Wisconsin card sorting test. *Archives of General Psychiatry* 1987; 44, 1008-1014.

Gould E. Neurogenesis in adulthood: a possible role in learning. *Trends in Cognitive Sciences.* 1999; 3(5): 186-191.

Green MF, Nuechterlein KH. Should Schizophrenia be Treated as a Neurocognitive Disorder? *Schizophrenia Bulletin* 1999; 25(2):308-318.

Green MF, Kern RS, Braff DL, Mintz J. Neurocognitive deficits and functional outcome in schizophrenia: Are we measuring the "right stuff?" *Schizophrenia Bulletin* 2000; 26(1):119-136.

Green MF. MATRICS: an example of government / industry / academic collaboration [online]. 2007 [cit. 2007-06-07]. From: <http://www.asent.org/meetings /documents /Green.ppt>.

Greig TC, Zito W, Wexler BE, Fiszdon J, Bell MD. Improved cognitive function in schizophrenia after one year of cognitive training and vocational services. *Schizophr. Res.* 2007;96(1-3):156-61.

Häfner, H. Psychiatric Rehabilitation: general issues. *European Psychiatry* 1996; 11 (2):39-50.

Heinrichs WR. In Search of Madness. New York: Oxford University Press 2001.

Heinrichs RW, Zakzanis KK. Neurocognitive deficit in schizophrenia: a quantitative review of the evidence. *Neuropsychology* 1998;12:426–445.

Helgason CM. Commentary on the significance for modern neurology of the 17th century B.C. Surgical Papyrus. Can J Neurol Sci. 1987 Nov;14(4):560-3

Hogarty GE, Flesher S, Ulrich R, Carter M, Greenwald DP, Pogue-Geile Mi, Kechavan M, Cooley S, DiBarry AL, Garrett A., Parepally H, Zoretich R: Cognitive Enhancement Therapy for Schizophrenia. *Arch. Gen. Psychiatry* 2004; 61: 866-876.

Hogarty GE, Greenwald DP, Eack SM. Durability and mechanism of effects of cognitive enhancement therapy. *Psychiatr. Serv.* 2006;57(12):1751-7.

Hoekert M, Kahn R, Pijnenborg M, Aleman A. Impaired recognition and expression of emotional prosody in schizophrenia: Review and meta-analysis. *Schizophrenia Research* 2007, 96: 135-145.

Hofer A, Baumgartner S, Bodner T, Edlinger M, Hummer M, Kemmler G, Rettenbacher MA, Fleischhacker WW. Patient outcomes in schizophrenia II: the impact of cognition. *Eur. Psychiatry* 2005;20(5-6):395-402.

Hogarty GE, Flesher S, Ulrich R, Carter M, Greenwald D, Pogue-Geile M, Kechavan M, Cooley S, Di Barry AL, Garrett A, Parepally H, Zoretich R. Cognitive enhancement therapy for schizophrenia: effects of a 2-year randomized trial on cognition and behavior. *Arch. Gen. Psychiatry* 2004, 61(9):866-76.

Hogarty GE, Anderson CM, Reiss DJ, Kornblith SJ, Greenwald DP, Ulrich RF, Carter M. Family psychoeducation, social skills training, and maintenance chemotherapy in the aftercare treatment of schizophrenia. II. Two-year effects of a controlled study on relapse and adjustment. Environmental-Personal Indicators in the Course of Schizophrenia (EPICS) Research Group. *Arch. Gen. Psychiatry* (United States) 1991; 48(4):340-347.

Hogarty GE, Flesher S. Practice Principles of Cognitive Enhancement Therapy for Schizophrenia. *Schizophrenia Bulletin* 1999; 25(4):693-708.

Hogarty GE, Greenwald DP, Eack SM. Durability and Mechanism of Effects of Cognitive Enhancement *Therapy Psychiatric Services* 2006; 57(12):1751-1757.

Huber TJ, Schneider U, Rollnik JD. Gender differences in the effect of repetitive transcranial magnetic stimulation in schizophrenia. *Psychiatry Res.* 2003; 30(120):103-105.

Huttenlocher, Peter R. Neural Plasticity : The Effects of Environment on the Development of the Cerebral Cortex. 2002; 1st edition. Chicago : Harvard University Press,. 286 s. *Perspective in Cognitive Neuroscience*. ISBN 13 978-0-674-007.

Jaeger J, Berns S, Loftus S, Gonzalez C, Czobor P. Neurocognitive test performance predicts functional recovery from acute exacerbation leading to hospitalization in bipolar disorder. *Bipolar Disord* 2007;9(1-2):93-102.

Johansson BB. Brain plasticity in health and disease: Review. *The Keio Journal of Medicine* 2004; 53(4):231-246.

Kennedy N, Foy K, Sherazi R, McDonough M, McKeon P.: Long-term social functioning after depression treated by psychiatrists: a review. *Bipolar Disord.* 2007;9(1-2):25-37.

Kolb B, Gibb R. Neuroplasticity and recovery of function after brain injury. In Stuss DT, Winocur G, Robertson IH. Cognitive Neurorehabilitation. 1999, Cambridge University Press, Cambridge.

Kopelowicz A, Liberman RP, Wallace ChJ. Psychiatric Rehabilitation for Schizophrenia. *International Journal of Psychology and Psychological Therapy* 2003; 3(2):283-298.

Kopřivová J, Brunovský M, Praško J, Horáček J. EEG biofeedback and its use in clinical practice. *Psychiatrie*, 2007;11(3):1-7.

Koren D, Seidman LJ, Goldsmith M, Harvey PD. Real-World Cognitive and Metacognitive-Dysfunction in Schizophrenia: A new approach for Measuring (and Remediating) More "Right Stuff." *Schizophrenia Bulletin* 2006; 32(2):310-326.

Kulišťák P. Využití počítačů v neuropsychologické diagnostice. Trendy v medicíně 2002; 4(1):37-47.

Kulišťák P. Neuropsychologie. 2003, Portál, Praha.

Kumari V, Gray JA, Geyer MA, Ffytche D, Mitterschiffthaler MT, Vythelingum GN, Williams SCR, Simmons A, Sharma T. Neural correlates of tactile pre-pulse inhibition: a functional MRI study in normal and schizophrenic subjects. *Psychiatry Res.* 2003a; 122(2): 99-113 New York.

Kumari V, Ettinger U. Prepulse inhibition deficits in schizophrenia: static or amenable to treatment? In: MV Lang (Ed). Progress in Schizophrenia Research; 2004, Nova Publishers, N.

Krabbedndam L, Aleman A. Meta-analyses of randomized controlled trials of social skills training and cognitive remediation. *Psychol. Med* .2003, 33 (4): 756-758.

Laes JR, Sponheim SR. Does cognition predict community function only in schizophrenia?: A study of schizophrenia patients, bipolar affective disorder patients, and community control subjects. *Schizophr. Res.* 2006;84(1):121-31.

Lewis, C., Mitchell, P. (Eds.). Children's early understanding of mind. 1994, Hillsdale, LEA.

Lezak MD. Neuropsychological assessment. 1995; Oxford University Press, Oxford. New York.

Lezak MD. Neuropsychological assessment (4er ed.). 2004; Oxford University Press, Oxford. New York.

Liberman RP, Wallace CJ, Blackwell G, Kopelowicz A, Vaccaro JV, Mintz J: Skills training versus psychosocial occupational therapy for persons with persistent schizophrenia. *Am. J. Psychiatry* 1998; 155:1087-1091.

Liberman RP, DeRisi WJ, Mueser KT. Social Skills Training for Psychiatric Patients. 1989; Pergamon Press, New York.

Lysaker P, Buck K. Neurocognitive as a barrier to psychosocial. Effects on Learning, Coping and Self-Concept. *Journal of Psychosocial Nursing*, Vol. 45, No. 7; 2007; 24-30.

Maj M, Sartorius N. Schizophrenia. 2nd edition. 2002; Willey, Chichester, England.

McGurk SR, Meltzer HY. The role of cognition in vocational functioning in schizophrenia. *Schizophrenia Research* 2000;45:175-184.

McGurk S. Twamley E, Sitzer D, McHugo G, Mueser Kim. A Meta-Analysis of Cognitive Remediation in Schizophrenia. Am J Psychiatry 164:1791-1802, December 2007

Medalia A, Richardson R. What Predicts a Good Response to Cognitive Remediation Interventions? *Schizophrenia Bulletin* 2005, 31(4):942-953.

Mohr P, Rodriguez M, Novák T, Kopeček M, Horáček J, Hendrychová Y, Záleský R, Kawaciuková R, Preiss M, Seifertová D. Repetitivní transkraniální magnetická stimulace a rehabilitace kognitivních funkcí u schizofrenie. *Psychiatrie* 2006;1, 1-9.

Mohr, P., Rodriguez, M., Novák, T., Kopeček, M., Horáček, J., Hendrychová, Y., Záleský, R., Kawaciuková, R., Preiss, M., Seifertová, D. Repetitive transcranial magnetic stimulation and rehabilitation of cognitive functions in schizophrenia. *European Psychiatry*, 2007, vol. 22, (1), p. S127.

Morgan K, David A, Murray R. Cognition and schizophrenia: improving real life function. Report based on a conference held at the institute of Psychiatry, London, UK on 16th – 17th September 2004. Cambridge Medical Communication, UK, 2006.

Moritz S, Birkner Ch, Kloss M, Jahn H, Hand I, Haasen Ch, Krausz M. Executive functioning in obsessive-compulsive disorder, unipolar depression and schizophrenia. *Archives on Clinical Neuropsychology* 2002, 17; 477-483.

Motlová L, Koukolík F. Schizofrenie: Neurobiologie, klinický obraz, terapie. 2004; Galén, Praha.

Nadler JD, Richardson ED, Malloy PF, Marran ME, Hosteller Brinson ME. The Ability of the Dementia Rating Scale to Predict Everyday Functioning. *Arch. Clin. Neuropsychol.* 1993;8(5):449-60.

Nelson CHA. Neural plasticity and human development. *Current Directions in Psychological Science* 1999;8(2):42-46.

Nuechterlein KH, Barch DM, Gold JM, Goldberg TE, Green MF, Heaton RK: Identification of separable cognitive factors in schizophrenia. *Schizophrenia research* 2004; 72, (1):29 – 39.

Palmer BW, Heaton RK: Executive dysfunction in schizophrenia. In: Sharma T, Harvey Ph: Cognition in Schizophrenia. Impairments, Importance and Treatment Strategies. 2000. Oxford University Press. New York. 51-73.

Park HS, Shin YW, Ha TH, Shin MS, Kim YY, Lee YO, Kwon JS. Effect of cognitive training focusing on organizational strategies in patients with obsessive-compulsive disorder. *Psychiatry and Clinical Neurosciences* 2006;60:718–726.

Penadés R, Boget T, Lomena F, Mateos J, Catalán R, Gasto C, Salamero M. Could the hypofrontality pattern in schizophrenia be modified through neuropsychological rehabilitation? *Acta Psychiatrica Scandinavica* 2002, 105: 202-208.

Penadés R, Boget T, Catalán R, Bernardo M, Gasto G, Salamero M. Cognitive mechanisms, psychosocial functioning, and neurocognitive rehabilitation in schizophrenia. *Schizophrenia Research* 2003; 63(3):219-227.

Penadés R, Catalán R, Salamero M, Boget T, Puig O, Guarch J, Gasto C. Cognitive remediation therapy for outpatients with chronic schizophrenia: a controlled and randomized study. *Schizophreniae Research* 2006;87(1-3):323-31.

Perglová P. Kognitivní rehabilitace u pacientů se schizofrenií. In Preiss M, Kučerová H et al. Eds. *Neuropsychologie v psychiatrii*. 2006; Grada, Praha.

Preiss M. Klinická neuropsychologie. 1998; Grada, Praha.

Preiss M, Kučerová H et al. eds. Neuropsychologie v psychiatrii. 2006; Grada Publishing, Praha.

Preiss M, Kucerova H, Dockalova E, Stepankova H, Sos P, Holubova M. Cognitive functions patients with unipolar depression in remission. *Psychiatrie* 2008; 12(suppl 3): 63-67.

Premack D, Woodruff G. Does the chimpanzee have a "theory of mind?" Behavioral and Brain Sciences 1978; 4:515 – 526 in: Brüne M. "Theory of Mind" in Schizophrenia: A Review of the Literature. *Schizophrenia Bulletin* 2005; 31:21– 42.

Prouteau A, Verdoux H, Briand C, Alain L, Lalonde P, Nicole L, Reinharz D, Stip E. Self-assessed cognitive dysfunction and objective performance in outpatients with schizophrenia participating in a rehabilitation program. *Schizophrenia Research* 2004; 69 (1):85-91.

Reeder C, Wykes T. A pilot study of a new computerised cognitive remediation program. Schizophrenia *Research 2008*, Volume 102, Issue 1, Pages 272-272

Roder V, Brenner HD, Kienzle N, Hodel B. Schizofrenie: Integrovaný psychoterapeutický program pro schizofrenní pacienty (IPT). 1993; Triton, Praha.

Rodriguez M, Preiss M, Mohr P. Computer-Assisted rehabilitation program of Cognitive Functions in Schizophrenia-Program počítačové rehabilitace kognitivních funkcí u schizofrenie. *Psychiatrie* 2002; 6(suppl. 4):42-45.

Rodriguez M, Mohr P, Preiss M, Krulišová O, Kawaciuková R. First Results of Computer-Assisted Rehabilitation of Cognitive Functions in Schizophrenia-První výsledky počítačové rehabilitace kognitivních funkcí u schizofrenie. *Psychiatrie* 2004;8 (Suppl. 3):71-75.

Rodriguez M. Úvod do problematiky neuropsychologické rehabilitace. In Preiss M, Kučerová H et al. eds. Neuropsychologie v psychiatrii. 2006; Grada, Praha.

Rodriguez M, et al. Augmentation of computer-assisted cognitive remediation with repetitive transcranial magnetic stimulation. In Polišenská V, Šolc M, Kotrlová J eds. Mapping of Psychological Knowledge for Society : 10th European Congress of Psychology : July 3-6, 2007, Prague.Union of Psychologists Associations of the Czech Republic, 2007.

Rodriguez M, Kawaciuková R, Bankovská-Motlová L, Mohr P, Dragomirecká E, Novák T, Preiss M, Šedivá J. Effects of cognitive remediation in schizophrenia patients. European Neuropsychopharmacology 2009;19(Suppl.3):S484-S485.

Rollnik JD., Huber TJ., Mogk H., Siggelkow S., Kropp S., Dengler R., Emrich HM., Schneider U. High frequency repetitive transcranial magnetic stimulation (rTMS) of the dorsolateral prefrontal cortex in schizophrenic patients. *Cognitive Neuroscicence* 2000; 11:4013-4015.

Sachs G. Cognitive Dysfunction and Psychosocial Impairments in Schizophrenia: Non-Pharmacological Aspects of Treatment of Cognitive Deficits. *Journal of Advances in Schizophrenia and Brain Research* 2000; 3(1):2-8.

Sharma T, Harvey Ph: Cognition in Schizophrenia. Impairments, Importance and Treatment Strategies. 2000. Oxford University Press. New York.

Singh S , McDonald P, Murphy B, O'Reilly R. Incidental neurodevelopmental episodes in the etiology of schizophrenia: An expanded model involving epigenetics and development. Minireview. *Clinical Genetics* 2004; 65(6):435-440.

Solé-Padullés C., Bartrés D., Junque C., Clemente I., Molinuevo J., Bargallo N., Sánchez J., Bosch B., Falcon C., Valls-Solé J. Repetitive Transcranial Magnetic Stimulation Effects on Brain Function and Cognition among Elders with Memory dysfunction. A Randomized Sham-Controlled study. *Cerebral Cortex* 2006; 16:1487-1493.

Sternberg RJ. Kognitivní psychologie. 2002; Portál, Praha.

Strakowski SM, Adler CM, DelBello MP. Volumetric MRI studies of mood disorders: do they distinguish unipolar and bipolar disorder? *Bipolar Disord* 2002;4(2):80-8.

Švestková O, Angerová Y. Rehabilitation in CZ - Rehabilitace v ČR. Florence: časopis moderního ošetřovatelství [online] – 2006, č. 3, [cit. 2007-04-08] www.florence.cz/cislo.php?stat=118.

Thatcher RW. EEG operant conditioning (biofeedback) and traumatic brain injury. *Clinical Electroencephalography* 2000;31:38-44.

Torres IJ, Boudreau VG, Yatham LN. Neuropsychological functioning in euthymic bipolar disorder: a meta-analysis. *Acta Psychiatr. Scand. Suppl.* 2007;434:17-26.

Trojan S, Pokorný J. Theoretical aspects of neuroplasticity (Minireview). *Physiological Research* 1999; 48(1): 87-97.

Tůma I, Lenderová Z. Schizofrenie a kognitivní funkce. *Psychiatrie* 2001; 5(4): 275-284.

Twamley EW, Jeste DV, Bellack AS. A Review of Cognitive Training in Schizophrenia. *Schizophrenia Bulletin* 2003; 29(2):359-381.

Van der Gaag M., Kern R.S., Van den Bosch R.J., Liberman, R.P. A controlled trial of cognitive remediation in schizophrenia. *Schizophrenia Bulletin* 2002; 28, 167-176.

Velligan, DI, Bow-Thomas CC, Huntzinger BA, Ritch J, Ledbetter MA, Prihoda TJ, Miller AL. Randomized Controlled Trial of the Use of Compensatory Strategies to Enhance Adaptive Functioning in Outpatients With Schizophrenia. *American Journal of Psychiatry* 2000; 157 (8):1317-1323.

Vernon DJ. Can neurofeedback training enhance performance? An evaluation of the evidence with implications for future research. *Applied Psychophysiology and Biofeedback* 2005;30:347-364.

Wallace CJ, Liberman RP, MacKain SJ, Blackwell G, Eckman TA. Effectiveness and replicability of modules for teaching social and instrumental skills to the severely mentally ill. *Am. J. Psychiatry* 1992; 149:654-658.

Wexler BE, Bell MD. Cognitive Remediation and Vocational Rehabilitation for Schizophrenia. *Schizophrenia Bulletin* 2005; 31(4):931-941.

Wexler BE, Anderson M, Fulbright RK, Gore JC. Preliminary Evidence of Improved Verbal Working Memory Performance and Normalization of Task-Related Frontal Lobe Activation in Schizophrenia Following Cognitive Exercises. *Am. J. Psychiatry* 2000; 157:1694–1697.

Wieloch T, Nikolich K. Mechanisms of neural plasticity following brain injury (Review). *Current Opinion in Neurobiology* 2006; 16(3):258-264.

Wölwer W, Frommann N, Halfmann S, Piaszek A, Streit M, Gaebel W. Remediation of impairments in facial affect recognition in schizophrenia: Efficacy and specificity of a new training program. *Schizophrenia Research* 2005; 80:295 – 303.

Woonings F, Appelo M, Kluiter H, Slooff C, van den Bosch R. Learning (potential) and social functioning in schizophrenia. *Schizophrenia Research* 2002; 59(2-3):287-296.

Wykes T. Cognitive Rehabilitation and Remediation in Schizophrenia. In Sharma T, Harvey P. Cognition in Schizophrenia. 2000; Oxford University Press, New York.

Wykes T, Brammer M, Mellers J, Bray P, Reeder C, Williams C, Conner J. Effects on the brain of a psychological treatment: cognitive remediation therapy. *Brit J. Psychiatry* 2002;181:144-152.

Wykes T, Williams C, Corner J, Rice C, Everitt B. Are the effects of cognitive remediation therapy (CRT) durable? *Schizophrenia Research.* 2003, vol. 61, is. 3, s. 163-174.

Wykes T., Reeder C.: Cognitive remediation therapy for schizophrenia. Theory and practice. 2005; Routledge Taylor and Francis Group.

Wykes T, Reeder C. Translating cognition to action: Improving function in people with schizophrenia [online]. 2005 [cit. 2007-07-13], <http://www.lit.kyushu-u.ac.jp/ito/paper/paper_Wykes.pdf>.

Wykes T, Reeder C., Greenwood K. Improving cognition will improve functioning but only with therapy—cognitive remediation therapy (CRT). In: Morgan K, David A, Murray R. Cognition and schizophrenia: improving real life function. Report based on a conference held at the institute of Psychiatry, London, UK on 16th – 17th September 2004. Cambridge Medical Communication, UK, 2006; 103-109.

Wykes T, Newton E, Landau S, Rice C, Thompson N, Frangou S. Cognitive remediation therapy (CRT) for young early onset patients with schizophrenia: an exploratory randomized controlled trial. *Schizophrenia Research* 2007;94(1-3):221-30.

Wykes T, Reeder C, Landau S, Everitt B, Knapp M, Patel A, Romeo R. Cognitive remediation therapy in schizophrenia: randomized controlled trial. *Br. J. Psychiatry* 2007;190:421-7.

Wykes T, Reeder C, Landau S, Mathiasson P, Hworth E, Htuchinson Ch. Does age matter? Effects of cognitive rehabilitation across the age span. Schizophrenia Research, 2009: 113(2-3):252-8

Yecker S, Borod J, Brozgold A, Martin C, Alpert M, Welkowitz J. Lateralization of Facial Emotional Expression in Schizophrenic and Depressed Paitents. *J. Neuropsychiatry Clin. Neurosciences* 1999; 11 (3): 370-379.

www.baobab.cz

http://www.nimh.nih.gov/health/publications/the-numbers-count-mental-disorders-in-america

www.lumosity.com/guardian.

Part 2. Neuropsychology in Neurology

In: Cognitive Deficit in Mental and Neurological Disorders ISBN: 978-1-60741-957-0
Editors: H. Kucerova, M. Preiss

Chapter VIII

Alzheimer's Disease

Ales Bartos, Miloslava Raisova and Daniela Ripova

Abstract

The neuropsychological examination should support a correct and early diagnosis of Alzheimer's disease by fulfilling the international criteria of the disease. A comprehensive neuropsychological assessment includes examination of global cognitive ability, memory, verbal abilities and language, executive functions and visuospatial functions. These cognitive domains may be examined by physicians using simple and concise tests and by psychologists using more complex methods. Their basic description and appropriate usage in diagnosing Alzheimer's disease and related diseases are given.

Introduction

Dementia is an acquired loss of cognitive abilities that interferes with social, working, and common everyday activities. It is defined in more detail in the diagnostic criteria of the *Diagnostic and Statistic Manual of the American Psychiatric Association* (DSM-IV-TR) (Table 1) (American Psychiatric Association, 2000) or the *International Classification of Diseases, Revision No. 10* (ICD-10). Global deterioration of cognitive functions in dementia always includes a decline in at least two cognitive areas and memory impairment must also always be present. Change in a single cognitive domain is not sufficient for the dementia syndrome. It could correspond to a single-focus brain lesion and not diffuse or multiple processes. Dementia is sometimes considered, in a narrower sense, as a cognitive deficit that is established by neuropsychological tests. However, these tests do not assess impact on the patient's everyday life, which is unavoidable when an obvious cognitive impairment is present.

The most common dementia is Alzheimer's disease (AD), which is the seventh-leading cause of death for people of all ages and the fifth-leading cause of death for those aged 65 and over (2008 AD Facts and Figures).

Table 1. Diagnostic criteria for Dementia (DSM-IV-TR)

Dementia syndrome is characterized by:
1. MEMORY IMPAIRMENT—impaired ability to learn new information or to recall previously learned information.
2. And at least one of the following: a) Language disturbance—APHASIA b) Loss of ability to perform complex tasks involving motor activities despite intact motor function—APRAXIA c) Loss of ability to recognize and use familiar objects— AGNOSIA d) Loss of ability to plan, organize, and execute normal activities—DYSEXECUTIVE SYNDROME
3. Substantial decline from previous abilities cause significant problems in everyday functioning (work, social activities, activities of daily living)
5. The disorder of consciousness (incl. delirium) is not present
6. The course is characterized by gradual onset and continuing cognitive decline.

(Adapted from the American Psychiatric Association. Diagnostic and statistical manual of mental disorders, 4th edition-text revised. (DSM-IV-TR), Washington, DC: 2000.)

It is a disease with an insidious onset and continuous deterioration of memory and other cognitive abilities affecting ability to work and social activities.

1. A definite diagnosis of AD is established on histopathological hallmarks of the disease that are present in individuals who suffered from dementia before their death. The gold standard for determining the etiology of dementia in an individual patient is still histopathological examination of the brain. The clinical diagnosis of AD is based on some degree of probability. AD is correctly diagnosed in 60 to 80% of cases according to clinical-pathological studies (Mendez et al., 1992). In other words, autopsy shows that 20 to 40% of the cases are caused by diseases other than AD, and these patients had been misdiagnosed as AD patients during their life. As a result, guidelines have been developed to increase the likelihood of a correct diagnosis. There are currently four international diagnostic criteria for AD: DSM-IV-TR criteria (APA, 1994) (Table 2)
2. NINCDS-ADRDA criteria (McKhan et al., 1984) (Table 3)
3. ICD-10 criteria (WHO, 1992)
4. New, revised criteria (Dubois et al., 2007) (Table 4)

Table 2. Diagnostic criteria for Dementia of the Alzheimer's type (DSM-IV-TR)

A. The development of multiple cognitive deficits manifested by both (1) memory impairment (impaired ability to learn new information or to recall previously learned information)
(2) one (or more) of the following cognitive disturbances:
(a) aphasia
(b) apraxia
(c) agnosia
(d) dysexecutive syndrome

B. The cognitive deficits in Criteria A1 and A2 each cause significant impairment in social or occupational functioning and represent a significant decline from a previous level of functioning.

C. The course is characterized by gradual onset and continuing cognitive decline.

D. The cognitive deficits in Criteria A1 and A2 are not due to any of other central nervous system or systemic conditions known to cause dementia nor substance-induced conditions

E. The deficits do not occur exclusively during the course of a delirium.

(Adapted from the American Psychiatric Association. Diagnostic and statistical manual of mental disorders, 4th edition-text revised. (DSM-IV-TR), Washington, DC: 2000.)

Table 3. Diagnostic criteria of Alzheimer's disease according to NINCDS–ADRDA (National Institute of Neurological and Communicative Disorders and Stroke and the Alzheimer's Disease and Related Disorders Association)

Criteria for Diagnosis of Probable Alzheimer's Disease:
Dementia established by clinical examination and documented by a standard test of cognitive function (e.g., Mini-Mental State Examination, Blessed Dementia Scale, etc.), and confirmed by neuropsychological tests.
Significant deficiencies in two or more areas of cognition, for example, word comprehension and task-completion ability.
Progressive deterioration of memory and other cognitive functions.
No loss of consciousness.
Onset from age 40 to 90, typically after 65.
No other diseases or disorders that could account for the loss of memory and cognition.
A Diagnosis of Probable Alzheimer's Disease is Supported by:
Progressive deterioration of specific cognitive functions: language (aphasia), motor skills (apraxia), and perception (agnosia).
Impaired activities of daily living and altered patterns of behavior.
A family history of similar problems, particularly if confirmed by neurological testing.
The following laboratory results:
Normal cerebrospinal fluid (lumbar puncture test).
Normal electroencephalogram (EEG) test of brain activity.
Evidence of cerebral atrophy in a series of CT scans.
Other Features Consistent with Alzheimer's Disease
Plateaus in the course of illness progression.
CT findings normal for the person's age.
Associated symptoms, including: depression, insomnia, incontinence, delusions, hallucinations, weight loss, sex problems, and significant verbal, emotional, and physical outbursts.
Other neurological abnormalities, especially in advanced disease, including increased muscle tone and a shuffling gait.
Features That Decrease the Likelihood of Alzheimer's Disease:
Sudden onset.
Such early symptoms as seizures, gait problems, and loss of vision and coordination.

Table 4. New research criteria for the diagnosis of Alzheimer's disease

Probable Alzheimer's disease is characterized by:
A plus one or more supportive features **B, C, or D**

Core diagnostic criteria

A. Presence of an early and significant episodic memory impairment that includes the following features:

1. Gradual and progressive change in memory function reported by patients or informants over more than six months
2. Objective evidence of significantly impaired episodic memory on testing: this generally consists of recall deficit that does not improve significantly or does not normalize with cuing or recognition testing and after effective encoding of information has been previously controlled
3. The episodic memory impairment can be isolated or associated with other cognitive changes at the onset of AD or as AD advances

Supportive features

B. Presence of medial temporal lobe atrophy

Volume loss of hippocampi, entorhinal cortex, amygdala evidenced on magnetic resonance imaging (MRI) with qualitative ratings using visual scoring (referenced to well-characterized population with age norms) or quantitative volumetry of regions of interest (referenced to well-characterized population with age norms)

C. Abnormal cerebrospinal fluid biomarker

Low amyloid β1–42 concentrations, increased total tau concentrations, or increased phospho-tau concentrations, or combinations of the three

D. Specific pattern on functional neuroimaging with PET

Reduced glucose metabolism in bilateral temporal parietal regions

Exclusion criteria

History

- Sudden onset
- Early occurrence of the following symptoms: gait disturbances, seizures, behavioral changes

Clinical features

- Focal neurological features including hemiparesis, sensory loss, visual field deficits
- Early extrapyramidal signs

Other medical disorders severe enough to account for memory and related symptoms

- Non-AD dementia
- Major depression
- Cerebrovascular disease
- Toxic and metabolic abnormalities, all of which may require specific investigations
- MRI FLAIR or T2 signal abnormalities in the medial temporal lobe that are consistent with infectious or vascular insults

Criteria for definite AD

AD is considered definite if the following are present:
Both clinical and histopathological (brain biopsy or autopsy) evidence of the disease, as required by the NIA-Reagan criteria for the post-mortem diagnosis of AD; criteria must both be present

(Modified from Dubois B., Feldman H., et al. Research criteria for the diagnosis of Alzheimer's disease: revising the NINCDS-ADRDA criteria. *Lancet Neurology* 2007; 6: 734-46).

The presence of memory impairment is required in all criteria (in DSM-IV and NINCDS-ADRDA within the definition of dementia). The NINCDS-ADRDA criteria (McKhan et al., 1984) have been, to date, the most frequently used. They underlie the progressive course of multiple cognitive functions (Table 3). New, revised criteria (Dubois et al., 2007) are under debate, if they can be feasibly used worldwide. Memory impairment is again the principal clinical feature. One of the new elements is a combination of typical symptoms together with biological indicators of the disease (mediotemporal atrophy as shown by magnetic resonance imaging of the brain, changes in concentrations of certain proteins in cerebrospinal fluid, and hypometabolism found by positron emission tomography) (Table 4). Thus an early identification of AD may be based on isolated memory impairment without deficits in other cognitive domains. The absence of multiple cognitive deficits is compensated for by the presence of certain biomarkers of AD. Another new feature is reflected by relatively typical memory impairment. It is characterized by a gradual and progressive decline in episodic memory reported by the patient or family members over a period of more than six months. Failure of episodic memory must be objectively demonstrated by testing. Encoding is enhanced by focused attention. Recall deficit does not improve significantly or does not normalize with cuing or recognition testing. Memory impairment in AD will be explained in more detail in other parts of the chapter. The new criteria do not include impairment of self-sufficiency due to dementia.

The neuropsychological examination should, therefore, seek to confirm AD based on the following findings:

1) Memory impairment, especially episodic type
2) Deficit of other cognitive functions: a) aphasia, b) apraxia, c) agnosia, d) alteration of executive functions (e.g., planning, organizing, abstraction)
3) Progressive impairment of memory and other cognitive functions over a course of at least six months

In addition, it is also advisable to assess the global intellectual abilities, attention, and visuospatial abilities. All of these cognitive functions will be discussed in detail in the following sections.

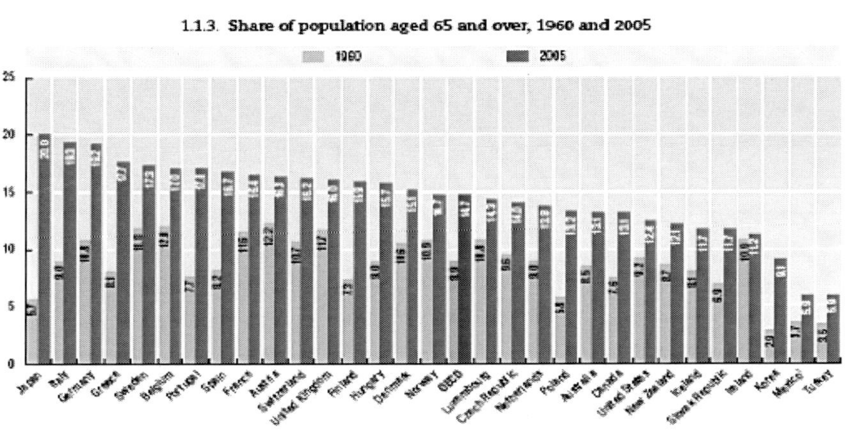

Figure 1. Share of population aged 65 and over, 1960 and 2005 (source: OECD Health Data 2007).

Prevalence

The percentage of the population aged 65 and over in 1960, and in 2005, is shown in Figure 1. The number of Americans with Alzheimer's and other dementias is increasing every year because of the steady growth in the older population. The prevalence of AD is estimated to double every five years between the ages of 65 and 85, starting from 1% of the population at age 60 to 65 years. A half of the population over 95 years is affected. An estimated 5.2 million Americans of all ages had AD in 2008. This figure includes five million people aged 65 and over and 200,000 individuals under age 65. One in eight persons aged 65 and over (13%) has AD. Every 71 seconds, someone in America develops AD (Alzheimer's Disease Facts and Figures, 2008). Women are more likely than men to have AD and other dementias. Fourteen percent of all people age 71 and over have some type of dementia. This includes 16% of women and 11% of men in that age group. Women are more likely to have AD and other dementias because they live long enough to develop these conditions. Additionally, people with fewer years of education are more likely to develop AD (Plassman et al., 2007). The number of Americans surviving into their 80s and 90s is expected to grow because of advances in medicine, social, and environmental conditions. Since the incidence and prevalence of AD increase with age, the number of people with AD will also grow rapidly. By 2050, the number of individuals in America, age 65 and over, with AD could range from 11 million to 16 million (Alzheimer's Disease Facts and Figures, 2008).

Principal Domains of Cognitive Functions

At present, there are a number of different approaches to the measurement of cognitive domains based on: (a) the character of the disease, (b) definitions of Alzheimer's disease, and (c) differential diagnostic purposes. The following cognitive functions should be examined during the neuropsychological examination of patients with suspicion of AD or with AD:

1. Global cognitive ability, general ability, and intelligence
2. Memory functions
3. Language and other instrumental functions
4. Executive functions
5. Visuospatial skills, construction

This categorization of cognitive domains is used to facilitate the description of the different components of brain function. It is obvious that each component is mutually linked with and influences the others (e.g., good memory depends on attention) and a change in a single domain may also affect other domains.

Global Cognitive Ability

Description

General cognitive capacity reflects all cognitive domains together. Based on all available information about the client and results of the neuropsychological examination, we can classify clients into one of the following three levels of performance:

1. *Physiological aging* with normal cognitive abilities within the extent of ±1 standard deviation from the norm.
2. *Mild cognitive impairment,* characterized by weaker performance than that corresponding to the age-matched average performance reduced by 1.5 standard deviation (less than the seventh percentile).
3. *Dementia,* characterized by a performance that is two or more standard deviations below the normal population standard with respect to age and also, optimally, to education (less than the fifth percentile).

We examine the global intellectual capacity of an individual and compare the current state with the premorbid state (level of intellectual abilities prior to disease or brain damage). Cognitive deterioration may be suspect if there is a difference between actual performance and past ability estimates (Table 5). To describe the intellectual abilities of an individual, we assess both verbal and non-verbal components of intellect, mental flexibility (rate of information processing), and executive functions, consisting of logical thinking ability, the ability to draw conclusions, and the ability to solve problems.

Intellect Deterioration in Alzheimer's Disease

In AD, an insidious onset is followed by a slow and irreversible deterioration of all cognitive functions. At the beginning, it is primarily manifested by memory impairment. Since memory is the cornerstone of the entire cognitive system, all other cognitive functions deteriorate as a result of its impairment.

Global intellectual deterioration should be demonstrated through neuropsychological tests. In this sense, diagnostic procedures to assess AD do not differ from those used to assess cognitive deterioration occurring in other brain diseases (e.g., after a stroke).

Memory

Since memory impairment is a typical and the most common sign of AD, it is discussed in more detail.

General Description of Memory Classification

Memory is defined as an ability to accept, process, store, and recall information. Three phases of memory processing may be distinguished for clinical purposes:

a) encoding—receiving information
b) consolidation—processing and maintenance of information
c) retrieval—which can take the form of either:

- immediate recall—related to encoding
- delayed recall

Memory is closely linked to the ability to learn new information. In fact, the basic indicator of brain damage is a failure to learn and the inability to improve one's own performance while repeating this new information. Therefore, the so-called *learning curve* is assessed in memory tests. The curve of patients with a brain disease is pathological (i.e., a flat one with subnormal performances). The curve is fluctuating in patients with pseudodementia, i.e., influenced by a depressive episodes, increased anxiousness, fatigue, etc. Thus, in these patients, performance may be within normal standards, subnormal or above normal. The learning curve in healthy persons without any brain disease has an increasing trend.

Several types of memory are covered under the general term "memory." The different types are classified based on various viewpoints. With respect to AD and from the viewpoint of clinical practice, it is suitable to classify memory with respect to (1) content, (2) time, and (3) recall strategy.

Memory Classification by Content

1. *verbal memory*
2. *visuospatial memory (non-verbal)*

Other Classification by Content (Squire, 1988)

1. *Declarative (explicit) memory* contains material that is accessible to conscious recall. In turn, it is divided into two subtypes:
    a. Episodic memory is related to experienced events (= episodes) from personal history (memories of experiences, autobiography, etc.).
    b. Semantic memory is used for factual material (facts, data, encyclopedic knowledge, etc.).
2. *Non-declarative (procedural, implicit) memory* provides motor skills and automated activities (e.g., sewing, cycling, or playing a musical instrument). Its activity is not related to language, cannot be described by words (therefore, it is called non-declarative) and recall is not conscious.

Memory Classification by Time

1. *Anterograde memory* = ability to learn new information for the future
2. *Retrograde memory* = ability to recall older information from the past (well-known events, autobiographic experience, etc.).
    a. Information obtained recently (short-term memory)
    b. Information obtained a long time ago (remote memory, long-term memory)

Memory Classification by Recall Strategy

1. *Free recall*—most difficult type of recall, involving unaided recall of information
2. *Cued recall*—moderately difficult; a cue is offered to assist recall, either by category, to which the information being recalled belongs (semantic cue, e.g., the recalled word/picture belongs to the category of animals), or the first letters of the word to be recalled are offered (lexical cue, e.g., mo-.. mother).
3. *Recognition*—easiest; a list of options is provided, from which the information to be recalled is selected.

Memory Changes in Alzheimer's Disease

Memory impairment is called amnesia. In AD, both memory storage *(encoding)* and reproduction *(recall)* are affected. AD patients have reduced *free recall* (can only recall a limited number of items), use of *cues are only partially helpful* and *confabulations occur.* Episodic and semantic memories are also affected. On the other hand, implicit memory is usually preserved (e.g., motor skills). Memories of the distant past (e.g., life experiences from childhood) are preserved best. *Problems with orientation in time* are a frequent and prominent symptom of AD. Therefore, all screening tests for AD contain questions pertaining to this symptom (date, day of the week, month, season, and year).

Memory changes in AD are manifested by several typical features.

Impairment of anterograde memory in Alzheimer's disease

This impairment is the most common in AD. It is manifested by the inability to remember recent events, new names, etc. Due to some specialization of the hemispheres, we can identify either an *impairment in verbal memory* (the left hemisphere—decreased ability to remember written/auditory information) or an *impairment in visual memory* (right hemisphere—impaired recall of naming of people, impaired memory of faces, problems with spatial orientation, etc.).

An impairment of anterograde memory in separate phases of the memory process is manifested by the following characteristic symptoms of AD:

a. *Encoding*—dysfunction is manifested in the latter stages of the disease, after the alteration of recall; it occurs in an advanced stage of memory impairment (the patient is unable to store information).
b. *Consolidation and storage*—relatively quick forgetfulness and loss of information, which means that the patient cannot keep new information in his/her memory for extended periods of time.
c. *Recall*
   - *delayed* recall is affected more and earlier than free recall
   - poor *free* recall
   - *cue* or *recognition*—an item from a list is either only partially effective or ineffective
   - *confabulations* occur (filling of gaps in the patient's memory with false information that the patient believes is accurate and true)

Impairment of the Retrograde Memory in Alzheimer's Disease

In patients with AD, a phenomenon called temporal gradient, or Ribot's rule (Ribot described this phenomenon as early as 1882) occurs. Patients with AD first forget recent events and information while their recall of information from the distant past is well preserved. Patients can remember their experiences from many years ago but are unable to describe what happened just a short while before. Long-term memory is impaired with further advancement of the disease (Kopelman, 2001).

Verbal Abilities and other Instrumental Functions and their Impairment in Alzheimer´s Disease

Language, praxis, and gnostic function are closely linked with the activity of the brain's grey cortex and, therefore, they are present in cortical dementias. A typical cortical dementia is represented by Alzheimer's disease. Such impairment is part of the diagnostic criteria of dementia according to DSM-IV.

The first problems include difficult recall of words that are replaced with circumlocution (anomia, anomic or amnestic aphasia). Speech becomes more vague and content poor. The inability to express one's self adequately is disguised by social or trite phrases. Patients often use various categories, for instance "that animal" and substitute pronouns (e.g., he, it, that) for names. Paraphasia may occur (speech impairment manifested by incorrect substitution of one letter/word for another). Difficulty in comprehension is often wrongly considered to be a hearing impairment, which is also common in seniors. Conversation difficulties significantly affect coexistence with close relations (sometimes more than the memory disorder). Repetition is usually relatively well preserved, unless memory impairment is already present. Language abilities gradually deteriorate to a stage of total aphasia.

Patients with AD often show *alexia, agraphia, and acalculia. Prosopagnosia* (inability to identify familiar faces) and *visual object agnosia a*re common. *Anosognosia* is a typical early sign. *Apraxia* (the inability to perform a movement with a body part despite intact sensory and motor function) is another clinical feature of AD.

Executive Functions and their Impairment in Alzheimer's Disease

An impairment of executive functions is called *dysexecutive syndrome* or *executive dysfunction*. It is an *impairment of understanding, planning, and organization of actions* (the working memory is the base for such activities). Dysexecutive syndrome occurs in various dementias and forms a part of the diagnostic criteria of dementia. Dysexecutive syndrome includes the following symptoms: impairment of working memory, problems with drawing-up a plan and its implementation, difficulties in problem-solving (especially if it is necessary to use new combinations of existing knowledge), problems in action planning, in abstraction and cognitive flexibility, and difficulties with attention and concentration. Typical signs include, for instance, low verbal fluency, scant use of language, verbal stereotypes and echolalia, perseverance, recall impairment, attention disorders, specific thinking, disinhibition, inability of adaptation, and uncontrolled behavior (Waldemar et al., 2007).

In AD, dysexecutive syndrome is not usually prominent; however, it is rather typical in the moderate and advanced stages of AD.

Visuospacial Functions and their Impairment in Alzheimer's Disease

Visuospatial abilities guarantee orientation in space and contribute to maintenance of proper spatial relations. In patients with AD, problems with visuospatial functions occur relatively early. They are manifested by so-called **topographic disorientation.** At first, disrupted orientation occurs in unknown or less-known environments; later, patients become lost in formerly well-known environments and, finally, disorientation occurs at home.

In the neuropsychological examination, we use tests that are sensitive to spatial relations, right-left orientation, or orientation in body scheme. AD patients show signs of *visuoconstructional apraxia*. In the clinical settling, such abilities are well evaluated by various drawing tests.

Examination and Tests

A natural part of every examination is a detailed interview and case history, including education and age. If the patient suffers from dementia, such information should be obtained from a person who knows the patient well. A patient with mild cognitive impairment (MCI, see later) is able to provide such information themselves. The MCI patients often complain of difficulties in cognitive functions, most frequently with regard to the memory. However, they are capable of normal activities of daily living. Therefore, MCI and dementia patients differ in their abilities to carry out normal everyday activities. Patients with minor dementia are often able to provide relevant information regarding their lives. However, confirmation by? a close relation is usually a good idea in such cases.

Only some of the most frequently used methods of neuropsychological testing used in AD are given in this section. The text is divided into the same cognitive areas as previously described. Each section has been divided to a part for physicians—non-psychologists—containing short tests, and a part for psychologists, containing formal neuropsychological assessments. We have chosen the most suitable tests for practical use from the list of various tests. A detailed review of all neuropsychological testing for Alzheimer's disease is beyond the scope of this chapter, but is readily available from other sources (Lezak et al., 2004; Spreen, 1998).

Global Cognitive Ability

Tests Suitable for Physicians and Psychologists

In practice, there are several brief tests that can quickly, easily, and informatively determine global cognitive capacity in AD patients. They are routinely used by non-psychologists (e.g., physicians or nurses) because of their ease and speed of administration.

Mini-Mental State Examination (MMSE)

The Mini-Mental State Examination (MMSE) (Folstein et al., 1975) is the most frequently used method for the determination of global cognitive function and for detection of the presence and severity of dementia syndrome. The test consists of ten subtests that assess the patient's orientation in time/space, short-term memory, calculation abilities, attention, reading, writing, language, and construction-practical skills. Administration of the test takes five to ten minutes. The maximal score on the MMSE is 30 points; the higher the score, the better the performance. A score of 26 to 25 points is a borderline finding; dementia begins at 24 (mild dementia 24 to 18, moderate dementia 17 to 6, severe dementia < 6). Moderate dementia from normal aging can be reliably separated using the test. Since the tasks are relatively undemanding, those with MCI cannot be reliably identified with the test (patients with MCI have scores similar to healthy individuals). The advantage of the MMSE rests in its convenient administration without any complex aids, short administration, and quantification of the deficit. Its disadvantages are that it lacks testing of executive functions and its dependence on age and education. Thus, patients with higher levels of education may reach normal values despite the presence of dysfunction. On the other hand, people with lower levels of education may score lower despite the absence of impairment. The MMSE should be considered a basic method that should be evaluated with respect to other test results. The test is suitable for general physicians, neurologists, psychiatrists, and geriatricians for initial evaluation, monitoring of progression of AD, and the effect of treatment.

Clock Drawing Test (CDT)

The patient is asked to draw a clock face with numbers and place the hands so that the requested time is shown. It is a popular, informative, and simple test that covers several cognitive functions—from spatial memory through the visuomotor coordination up to semantic memory and the ability to plan and concentrate. The CDT is a complex task requiring little time (one to three minutes). The CDT provides a relatively broad assessment of information with respect to cognitive functions. Because of an indefinite number of test variations, its disadvantage lies in inconsistent and often difficult scoring, regardless of which scoring system is used. The following assessment scales are frequently used: Hendriksen's five- to three-point scale, Sunderland's ten-point scale, and Shulman's five-point scale (Hendriksen et al., 1993; Sunderland et al., 1989; Shulman et al., 1986). The CDT is an informative test but must be complemented with other tests. Its use with the MMSE is common. In this case, an examination of cognitive functions is completed with an assessment of frontal and visuospatial functions. It may be administered by physicians or other health care workers in everyday practice.

Seven-Minute Screen Test (7 MST)

A short battery called the Seven-Minute Screen Test (7MST) has been developed using new neuropsychological knowledge to improve detection of dementia (Solomon et al., 1998). It consists of four brief subtests that assess various, typically impaired, cognitive domains in AD: 1) orientation in time, 2) memory, 3) visuospatial abilities and visuoconstruction, and 4) verbal fluency. Its administration takes longer than the name of the test suggests (about ten minutes). A complicated calculation involving all four subscores results a number that reflects the probability of AD. Individuals with values of 0.7 to 1.0 have a high probability of having AD. On the other hand, a low probability is indicated by values between 0 to 0.3. The zone between these extremes is ambiguous and requires follow-up and retesting. The test is useful as part of a rapid evaluation and aims to assess typical deficits in AD with patient-friendly administration. It requires no clinical judgment and minimal training. The use of the test is limited by the need for a pre-prepared set of standard pictures and final calculation of probability that requires a computer. The test may be administered by a physician or other health care worker after a short training period.

Addenbrooke's Cognitive Examination—Revised (ACE-R)

A new short test called the Addenbrooke's Cognitive Examination-Revised (ACE-R) is a simple bedside test battery containing improved psychometric features that are not included in the MMSE (Mioshi et al., 2006).

The test contains the MMSE, which is extended by other tasks evaluating additional cognitive functions in more detail. Generally, it consists of 18 subtests that assess five basic cognitive functions: 1) attention and orientation, 2) memory (short-term memory and delayed recall), 3) verbal fluency, 4) language, and 5) visuospatial abilities. The administration of the test takes approximately 20 to 30 minutes, depending on cognitive deficit. The maximum score is 100 points; the higher the score, the better the patient's cognitive functions. The cut-off values are usually between 82 to 88 points. The benefit of the test includes a more detailed examination of different memory types and visuospatial skills, subtests for executive functions, , and more complex language assessment. In addition to the total score, the cognitive profile may be obtained using the subscores of the five cognitive domains.

However, the benefits of the test are counterbalanced by a longer administration time and are, therefore, not suitable for monitoring cognitive deterioration in everyday practice. The principal value of the ACE-R rests in its differential diagnosis of dementias and detection of early impairment of cognitive functions, especially in Alzheimer's disease and frontal-temporal dementia. It may be administered by physicians or other health care workers.

Alzheimer's Disease Assessment Scale (Adas)

The Alzheimer's Disease Assessment Scale (ADAS-Cog., ADAS-Non-Cog.) (Rosen et al., 1984) is a complex scale that is focused on cognitive and non-cognitive (behavioral) changes specific for AD. It consists of 21 items; 11 cognitive items and 10 non-cognitive items. The cognitive part includes assessment of memory, language, praxis, and orientation. The non-cognitive part contains items related to psychiatric symptoms (e.g., mood, perception, and thinking). The administration of the ADAS takes approximately 20 minutes. The maximum score of the cognitive part is 70 points; the higher the score, the more pronounced the cognitive deficit. Values between 0 to 10 points are normal findings, which is typical for healthy people. Scores between 11 to 21 points are ambiguous and may indicate patients at risk of developing AD (possible mild cognitive impairment) and scores greater than 22 points indicate suspected dementia. In the non-cognitive part of the test, the maximum score is 50 points. An advantage of this test is a more complex evaluation of cognitive functions within a relatively short period of time. The disadvantage is that the scores are approximate. The test has not yet been standardized. Several standardized tools (e.g., envelope, card, pencil, watch, comb, flower, and whistle) must be available for testing. The test may by administered by a physician or a health care worker after training. The test is most frequently used in clinical trials for evaluation of therapeutic effects.

Dementia Rating Scale (DRS)

The Dementia Rating Scale (DRS) (Mattis, 1988) is a screening test consisting of 37 tasks. Five cognitive areas can be assessed: 1) attention, 2) initiation and perseveration (ability to start and independently complete certain activities), 3) construction (drawing of geometric/other shapes), 4) conceptualization (ability of abstraction), and 5) memory.

The DRS-2 incorporates the original 36 DRS tasks and 32 stimuli, yielding five subscale scores together with an assessment of the patient's overall level of cognitive functioning. The five DRS-2 subscales provide additional information on specific abilities including Attention (8 items), Initiation/Perseveration (11 items), Construction (6 items), Conceptualization (6 items), and Memory (5 items). Stimulus items consist of material familiar to most individuals.

The administration of the test takes approximately 20 to 30 minutes. The highest score on the DRS is 144 points; the higher the score, the better the cognitive function. The definition of the cut-off score for incipient dementia varies according to various authors. Mattis recommends a cut-off score of 137 for the evaluation of dementia. Most healthy, elderly people reach a score within the range 140 to 144 points. Cut-off scores have also been proposed for each of the five cognitive areas. Mattis recommends the norms of Montgomery and Costa, who suggest the following values for cut-offs (two standard deviations below the average): attention = 32 points, initiation = 29 points, construction = 4 points, concept = 32 points, memory = 19 points. The DRS is a suitable scale to detect cognitive decline and provides a profile of cognitive domains. One may benefit from shortening the administration by skipping of some tasks in individuals who can cope with similar but even more difficult tasks. It also provides better evaluation of subcortical cognitive functions. The test is not overly difficult to administer and evaluate. However, standard tools should be used for its administration. It may also be used by non-psychologists after training.

Tests for Psychologists

Wechsler Adult Intelligence Scale-Revised (Wais-R)

The Wechsler Adult Intelligence Scale-Revised (WAIS-R) (Wechsler, 1981) is a well-known test, and thus it is described only briefly. The WAIS-R test assesses: 1) the current intellectual capacity of an individual, 2) his/her premorbid intellectual abilities, and 3) information on the structure of mental capacity. Deterioration of global cognitive abilities may be evaluated according to the following indicators:

1. **Overall IQ**
   An intellectual capacity less than IQ 70 is suggestive of dementia.

2. **Comparison of premorbid intellectual performance (subtests Information and Vocabulary) with the current intellectual level** (Table 5)
3. **Differences between verbal and non-verbal IQs** (Table 6)

Table 5. Differences between premorbid and current intellectual level

The difference in points	Level of deterioration
0 to 12	Without deterioration
13 to 19	Mild deterioration
20 to 34	Moderate deterioration
35 and higher	Severe deterioration

Table 6. Differences between verbal and nonverbal IQ

The difference in points	Level of deterioration
0 to 12	Normal, healthy individuals
13 to 14	Suspected difference
15 and higher	Probable deterioration

The WAIS-R is an essential part of the neuropsychological examination in cases where cognitive decline is suspected. Because of the level difficulty, the test is not used with patients having advanced dementia. It is not appropriate to use it in patients with an MMSE of less than about 20 points. The test provides comprehensive information on the level of all cognitive functions, comparison of performance of the examined patient with population norms, and comparison of the current cognitive state compared with the premorbid state. However, the administration and evaluation is lengthy (it takes about one to two hours). This test is exclusively used by psychologists.

Memory Tests

The following is a brief overview of some neuropsychological tests used to assess memory in AD. The majority of memory tests are based on repeated presentation of stimuli (words, pictures) that the patient is to remember. Then the patient is asked to recall (immediately or later), both by free recall and cued recall or by recognition from a list of items. When we evaluate memory, we assess it as a whole, its different subtypes, and the "learning curve."

Tests Suitable for Physicians or Psychologists

In AD, the first memory assessment can be carried out using the following simple tests:

1) Anterograde memory—to remember three words, an address or a sentence and then to recall the information after a short time.
2) Retrograde memory

2a) Recent memory—orientation in time, place, and close contacts; type of last meal that the patient had; patient's last activity; main events in the country or in the family; time sequencing and moving from one place to another, etc.

2b) Long-term memory—important information from the distant past (e.g., date of birth, date of marriage, the place where one worked, recent presidents, etc.).

An elementary assessment of memory is also contained in tests for assessment of global cognitive abilities, such as the MMSE, 7MST, ACE-R, and ADAS, DRS.

Logical Memory Test

This test is sometimes referred to as "Stories." It is a part of the Wechsler Memory Scale (Wechsler, 1997). The test contains two stories (A and B), which are read to the patient (story A is read once and then story B is read twice). The patient then recounts what he/she remembers from the stories. The patient is asked to recall both stories after 25 to 35 minutes. Then a total score of retention is recorded (sum of the correctly recalled items of stories A and B) and scores of correctly recalled items separately in each story (logical memory I and II). The test may be completed with recognition. The test determines the level of auditory episodic short-term (immediate recall) and long-term memory (delayed recall), ability to "learn something new" and quality of consolidation and retention of information. The administration of the test takes about 15 minutes. The evaluation may be done both quantitatively and qualitatively. The performance of an individual may be compared with age-matched population norms available for the WMS-III (1997). The average performance in persons between 55 to 89 years of age on Logical memory test I is about 32 points (the pathologic value is about 20 points or less), the average performance for Logical memory test II is about 16 points (the pathological value is about 7 points or less) and the total retention score is about 24 points (the pathological value is about 14 points or less). The interpretation of the test is unfortunately dependent on age and education. On the other hand, memory is assessed in detail, and it can be carried out by non-psychologists. A data sheet is necessary for the test.

Tests for Psychologists

Wechsler Memory Scale (WMS)

The Wechsler Memory Scale (WMS-III) (Wechsler, 1997) is a complex, standardized and well-known test. It consists of seven subtests (information, orientation, calculation, logical memory—stories, number repetition, visual reproduction, and associative learning) and their result is a memory quotient (MQ), which is comparable with the IQ score of the WAIS-R (an average of 100, SD 15). The test assesses auditory and visual memory, both short-term (immediate recall) and long-term (delayed recall). Its administration is relatively lengthy (about one hour), which is a disadvantage of the test. Therefore, only certain isolated subtests are used during the evaluation of patients with AD in neuropsychological practice. The most common is the "Logical Memory" (Stories) or the "Visual Reproduction" subtest. The WMS-III is difficult and unsuitable for patients with advanced cognitive deficits. The advantage of the test is its comprehensive evaluation of all memory types and MQ. It enables a comparison of the memory ability of the patient with a standard. It is exclusively used by psychologists.

California Verbal Learning Test (CVLT)

The likely inspiration for the California Verbal Learning Test (CVLT) (Delis et al., 1987) is the well-known RAVLT (Rey Auditory Verbal Learning Test) (Rey, 1958). Both tests are quite similar in their principles and structures, and they both assess verbal learning. The CVLT differs mainly in the areas of categorical recall, recognition, and arrangement of testing material, i.e., association and category links between words, which are not present in the RAVLT. The objective of CVLT is to remember and subsequently recall a set of words that is presented in both written and verbal forms. This list is repeated several times and learning is monitored ("learning curve"). The first part of the test involves immediate recall of the submitted words. Then delayed recall after interference (distraction or other testing) is assessed. Lastly, delayed recall after longer interval and recognition are also examined. In cases of decreased free recall, cues are provided and any improvement is noted. The CVLT has several alternatives that differ from each other in administration and assessment criteria. Its administration takes about 20 to 25 minutes. However, if the latency phase is added, the whole test takes 45 to 50 minutes in healthy persons and slightly more in persons having memory deficits. The test is an instrument for accurate and detailed memory evaluation. Its disadvantage is that it is time-consuming and complex to administer. The CVLT is one of the most frequently used neuropsychological tests in the North America and one of the most common diagnostic tools used by clinical psychologists (Woods et al., 2006).

Benton's Visual Retention Test (VRT)

The Visual Retention Test (Benton, 1972), first published in 1945, is one of best-known and commonly used examinations in psycho-diagnostic practice. It is a test of non-verbal, immediate (recent) memory for visuospatial inputs. Visuomotor coordination is another component. It is an important part in determination of cognitive deficits in patients with organic brain damage. Because of its general familiarity, it's not essential to give a detailed description at this point. It is only used by psychologists.

Assessment of Language and Instrumental Functions

Language should be evaluated throughout the entire examination. Attention should be paid with regard to verbal fluency and methods of expression, content, ability to use appropriate words, and whether the patient is struggling to fine words or paraphasia occurs. Extensive use of pronouns (this, that, it, etc.) and general categories ("that animal") may indicate a language deficit. Comprehension should be also assessed (e.g., pointing to an object, questions with yes-no answers, naming of objects, or responses to complex commands). In AD, information gained from interviews and short tests are sufficient to evaluate language and instrumental functions. The patient should tell a story or describe a period of his/her life (e.g., professional career, childhood, place where he/she was born, a recent story, etc.). Language is assessed during all screening tests, and such tests also usually contain subtests related to other instrumental functions. The following tests offer detailed assessments of language impairment: Western Aphasia Battery (Kertesz, 1979), Token Test (De Renzi, 1962) or Boston Naming Test (Kaplan et al., 1983).

The Individual Instrumental Functions and Their Examination:

Alexia: The patient should read a sentence or follow directions in accordance with written instructions (MMSE) or should read an extract from a book or magazine.

Agraphia: The patient should write down a sentence (MMSE) or a short message, or signature.

Acalculia: repeated subtractions of seven starting from 100 (MMSE), perform simple calculations, simple addition either by mental arithmetic or counting the things on a table, etc.

Apraxia: The patient should perform certain task, e.g., to write an address on an envelope, insert a letter and prepare for dispatching (ADAS); the patient is encouraged to show certain operations. The order and way they carry out the operation or task is observed (e.g., to salute, take off their hat, light a cigarette, brush their teeth, hammer a nail into the wall, etc.).

Testing of Executive Functions

In the assessment of frontal functions, it is important to know that mild dysexecutive syndrome may occur even in healthy people of advanced age. Therefore, test results should be interpreted with caution. Minor executive dysfunction may not be noticed during normal examination.

Tests for Physicians and Psychologists

Frontal Assessment Battery

The Frontal Assessment Battery (FAB) (Dubois et al., 2000) is a short, bedside, cognitive and behavioral battery used to assess frontal lobe functions. The battery consists of six subtests exploring the following: conceptualization, mental flexibility, motor programming, sensitivity to interference, inhibitory control, and environmental autonomy. The third subtest (sequence of movements) is a sensitive frontal test also known as *Luria's sequences.* This test assesses motor programming and is often used separately. The patient is instructed to repeat a series of three hand movements (fist – edge – palm). The administration of the whole FAB test is relatively short, between five and ten minutes. A cut off score for AD is approximately 13 and for frontotemporal dementia the cut off is eight points. The FAB is easy to administer at bedside and is sensitive to frontal lobe dysfunction. The advantage of the FAB lies in its ease of administration and evaluation. However, it is only an elementary assessment, requiring further, more detailed examinations. The test is suitable both for physicians and psychologists.

4.4.1.2. Verbal Fluency Test (VFT)

The patient is asked to name as many words as possible according to a certain rule in a limited period of time, usually one minute. VFT is a test with overlap between executive and memory abilities (semantic memory) and also includes attention. Two principal types are used: 1) phonetic VFT (naming as many words beginning with certain letter, e.g., with F, A, or S as possible) and 2) category (semantic) VFT (e.g., animals, fruits, etc.). Young adults can produce 20 animals, 15 animals is low average, and less than 10 is definitely impaired. Letter fluency is usually more difficult (a score of 15 words per letter is normal) (Kipps, 2005). In addition to total production of words, the number of repetitions and presence of confabulations are also determined. VFT is significantly reduced in patients with AD in comparison with healthy individuals and both repetitions and confabulations are more frequent. The test of production of as many animals in one minute as possible is a classical test of executive functions and semantic memory. This test is not based on episodic memory and deteriorates relatively early in the course of AD (Vandeberghe, 2005). In patients with AD, semantic fluency is disproportionately more affected than phonetic fluency (words beginning with a certain letter) (Duff et al., 2004; Kipps, 2005). A result of less than 12 animals is almost always abnormal (Vandeberghe, 2005). Animal fluency scores of less than 15 animals were 20 times more likely in a patient with AD than in controls subjects without dementia. Animal naming is also reduced in patients with MCI (Duff et al., 2004). Therefore, a one-minute semantic fluency test can assist in early detection of dementia in the memory clinic setting. On the other hand, the VFT of words beginning with certain letter and vocabulary (Vocabulary part of the WAIS-R) is stable in the preclinical phase and even in the early stages of AD (Saxton et al., 2004).

Tests for Psychologists

4.4.2.1 Trail Making Test (TMT)

The Trail Making Test (TMT) is a classic, simple, and short test of executive functions, psychomotor speed, and working memory. It has two variants. In version A (TMT-A) there are rings containing numbers 1 to 25 randomly placed on a paper, and the patient is to link all the rings with lines. The duration of this task is measured. An analogical version B (TMT-B) is more complex since it is necessary to alternate a number and a letter following the principle of step-wise increase (1-A, 2-B, 3-C, etc.). The second variant of the test is particularly sensitive to organic brain damage, and patients with cognitive deficits usually fail. This test is difficult for patients with moderate or advanced AD. An advantage of the test is the existence of standards and an opportunity to compare an individual's performance with age-matched norms. The test is influenced by education. This fact should be taken into account during interpretation of the time required to complete it. TMT is used by psychologists.

Testing of Visuospatial Functions

A part of visuospatial ability is topographic orientation and involves assessment of orientation in unknown/known places in the neighborhood of the patient's home and in the home environment. The patient is questioned regarding details of his/her current location (e.g., town, floor, etc.). In addition, the patient is questioned regarding the course of common activities of daily living (traveling, dressing, meal preparation, writing, and posting a letter, etc.).

In the neuropsychological examination, visuospatial functions are mainly assessed using various drawing tests. It is useful to distinguish between constructional apraxia (if cues or a model of a picture does not help to copy it) and impairment of semantic memory or imagination (e.g., the patient does not know what a cube looks like but, after seeing a picture of a cube, can draw it).

Drawing of interlocking pentagons or a wire cube, or the Clock Drawing Test, are classical tests of constructional apraxia. It is also possible to use isolated subtests of the WAIS-R ("Block Design" and "Picture Arrangement"). Benton's visual retention test or the Trail Making Test are often used for assessment of visuospatial abilities.

Overview of Tests for Assessment of Cognitive Domains

In conclusion to the section of test methods, we summarized all tests divided according to separate cognitive domains in Table 7. Simple tests for non-psychologists (e.g., physicians) and comprehensive batteries for psychologists are proposed for each domain.

Table 7. Psychological assessment of cognitive domains

Cognitive domains	Tests for psychologists	Options for non-psychologists
GLOBAL COGNITIVE ABILITY		
Deterioration of cognitive functions	WAIS-R (WAIS-III)	
Premorbid level of intellect	1. WAIS-R (WAIS-III) 2. Subtests from WAIS-R "Information" or "Vocabulary"	Judgment according to the level of education and profession.
Current level of intellect	1. WAIS-R 2. Raven's Progressive Matrices (suitable for language Disorders)	
Screening of dementia	1. MMSE, ACE, ADAS cog, 7MST, DRS 2. Clock Drawing test	1. MMSE, ACE, ADAS cog, 7MST, DRS 2. Clock Drawing test
MEMORY		
Global assessment of memory	WMS	
Immediate Memory	1. MMSE, ACE, 7MST, DRS, ADAS cog. 2. subtest from WAIS-R "Digit Span" 3. subtest from WMS "Visual Recall" 4. Benton Visual Retention Test	1. MMSE (subtraction of number 7 from number 100 – repetition 5 times) and remembering words "shovel – scarf – vase" 2. Repetition of short lines of numbers (forward and backwards direction)
Delayed Recall	1. WMS 2. subtest from WMS "Logical Memory" (Stories) 3. CVLT 4. DRS 5. Rey-Osterrieth Complex Figure Test	Repetition of 3 words in MMSE ("shovel – scarf – vase") after a longer time interval (e.g., after 20 minutes) or repetition address in ACE.
Cued Recall	1. CVLT 2. 7MST 3. Memory Capacity Test (Buschke)	1. 7MST
Episodic Memory	Questions such as: What did you have for dinner last night? Who did you meet yesterday? What channel did you watch yesterday?	The same as "Tests for psychologists."
Semantic Memory	1. WAIS-R 2. 7MST 3. Verbal Fluency Test 4. Questions about general knowledge, e.g., "How many months does a year have?"	General information – questions such as: How many months are there in one year? Where is London? What is the capital of Japan? Who wrote a book ... ?

Table 7. (Continued)

Cognitive domains	Tests for psychologists	Options for non-psychologists
LANGUAGE AND OTHER INSTRUMENTAL FUNCTIONS	1. Western Aphasia Battery 2. Token test 3. Screening Assessment of Aphasia 4. Interview with the patient 5. Spontaneous discussion about certain topics (e.g., employment, city of birth…)	1. Interview with the patient 2. Spontaneous discussion about certain topics (e.g., employment, city of , birth, childhood, hobbies...)
Aphasia		
Alexia	1. MMSE 2. Reading of short story	The same as "Tests for psychologists."
Agraphia	1. MMSE 2. Writing of short paragraph, short sentence, signature	The same as "Tests for psychologists."
Acalculia	1. WAIS-R (subtest "Arithmetic") 2. MMSE (subtraction of number 7 from number 100 – repetition (5 times)	1. MMSE (subtraction of number 7 from the number 100 - five times) 2. Counting simple examples
Apraxia	1. Writing a letter and getting ready to mail it out (subtest from ADAS cog.) 2. Specific questions about certain everyday activities (dressing up, preparing meals) 3. Demonstration of certain tasks (taking hat off, light up a cigarette…)	The same as ""Tests for psychologists."
EXECUTIVE FUNCTIONS Dysexecutive Syndrome	1. Verbal Fluency test 2. Trail Making Test 3. DRS (subtests "Alternating Movements") 4. Luria's Fist-Edge-Palm test 5. Wisconsin Card Sorting Test 6. Design Fluency Test	1. Luria's Fist-Edge-Palm test 2. DRS (subtests "Alternating Movements") 3. Verbal Fluency Test
VISUOSPACIAL FUNCTIONS	1. Clock Drawing Test 2. MMSE (drawing of pentagons) 3. 7MST (subtest Clock Drawing Test) 4. ACE, ADAS cog., DRS 5. Rey-Osterrieth Complex Figure Test 6. Benton Visual Retention Test 7. WAIS-R subtests "Block Design" and "Digit Symbol" 8. Trail Making Test	1. Clock Drawing Test 2. MMSE (drawing of pentagons) 3. 7MST (subtest Clock Drawing Test) 4. ACE, ADAS cog., DRS

Course of the Cognitive Deficit

Concept of Mild Cognitive Impairment

Mild cognitive impairment (MCI) is a transient phase between cognitive changes during normal aging and early dementia. Individuals with MCI are at an increased risk of conversion to probable AD (15% a year) (Petersen et al., 1999). Patients with MCI are, however, a heterogeneous group. From the point of view of a prognosis, some MCI subjects may become AD patients, while cognitive capacity of other MCI subjects does not change for many years or even slightly improves. In terms of a cognitive profile, two groups of MCI subjects can be identified: 1) patients with purely memory deficits without impairment in other cognitive domains, and 2) patients who also suffer from impairment of other cognitive domains in addition to amnestic syndrome. MCI patients in the second group show a higher risk of AD development than patients with amnestic MCI (Tabert et al., 2006).

Early Neuropsychological Changes in the Old Age with Risk of Alzheimer's Disease Development

In recent years, an intensive effort has been directed toward identifying neuropsychological changes, even in normal aging, which suggest future deterioration to AD. Some cognitive dysfunctions are associated with a more probable development of AD in 2 to 15 years. The earliest signs include impairment in the following domains (Saxton et al., 2004; Tabert et al., 2006; Tirney et al., 2005; Vandenberghe 2005): episodic memory, semantic memory, verbal memory—immediate and delayed verbal recall, executive functions/psychomotor speed, abstract thinking, and visual memory.

Individuals show cognitive changes in neuropsychological tests as early as 1.5 to 8 years before the onset of AD. The worst results were found in the group of individuals closest to AD development: verbal, visual and global memory and delayed recall (WMS), lower number of fruits named in one minute (fVFT), and Trail Making Test A (TMT-A). Impaired performance in four tests (global memory and delayed recall in the WMS, fVFT, and TMT-B) was significantly associated with the onset of AD within 3.5 to 8 years. The deficits in two memory tests (verbal memory and delayed recall) preceded AD development by five to eight years (Saxton et al., 2004).

Unfortunately, nearly half of the individuals with preclinical AD (46%) did not show any cognitive impairment during the years preceding AD. Patients in this group were among the most educated. They were able to compensate for their deficits thanks to their higher education. On the other hand, some individuals who suffered from various cognitive deficits did not go on to develop AD. Subjects in this group were the oldest and least educated. Therefore, it may be assumed that those individuals exhibited lower intellectual performance throughout their entire lives and were not demented (Saxton et al., 2004).

Deficits in verbal memory, psychomotor speed, and executive functions in patients with MCI suggest probable conversion to AD (Tabert et al., 2006).

Cognitive functioning shows the successive emergence of deterioration long before the typical symptoms of AD are evident. The first decline in cognitive performances appears as early as 12 years before dementia and involves semantic memory and conceptual knowledge. They are followed by more global congitive deficits that are concomitant with an increase in memory complaints and depressive symptoms (Amieva et al., 2008).

In conclusion, cognitive impairment may appear many years before the onset of AD, which supports the concept of a long preclinical phase in AD.

Proposal for a Standardized Examination

Neuropsychological examination is different for patients with MCI and patients with expected dementia. It is sometimes possible for patients with mild or incipient dementia to use the same tests as those used for the patients with MCI. The selection of tests always depends on careful consideration of the individual patient and assessment by a psychologist. We usually choose short and simple tests in patients with dementia. Only after an initial interview, history and screening examination should take place and decisions regarding which tests are appropriate should be made.

The most frequently used tests to guide further cognitive assessment are the MMSE (or ACE-R), which quite reliably differentiate healthy performance from obviously pathological ones.

If the patient suffers from advanced dementia, it is necessary to consult with the caregiver to obtain important information about the patient. Hand dominance should also be determined. The following suggested neuropsychological examination is only one of many options.

The classic memory tests (e.g., WMS, CVLT) may only be used in patients with MCI or in patients in the initial phase of AD. If dementia is more advanced, changes in memory abilities are generally assessed using easier tests (e.g., MMSE, 7MST, ACE-R, ADAScog., DRS).

Proposal for a Standardized Examination

According to the degree of cognitive deficit and results on the *MMSE/ACE-R* tests, other examinations are added. The following cognitive tests are proposed for a standardized examination. However, it is always necessary to assess the global and other mental states of the patient (e.g., Beck Depression Inventory-BDI, Geriatric Depression Scale-GDS) and activities of daily living. Several questionnaires are available for such purposes, e.g., Functional Activities Questionnaire (FAQ), the Disability Assessment in Dementia (DAD), or the Bristol Activities of Daily Living Scale (BADLS) (Waldemar et al., 2007).

A. Patients with MCI (MMSE 30 to 25 points):

1. Wechsler Adult Intelligence Scale-Revised (WAIS-R)
2. California Verbal Learning Test (CVLT)
3. Benton Visual Retention Test (VRT)
4. Verbal Fluency Test (VFT) —verbal and semantic fluency
5. Rorschach test

B. Patients with mild form of dementia (MMSE 24 to 18 points):

1. WAIS-R (depending on the consideration of a psychologist), another alternative is one subtest from WAIS-R ("Information") and Raven's Progressive Matrices
2. Seven-Minute Screen Test (7 MST) (contains Clock Drawing Test and semantic fluency)
3. Trail Making Test (TMT)
4. Verbal fluency test (VFT)
5. Rorschach test

C. Patients with moderate or severe dementia (MMSE 17 points or less):

1. Dementia Rating Scale (DRS)
2. Subtests from WAIS-R "Block Design" and "Digit Span"
3. 7MST (includes Clock Drawing Test and semantic fluency)

Close cooperation is necessary with the caregiver for patients with moderate or severe dementia. The psychologist is essential to identify subtle cognitive changes. Physicians usually do not have enough time or access to the detailed tests needed to distinguish initial cognitive deficits from normal aging.

Rehabilitation and Therapy in Alzheimer's Disease

A complex approach in the treatment of Alzheimer's disease includes pharmacological, psychotherapeutic treatment and rehabilitation. Close cooperation between the physician and the caregiver (including also other relatives) is a necessary condition for successful therapy and rehabilitation for patients with AD dementia. The assistance of close contacts of the patient are an indispensable part of AD management. Unfortunately, caregivers often become exhausted with each passing day and often need targeted therapeutic care themselves.

No efficient causal therapy of AD is known yet. Present pharmacological therapy (cognitive enhancers) for AD only provides temporary improvement of symptoms in the initial stages of the disease. Although none of the drugs stops the mental decline, their early administration can delay the need of institutional help and prolongs the self-sufficiency of the patient.

Non-pharmacological therapy is based on knowledge of the principal problems of patients with AD and, therefore, is mostly focused on the field of cognitive-behavior. The aim is to consolidate/modify behaviors in patients such that they can live independently as long as possible. There is a wide range of techniques aimed at the practical aspects of the patient's activities of daily living. The main objective is to introduce regimen and order into the life of the patient with the goal of simplifying everyday tasks and making them more transparent. It is important to properly balance periods of activity with those of relaxation during the day. Patients learn to use various methods and aids to facilitate daily activities. Practical advice includes the following: e.g., to place clocks in all rooms, to place all important phone numbers near the telephone, to have spare keys available, to put down all tasks for each day and to check task completion each evening, to minimize exposure to sharp edges on furniture and other dangerous items, to leave some lights on at night and to secure valuable things, e.g., financial items, and records. Patients should practice specific everyday activities during therapy, e.g., shopping, visits, dressing, self-assistance, or personal hygiene. They learn to work on their daily schedules (to put everything down on a calendar, utilize their daily diaries). They also acquire principles that need to be followed during everyday life. For instance, it is very important to take breaks during the day and undertake complicated tasks during daytime hours when the patient feels best. It is also important to reserve time enough for each activity in order to avoid stress and anxious feelings of time pressure and being hurried. Everyday training of cognitive functions is also important (e.g., playing puzzles, cards, chess, doing crosswords, everyday reading, writing and calculating—at least a little bit).

Previously acquired abilities should also be practiced during therapy in addition to the development of new skills. Skills that have been partially preserved should be routinely practiced; however, trying to relearn lost skills can be traumatic for the patient.

Caregivers should be informed during therapy that it is necessary to speak slowly and clearly to the patient and to ask them several times whether they completely understand what they have been asked to do. It is good to allow the patient to work as independently as possible. However, supervision becomes more and more essential as the disease advances. Involvement of the entire family, as well as acquaintances, in caring and working with the patient is optimal.

Besides cognitive-behavioral therapy, other types can be chosen. Such therapy may be mainly directed at coping emotionally with the personal trauma of AD (the awareness of the disease and its inevitable progression toward dementia and death). This especially applies to patients in the initial phase of the disease, when the awareness and understanding of the disease is preserved.

Conclusion

The expected population aging will make ever higher demands on accurate and early diagnosis of Alzheimer's disease. An essential part of the diagnostic procedure involves psychometric assessments. The appropriate use of tests is based on good knowledge of what tests are available and which ones are best suited to specific situations. The aim of this chapter has been to provide assistance in both these areas.

Acknowledgments

The chapter was supported by the research projects KAN200520701 and MZ0PCP2005.

References

Alzheimer's Disease Facts and Figures – statistical abstract of U.S. data on Alzheimer's disease. Alzheimer's Association, 2008.

Amieva H, Le Goff M, Millet X, Orgogozo JM, Pérès K, Barberger-Gateau P, Jacqmin-Gadda H, Dartigues JF. Prodromal Alzheimer's disease: successive emergence of the clinical symptoms. *Ann Neurol,* 2008; 64(5):492-8.

Benton AL. Der Benton – Test. Huber, Bern, 1972.

Delis DC, Kramer JH, Kaplan E, Ober BA. California Verbal Learning Test. San Antonio: The Psychological Corporation. A Harcourt Assessment Company, 1987.

De Renzi E, Vignolo LA. The Token test: a sensitive test to detect receptive disturbances in aphasics. *Brain*, 1962; 85: 665-678.

Diagnostic and Statistical Manual of Mental Disorders. Fourth Edition (DSM-IV), American Psychiatric Association, 1994.

Dubois B, Slachevsky A, Litvan I, Pillon B. The FAB: a Frontal Assessment Battery at bedside. *Neurology*, 2000; 55:1621-1626.

Dubois B, Emre M, Georges J, McKeith IG, Rossor M, Scheltens P, Tariska P, Winbland B, Waldemar G. Recommendations for the diagnosis and management of Alzheimer's disease and other disorders associated with dementia: EFNS guideline. *European Journal of Neurology*, 2007; 14: e1-e26.

Duff Canning SJ, Leach L, Stuss D, Ngo L, Black SE. Diagnostic utility of abbreviated fluency measures in Alzheimer disease and vascular dementia. *Neurology*, 2004; 62:556-562.

Folstein MF, Folstein SE, McHugh PR. Mini-Mental State: A practical method for grading the cognitive state of patients for the clinician. *Journal of Psychiatric Research*, 1975; 12:189–198

Hendriksen CH, Meier D, Klitzing W, Krebs M, Ermini-Funfschilling D, Stahelin HB. Early Dementia and the clock drawing test. Memory Clinic. Geriatric University Clinic, Basel, Switzerland – Internal Press, 1993.

Kaplan EF, Goodglass E, Weintraub S. Boston naming test. The Psychological Corporation, 1983.

Kertesz A. Aphasia and associated disorders. Taxonomy, localization and recovery. Grune and Stratton, New York, 1979.

Kipps CM, Hodges JR. Cognitive Assessment for Clinicians. Journal of Neurology Neurosurgery and Psychiatry, 2005; 76:i22-i30.

Kopelman MD, Kapur N. The loss of episodic memories in retrograde amnesia: Single-case and group studies. *Philos. Trans. R Soc. Lond B Biol. Sci.,* 2001; 356:1409-1421.

Lezak MD, Howieson DB, Loring D.W. Neuropsychological Assessment. Fourth Edition. Hardcover, New York, Oxford University Press, 2004.

Mattis S. Dementia Rating Scale. Professional Manual. Florida: *Psychological Assessment* Resources, 1988.

McKhan G, Drachman D, Folstein M, Katzman R, Price D, Stadlan E. Clinical diagnosis of Alzheimer's disease: report of the NINCDS-ADRDA work group. *Neurology*, 1984; 34:939-944.

Mendez MF, Shapira JS, McMurtray A. Alzheimer's Disease Diagnosis and Treatment Centers. *Neurology*, 1992; 42:473-480.

Mioshi E, Dawson K, Mitchell J, Arnold R, Hodges JR. The Addenbrooke's Cognitive Examination Revised (ACE-R): a brief cognitive test battery for dementia screening. *Int. J. Geriatr. Psychiatry*, 2006; 21:1078-1085.

Petersen RC, Smith GE, Waring SC, Invik RJ, Tangalos EG, Kokmen E. Mild cognitive impairment: clinical characterization and outcome., *Arch. Neurol.*; 1999; 56:303-8

Plassman BL, Langa KM, Fisher GG, Heeringa SG, Weir DR, Ofstedal MB, Burke JR, Hurd MD, Potter GG, Rodgers WL, Steffens DC, Willis RJ, Wallace RB. Prevalence of dementia in the United States: the aging, demographics, and memory study. *Neuroepidemiology*, 2007; 29: 125-132.

Rey, A. L`Examen Clinique en Psychologie. Paris, Presses Universitaries 1958:140–153.

Rosen WG, Mohrs RC, Davis KI. A new rating scale for Alzheimer's disease. *Am. J. Psychiatry*, 1984; 141:1356–64.

Saxton J, Lopez OL, Ratcliff G, Phil D, Dulberg C, Fried LP, Carlson MC, Newman AB, Kuller L. Preclinical Alzheimer disease Neuropsychological test performance 1.5 to 8 years prior to onset. *Neurology*, 2004; 63:2341–2347.

Shulman KL, Shedletsky R, Silver IL. The challenge of time: Clock-drawing and cognitive function in the elderly. *Int. J. Geriatr. Psychiatry,* 1986; 1:135–140.

Solomon PR, Hirschoff A, Kelly B, Relin M, Brusch M, deVeaux RD, Pendlebury WW. A 7 minute neurocognitive screening battery highly sensitive to Alzheimer's disease. *Arch. Neurol.*, 1998; 55: 349–355.

Spreen O, Strauss E. A compendium of neuropsychological tests. Administration, Norms and Commentary. New York, Oxford University Press, 1998.

Squire LR, Shimamura AP. Long-term memory in amnesia: Cued recall, recognition memory, and confidence ratings. *Journal of Experimental Psychology Learning Memory and Cognition*, 1988; 14:763-770.

Sunderland T, Hill JL, Mellow AM, Lawlor BA, Gunderscheimer J, Newhouse PA, Grafman JH. Clock drawing in Alzheimer's disease: A novel measure of dementia severity. JAGS 1989; 37: 725–729.

Tabert MH, Manly JJ, Liu X, Pelton GH, Rosenblum S, Jacobs M, Zamora D, Goodkind M, Bell K, Stern Y, Devanant DP.

Neuropsychological prediction of conversion to Alzheimer disease in patients with mild cognitive impairment. *Arch. Gen. Psychiatry* 2006; 63: 916-924.

Tirney MC, Geslani DM, Herrmann N, Szalai JP. Mild cognitive impairment: an operational definition and its conversion rate to Alzheimer's disease. *Dement. Geriatr. Cogn. Disord., 2005;*19:383-389.

Vandenberghe R, Tournoy J. Cognitive aging and Alzheimer's disease, *Postgrad. Med. J.*, 2005;81: 343 – 352.

Waldemar G, Dubois B, Emre M, Georges J, McKeith IG, Rossor M, Scheltens P, Tariska P, Winbland B. Recommendations for the diagnosis and management of Alzheimer's disease and other disorders associated with dementia: EFNS guideline. *European Journal of Neurology* 2007; 14:1-26.

Wechsler D. Wechsler Adult Intelligence Scale-Revised (WAIS-R) New York, NY: *Psychological Corporatio*n, 1981.

Wechsler D. Wechsler Memory Scale-Revised (WMS-R). San Antonio: *The Psychological Corporatio*n, 1987.

Wechsler D. Wechsler Memory Scale - Third edition (WMS-III). San Antonio, TX: Harcourt Assessment, 1997.

Woods SP, Delis DC, Scott CJ, Kramer JH, Holdnack JA. The California Verbal Learning Test – second edition: Test-retest reliability, practice effects, and reliable change indices for the standard and alternate forms. *Archives of Clinical Neuropsychology*, 2006; 21: 413–420.

World Health Organization. The ICD-10 classification of mental and behavioural Disorders: Clinical description and diagnostic guidelines. Geneva: World Health Organization, 1992.

In: Cognitive Deficit in Mental and Neurological Disorders ISBN: 978-1-60741-957-0
Editors: H. Kucerova, M. Preiss

Chapter IX

Epilepsy

Jan Preiss

Abstract

Not only one disease is concerned but a number of markedly various syndromes. It is better to talk about epilepsies rather than about epilepsy itself. There is no uniform profile of cognitive functions. On the one hand, there are special disorders that occur, especially in early childhood, and that cause severe cognitive deficits. On the other hand, there are a considerable number of people with compensated disease who are well adapted to work and social life.

A summary of classifications of seizure disorders, neuropsychological impacts of localization and epileptogenic factors, impacts of ethiological factors and EEG abnormalities on neuropsychological performance is provided.

The prevalence in the population is 0.5 to 1%. Compared to the current prevalence, the lifetime prevalence is higher (2 to 5%), which means that most patients have a chance for long-term remission.

Characteristics of changes in the main domains of measurable cognitive functions are provided. Important factors include etiology, heredity, disposition, age of disease onset, duration of disease, type and intensity of seizures, frequency of seizures, pharmacotherapy and status epilepticus. The most common subjective complaints and objective finding in adults include memory disorders, mental retardation and attention disorders. In children, cognitive disorders cause speech difficulties, learning disorders, poor school results, behavioral problems, and unfavorable social and vocational prognosis. Except for cognitive disorders, the following disorders are common: behavioral disorders, mental difficulties in adults—especially depressions, dysphorias and increased anxiety—and, according to some authors, personal specificities, and learning disorders in children. Cognitive performance can especially be affected by depressive disorders and anxiety.

Neuropsychological methods designed especially for epilepsy, such as the Neuropsychological Battery for Epilepsies (NBE), FePsy Battery, Washington Psychosocial Seizure Inventory (WPSI), memory test as a part of the Wada Test, Quality of Life in Epilepsy Inventory (QOLIE-89) and others are described.

The course of cognitive deficits is described in subsections of the longitudinal follow-up and includes the question of dementia, monitoring of concomitant factors, effects of neurosurgery, prediction of surgical results, quality of life, and antiepileptic medication.

The proposal for a standardized examination of cognitive functions is divided into examinations performed at the standard clinics and at specialized clinics for the treatment of epilepsy. Detailed examinations are performed in relation to brain surgeries in response to pharmacoresistant epilepsy. Except for cognitive areas, neuropsychological examinations should also describe psychosocial problems of patients, personality, disease adaptation, subjective quality of life, possible psychopathology, or suicidal tendencies.

Methods of psychotherapy and rehabilitation of cognitive deficits are subdivided according to the type of intervention and the declared target for psychological-educative, relaxation, behavioral and methods aimed at social psychological adaptation and cognitive rehabilitation.

The main emphasis is transferred from diagnostics and localization to the description of weak and strong cognitive features and to cognitive and psychosocial rehabilitation.

1. Introduction

1.1. Classification of Seizure Disorders

Epilepsy can affect cognitive functions as well as behavior, psychological adaptation, and psychopathology. Cognitive functions can be affected by three different factors: seizures, primary disease, interictal discharges and possibly by epilepsy itself. Three combined factors contribute to cognitive impairment: syndrome (that often includes etiology), seizures, and "central" side effects of the therapy (Aldenkamp, 2006). In other words, based on the conceptual model of Hermann and Whitman (1984), variables associated with cognitive and behavioral impairment can be classified as seizure-related variables (such as etiology, syndrome, severity and frequency of seizures, epileptiform discharges, age at onset of the disease, etc.), variables related to therapy (antiepileptics, surgery that may provide improvement but also risks), and non-seizure-related variables (comorbid psychiatric difficulties, intellectual level of parents, psychiatric disorder in the family history, socioeconomic status, attitude towards epilepsy).

Epileptic seizures are caused by abnormal electric paroxysmal discharges of brain neurons. It is manifested by transient motor, sensory, or vegetative symptoms or alteration of consciousness. They are often combined with symptoms in several areas. Each person has a predisposition to an epileptic seizure. If epileptic seizures occur within the scope of acute neurological injury (e.g., cerebral contusion, ictus, etc.) or shortly after such an injury (within two weeks of the injury) we are talking about early epileptic seizures and do not classify the event as epilepsy. Epilepsy usually involves at least two unprovoked seizures. Epileptic seizures are only a symptom of a neurological disease. It may be the only symptom, as in some idiopathic epilepsy. In such cases, no other neurological signs of central nervous system impairment are present. Except for epileptic seizures, some neurological diseases (e.g., tumors) can come out as another neurological symptomatology (e.g., pareses) and neuropsychological deficit. Especially in pediatric epilepsies, we may define an epileptic syndrome according to family history, onset of the disease, semiology of the seizures, EEG, and results of neuroimaging examinations. Currently, there 30 to 40 defined epileptic syndromes. Diagnosis of the syndrome is an important step in making a meaningful prognosis.

There are many classification systems for seizures. Some of them focus on the seizure type, while the others focus on the type of epilepsy. Classification of seizures according to the clinical manifestation and EEG is important for selection of antiepileptics. However, if we want to provide the patient with more information, e.g., prognostic information, we must use other information (genetics, age of the onset of seizures, neuroimaging examinations, etc.) and classify the type of epilepsy or even the epileptic syndrome.

According to the international classification of seizures (The International Classification of Epileptic Seizures, ICES, 1981) —which however, does not take into account the anatomic background of seizures, age and gender—epileptic seizures are classified as follows: 1. Partial: initial clinical symptoms or EEG indicates that the seizure is initiated in one area of the brain. Simple partial seizures (without alteration of consciousness) are classified as follows: motor, somatosensory with autonomous symptoms and with mental symptoms (dysphatic, dysmnestic, cognitive, affective symptoms, illusions, and structured delusions). Complex partial seizures (with alteration of consciousness) are classified (presented here in a simplified form) as seizures with complex symptomatology with initial simple symptoms and subsequent alteration of consciousness, seizures with complex symptomatology with initial alteration of consciousness and to partial seizures, which switch to generalized seizures. 2. Generalized seizures: the first clinical changes indicate that both sides of the brain are initially involved, consciousness is often impaired, motor symptoms are bilateral and ictal EEG patterns are bilateral from the beginning. The following types of seizures (presented here in a simplified form) are defined: absence seizures (previously called petit mal), atypical absences, myoclonic seizures, clonic seizures, tonic-clonic seizures (previously called grand mal), and atonic seizures. 3. Non-classified epileptic seizures: all seizures that cannot be classified due to insufficient or incomplete data.

Paroxysmal events are seizures in which the epileptic origin is unclear. Except for seizures that will ultimately be classified as epileptic, this group also includes conditions without an epileptic origin. They are often classified as "non-epileptic seizures" or inaccurately "pseudoseizures." They can be of somatic or psychogenic origin. It is particularly difficult to differentiate epileptic seizures from non-epileptic, psychogenic seizures, since both types may occur in the same person, although this is not the only reason. Reduced cognitive performance and neuropsychological deficits that are quite common are often detected in groups of people with undoubtedly non-epileptic psychogenic seizures as well as in patients with epilepsies.

According to the International Classification of Epilepsies and Epileptic syndromes (ICES, 1989), we distinguish (as in the case of epileptic seizures): partial epilepsies (and epileptic syndromes) and generalized epilepsies (and epileptic syndromes). Apart from this localization dichotomy, this classification applies a second type of ethiological dichotomy. Epilepsies and epileptic syndromes are classified as: symptomatic (secondary) with exactly defined and known causes and idiopathic (primary) whose etiology is not known and where a genetic basis for the disease is likely. In cases of idiopathic epilepsy, patients with similar disorders can be found in the family history. The disease usually starts in childhood without structural abnormalities and EEG backgrounds are often normal; cryptogenic epilepsy is often placed in this classification if the epilepsy or epileptic syndrome is likely to have a "symptomatic," although unknown, cause. Idiopathic epilepsies have more benign courses compared to cryptogenic and symptomatic epilepsies. Both partial and generalized seizures may be included in both categories (idiopathic or symptomatic).

According to the new diagnostic scheme of epileptic seizures and epilepsies from 2001 (Engel, 2001), the classification of seizures based on the existence or non-existence of consciousness disorders is not considered satisfactory. It is recommended that the word "partial" be replaced by "focal" and the words "convulsion" and "convulsive" be omitted. The word "anti-convulsives" as the synonym for antiepileptics is also considered inappropriate; and the term "possibly symptomatic" is now recommended instead of "cryptogenic." The proposed new classification includes five levels (Axis 1 - 5). Level 1 consists of the description of ictal semiology, using a standardized glossary of descriptive terminology; Axis 2 classifies the type of epileptic seizure; Axis 3 defines epileptic syndrome; Axis 4 allocates etiology to the relevant syndrome; and Axis 5 completes the degree of impairment caused by the epileptic condition. The proposal has not yet been generally accepted and it is still under discussion (Engel, 2006).

1.2. Neuropsychological Impacts of Localization of the Epileptogenic Zone

Numeric data in this part of text (and in the section describing impacts of etiological factors) are based on the work of the Swiss authors (Jokeit and Schacher, 2004).

Idiopathic Generalized Epilepsies

Epilepsy with generalized tonic-clonic seizures (23%), with absences (6%) and myoclonic epilepsies (3%) belong to the most common idiopathic generalized epilepsies. Generalized tonic-clonic seizures possibly reduce cognitive functions more than simplex or complex partial seizures, and higher risks are present only if status epilepticus is present (Dodrill, 1986). Neuropsychological tests show weakening of prefrontal functions such as working memory and mental flexibility. However, these frontal deficits are not pathognomic for generalized epilepsies. Temporal, parietal, and frontal focal epilepsies may cause similar or even more significant weakening of frontal functions.

Based on the localization of the epileptogenic zone, we distinguish four localizable epilepsies: temporal, frontal, parietal and occipital.

Temporal Lobe Epilepsies

Temporal epilepsy is the most common focal epilepsy. Most patients with temporal epilepsy (70%) have hippocampal sclerosis (HS). Mesiotemporal epilepsy is only rarely controlled by antiepileptics, and these patients are therefore the most probable candidates for neurosurgery. They also most often undergo neuropsychological examinations. The main symptoms in these patients include material-specific or nonspecific weakening of episodic memory, corresponding to structural lesions of the hippocampal formation. The main difference between the two temporal lobes is that the dominant lobe (usually the left one) mediates memory for verbal information such as names, lists of words, stories or series of numbers, and the right lobe mediates memory for information that cannot be easily verbalized such as faces, places, music or abstract forms (Hermann et al., 1992; Seidenberg et al., 1993). It appears that the focus of seizures in the nondominant mesiotemporal lobe causes learning deficits that are characterized by memory dysfunction, while reduced retention is the most distinct feature of the epileptic focus in the dominant temporal lobe (Djordjevic and Jones-Gotman, 2004).

In patients with HS in the speech dominant hemisphere, the most marked symptom is usually a deficit in finding words, although some patients also think their memory has deteriorated (Mayeux et al., 1980; Mungas et al., 1985). We may assume that it is caused by frequent propagation of epileptic activity to the temporolateral areas.

Mesial temporal epilepsy is often associated with a mild impairment in intelligence, school results, speech and visual-spatial functions (Hermann et al., 1997). Prefrontal functions, such as attention and executive functions, are often intact. Absence and myoclonic seizures do not reduce cognitive functions. However, patients with secondary generalized tonic-clonic seizures have a clear risk of generalized intellectual weakening and specific weakening with regard to prefrontal functions (Jokeit et al., 1997). Opinions differ on whether chronic refractory temporal epilepsy represents an increased risk of progressive cognitive deterioration. Dementia is, however, very rare.

Frontal Lobe Epilepsies

This is the second most common localized type of epilepsy. Part of the known functions in this area of brain are associated with planning, organizing, self-monitoring and self-regulation, and decision-making; the definitions of executive functions involved are not uniform. Problem-solving tests, fluency, propensity for disturbing, planning, and motor skills are all used to investigate possible impairments of the frontal lobes. In comparative neuropsychological studies, patients with frontal epilepsy had reduced attention and reduced psychomotor speed, while patients with temporal epilepsy had reduced episodic memory. Helmstaedter (2002) found a lower level of education in patients with mesial temporal epilepsy compared with frontal epilepsy (with statistically significant difference regarding lowest and highest levels of education), while the employment levels remained the same. The age at onset of the disease may have an important effect on the presence of specific deficits (Boone et al., 1988; Upton and Thompson, 1996).

Parietal and Occipital Lobe Epilepsies

These cases are rather rare. There are various opinions regarding the direct role of the parietal lobe in spatial and verbal functions. Massive lesions in the non-dominant parietal lobe may markedly reduce performance on almost all nonverbal intellectual tests (Sands et al., 2000). Lesions in the dominant speech hemisphere may cause severe receptive aphasia. Cognitive symptoms in patients with parietal lobe epilepsy are markedly different based on lateralization and localization, age at the time of damage, and age at the beginning of epilepsy. The profile of neuropsychological functions in patients with idiopathic epilepsy of the occipital lobe probably does not systematically differ from other types of epilepsy. The disorders were present when compared with the controls relative to attention, memory, and intellectual performance (Gülgönen et al., 2000).

1.3. Neuropsychological Impacts of Ethiological Factors

Seizures may appear due to any brain pathology that increases excitability of brain tissue.

Cerebrovascular Diseases

Cerebrovascular accident is the main cause of acquired epilepsy in western countries. It is responsible for half of epilepsies that occur in people above 60 years of age. One year after the event, a considerable percentage of patients have visual-spatial, memory and psychomotor speed deficits, and reduced mental flexibility. The specific nature of the deficits depends on lateralization, site, and extent of the lesion. Left-sided lesions usually cause speech disorders, while perception and visual-spatial deficits are common with right-sided lesions (Details: Mahalick et al., 1991; Ogden et al., 1993; Lezak, 1995; Lezak et al., 2004).

Traumatic Brain Injury

Traumatic brain injuries cause epilepsy in 3 to 4% of patients. Patients who survive serious traumatic brain injuries have cognitive deficits of various grades in each aspect of cognitive functions. The main areas of damage are memory and attention, speed of processing and use of information. Prolonged reaction times in experiments involving two test tasks indicate pronounced deficits in fractional attention (Leclerq et al., 2000). Speech and perception skills tend to remain relatively intact. Deficits associated with frontal lobe impairment often result the most severe handicaps by affecting the patient's ability to use knowledge and skills fluently, adequately, and adaptively (Lezak, 1995, 2004).

Prospective studies in patients with severe brain injuries indicate a negative effect of epilepsy on behavioral disorders such as disinhibited behavior, irritability, aggressive, and agitated behavior (Mazzini et al., 2003). However, according to some studies, the risk factors are linked to hydrocephalus and hypoperfusion and not epilepsy.

Central Nervous System Infections

CNS infections are responsible for 2 to 3% of all epilepsies. This etiology belongs to the most common causes of epilepsy in small children, the second peak being in older aged children. Encephalitides, in particular, causes extraordinarily severe memory deficits with deep anterograde amnesia and marked retrograde amnesia. Severe behavioral changes such as loss of fear, social responsibility, social and personal inhibitions are described as well as reduced discrimination ability (Lezak, 1995, 2004).

Brain Tumors

Brain tumors are responsible for 4% of all cases of epilepsy and for 12% of acquired epilepsies. The highest incidence is between 25 and 64 years of age. If intracranial pressure is increased, it can reduce intellect and cause confusion and memory difficulties. Impairment of executive functions has been observed in 78% of patients, impairment of memory and attention in more than 60% of patients (Tucha et al., 2000).

Degenerative Cns Diseases

Epilepsy associated with degenerative diseases is responsible for approximately 2% of all cases of epilepsy. Patients with Alzheimer's disease have a 10 times higher risk of epilepsy with generalized, tonic-clonic seizures. Loss of memory function is the earliest symptom. Furthermore, visual perception deficits (visual discrimination, analysis, spatial perception, perceptive organization) and attention deficits are common. Deterioration in quality, quantity, and meaningfulness of speech, as well as understanding, is typical for most patients in early stages of Alzheimer's disease. Patients have reduced understanding of read text and reduced scores on tests of verbal fluency (Pasquier, 1999). Patients with Alzheimer's disease and seizures show a more rapid decline in language skills (Volicer et al., 1995).

1.4. The Impact of EEG Abnormalities on Neuropsychological Performance

Neuronal discharges are the determining sign of epilepsy. The epileptiform patterns captured during a clinically manifest seizure and EEG seizures patterns that correlate with epileptic seizures can be seen on the EEG. The first EEG associations with a number of different seizure types were detected early after the first EEG recordings in humans (Berger, 1929); shortly thereafter, investigations began on the effects of these abnormal discharges on neuropsychological functions.

The work describing the effects of abnormal discharges on cognitive performance (Schwab, 1939) was one of the founding studies for a new branch of neuropsychological EEG research, i.e., monitoring the effects of subclinical discharges on performance on tests of cognitive abilities.

The second line of neuropsychological literature associated with EEG investigated the effects of a number of abnormal features of EEGs, such as frequencies, distribution, and amount of abnormal discharges on various qualitative and quantitative parameters.

Dodrill and Wilkus (1976) monitored the effects of discharges, their average quantity and topographic distribution on performance on the WAIS. Lower intellectual performances were associated with more generalized than focal discharges, and with more than one discharge per minute. Later on, the authors monitored the effects of such discharges on performance on the Halstead-Reitan battery, relative to other abnormal EEG patterns and neuropsychological performances. Similar debilitating impacts, of epileptiform activity on neuropsychological performance, were detected during intraictal EEG recordings using deep electrodes. The development of epilepsy centers that perform neurosurgical procedures along with the use of intracranial EEGs provided further information. Some authors use the term transitory cognitive impairment to describe the effects of interictal epileptiform discharges (Binnie, 1987; Aldenkamp, Arend, 2004; Holmes and Lenck-Santini, 2006).

2. Prevalence

Epilepsy is a relatively common neurological disorder. The incidence ranges between 24 to 53/100,000 people per year in industrial countries, and it is considerably higher in developing countries. People under 18 years of age represent approximately 30% of the overall incidence. The incidence is slightly higher in men than in women, possibly due to the greater number of risk factors in males (injuries, alcohol, and stroke). In industrial countries, age-specific incidence is highest during the first several months of life with a subsequent marked reduction after the first year of life, with a generally stable level during the first decade and another marked reduction during adolescence. Incidence values remain low during adulthood followed by a marked increase during later years. Based on some studies, incidence after 70 is the same as during the first decade. The reduction of incidence in pediatric epilepsy and its increase in the elderly have been reported in the last decades.

Prevalence (i.e., relative number of patients who have experienced at least one epileptic seizure in the preceding five years) ranges between 0.5 to 1% of the population. Most individuals who suffer from epilepsy have a chronic form that requires therapy. Compared to the actual prevalence, the lifelong prevalence is significantly higher (2 to 5%), which means that most patients can achieve long-term remission.

Epilepsy, therefore, is more common than all psychotic disorders put together; with 2 to 5% of the population experiencing at least one epileptic seizure during their lives.

Although seizures and specific EEG patterns disappear over time in most patients, approximately 20 to 30% of patients never become seizure free, despite adequate therapy. The prevalence of pharmacoresistant epilepsy is estimated between 0.2 to 0.3%. Other epidemiological data indicate a higher risk of suicide, which accounts for 5 to 7% of deaths in epileptics, compared to 1.4% in general population. The risk is especially high in people with comorbid psychiatric disease or those receiving antipsychotic therapy (Nilson et al., 2002).

3. Principal Domains of the Measured Cognitive Functions

3.1. Intellectual Performances

Assessment of cognitive abilities developed concurrently with the development of psychometric methods. The first studies that used new intelligence tests appeared prior to 1920. Most of these early works provided total IQ values and concluded that a significant percentage of patients suffered cognitive deterioration. Because most of the works involved patients who were hospitalized in various long-term care institutions, below-average IQs were frequently observed.

A 1924 study, involving 150 children, found an average IQ (using the Binet-Simon test) of 71 in boys and 65 in girls (Fox, 1924, according to Hermann, 1991).

In the 1940s, some researches began to point out that these studies were not representative of the general population of epileptic patients.

A 1947 study involving patients in the care of private general practitioners' found that among 100 children, the average IQ was 104 (Stanford-Binet, form L), and among 200 adults the average IQ was 111 (Wechsler-Bellevue) (Collins and Lennox, 1947).

There are still discussions regarding the possibility of cognitive deterioration in patients with a persistent form of the disease. Intellectual disorders are often overestimated and the majority of patients show normal intelligence (Preiss, Haas, 2001, 2002, *Graph 1)*.

3.2. Memory and Learning

An association between epilepsy and memory disorders *(Table 1)* has been observed for centuries. It was perceived as one of the first signs of a presumed inevitable breakdown of intellectual abilities. Even today, complaints of impaired memory are the most common complaints about cognitive problems. For example, out of 760 epileptic patients, 54%

evaluated their memory as moderately or seriously impaired compared to 23% of the control group patients (Thompson and Corcoran, 1992).

Reduced verbal memory associated with left temporal lobe lesions takes various forms, including episodic, short-term and learning, semantic and remote. Vecchio et al. (2004) describe dissociation between reduced explicit and normal implicit memory. Non-verbal disorders (i.e.,, auditory, tactile and visual) appear during resections of the right temporal lobe and in right-side lesions, i.e., where perception or knowledge cannot be easily transferred into words. Nevertheless, it appears that the relationship between the type of information (verbal or non-verbal) and the hemisphere involved is not simple. Because of this, it is also difficult to design information-specific tests that would be strictly non-verbal and would not involve a verbal component as part of the solution. For example, functional magnetic resonance demonstrates that both hemispheres can be activated when solving verbal tasks (Dupont et al., 2002).

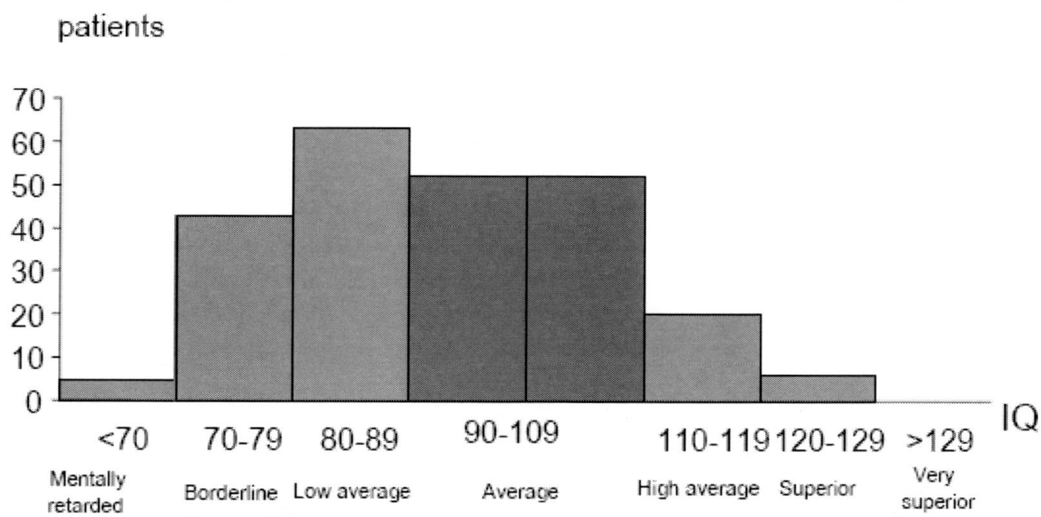

Figure 1. Intellectual level (WAIS-R) according to so-called "intelligence ranges," sample of 241 patients (Preiss, Haas, 2001).

The factors that affect memory and learning disorders also include age at onset of the disease and duration of disease; the findings are not uniform and these variables are affected by other factors such as etiology and the level of seizure control. Furthermore, the seizures that demonstrate their effect, especially at high seizure rate (several times daily), are concerned when it is possible to assume that the ability to register information and remember current events is impaired. "Subclinical" seizures, detected during EEG monitoring, also have similar effects.

3.3. Attention

Patients with temporal epilepsy are less able to maintain attention, for example in the Continuous Performance Test (Fleck et al., 2002). Weak performance in subtests Speech-

Sounds Perception Test and Rhythm Test, which are subtests of the Halstead-Reitan Neuropsychological Battery (HRNB) or Dodrill Neuropsychological Battery for Epilepsies, are very probably affected most by attention and concentration disorders.

Table 1. Memory performances in a sample of 197 epileptic patients according to WMS-R (Preiss, Haas, 2004)

Index	N	Average	SD	Min	Ma
General Memory (MQ)	197	83.12	18.74	50	137
Attention/Concentration	197	84.10	17.57	50	134
Verbal Memory	197	87.84	16.77	50	128
Visual Memory	197	85.26	19.20	50	128
Delayed Recall	197	84.12	18.00	50	138

According to clinical studies, the prevalence of personality disorders and attention deficits with hyperactive disorder (ADHD) in children with epilepsy is estimated to be 30 to 40%; impairment of attention is more common than hyperactivity and impulsivity (Dunn, Kronenberger, 2005).

Speech

Patients with epilepsy may have language problems. These problems have an adverse effect on performance at school or on the job and in social adaptation. Assessment of language skills should include examination of six verbal functions: speech spontaneity, repeating of words, verbal understanding, confrontation naming, reading, and writing. Peng (1995) provided a summary of speech disorders in epilepsy, empirical data were provided by Seidenberg (1989), *Table 2.*

The highest risk is in individuals whose seizures are located in the speech-dominant hemisphere. Patients with epilepsy often have atypical speech dominance, in which speech functions are located mainly in the right hemisphere or bilaterally.

Table 2. Academic underachievement of male and female children with epilepsy (Seidenberg, 1989, adapted)

Variable	Percentage significantly underachieving[a]	
	Males (n = 54)	Females (n = 68)
Word recognition	10.5	10.1
Spelling	33.3	15.9
Arithmetic	28.1	31.9
Reading comprehension	22.8	13.0

academic score was 1 SD below (12 points) than expected score based on WISC-R Full-Scale IQ level.
[a] Children were classified as significant underachievers of their obtained

Early brain injuries in the left hemisphere, early onset of repeated seizures, pathological left-handedness, and less marked right-handedness may be contributing factors. Patients with left-sided epilepsy whose speech functions were shifted contralaterally have verbal memory deficits to a lesser degree when compared to patients whose speech functions remain lateralized in the left hemisphere (Rausch and Langfitt, 1991).

Expressive functions are most likely to be impaired if the seizure focus is located in the frontal-temporal areas. Patients with the epileptogenic zone in the dominant temporal lobe often have verbal memory defects and difficulties in finding words that may present clinically as dysnomia (Mayeux et al., 1980). Prosodic speech elements, i.e., rhythm, intonation and others, are often affected in cases where the epileptogenic zone is in the non-dominant temporal lobe.

Comprehension may be impaired in more posterior lesions.

Reading and spelling may be impaired in parietal lesions.

3.5. Executive Functions

With regard to executive functions, the clinical picture is not uniform. Reduced programming and coordination of motor procedures, reduced work memory, and inhibition of reactions can be found in studies. Deficits of executive functions are more apparent in individuals with bilateral impairment or more extensive frontal impairment. Individuals with late onset of secondary seizures after acquired pathology (tumors and head injuries) represent another risk group. If seizure activity expands into the temporal areas, memory deficits characteristic of temporal epilepsy can be seen.

Visual Perceptions

The nondominant temporal lobe is considered to be a mediator of visuospatial processing and perceptive functions. Visual perception is usually reduced (together with visual memory) in lesions located in the non-dominant (mostly right) hemisphere (Delaney et al., 1980; Mayeux et al., 1980; Smith & Milner, 1981; Hermann et al., 1987; Jones-Gotman, 1991; Matkovic, 1995).

Inconsistent findings may be affected by the lack of good methods for evaluation of non-verbal perception.

Non-Verbal Auditory Perception

The Speech-Sounds Perception Test (involving discrimination between nonsense syllables) and the Seashore Rhythm Test (a test of rhythm) and other Seashore tests of musical talent are used. Although the rhythm test was originally considered sensitive to right hemisphere dysfunction, it is actually more a measure of attention and concentration.

In relation to the monitoring of amusia (defect of perception of music or its components), some findings show that perception of melody is reduced primarily in lesions in the right temporal lobe, while rhythm resolution may be affected by lesions regardless of the side.

Motorics

Evaluation of motor functions is usually limited to upper limbs; relative weakening of one side may be a supplemental marker indicating lateralization of the lesion. Patients with epilepsy have generally weak performances, e.g., on the Finger Tapping Test.

4. Measurements

This section describes examination methods intended exclusively for epileptic patients.

Neuropsychological Battery for Epilepsy (NBE)

Dodrill (1978) designed a battery based on the HRNB. By adding memory tests, motor control, and concentration as well as other modifications, he ensured greater sensitivity of the battery relative to epileptic patients. We found the NBE to also be good in monitoring the effect of antiepileptic drugs (Kolínová and Preiss, 1991; Preiss, 1998).

FePsy Battery

The FePsy is a computerized battery (Moerland et al., 1988; Alpherts, Aldenkamp, 1990) extensively used with epileptic patients. It includes tests of single and selective reaction times, distinction of rhythms, finger tapping, visual search, measures of attention, spatial and verbal memory test, tests similar to the WCST (Wisconsin Card Sorting Test) and others. It is especially useful in evaluation of cognitive effects of drugs and in monitoring relationships between EEG changes and cognitive performance.

Washington Psychosocial Seizure Inventory (WPSI)

The authors are Dodrill et al. (1980). This method enables the acquisition of information about psychological and social problems and less precise information regarding the level of intellectual and neuropsychological impairment. It has 132 items (separate questions expressed in the form of single sentences), 10 clinical scales, and three control scales to verify the validity of answers. Better preoperative psychosocial performance according to the WPSI predicts better seizure control after surgery (Wheelock et al., 1998). Increased preoperative values on the scale associated with problems involving emotional adaptation may be an indicator of possible postoperative depression (Derry and Wiebe, 2000).

Epilepsy Surgery Inventory (ESI-55)

In 1990, the National American Conference recommended the creation of tools for measuring the quality of life in epileptic patients after neurosurgery. The first such method was the Epilepsy Surgery Inventory—ESI-55 (Devinski et al., 1995). It contains 55 items (questions) and provides the scores on 11 dimensions.

Quality of Life in Epilepsy Inventory-89 (QOLIE-89)

During further development, a psychometrically better documented method called the QOLIE-89 (Vickrey et al., 1993a, b) was created and includes 17 partial scales and total scores, QOLIE-31 (Cramer et al., 1998) and QOLIE-10 (Cramer et al., 1996). Postoperatively, patients without seizures have better scores compared to those that are not seizure free (Birbeck et al., 2002; Markand et al., 2000; Preiss & Vojtěch, 2007). The clinically important change in the current quality of life is reflected by the change of 10.1 for QOLIE-89, 11.8 for QOLIE-31 (Wiebe et al., 2002).

Interesting work has been done (by Leidy et al., 1999) on getting reliable QOLIE-89 values by telephone.

Epilepsy and Learning Disabilities Quality of Life (ELDQOL)

This newly redesigned and psychometrically verified method (Buck et al., 2007) contains 70 items for the evaluation of the quality of life in children and adolescents with concomitant learning disorders.

Bear-Fedio Inventory (BFI)

The questionnaire (Bear & Fedio, 1977) contains 100 items. The answers provide 18 personality characteristics and a scale quality of life according to the MMPI. Single features include humorlessness, dependence and circumstantiality, sense of personal destiny, obsessionalism, viscosity, emotionality, guilt, philosophic interest, anger, religiosity, altered sexual interest, hypermoralism, paranoia, sadness, hypergraphia, elation-euphoria, and aggression. This tool has been used to explore the relationship to lateralization, to compare various ethiological groups of epilepsy and to investigate the personalities of patients. There is still controversy regarding Gestaut-Geschwinn syndrome in temporal epilepsy with hypergraphia, hyperreligiosity, and hyposexuality as the main three symptoms.

Intracarotid Amytal Procedure (IAP, Wada Test)

The Wada Test (Wada and Rasmussen, 1960) is used especially for preoperative evaluation of patients indicated for resection in one temporal lobe. The most important finding is determining, in a particular patient, whether the right or left hemisphere is dominant regarding preservation of memory and speech functions. During the test, amobarbital sodium, which is commonly used, is injected (transfemoral) into the carotid artery. The rationale of the test is based on the assumption that the patient uses only the hemisphere that is not pharmacologically anesthetized to speak and to remember material presented during barbiturate application. The test requires close cooperation among a team of specialists (neuropsychologist, neurologist, radiologist, EEG technician). Most protocols are based on procedures developed in the Montreal Neurological Institute or in the Mayo Clinic. Good storage of pictures presented after barbiturate injection into the epileptogenic hemisphere is associated with the absence of amnesia after removal of the temporal lobe (Blume et al., 1973). Weak memory performance after injection into the epileptogenic hemisphere may predict poorer results following surgery (Jones-Gotman, 1992; Wyllie et al., 1991). If memory performance with regard to images after injection into the non-epileptic hemisphere is better, it indicates that the epileptogenic hemisphere plays a significant role relative in memory, and ablation in such cases may result in a deterioration of memory (Kneebone et al., 1995). Absence of aphasia following the injection into the epileptogenic hemisphere suggests an absence of postoperative aphasia. Development of aphasia after injection may lead to the recommendation to limit the extent of surgery in order to avoid postoperative language impairment (Blume et al., 1973). Besides the determination of speech lateralization and prediction of mnestic problems, it also enables determination of lateralization of the epileptogenic zone, i.e., determination of the lateralization of the onset of seizures (Perrine et al., 1995; Wyllie et al., 1991). Prediction of the results of surgery, i.e., rate of seizures after surgery, is carried out on the basis of differences in performances following injections into the hemispheres (Loring et al., 1992). It is possible that in time, the method will be replaced by functional magnetic resonance (fMRI). However, the Wada Test has an advantage in that it models the situation after surgery, including memory performance.

A-B Neuropsychological Assessment Schedule (ABNAS, Aldenkamp et al., 1995)

This self-assessment method contains 24 questions regarding the unfavorable affects of antiepileptic medication on cognitive functions.

Epilepsy Foundation of America (EFA) Concern Index (Gilliam et al., 1997)

This scale uses 20 questions to monitor specific effects of the disease on quality of life. Loring et al. (2005) underline the difference of single dimensions of the method.

Liverpool Assessment Battery (Baker et al., 1993)

The battery uses eight methods associated with the quality of life related to health. Four methods were developed earlier for use with a variety of populations. The other four methods were designed by the authors and are focused strictly towards epilepsy. The newly developed methods include the Severity-PERCEPT and Seizure Severity–ICTAL tests, which ask patients to evaluate physical perception of the seizure severity and actual seizures severity (Baker et al., 1991). The Adverse Events Profile scale identifies side effects of medication, and the Impact of Epilepsy scale is focused on social effects of epilepsy and therapy on everyday performance (Jacoby et al., 1993). Individual parts of the battery are used in various combinations.

Side Effects and Life Satisfaction (SEALS, Gilham et al., 1996)

Quality of Life in Childhood Epilepsy Questionnaire (USQOLCE, Sabaz et al., 2003).

The USQOLCE is an adaptation of the original Australian questionnaire with adjustments and validation for the United States. It has 79 items with 16 subscales intended for children between 4 and 18 years of age. It correlates with independent evaluations of severity of seizures and an independent scale of postoperative control of seizures.

Neurological Disorders Depression Inventory for Epilepsy (NDDI-E)

According to the authors (Gilliam et al., 2006), the questionnaire, which includes 46 questions, provides rapid detection of major depression without affection by cognitive deficits or undesirable effects of antiepileptics.

5. Course of Cognitive Deficits

The reports on unfavorable findings in epilepsy, deterioration, and dementia used to be typical findings over long periods. The distortion was due to the selection of mainly hospitalized patients or patients placed in long-term care institutions with inadequate treatment. Compared to the past, more recent works offer more optimistic conclusions and a variety of courses relative to cognitive changes is apparent.

5.1. Cross-Sectional and Longitudinal Monitoring

Impairment of cognitive performance can be found in relation to a number of factors such as basic pathology, seizure, and medication.

New cross-sectional studies provide some evidence concerning the relationship between the rate of seizures and cognitive impairment (besides others, Dikmen & Matthews, 1977; Dodrill, 1986). Prolonged duration of the disease is associated with higher cognitive deficits (Jokeit, Ebner, 1999; Stefan & Pauli, 2002, Oyegebile et al., 2004), see also *Graph 2*. One study found that cognitive impairment (based on the language abilities) was not related to the rate but to the severity of seizures (Thompson et al., 1987), and another study has found that duration of the disease is the best predictor of cognitive impairment (Jokeit, Ebner, 2002).

In a summary of nine longitudinal studies, in children (follow-up period up to four years), Dodrill (2004) found an impairment in performance and suggested that poorly controlled seizures were a possible cause. Seidenberg et al. (1981) reported intellectual improvement with better seizure control. Several studies have found that stable cognitive performance in groups with good seizure control (Äikiä et al., 1999; Dodrill, Wilenski, 1992). Other studies found poorer cognitive performance in patients with persistent seizures (Helmstaedter et al., 2003; Anderson-Roswall et al., 2004). However, some studies have found no cognitive changes in groups of patients with persistent seizures (Selwa et al., 1994; Holmes et al., 1998).

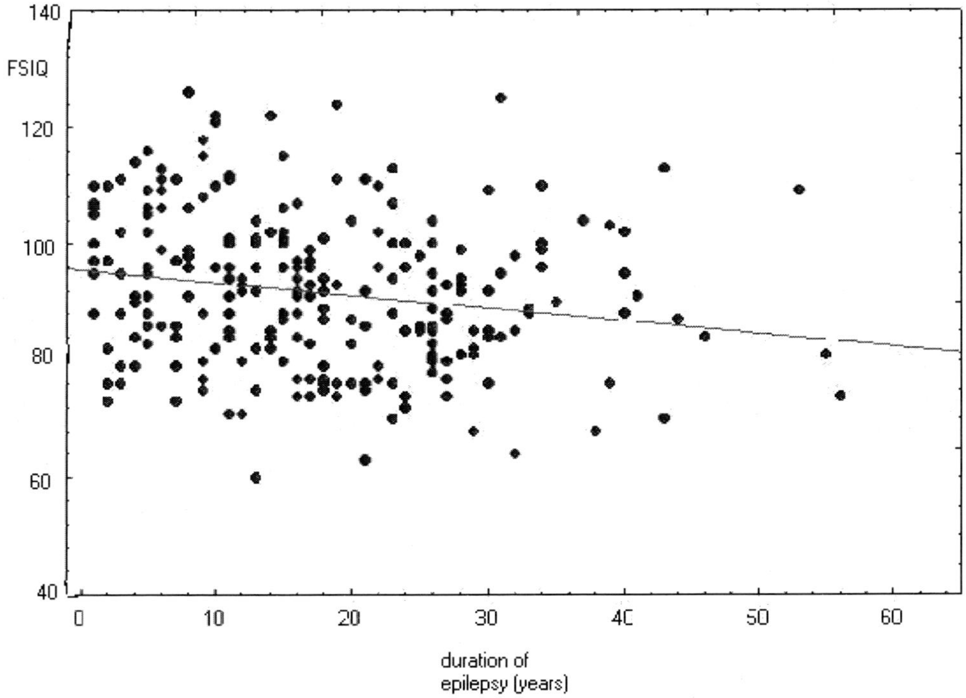

Figure 2. Duration of epilepsy and General IQ (FSIQ, WAIS-R). Correlation $r = -0.190$, $p < 0.05$, $N = 241$ (Preiss, Haas, 2002).

During 10 years of monitoring, Dodrill (2002) found a number of symptoms of cognitive decline in patients compared to healthy controls. Over a 10-plus year interval, Thompson and Duncan (2005) found severe cognitive impairment in a wide extent of cognitive functions.

Generalized tonic-clonic seizures were the strongest predictor of this impairment. Good seizure control had a favorable impact on cognitive prognosis even after years of the disease being poorly controlled.

Nevertheless, neither the cross-sectional studies nor relatively short longitudinal studies have found a convincing relationship between psychometrically detected intelligence and duration of epilepsy in adult patients. On one hand, this shows that no dramatic changes probably occur over a time period of several years. On the other hand, it is possible that methodological limitations (e.g., limited time span of longitudinal studies, which have only rarely exceeded 10 years) and mistakes in compiling groups for cross-sectional studies could obscure the possible effects of duration of the disease. Small groups can easily cause type II mistakes (a non-significant result has been identified despite the fact that the null hypothesis is, in reality, not valid). According to some studies, only in the event of intractable temporal epilepsy for more than 30 years is it possible to expect a significant relationship between the duration of the disease and intelligence (Jokeit & Ebner, 1999). Higher achieved education as an indicator of higher cognitive reserve may postpone the onset of measurable cognitive impairment.

5.2. The Question of Dementia

The original ideas about the development of dementia in a substantial percentage of epileptic patients were associated with prejudices and social stigmatization of patients. Recent works provide more encouraging results, and Helmstaedter and Elger (1999) even talk about the "phantom of dementia." Brown (2002) concluded that real intellectual deterioration is relatively rarely linked with epilepsy. When it occurs, it is usually connected with another etiology (e.g., concomitant degenerative brain disease, some epileptic syndromes) or as a result of therapy. Direct effects of seizures (usually tonic-clonic) and transitory cognitive impairment due to interictal epileptiform discharges are possibly less important. In some cases, temporal lobe focus during the critical period of development may adversely affect maturation, which may cause a clinical picture of damage or deterioration. However, Brown described some patients who experienced cognitive problems that were not caused by the above-stated reasons. They occurred more often in males compared to females and in those with a long-term history of insufficiently controlled temporal epilepsy. An epidemiological study (Breteler et al., 1995) found total relative risk of dementia of 1.5 in people between 50 and 75 years with a diagnosis of epilepsy, which is a moderately increased risk compared with expected values. Griffith et al (2006) found cognitive impairment in elderly people with epilepsy that was comparable with patients with mild cognitive impairment. Carter et al. (2007) found anti-epileptics as risk factors of dementia in elderly people.

Temporal negative effects, e.g., increased frequency of seizures, irrational polypharmacotherapy, insufficient cooperation (non-compliance), intoxication with antiepileptics or personality changes during psychosocial stress or psychopathological symptoms (frequent depression) must be differentiated. Therefore, it is suitable to perform repeated control assessment of cognitive functions.

5.3. Monitoring of Concomitant Factors

Cognitive performance studies mostly address only one or a small number of variables. New interpretation possibilities are provided using multidimensional analysis of potential predictors of cognitive performance that have been used by a number of recent studies.

5.4. Effects of Neurosurgery on the Cognitive Status

In spite of the development of modern pharmacotherapy for epilepsy, a percentage of patients still do not respond to medication to the point that they are seizure free. Most of these patients suffer from focal epilepsies. Current advances achieved, especially in neuroimaging and electrophysiological examination methods, provide for localization of the epileptogenic zone in a considerable number of these patients. As a result, these patients are potential candidates for neurosurgery, which has been able to treat epilepsy in many of them (Engel et al., 1998; Wiebe et al., 2001).

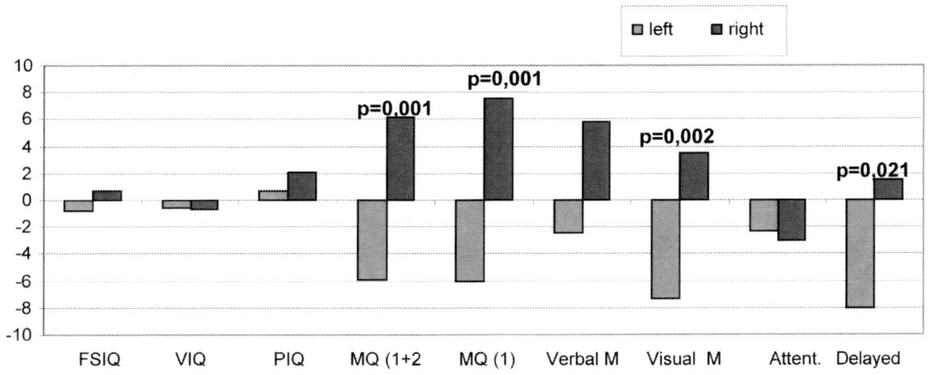

FSIQ = Full-Scale IQ, General IQ (WAIS-R)
VIQ = Verbal IQ (WAIS-R)
PIQ = Performance IQ (WAIS-R)
MQ 1+2) = General Memory Quotient, summary of results for WMS-R and WMS.
MQ (1) = General Memory Quotient, WMS-R only.
Verbal M = Verbal Memory (WMS-R)
Visual M = Visual Memory (WMS-R)
Attent. = Attention/Concentration (WMS-R)
Delayed = Delayed Recall (WMS-R)

Figure 3. Changes after resection surgery of temporal epilepsy in relation to the side of surgery (left = 18, right = 23) (Preiss, Vojtěch, 2006b).

However, epilepsy surgery includes surgical, general medical, neurological, and neuropsychological risks.

In principal, the results are very favorable with regard to seizure control (up to 80% of patients are seizure-free over the long term). Cognitive status is usually unchanged or with slight improvements. Only a small proportion of patients experience mild deterioration; such events usually take the form of impairment of verbal memory or intellectual performances and are associated with left hemisphere surgeries, with less marked impairments of non-verbal performances in the right hemisphere surgeries; and in a large number, these impairments are only transient (Gleissner et al., 2002; 2004), see also Preiss, Vojtěch, 2006a,

Graph 3. Subjective quality of life is usually improved, although only in seizure-free cases or in cases where the seizure reduction is at least 75%.

We provide examples of several studies to illustrate cognitive results. Hermann and Wyler (1988) provide results through the use of an extensive battery of 23 neuropsychological tests, which provide 64 cognitive indices (38 patients were tested before surgery and at six months after surgery). Seventy-seven percent of the measures remained unchanged following anterior temporal lobectomy. In the event of changes, 58% reflected significant cognitive improvement and 42% relative cognitive losses. Only memory/learning showed more cognitive losses than gains. Problem-solving ability showed the greatest improvement. Details are provided in *Table 3.*

Paglioli et al. (2004) had postoperative neuropsychological tests available from 65 patients out of 134 successive patients with temporal epilepsy and hippocampal sclerosis who were prospectively monitored.

Table 3. Cognitive changes after anterior temporal lobectomy (Hermann, Wyler, 1988)

Cognitive domain	Direction of change Stability %	Change %	Improvement %	Decline %
Psychometric intelligence	85	15	63	37
Academic achievement (WRAT-R)	97	3	0	100
Language function	80	20	62	38
Visuoperceptual and visuospatial ability	72	28	56	44
Memory and learning ability	63	37	45	55
Problem-solving skills	61	39	93	7
Auditory-perceptual function	84	16	83	17
Sensorimotor ability	83	17	61	39
Complex attention/concetration skills	72	28	60	40

Impairment of performance by more than 1 SD was present in verbal memory in 26% of patients with left-side surgery and in visual memory in 22% of right-side surgery patients. Preiss and Vojtěch (2006b) reported similar results, *Graph 4.*

One problem that makes evaluation of changes over time more difficult, includes artifacts associated with repeated tests, either by the same method or by its variants. Martin and Grote (2002) proposed the procedures and standards for evaluation of reliability of change, both for individuals and groups using the WAIS-III and WMS-III. Chelune et al. (1991; 1993) and Franzen and Iversen (2000) provide important data. Martin et al. (2006) provided data evaluating reliability of cognitive questionnaires.

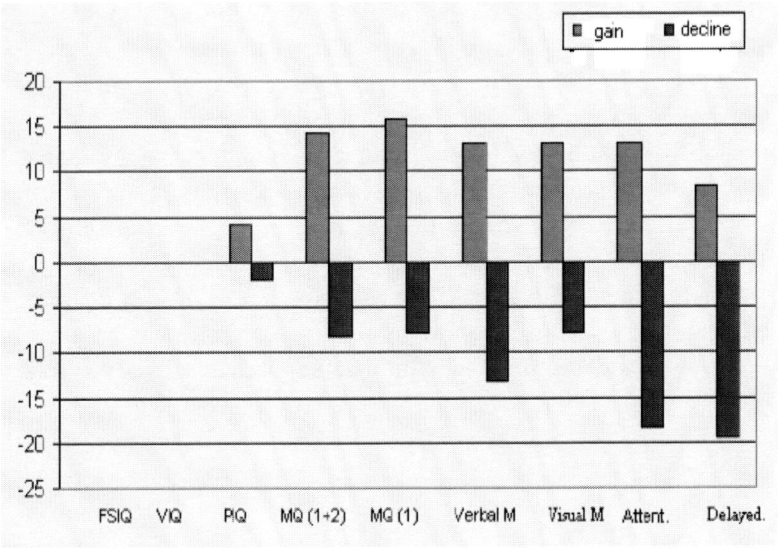

Figure 4. Cognitive changes > 1 SD after resection surgery in mixed sample (percentage of the sample, N = 49) (Preiss, Vojtěch, 2006a).

5.5. Prediction of the Results of Surgery

Rausch (1991), Chelune (1991), Dodrill et al. (1993), Chelune et al. (1998), Davies et al. (1998) and Lee et al. (2002) summarize the issue of prediction. The area of prediction can be divided to (a) seizure control predictions, (b) cognitive status, and (c) psychosocial impacts, or quality of life. Prediction tools may include (except for neurological aspects): (1) cognitive neuropsychological tests alone or in relation to neurological findings, (2) the Wada test results, and (3) psychosocial findings.

(a) Seizure control prediction: The possibility of eliminating seizures is higher if the side of the surgery is in line with the localization of the dysfunction based on neuropsychological tests. It is not suitable to rely on one type of assessment (e.g., impairment index or overall intelligence) for reliable seizure predictions following surgery based on performances in neuropsychological tests. A multivariant approach using various types of supplemental predictors is more appropriate (Dodrill et al., 1986).

An extensive study focused on the issue of whether preoperative IQ can predict results of temporal lobotomies with regard to the rate of postoperative seizures (Chelune et al., 1998). The data involved 1,034 patients from eight epileptic centers. Patients with unabated postoperative seizures had statistically significant lower preoperative IQs. Postoperative seizures occurred in 32.8%, 23.8%, and 16.9% in patients with IQ < 75, 76-109 and IQ > 109, respectively. Preoperative IQ is not a good predictor of results for postoperative seizure-free periods and should not be used to exclude patients as potential candidates for surgery; however, IQ scores could be a useful guide for patients and their families regarding relative surgical risks and outcomes.

Several studies (e.g., Bjørnæs et al., 2004) have shown that good results for both postoperative seizure control and cognitive and psychosocial performance can be obtained even in people with preoperative IQs below 70, especially if the surgery of intractable focal epilepsy was performed relatively quickly after the onset of the disease (with the duration of the disease less than 12 years). A history of status epilepticus was the only significant predictor of failure of surgery in pathologically verified mesial temporal scleroses in a set of 118 patients (Hardy et al., 2003). More recently, van Roost et al. expressed their opinion on the prediction of results for seizures relative to the use of the Wada test (2007).

(b) Prediction of the cognitive status: It can be expected that as a group. patients show no deterioration and a mild improvement of the intellectual results, especially if the resection was on the side not associated with speech (Lee et al., 2002), and if they are seizure free. The greatest risk of memory impairment is in patients whose memory function was most intact prior to surgery (Chelune et al., 1991), and where the onset of seizures occurred after the age of fifty (Saykin et al., 1989). Risks factors sometimes include older age at the time of surgery (Hermann et al., 1995) —although not all findings support this (Acosta et al., 2008)—and male gender (Trenerry et al., 1995).

If evidence of intact performance, in the expected epileptogenic temporal lobe, is indicated, the chances that postoperative selective performance will be reduced are higher. A neuropsychological finding of functional system integrity out of the area of the expected origin of seizures is positive as far as the prediction is concerned. Evidence of reduced performance outside the expected area (either focal or diffuse) is significant, and it indicates reduced potential for postoperative seizure control. Neuropsychological findings of significant dysfunction in the hemisphere contralateral to the expected focus indicates that the seizure focus has not been adequately identified. However, it may also indicate that the contralateral hemisphere has reduced and insufficient ability to compensate for postoperative cognitive deficits. If an apparent dysfunction of memory in the contralateral hemisphere to that of the seizure focus is observed, amnestic syndrome should be considered a possibility if the temporal lobe, with expected seizure focus, is resected. Although the Wada test (IAP) is used to answer these questions, it is newly recommended to integrate the results of the Wada test with findings of neuropsychological assessment due to technical complications during the IAP and controversial efficacy of various protocols of the Wada test, which should improve prediction accuracy regarding postoperative amnesia. Questions involving the suitability of the Wada test to predict memory impairment after surgery are summarized by Martin and Grote (2002). Alpherts et al. (2008) describes various cognitive results in relation to the radicality of resection of left temporal lobe surgeries (2008).

(c) An improvement in mentally stable people (with no or mild psychopathology), which has been strongly supported by the family members, a preoperative independent personality profile (at least partial employment before the surgery), and successful seizure control after surgery is a good predictor of psychosocial results. Evaluation of psychosocial adaptation to the disease may be a predictor of results: good preoperative adaptation to the disease indicates that an individual will also cope well with postoperative changes. Patients who had mental problems prior to surgery have a tendency to show postoperative psychosocial problems, even if the surgery provides seizure control.

5.6. Quality of Life Generally and in Relation to Neurosurgery

Epilepsy is an example of a disorder in which the quality of life in relation to health plays an important role. While seizures represent only a fragment of the patient's life, their practical consequences (life regiment, limitation, social stigmatization together with adverse drug effects) are long term. Depressive and dysphoric disorders undoubtedly play a significant role in subjectively perceived reduction in the quality of life (Blumer, 2002). Lateralization of the lesion may possibly have some effect in patients with right-side lesions who overestimate their own performance and underestimate their own deficits (Bear & Fedio, 1977; Andelman et al., 2001) and in patients with left-side lesions with the possibly of more frequent effects of depression (Paradiso et al., 2001).

In patients treated only pharmacologically, it has been identified through the use of QOLIE-89 and QOLIE-31 (Birbeck et al., 2002) that even a 50% seizure reduction does not result in any subjectively perceived change in the quality of life and that apparent change comes only after of the patient is seizure free.

The quality of life in relation to health is affected, among others, by seizure frequency, onset of the disease, duration of the disease, generalized seizures, and polytherapy. Compared to the general population, epileptics have more psychosocial problems, including stigmatization, higher unemployment, reduced self-esteem, interpersonal problems, including social isolation, and low social competence (Baker et al., 1997, 1998). However, epileptic patients do not represent a homogenous group and some studies, in well–controlled, uncomplicated epilepsy with long seizure-free periods, have not identified a reduction in the quality of life (Engelberts et al., 2002c; Räty & Wilde Larson, 2007).

It is appropriate to use a variety of methods that address changes in the quality of life and psychosocial area at the same time and to determine the validity of the patient's responses.

Postoperative seizure-free periods are important; however, they are not the only factor that determines postoperative improvement in the quality of life. Monitoring of subjective quality of life may help to prevent psychosocial postoperative complications.

Cases of nonepileptic psychogenic seizures, which occur shortly after surgery due to epilepsy and which are extremely difficult to diagnose, deserve special attention (Parra et al., 1988; Davies et al., 2000). Repeated findings of significantly increased numbers of suicidal attempts and suicides following successful surgeries (patient was seizure free) and in patients with chronic epilepsy, is alarming (Blumer, 2002). Monitoring subjective quality of life and preoperative and early postoperative neuropsychiatric monitoring may help in early detection of psychiatric complications. It is then possible to address complications due to the "burden of normality" by initiation of appropriate therapy (Wilson et al., 2004).

5.7. Antiepileptic Medication

Neuropsychological methods help monitor the effects of anti-epileptic therapy and changes in the clinical status of the patient. Anti-epileptic drugs may affect cognitive performance and behavior (e.g., irritability, hyperactivity, or positive psychotropic effects on mood).

During monotherapy, the maintenance of therapeutic drugs levels limits the significance of adverse side effects. The risk increases with higher doses of drugs (and therefore higher blood levels) and when drugs are used in combination. Neuropsychological functions, such as psychomotor speed, attention, memory, and mood, are affected most often. The most marked adverse side effects involve the use of barbiturates and benzodiazepines, which belong to an older therapeutic class. However, individual effects can vary widely. While some patients report problems at very low dose levels, others tolerate very high levels without any complaints.

The cognitive profiles of newer anti-epileptic drugs are under investigation. However, they are probably more favorable compared to older drugs (Dodrill et al., 1989; Leach et al., 1997; Marciani et al., 1998; Meador et al., 2001; Ortinski & Meador, 2004; Lagae, 2006; Weintraub et al., 2007). Nevertheless, the risk of impairment in cognitive performance with the majority of these substances still remains (Loring et al., 2007). Topiramate, with its adverse effect on verbal fluency, is an exception. Anatomical and cognitive effects of anti-epileptic drug exposure during prenatal development are being increasingly investigated. It is very important to separate motor speed from other cognitive measures during evaluation of cognitive changes (Dodrill & Temkin, 1989; Dodrill & Troupin, 1991).

6. Draft on Standardized Examination of Cognitive Functions

Neuropsychological methods are under development, recent studies have changed the evaluation of established methods and the new experimental methods are being designed. Standards are specified and interpretations are added or challenged; additionally, discussions are underway regarding information-specific theory in relation to memory, verbal and non-verbal disorders, and the side of the epileptogenic focus (Bell, Giovagnoli, 2007). The need for standardization is illustrated by differences seen between centers in one country, and these differences increase further between countries.

Neuropsychological tests generally do not measure single cognitive operations but complex ones (e.g., the Stroop test requires attention and ability to name things but also mental flexibility, and it reflects sensitivity to disturbances). It is, therefore, necessary to search for mutually convergent qualitative and quantitative signs when creating diagnostic hypotheses or conclusions and not to start from single markers or one test.

Reitan (1976), Dodrill & Matthews (1992), Rausch et al. (1997), and partially Lezak et al. (2004) discuss suitable arrangements for neuropsychological examination in epileptic patients. Preoperative examination is summarized in the findings of Jones-Gotman (1987, 1991, 1992); Rausch (1991a); Chelune (1991); Oxbury (1997); Jones-Gotman et al., (2003); Djordjevic & Jones-Gotman (2004); Fanfrdlová, Javůrková (2004); Andelman et al. (2004); Helmstaedter (2004); Raspall et al. (2005).

The selection of the battery is very important, because only after some time does the psychologist get experience with different types of patients; therefore, it is important to adhere to the selected arrangement for a sufficient amount of time (Oxbury, 1997).

Although the literature does not recommend testing before 12 hours post-seizure, most patients come back to the baseline levels within two or three hours (Helmstaedter, 2004). Although the presence or absence of depression should always be evaluated, it appears that in most cases, depression and cognitive weakening are independent symptoms of epilepsy. However, depression significantly affects complaints of patients regarding subjectively perceived performance and quality of life. It is important to recognize the possible impact of drug therapy on identifiable neuropsychological profiles.

Baker and Goldstein (2004) focus on practical points of the neuropsychological evaluation in epilepsy. They discuss the following three areas: assessment of cognitive abilities of the candidates for neurosurgery, detailed description of memory weakening relative to needs of rehabilitation, and documentation of the effects of specific anti-epileptic drugs on routine clinical conduct. They refer to the most common mistakes.

6.1. Examination Outside the Specialized Epileptologic Centers

The first assessment after the initial diagnosis of epilepsy should provide baseline measurements that can be used as a reference during future examinations. Therefore, it should provide an evaluation of a wide range of cognitive abilities. A proposal for neuropsychological examinations outside the scope of specialized centers is provided in *Table 4.*

Table 4. The proposal of neuropsychological evaluation out of special centers

Domain	Tests (alternatives)
Intelligence	Wechsler Adult Intelligence Scale III –WAIS-III
Dexterity	Edinburgh Handedness Inventory (Grooved Pegboard Test, Finger Taping Test, Hand Dynamometer)
General memory	Wechsler Memory Scale III – WMS-III
Verbal memory	Logical Memory I (immediate), WMS-III Logical Memory II (delayed), WMS-III
Nonverbal memory	Faces I (immediate), WMS-III Faces II (delayed), WMS-III
Psychosocial problems, personality	Beck Depression Scale II, (WPSI, MMPI)

6.2. Examinations at Specialized Epileptologic and Neurosurgery Centers

Direct contact for six to eight hours between the patient and neurosurgeon is recommended for a preoperative neuropsychological examination (Djordjevic, Jones-Gotman, 2004). Testing should preferably be performed prior to withdrawal of anti-epileptic therapy, done to provoke a seizure. Topiramate, which considerably affects neuropsychological results, is an exception. It should be quickly withdrawn prior to the examination (Helmstaedter, 2004).

Postoperative control evaluations, preferably repeated, are very important. The impact of demographic factors, such as age and gender, and factors related to epilepsy, such as age at disease onset, disease duration, frequency of seizures, and their severity must be taken into account during interpretation of results. A number of tests focused on lateralization are based on findings from patients with different types of pathology, and the transfer to epileptic patients may not be adequate (Djordjevic, Jones-Gotman, 2004). The pathological substrate is often heterogeneous, even in epileptogenic lesions themselves (e.g., not only the most common finding in the hippocampal sclerosis in temporal epilepsy but also tumors, malformations, etc.). There are not enough reliably comparable verbal and especially non-verbal tests available that enable direct comparison of functional ability of both hemispheres in single patients. The tests may distinguish between groups of patients. However, there is still a question of their sensitivity and specificity in single patients (Djordjevic, Jones-Gotman, 2004). It is necessary to develop parallel forms of single tests for repeated measurements and to have confidential intervals for spontaneous changes after repeated testing. New methodological approaches were provided in the concept of significant individual change (Hermann et al., 1996; Sawrie et al., 1996; Martin et al., 2002), which use either reliable change indices (RCI) or methods based on standardized-regression (SRB).

In temporal epilepsies, discussions continue what part of patients should undergo examination of speech lateralization, using the sodium-amytal test (the Wada test—described in the section on measuring). Some centers perform the speech lateralization examination based on dichotic hearing, in which atypical speech lateralization is suspected if a patient does not show preferable performance (normal) of the right ear (Strauss et al., 1987; Zatorre, 1989).

There is relatively extensive experience with neuropsychological examination of temporal epilepsies with an emphasis on memory functions and speech, and in frontal epilepsies with the focus mainly on executive abilities. Most patients with parietal lobe epileptic foci have only small abnormalities that cannot be unambiguously detected. Visual construction tests and tests of visual spatial functions, reading and somatosensory functions can be used in these cases. Patients with seizures that originate in the occipital lobes are rare; accordingly, there is a lack of information about profiles for such patients and the examination is focused on the visual perception system. *Table 5* shows a proposal for examinations in specialized centers.

7. Rehabilitation and Psychotherapy of the Cognitive Deficit

This part is not focused on neurophysiological approaches such as biological feedback in combination with EEG (e.g., Lantz & Sterman, 1988, 1992; Kotchoubey et al., 1999; Strehl et al., 2005) and vagal stimulation (e.g., Ergene et al., 2001; Boon et al., 2006), although they also include psychotherapeutic aspects. The referred approaches will be divided based on the type of psychological intervention and declared target. Critical summaries of psychological interventions in epilepsy are provided by Mostofsky and Balashak (1977), Goldstein (1997, 1990) and Engelberts et al. (2002b).

7.1. Psychological-Educative Approaches

Efficacy of educative programs were reported by Helgeson et al. (1990) and May Pfäfflin (2002).

Table 5. The proposal of neuropsychological evaluation for special centers for epilepsy and neurosurgery

Domain	Tests (alternatives)
Neuropsychological evaluation of temporal lobes and hippocampus function	
Inteligence	WAIS-III
General memory (Warrington Recognition Memory Test –RMT)	WMS-III
Dexterity Dynamometer	Grooved Pegboard Test (Finger Taping Test, Hand)
Verbal memory	Logical Memory I (immediate), WMS-III Logical Memory II (delayed), WMS-III California Verbal Learning Test –CVLT (Warrington Recognition Memory Test-RMT) (Rey Auditory-Verbal Learning Test –RAVLT) (Buschke Selective Reminding Test)
Visual memory	Faces I (immediate), WMS-III Faces II (delayed), WMS-III Rey-Osterrieth Complex Figure Test -CFT (Benton Visual Retention Test -BVRT) (Hodges elements) (Brown-Peterson interference task) (Denman Face Recognition test)
Language	Boston Naming test -BNT (Token test) (Semantic fluency) (Controlled Oral Word Association test –COWAT)
Auditory function (Auditory Reception Test)	Tonal Memory Test -Seashore Tests of Musical Talent
Visual perception	Hooper Visual Organization test - HVOT (Benton Judgment of Line Orientation) (Benton Face Recognition Test)

Table 5.(continued)

Domain	Tests (alternatives)
Neuropsychological evaluation of frontal lobes	
Problem-solving	Wisconsin Card Sorting Test -WCST[1]
	(Modified Cart Sorting Test- MCST)
	(Left-Right Orientation)
Neuropsychological evaluation of occipital lobes	
Visual perception	Rey-Osterrieth Complex Figure
	(Facial Recognition test)
	(Benton Judgment of Line Orientation -JLO)
	(Overlapping Figures Test)
	(Visual Object and Space Perception Battery- VOSP)
	(Hooper Visual Organization Test- HVOT)

The educative program MOSES for adults (Ried et al., 2001) and "famoses" program, were prepared partly for epileptic children and partly for parents or caregivers in German language areas (Wohlrab et al., 2007). Educative programs for adult patients, in Nigeria, including a control group were described by Olley et al. (2001).

7.2. Approaches Focused on Relaxation Programs

They include studies that use muscle relaxation (e.g., Rousseau et al., 1985; Dahl et al., 1987; Whitman et al., 1990; Puskarish et al., 1992), using breathing to influence the patterns of relaxation (Goldstein, 1990), with a combination of relaxation with systematic desensitization and imaginative techniques (Brown & Fenwick, 1989), and application of aromatherapy in combination with relaxation techniques (Betts et al., 1995). The application of yoga was reported by Ramaratnam (2001).

7.3. Approaches of Behavioral or Cognitive-Behavioral Therapy

Cognitive-behavioral approaches focused on self-control and based on findings between stress situations and seizures; they describe cognitive restructuralization and seizure control, and they are sometimes similar to approaches that focused on psychological and social adaptation (Tan & Bruni, 1986; Au et al., 2003; Strehl et al., 2005).

7.4. Approaches Focused on Psychological and Social Adaptation

These approaches don't have seizure frequency as the primary focus; however, their effectiveness cannot be completely dismissed, especially since they may achieve better compliance with the therapeutic regimen. They are oriented mainly on psychosocial problems, and they often use a series of interventions that often makes evaluation of efficacy more complicated. Included are various psychological approaches, both individual and group (Gillham, 1990; Andrews & Schonfeld, 1992; Preiss, 1994; Spector et al., 1995, 1999), for pediatric use summarizing the work of Wagner and Smith (2006, 2007) and various psychotherapeutic approaches, especially dynamic orientations but also for example physical training (McAuley et al., 2001).

They are prepared by special rehabilitation programs for adaptation to postoperative conditions following epilepsy surgery when new problems appear during adaptation to life without seizures (Fraser et al., 1993; Fraser, Thorbecke, 1997; Langfitt et al., 1999; Wilson et al., 2001, 2004).

Cognitive Rehabilitation

A number of works are based on the fact that programs of learning compensation mechanisms (specific for individual's performance level) aimed at minimizing the effects of cognitive impairment have been found (Bennet, Krein, 1988; Thompson, 1997; Hendriks, 2001; Wilson, 2002). Even a small improvement may cause a significant increase in the patient's independence (Aldenkamp, Vermeulen, 1991). Assessment for rehabilitation training should include a wide range of memory measures but also other aspects of cognitive performance. Determination of memory deficits may help the patient and his/her family to achieve realistic life goals (Thompson, 1997). However, complaints about memory do not necessarily indicate memory deficits. Only mild correlations between self-assessment of memory and objective test results have been found (Vermeulen et al., 1993; Elixhauser et al., 1999; Preiss and Vojtěch, 2008), and they are related to emotional problems, which in such cases should also be targeted.

External memory aids are most valuable for epileptic patients. Training in using diaries may be significantly beneficial for everyday life. Computer diaries or personal organizers and other reliable drug-dosing devices may provide similar benefits.

Cognitive rehabilitation in epilepsy, program-planning and selection of participants must take into account certain differences (Ponds, Hendriks, 2006). Memory deficits in epilepsy are less serious compared to patients with severe brain injury or dementia. In contrast to patients with closed head injuries or vascular brain accidents who will get better in time, epilepsy is a chronic condition without a tendency toward gradual improvement. Patients with epilepsy retain their awareness regarding their limitations, abilities, and daily problems (in contrast to patients, e.g., with frontal lobe injury or anosognosia).

Neuropsychological memory rehabilitation in patients with epilepsy was described by Aldenkamp and Vermeulen (1991). Compensation strategies in memory deficits were addressed by Hendriks (2001) and Ponds and Hendriks (2006), who describe in detail the procedures used in the Epilepsy Centre, Kempenhaeghe, The Netherlands.

Engelberts et al. (2002a) applied two cognitive rehabilitation methods for attention deficits that are commonly used in patients with central nervous system lesions but not yet in epileptic patients. The methods included training (retrained) and compensation. A control performed after six months found both programs effective in patients with focal seizures. Patients with active epilepsy showed greater benefits from both programs compared to seizure-free patients. Authors recommend including both methods in patient care programs.

Other well-controlled studies appear, even though they are scarce in the field of epilepsy compared to other diagnoses.

Conclusion

Impacts of epilepsy are often the same or even more serious than the disease itself, and diminished cognitive performance is especially important. The most common cognitive disorders associated with epilepsy in adults are deterioration in memory, mental retardation, and attention deficits. Cognitive problems in children are more diffuse and are responsible for speech problems, learning disorders, poor school results, behavioral problems, and unfavorable social and job prospects (Fatenau et al., 2004; Dunn & Kronenberger, 2005; Rijskevorsel, 2006). In addition, some malign disorders with severe cognitive deficits occur in childhood. On the other side of the age range, older aged patients with chronic epilepsy have more severe cognitive deterioration, especially those on polytherapy, compared to controls (Griffith et al., 2006). The prevalence of epilepsy in adults with intelligence disorders is probably higher compared to the general population (McGrother et al., 2006).

The number of patients with well-controlled epilepsy is growing. Successful therapy (pharmacological, neurosurgical or vagal stimulation) may significantly increase cognitive performance and improve the quality of life. Psychosocial and rehabilitation procedures that have gradually become more sophisticated and are based more on controlled studies may also provide benefits.

Social attitudes toward epilepsy vary considerably among cultures. Many patients perceive the disease as a stigma; they experience discrimination, chronic emotional stress, and social isolation. Cooperative patient societies and, more recently, internet–based support groups, can play an important role (Hoch & Ferguson, 2005http://www.plosmedicine.org/). New neuroimaging methods (e.g., Vingerhoets et al., 2004) enable the transfer of focus from neuropsychology, in the area of epilepsy, from diagnostics and localization, to more accurate descriptions of weak and strong aspects of the patient's cognitive status and to psychosocial and cognitive rehabilitation.

References

Acosta I, Vale F, Tatum WO IV, Benbadis SR. Epilepsy surgery after age 60. *Epilepsy and Behavior* 2008; 12:324-325.

Äikiä M, Kälviäinen R, Mervaala E, Riekkiner Sr PJ. Predictors of seizure outcome in newly diagnosed partial epilepsy: memory performance as a prognostic factor. *Epilepsy Research* 1999; 37:159-167.

Aldenkamp AP. Cognitive impairment in epilepsy: state of affairs and clinical relevance. *Seizure* 2006; 15:219-220.

Aldenkamp AP, Arend J. Effects of epileptiform EEG discharges on cognitive function: Is the concept still valid? *Epilepsy and Behavior* 2004; 5(Suppl 1):S25-S34.

Aldenkamp AP, Baker G, Pieters MS, Schoemaker, HC, Cohen AF, Schwabe G. The Neurotoxicity Scale: The validity of patients-scale, assessing neurotoxicity. *Epilepsy Research* 1995; 20:229–239.

Aldenkamp AP, Vermeulen J. Neuropsychological rehabilitation of memory function in epilepsy. *Neuropsychological Rehabilitation* 1991; 1:199–214.

Alpherts WCJ, Aldenkamp AP. Computerized neuropsychological assessment of cognitive functioning in children with epilepsy. *Epilepsia* 1990; 31(Suppl 4):S35–S40.

Alpherts WCJ, Vermeulen J, van Rijen PC, da Silva L, Veelen CWM. Standard versus tailored left temporal lobe resections: Differences in cognitive outcome? *Neuropsychologia* 2008; 46:455-460.

Andelman F, Fried I, Neufeld MI. Quality of life self-assessment as a function of lateralization of lesion in candidates for epilepsy surgery. *Epilepsia* 2001; 42:549–555.

Andelman F, Neufeld MY, Fried I. Contribution of neuropsychology to epilepsy surgery. *Isr. J. Psychiatry Relat Sci.* 2004; 41:125–132.

Anderson-Roswall L, Engman E, Samuelsson H, Sjörberg-Larsson Ch, Malmgrem K. Verbal memory decline and adverse effects on cognition in adult patients with pharmacoresistant partial epilepsy. *Epilepsy and Behavior* 2004; 5:667-686.

Andrews DJ, Schonfeld WH. Predictive factors for controlling seizures using a behavioural approach. *Seizure* 1992; 1:111–116.

Au A, Chan F, Li K, Leung P, Li P, Chan J. Cognitive-behavioral group treatment program for adults with epilepsy in Hong Kong. *Epilepsy and Behavior* 2003; 4:441-446.

Baker GA, Gagnon D, McNulty P. The relationship between seizure frequency, seizure type and quality of life: Findings from three European countries. *Epilepsy Research* 1998; 30:231-240.

Baker GA, Goldstein LH. The dos and don'ts of neuropsychological assessment in epilepsy. *Epilepsy and Behavior* 2004; 5:77–80.

Baker GA, Jacoby A, Buck D, Stalgis C, Monnet D. Quality of life of people with epilepsy: a European study. *Epilepsia* 1997; 38:353-362.

Baker GA, Smith DF, Dewey M, Morrow J, Crawford PM, Chadwick W. The development of a seizure severity scale as an outcome measure in epilepsy. *Epilepsy Research* 1991; 8:245–251.

Baker GA, Smith DF, Dewey M, Jacoby A, Chadwick, DW. The initial development of health-related quality of life model as an outcome measure in epilepsy. *Epilepsy Research* 1993; 16:65–81.

Bear D, Fedio P. Quantitative analysis of interictal behavior in temporal lobe epilepsy. *Arch. Neurol.* 1977; 34:454–467.

Bell, BD, Giovagnoli AR. Recent innovative studies of memory in temporal lobe epilepsy. *Neuropsychology Review* 2007; 17:455-476.

Bennet TL, Krein LK. The neuropsychology of epilepsy: Psychological and social impact. In: Reynolds CR, Fletscher-Janzen, eds. Handbook of clinical child neuropsychology. New York: Plenum Press, 1988; 419–441.

Berger H. Über das Elektrenkephalogramm des Menschen. *Arch. Psychiat. Nervenkr.* 1929; 87, 527–570.

Betts T, Fox C, MacCallum R. An olfactory countermeasures treatment for epileptic seizures using a conditioned arousal response to specific aromatherapy oils. *Epilepsia* 1995; 36(Suppl 3):S130–S131.

Binnie CD. Seizure, EEG discharges and cognition. In: Trimble MR, Reynolds EH, eds. Epilepsy, behaviour and cognitive function. New York: Willey, 1987; 45-51.

Birbeck GL, Hays RD, Cui X, Vickrey BG. Seizure reduction and quality of life improvement in people with epilepsy. *Epilepsia* 2002; 43:535–538.

Bjørnæs H, Stabell KE, Heminghyt E, Røste GK, Bakke SJ. Resective surgery for intractable focal epilepsy in patients with low IQ: Predictors for seizure control and outcome with respect to seizures and neuropsychological and psychosocial functioning. *Epilepsia* 2004; 45:131–139.

Blume WT, Grabow JD, Darley FL, Aronson AE. Intracarotid amobarbital test of language and memory before temporal lobectomy for seizure control. *Neurology* 1973; 23:812-819.

Blumer D. Epilepsy and suicide: a neuropsychiatric analysis. In: Trimble MR, Schmitz B, eds. The neuropsychiatry of epilepsy. Cambridge: Cambridge University Press, 2002; 107–116.

Boon P, Moors I, Herdt VD, Vonck K. Vagus nerve stimulation and cognition. *Seizure* 2006; 15:259-263.

Boone KB, Miller BL, Rosenberg L, Durazo A, McIntyre H, Weil M. Neuropsychological and behavioural abnormalities in an adolescent with frontal lobe seizures. *Neurology* 1988; 38:583–586.

Breteler MM, de Groot RR, Van Romunde IK, Hofman A. Risk of dementia in patients with Parkinson's disease, epilepsy, and severe head trauma: a register-based follow-up study. *Am. J. Epidemiol.* 1995; 142:1300–1305.

Brown SW. Dementia and epilepsy. In: Trimble M, Schmitz B, eds. The neuropsychiatry of epilepsy. Cambridge: Cambridge University Press, 2002; 135–151.

Brown SW, Fenwick PBC. Evoked and psychogenic epileptic seizures: II. Inhibition. *Acta Neurologica Scandinavica* 1989; 80:541–547.

Buck D, Smith M, Appleton R, Baker GA, Jacoby A. The development and validation of the Epilepsy and Learning Disabilities Quality of Life (ELDQOL) Scale. *Epilepsy and Behavio*r 2007; 10:38-43.

Carter MD, Weaver DF, Joudrey HR, Carter AO, Rockwood K. Epilepsy and antiepileptic drug use in elderly people as risk factors for dementia. *Journal of Neurological Sciences* 2007; 252:169-172.

Collins AL, Lennox WG. The intelligence of 300 private epileptic patients. *Assoc. Res. Nerv. Men. Dis.* 1947; 26:586–603.

Cramer JA, Perrine K, Devinski O, Meador K. A brief questionnaire to screen for quality of life in epilepsy: the QOLIE-10. *Epilepsia* 1996; 37:577–582.

Cramer J, Perrine K, Devinski O, Bryant-Comstock L, Meador K, Hermann B. Development and cross-cultural translations of a 31-item quality of life in epilepsy inventory. *Epilepsia* 1998; 39:81–88.

Dahl J, Mellin L, Lund L: Effects of a contingent relaxation treatment program on adults with refractory epileptic seizures. *Epilepsia* 1987; 28:125–132.

Davies KG, Bell BD, Bush AJ, Wyler AR. Prediction of verbal memory loss in individuals after temporal lobectomy. *Epilepsia* 1998; 39:820-828

Davies KG, Blumer DP, Hermann BP, Phillips BLB, Montouris GD. De novo nonepileptic seizures after cranial surgery for epilepsy: incidence and risk factors. *Epilepsy and Behavior* 2000; 1:436-443.

Delaney RC, Rosen AJ, Mattson RH, Novelly RA. Memory function in focal epilepsy: a comparison of non-surgical, unilateral temporal lobe and frontal lobe samples. *Cortex* 1980; 16:103-117.

Derry PA, Wiebe S. Psychological adjustment to success and to failure following epilepsy surgery. *Canadian Journal of Neurological Sciences* 2000; 27(Suppl 1):S116–S120.

Devinski O, Vickrey BG, Cramer JA, Perrine K, Hermann B, Meador K, Hays RD. Development of the quality of life in epilepsy inventory. *Epilepsia* 1995; 36:1089–1094.

Dikmen S, Matthews CG. Effect of major motor seizure frequency upon cognitive-intellectual functions in adults. *Epilepsia* 1977; 18:21-29.

Djordjevic J, Jones-Gotman M. Psychological testing in presurgical evaluation of epilepsy. In: Shorvon S, Perucca E, Dodson E, eds. The treatment of epilepsy. Oxford: Blackwell Science, 2004; 699–722.

Dodrill CB. A neuropsychological battery for epilepsy. *Epilepsia* 1978; 19:611–623.

Dodrill CB. Correlates of generalized tonic-clonic seizures with intellectual, neuropsychological, emotional, and social function in patients with epilepsy. *Epilepsia* 1986; 27:399–411.

Dodrill CB. Neuropsychological effects of seizures. *Epilepsy and Behavior* 2004; 5(Suppl 1): S21-S24.

Dodrill CB. Progressive cognitive decline in adolescent and adults with epilepsy. *Prog. Brain. Res.* 2002; 135:399-407.

Dodrill CB, Batzel LW, Queisser HR, Temkin N. An objective method for the assessment of psychological and social problems among epileptics. *Epilepsia* 1980; 21:123–135.

Dodrill CB, Herman B, Rausch R, Chelune, G., Oxbury, S.: Neuropsychological testing for assessing prognosis following surgery for epilepsy. In: Engel J, (ed). *Surgical treatment of epilepsies*. New York: Raven, 1993; 263–271.

Dodrill CB, Matthews CG. The role of neuropsychology in the assessment and treatment of persons with epilepsy. *Am. Psychol.* 1992; 47:1139–1142.

Dodrill CB, Temkin NR. Motor speed is a contaminating factor in evaluating the "cognitive" effects of phenytoin. *Epilepsia* 1989; 30:453–457.

Dodrill C, Troupin A. Neuropsychological effects of carbamazepine and phenytoin: a reanalysis. *Neurology* 1991; 41:141-143.

Dodrill CB, Wilensky AJ. Neuropsychological abilities before and after five years of stable antiepileptic drug therapy. *Epilepsia* 1992; 33:327-334.

Dodrill CB, Wilkus RJ. Relationships between intelligence and electroencephalographic epileptiform activity in adult epileptics. *Neurology* 1976; 26:525–531.

Dodrill CB, Wilkus RJ, Ojemann GA, Ward AA, Wyler AR, Van Belle G, Tamas L. Multidisciplinary prediction of seizure relief from cortical resection surgery. *Ann. Neurol.* 1986; 20:2–12.

Dunn DW, Kronenberger WG. Childhood epilepsy, attention problem and AHDD: review and practical considerations. *Seminars in Pediatric. Neurology* 2005; 12:222-228.

Dupont S, Samson Y, van de Moortele PF, Samson S, Poline J-B, Hasboun D, Lebiha D, Baulac M. Bilateral hemispheric alteration of memory processes in right temporal lobe epilepsy. *J. Neurol. Neurosurg. Psychiatry* 2002; 73:478–485.

Elixhauser A, Leidy NK, Meador K, Means E, William MK. The relationship between memory performance, perceived cognitive function, and mood in patients with epilepsy. *Epilepsy Research* 1999; 37:13–24.

Engel J Jr. A proposed diagnostic scheme for people with epileptic seizures and with epilepsy: Report of the ILAE Task force on classification and terminology. *Epilepsia* 2001; 42:796-803.

Engel J Jr. Report of the ILAE classification core group. *Epilepsia* 2006; 47:1558-1568.

Engel J Jr, Cascino GD, Shields WD. Surgically remediable syndromes. In: Engel J Jr, Pedley TA, eds. Epilepsy. A comprehensive textbook. Philadelphia-New York: Lippincott-Raven, 1998; 1687-1696.

Engelberts HJ, Klein M, Adèr HJ, Heimans JJ, Kasteleijn-Nolst Trenité DGA, van der Ploeg HM. The effectiveness of cognitive rehabilitation for attention deficits in focal seizures: A randomized controlled study. *Epilepsia* 2002a; 43:587-595.

Engelberts NHJ, Klein M, Kastelein-Nolst Trenité DGA, Heimans JJ, van der Ploeg HM. The effectiveness of psychological interventions for patients with relatively well-controlled epilepsy. *Epilepsy and Behavior* 2002b; 3:420–426.

Engelberts HJ, Klein M, van der Ploeg HM, Kasteleijn-Nolst Trenité, DGA. Cognition and health-related quality of life in well-defined subgroup of patients with partial epilepsy. *J. Neurol.* 2002c; 249:290-294.

Ergene E, Behr PK, Shih JJ. Quality-of-life assessment in patients treated with vagus nerve stimulation. *Epilepsy and Behavior* 2001; 2:284-287.

Fastenau PS, Shen J, Dunn DW, Perkins SM, Hermann BP, Austin JK. Neuropsychological predictors of academic underachievement in pediatric epilepsy: moderating roles of demographic, seizure, and psychosocial variables. *Epilepsia* 2004; 45:1261–1272.

Fanfrdlová Z, Javůrková A. Neuropsychologické vyšetření. (Neuropsychological examination). In: Brázdil M, Hadač M, Marusič P, eds. Farmakorezistentní epilepsie. Praha: Triton 2004; 140–147.

Fleck DE, Shear PK, Strakowski S. A reevaluation of sustained attention performance in temporal lobe epilepsy. *Archives of Clinical Neuropsychology* 2002; 17:399–405.

Fox JT. The response of epileptic children to mental and educational tests. *Brit. J. Med. Psychol.* 1924; 4:235–248.

Franzen MD, Iverson, GL. The Wechsler memory scales. In: Groth-Marnat, G, ed. Neuropsychological assessment in clinical practice. New York: John Wiley and Sons, Inc., 2000; 195-222.

Fraser RT, Thorbecke R. Postoperative rehabilitation. In: Engel J Jr, Pedley TA, eds. Epilepsy: a comprehensive textbook. New York: Raven Press, 1997; 1901–1910.

Fraser RT, Gumnit RJ, Thorbecke R, Dobkin BH. Psychosocial rehabilitation. A pre- and postoperative perspective. In: Engel J Jr, ed. Surgical treatment of epilepsies, 2nd ed. New York: Raven Press, 1993; 669–677.

Gillham R. Refractory epilepsy: an evaluation of psychological methods in outpatients' management. *Epilepsia* 1990; 31:427–432.

Gilham R, Baker G, Thompson P, Birbeck K, McGuire A, Tomlinson L, Eckersley L, Silveria C, Brown S. Standardisation of a self-report questionnaire for use in evaluating cognitive, affective and behavioural side-effects of anti-epileptic drug treatments. *Epilepsy Research* 1996; 24:47–55.

Gilliam FG, Barry JJ, Hermann BP, Meandor KJ, Vahle V, Kanner AM. Rapid detection of major depression in epilepsy: a multicenter study. Lancet Neurology 2006; 5:399-405.

Gilliam F, Kuzniecki R, Faugt E, Black L, Carpenter G, Schrodt R. Patient-validated content of epilepsy-specific quality-of-life measurement. *Epilepsia* 1997; 38:233–236.

Gleissner U, Helmstaedter Ch, Schramm J, Elger ChE. Memory outcome after selective amygdalohippocampectomy: a study in 140 patients with temporal lobe epilepsy. *Epilepsia* 2002; 43:87–95.

Gleissner U, Helmstaedter Ch, Schramm J, Elger ChE. Memory outcome after selective amygdalohippocampectomy in patients with temporal lobe epilepsy: one-year follow-up. *Epilepsia* 2004; 45:960-962.

Goldstein LH.: Effectiveness of psychological intervention for people with poorly controlled epilepsy. *J. Neurol. Neurosurg. Psychiatry* 1997; 63:137-142.

Goldstein LH. Behavioural and cognitive-behavioural treatments for epilepsy: a progress review. *British Journal of Clinical Psychology* 1990; 29:257–269.

Griffith HR, Martin RC, Bambara JK, Marson DC, Faught E. Older people with epilepsy demonstrate cognitive impairments compared with patients with amnestic mild cognitive impairment. *Epilepsy and Behavior* 2006; 8:161-168.

Gülgönen S. Demirbilek V, Korkmaz B, Dervent A, Townes BD. Neuropsychological functions in idiopathic occipital lobe epilepsy. *Epilepsia* 2000; 41:405–411.

Hardy SG, Miller JW, Holmes MD, Born DE, Ojemann GA, Dodrill CB, Hallam DK. Factors predicting outcome for intractable epilepsy with pathologically verified mesial temporal sclerosis. *Epilepsia* 2003; 44:565-568.

Helgeson DC, Mittan R, Tan SY, Chayasirisobhon S. Sepulveda epilepsy education: the efficacy of psycho-educational program in the treatment of medical and psycho-social aspects of epilepsy. *Epilepsia* 1990; 31:75-83.

Helmstaedter Ch. Behavioural and neuropsychological aspects of frontal lobe epilepsy. In: Trimble MR, Schmitz B, eds. The neuropsychiatry of epilepsy. Cambridge: Cambridge University Press, 2002; 164–185.

Helmstaedter Ch. Neuropsychological aspects of epilepsy surgery. *Epilepsy and Behavior* 2004; 5:S45-S55.

Helmstaedter C, Elger CE. The phantom of progressive dementia in epilepsy. *The Lance*t 1999; 354:2133-2134.

Helmstaedter C, Kurthen M, Lux S, Neuber M, Elger CE. Chronic epilepsy and cognition: a longitudinal study in temporal lobe epilepsy. *Ann. Neurol.* 2003; 54:425-432.

Hendriks M. Neuropsychological compensatory strategies for memory deficits in patients with epilepsy. In: Pfaflin M, Fraser RT, Thorbecke R, Spech U, Wolf P, eds. Comprehensive care for people with epilepsy. London: John Libbey, 2001; 87–94.

Hermann BP. Contributions of traditional procedures to an understanding of the neuropsychology of epilepsy. In: Dikmen S, Dodson WE, Kinsbourne M, Hiltbrunner B, eds. The assessment of cognitive function in epilepsy. New York: Demos Publication, 1991; 1-22.

Hermann BP, Seindenberg M, Haltiner A, Wyler AR. Relationship of age of onset, chronological age, and adequacy of preoperative performance to verbal memory change after anterior temporal lobectomy. *Epilepsia* 1995; 36:137–145.

Hermann BP, Seindenberg M, Schoenfeld J, Davies K. Neuropsychological characteristics of the syndrome of mesial temporal lobe epilepsy. *Arch. Neurol.* 1997; 54:369–376.

Hermann BP, Seindenberg M, Haltiner A, Wyler AR. Adequacy of language function and verbal memory performance in unilateral temporal lobe epilepsy. *Cortex* 1992; 28:423–433.

Hermann BP, Seidenberg M, Schoenfeld J, Peterson J, Leveroni C, Wyler AR. Empirical techniques for determining reliability, magnitude, and pattern of neuropsychological change after epilepsy surgery. *Epilepsia* 1996; 2:942-950.

Hermann BP, Whitman S. Behavioral an personality correlates of epilepsy: a review, methodological critique and conceptual model. *Psychol Bull* 1984; 95:451-497.

Hermann BP, Wyler AR. Neuropsychological outcome of anterior temporal lobectomy. *J. Epilepsy* 1988; 23:585–588.

Hermann BP, Wyler AR, Richey ET, Rea JM. Memory function and verbal learning ability in patients with complex partial seizures of temporal lobes origin. *Epilepsia* 1987; 28:547-554.

Hoch D, Ferguson T. What I've learned from E-patients. PLOS Medicine 2005; 2:e206.

Holmes MD, Dodrill CB, Wilkus RJ. et al.: Is partial epilepsy progressive? Ten-years follow-up of EEG and neuropsychological changes in adults with partial seizures. *Epilepsia* 1998; 39:1189-1193.

Holmes GL, Lenck-Santini P-P. Role of interictal epileptiform abnormalities in cognitive impairment. *Epilepsy and Behavior* 2006; 8: 504-515.

Chelune G. Using neuropsychological data to forecast postsurgical cognitive outcome. In: Lüders H, ed. Epilepsy surgery. New York: Raven 1991; 477–485.

Chelune GJ, Naugle RI, Hermann BP, Barr WB, Trenerry MR, Loring DW, Perrine K, Strauss E, Westerweld M. Does presurgical IQ predict seizure outcome after temporal lobectomy? Evidence from the Bozeman epilepsy consortium. *Epilepsia* 1998; 39:314–318.

Chelune GJ, Naugle RI, Luders H, Sedlak J, Awad IA. Individual change after epilepsy surgery: practice effect, and base-rate information. *Neuropsychology* 1993; 7:41-52.

Chelune GJ, Naugle RI, Lüders H, Awad IA. Prediction of cognitive change as a function of preoperative ability level among temporal lobectomy patients at six months follow-up. *Neurology* 1991; 41:399-404.

Jacoby A, Baker G, Smith D, Dewey M, Chadwick D. Measuring the impact of epilepsy: The development of a novel scale. *Epilepsy Research* 1993; 16:83–88.

Jokeit H, Ebner A. Effects of chronic epilepsy on intellectual functions. *Prog. Brain Res.* 2002; 135:455-463.

Jokeit H, Ebner A. Long-term effects of refractory temporal epilepsy on cognitive abilities: a cross sectional study. *Journal of Neurology, Neurosurgery and Psychiatry* 1999; 67:44-50.

Jokeit H, Schacher M. Neuropsychological aspects of type epilepsy and etiological factors in adults. *Epilepsy and Behavior* 2004; 5 (Suppl 1):14–20.

Jokeit H, Seitz RJ, Markowitsch HJ, Neumann N, Witte OW, Ebner A. Prefrontal asymmetric interictal glucose hypometabolism and cognitive impairment in patients with temporal lobe epilepsy. *Brain* 1997; 120:2283–2294.

Jones-Gotman M. Commentary: Psychological evaluation. Testing hippocampal function. In: Engel J Jr, ed. Surgical Treatment of the Epilepsies. New York: Raven Press 1987; 203–211.

Jones-Gotman, M. Presurgical neuropsychological evaluation for localization of seizure focus. In: Lüders H, ed. Epilepsy surgery. New York: Raven Press Ltds 1991; 469–475.

Jones-Gotman M. Neuropsychological techniques in the identification of epileptic foci. *Epilepsy Reseach* 1992; 5 (Suppl):87-94.

Jones-Gotman M, Smith M.-L, Zatorre R. Neuropsychological testing for localizing and lateralizing the epileptogenic region. In: Engel J Jr, ed. Surgical Treatment of the Epilepsies. 2nd ed. New York: Raven Press 2003; 245–261.

Kneebone AC, Chelune GH, Dinner DS, Naugle RI, Award IA. Intracarotid amobarbital procedure as a predictor of material-specific memory change after anterior temporal lobectomy. *Epilepsia* 1995; 36:875-865.

Kolínová M, Preiss J. Therapy and antiepileptic drug monitoring. 5th Epileptologic days, Abstracts, Prague 1991;

Kotchoubey B, Strehl U, Holzapfel S, Blankenhorn V, Fröscher W, Birbaumer N. Negative potential shifts and the prediction of the outcome of neuro feedback therapy in epilepsy. *Clinical Neurophysiology* 1999; 110:683-686.

Lagae L. Cognitive side effects of anti-epileptic drugs. The relevance in childhood epilepsy. *Seizure* 2006; 15:235-241.

Langfitt JT, Wood BL, Brand KL, Brand J, Erba G. Family interactions as targets for intervention to improve social adjustment after epilepsy surgery. *Epilepsia* 1999; 40:735–744.

Lantz D, Sterman MB. Neuropsychological assessment of subject with uncontrolled epilepsy: effects of EEG feedback training. *Epilepsia* 1988; 29:163–171.

Lantz D, Sterman MB. Neuropsychological prediction and outcome measures in relation to EEG feedback training for the treatment of epilepsy. In: Benett TL, ed. The neuropsychology of epilepsy. New York: Plenum Press 1992; 213–231.

Leach JP, Girvan J, Paul A, Brodie MJ. Gabapentin and cognition: a double-blind, dose-ranging, placebo-controlled study in refractory epilepsy. *J. Neurol. Neurosurg. Psychiatry* 1997; 62:372-376.

Leclercq M, Coullet J, Azouvi P, Marlier N, Martin Y, Strypstein E, Rousseaux M. Dual task performance after severe diffuse traumatic brain injury or vascular prefrontal damage. *J. Clin. Exp. Neuropsychol.* 2000; 22:339-350.

Lee TMC, Yip JTH, Jones-Gotman M. Memory deficits after resection from left or right anterior lobe in humans: a meta-analytic review. *Epilepsia* 2002; 43:283-291.

Leidy NK, Elixhauser A, Rentz AM, Beach R, Pellock J, Schachter S, Willian MK. Telephone validation of the Quality of life in epilepsy Inventory-89 (QOLIE-89). *Epilepsia* 1999; 40:97-106.

Lezak MD. Neuropsychological assessment. 3rd ed.. New York: Oxford University Press 1995;

Lezak MD, Howieson DB, Loring DW. Neuropsychological Assessment. 4th ed. New York: Oxford University Press 2004; 1016.

Loring DW, Kimford JM, Lee GP, King DW. Amobarbital effects and lateralized brain function. The Wada test. New York: Springer-Verlag 1992;

Loring DW, Marino S, Meador KJ. Neuropsychological and behavioral effects of antiepilepsy drugs. *Neuropsychology Review* 2007; 17:413-425.

Loring DW, Meador KJ, Lee GP. Dimensions of Epilepsy Foundation Concern Index.

Epilepsy and Behavior 2005; 6:348-352.

Mahalick DM, Ruff RM. Neuropsychological sequelae of arteriovenous malformations. *Neurosurgery* 1991; 29:351–357.

Marciani MG, Stanzione P, Mattia D. Lamotrigine add-on therapy in focal epilepsy: electroencephalographic and neuropsychological evaluation. *Clin. Neuropharmaco.* 1998; 21:41-47.

Markand ON, Salanova W, Whelihan E, Emsley CL. Health-related quality of life outcome in medically refractory epilepsy treated with anterior temporal lobectomy. *Epilepsia* 2000; 41: 749–759.

Martin R, Griffith HR, Sawrie S, Knowlton R, Faught E. Determining empirically based self-reported cognitive change: development of reliable change indices and standardized regression-based change norms for the multiple abilities self-report questionnaire in an epilepsy sample. *Epilepsy and Behavior* 2006; 8:239-245.

Martin RC, Grote ChL. Does the Wada test predicts memory decline following epilepsy surgery? *Epilepsy and Behavior* 2002; 3:4-15.

Martin R, Sawrie S, Gilliam F, Mackey M, Faught E, Knowlton R, Kuzniekcy R. Determining reliable cognitive change after epilepsy surgery: Development of reliable change indices and standardized regression-based change norms for the WMS-III and WAIS-III. *Epilepsia* 2002; 43:1551–1558.

Matkovic Z, Oxbury SM, Hiorns RW, Morris JH, Carpenter KN, Adams CBT, Oxbury JM.. Hippocampal neuronal density correlates with pre-operative non-verbal memory in patients with temporal lobe epilepsy. *Epilepsia* 1995; 36(Suppl 3):S93.

May TW, Pfäfflin M. The efficacy of an educational treatment program for patients with epilepsy (MOSES): results of a controlled randomized study. *Epilepsia* 2002; 43:539–549.

Mayeux R, Brandt J, Rosen J, Benson DF. Interictal memory and language impairments in temporal lobe epilepsy. *Neurology* 1980; 30:120–125.

Mazzini L, Cossa FM, Angelino E, Campini R, Pastore I, Monaco F. Posttraumatic epilepsy: neuroradiologic and neuropsychological assessment of long-term outcome. *Epilepsia* 2003; 44:569–574.

McAuley JW, Long L, Heise J, Kirby T, Buckworth J, Pitt C, Lehrman KJ, Moore JL, Reeves AL. A prospective evaluation of the effects of 12-week outpatient exercise program on clinical and behavioral outcomes in patients with epilepsy. *Epilepsy and Behavior* 2001; 2:284-287.

McGrother CW, Bhaumik S, Thorp C, Hauck A, Branford D, Watson JM. Epilepsy in adults with intellectual disabilities: Prevalence, associations and service implications. *Seizure* 2006; 15:376-386.

Meador KL, Gilliam FG, Kanner AM, Pellock JM. Cognitive and behavioral effects of antiepileptic drugs. *Epilepsy and Behavior* 2001; 2:SS1-SS17.

Moerland MC, Aldenkamp AP, Alpherts WCJ. Computerized psychological testing in epilepsy. In: Maarse FJ, Mulder LJM, Sjouw WPB, Akkerman AE, eds. Computers in psychology. Methods, instrumentation and psychodiagnostics. Lisse: Swet and Zeitlinger, 1988; 157–164.

Mostofsky D, Balashak BA. Psychobiological control of seizures. *Psychological Bulletin* 1977; 84:723-750.

Mungas D, Ehler C, Walton N, McCutchen CB. Verbal learning differences in epileptic patients with left and right temporal lobe foci. *Epilepsia* 1985; 26:340–345.

Nilsson L, Ahlbom A, Farahmand BY, Asberg M, Tomson T. Risk factors for suicide in epilepsy. *Epilepsia* 2002; 43:644-651.

Ogden JA, Mee EW, Henning M. A prospective study of impairment of cognition and memory and recovery after subarachnoid hemorrhage. *Neurosurgery* 1993; 33:572–586.

Olley BO, Osinowo HO, Brieger WR. Psycho-educational therapy among Nigerian adult patients with epilepsy: a controlled study. *Patient Education and Counseling* 42, 2001; 42:25-33.

Ortinski P, Meador KJ. Cognitive side effects of antiepileptic drugs. *Epilepsy and Behavior* 2004; 5(Suppl 1):S60-S65.

Oxbury S. Assessment for surgery. In: Cull Ch, Goldstein LH, eds. The clinical psychologist's handbook of epilepsy. London, New York: Rutledge 1997; 54–76.

Oyegbile TO, Dow C, Jones J, Bell B, Rutecki P, Sheth R, Seidenberg M, Hermann BP. The nature and course of neuropsychological morbidity in chronic temporal lobe epilepsy. *Neurology* 2004; 62:1736–1742.

Paglioli E, Palmini A, Paglioli E, da Costa JC, Portuguez M, Martinez JV, Calcagnotto ME, Hoefel JR, Raupp S, Barbosa-Countiho L. Survival analysis of the surgical outcome of temporal lobe epilepsy due to hippocampal sclerosis. *Epilepsia* 2004; 45:1383–1391.

Paradiso S, Hermann BP, Blumer D, Davies K, Robinson RG. Impact of depressed mood on neuropsychological status in temporal lobe epilepsy. *J. Neurol. Neurosurg. Psychiatry* 2001; 70:180–185.

Parra J, Iroiarte J, Kanner AM, Bergen DC. De novo psychogenic nonepileptic seizures after epilepsy surgery. *Epilepsia* 1998; 39:474–477.

Pasquier F. Early diagnosis of dementia: neuropsychology. *J Neurol* 1999; 246:6–15.

Peng FCC. Language impairment in epileptics. *Acta neurologica Sinica* 1995; 45:1–21.

Perrine K, Westerveld M, Sass KJ, Devinsky O, Digal IM, Spencer DD, Luciano DJ, Nelson PK. Wada memory disparities predict seizure laterality and postoperative seizure control. *Epilepsia* 1995; 36:851-856.

Ponds RWHM, Hendriks M. Cognitive rehabilitation of memory problems in patients with epilepsy. *Seizure* 2006; 15:267-273.

Preiss J. Srovnání tří forem psychosociální rehabilitace nemocných epilepsií. (Comparison of three forms of psychosocial rehabilitation of epileptic patients). *Čs Psychiat* 1994; 90:216-224.

Preiss J. Epilepsie a neuropsychologie. (Epilepsy and neuropsychology). In: Preiss M, a kol.: Klinická neuropsychologie. (Clinical neuropsychology). Praha: Grada 1998b; 194–218.

Preiss J, Haas T. Intelektová výkonnost v souboru 241 nemocných epilepsií podle WAIS-R. (The intellectual performance in a sample of 241 epileptic patients according WAIS-R). Čes a Slov Psychiat 2001; 97:23–26.

Preiss J, Haas T. Mnohorozměrná analýza intelektové výkonnosti nemocných epilepsií. (Multivariate analysis of intellectual functioning in epileptic patients). *Čs Psychol* 2002; 46:3–21.

Preiss J, Vojtěch Z. Jak měřit spolehlivě změnu? Kognitivní změny po resekčních operacích pro farmakorezistentní epilepsii. (How to measure change reliably? Cognitive changes after resection operation for farmacoresistent epilepsy). *Čs Psychol* 2006a; 50:349-360.

Preiss J, Vojtěch Z. Kognitivní změny po resekčních operacích pro farmakorezistentní epilepsii s ohledem na stranu operace. (Cognitive changes after resective surgery for medical refractory temporal epilepsy in relation to the side of surgery). *Čes a slov Psychiat.* 2006b; 102:406-415.

Preiss J, Vojtěch Z. Kvalita života po resekční operaci pro farmakorezistentní epilepsii. (The quality of life after resective surgery for medial refractory epilepsy). *Čes a slov Psychiat* 2007; 103:175-183.

Preiss J, Vojtěch Z. " Subjektivní paměť" ve vztahu k operacím pro farmakorezistentní epilepsii. (Subjective memory in relation to surgery for farmacoresistent epilepsy). *Čs Psychol* 2008; 52:225-239.

Puskarish CA, Whitman S, Dell J, Hughes J, Rosen AJ, Herrmann BP. Controlled examination of progressive relaxation training of seizure reduction. *Epilepsia* 1992; 33:675–680.

Ramaratnam S. Yoga for epilepsy: methodological issues. *Seizure* 2001; 10:3-6.

Raspall T, Doñate M, Boget T, Carreño M, Donaire A, Agudo R, Bargalló N, Rumià J, Setoain X, Pintor L, Salamero M. Neuropsychological tests with lateralizing value in patients with temporal lobe epilepsy: Reconsidering material-specific theory. *Seizure* 14; 2005:569-576.

Räty LKA, Wilde Larsson BM. Quality of life in young adults with uncomplicated epilepsy. *Epilepsy and Behavior*, 2007; 10:142-147.

Rausch R. Factors affecting neuropsychological and psychosocial outcome of epilepsy surgery. In: Lüders H, ed. Epilepsy surgery. New York: Raven Press Ltds., 1991; 487–492.

Rausch R., Le M.-T, Langfitt JT. Neuropsychological evaluation-adults. In: Engel J Jr, Pendley TA, eds. Epilepsy. A comprehensive textbook, vol.1. Philadelphia: Lippincott-Raven, 1997; 977–987.

Rausch R, Langfitt JT: Memory evaluation during the intracarotid sodium amobarbital procedure. In: Lüders H, ed. Epilepsy surgery. New York: Raven Press Ltds,1991; 507–514.

Reitan RM. Psychological testing of epileptic patients. In: Vinken PJ, Bruyn GW, eds. Handbook of clinical neurology: The epilepsies. Vol. IX and X. New York: North Holland Publishing Company,1976;

Ried S, Specht U, Thorbecke R, Goecke K, Wohlfarth R. MOSES: an educational program for patients with epilepsy and their relatives. *Epilepsia* 2001; 42 (Suppl 3):76-80.

Rijkevorsel K, van. Cognitive problems related to epilepsy syndromes, especially malignant epilepsies. *Seizure* 2006; 15:227-234.

Roost DV, Boon P, Vingerhoets G. Can the Wada test predict seizure outcome in epilepsy surgery patients. *Surgical Neurology* 2007; 68:202. doi:10.1016/j.surneu.2007.06.059

Rousseau A, Hermann B, Whitman S. Effects of progressive relaxation on epilepsy: analysis of a series of cases. *Psychological Reports* 1985; 57:1203–1212.

Sabaz M, Lawson JA, Cairns DR, Duchovny MS, Resnick TJ, Dean PM, Bye AME. Validation of the Quality of Life in Childhood Epilepsy Questionnaire in American epilepsy patients. *Epilepsy and Behavior* 2003; 3:680-691.

Sands S, Van Gorp WG, Finlay JL. A dramatic loss of non-verbal intelligence following a right parietal epyndymona: brief case report. *Psychooncology* 2000; 9:259–266.

Sawrie SM, Chelune GJ, Naugle RI, Lüders HO. Empirical methods for assessing meaningful neuropsychological change following epilepsy surgery. *J. Int. Neuropsychol. Soc.* 1996; 2:556-564.

Saykin AJ, Gur RC, Sussman NM, O'Connor MJ, Gur RE. Memory deficits before and after temporal lobectomy: effect of laterality and age of onset. *Brain Cogn.* 1989; 9:191-200.

Seidenberg M. Neuropsychological functioning of children with epilepsy. In: Hermann BP, Seidenberg M, eds. Childhood epilepsies: Neuropsychological, psychosocial and intervention aspects. Chichester: John Wiley and Sons, 1989; 41–81.

Seidenberg M, Hermann B, Haltiner A, Wyler A. Verbal recognition memory performance in unilateral temporal lobe epilepsy. *Brain and Language* 1993; 44:191–200.

Seidenberg M, O'Leary DS, Berent S, Boll T. Changes in seizure frequency and test-retest scores on Wechsler adult intelligence scale. *Epilepsia* 1981; 22:75–83.

Selwa LM, Beren S, Girodani B, Henry TR, Buchtel HA, Ross DA. Serial cognitive testing in temporal lobe epilepsy: Longitudinal changes with medical an surgical therapies. *Epilepsia* 1994; 35:743–749.

Schwab RS. A method of measuring consciousness in petit mal epilepsy. *J. Nerv. Ment. Dis.* 1939; 89:690–691.

Smith ML, Milner B. The role of right hippocampus in the recall of spatial location. *Neuropsychologia* 1981; 19:781–793.

Spector S, Foots A, Goldstein LH. Reduction in seizure frequency as a result of group intervention for adults with epilepsy. *Epilepsia* 1995; 36(Suppl 3):S130.

Spector S, Tranah A, Cull, C, Goldstein LH. Reduction in seizure frequency following a short group intervention for adult with epilepsy. *Seizure* 1999; 8:297-303.

Stefan H, Pauli E. Progressive cognitive decline in epilepsy: an indication of ongoing plasticity. *Prog. Brain Res.* 2002; 135:409-417.

Strauss E, Gaddes W, Wada J. Performance of free recall verbal dichotic listening test and cerebral speech dominance determined by carotide amytal test. *Neuropsychologia* 1987; 25: 747–753.

Strehl U, Kotchoubey B, Trevorrow T, Birbaumer N. Predictors of seizure reduction after self-regulation of slow cortical potentials as a treatment of drug-resistant epilepsy. *Epilepsy and Behavior* 2005; 6:156-166.

Tan S-Y, Bruni J. Cognitive-behavioral therapy with adults patients with epilepsy: a controlled outcome study. *Epilepsia* 1986; 27:225-233.

Thompson PJ. Epilepsy and memory. In: Cull Ch, Goldstein LH, eds. The clinical psychologist's handbook of epilepsy. London, New York: Rutledge, 1997; 35–53.

Thompson PJ, Corcoran R. Everyday memory failures in people with epilepsy. *Epilepsia* 1992; 33(Suppl 6):S18–S20.

Thompson PJ, Duncan JS. Cognitive decline in severe intractable epilepsy. *Epilepsia* 2005; 46:1780-1787.

Thompson PJ, Sander JWAS, Oxley JR. Intellectual deterioration in epilepsy, In: Dan M., Dreifus F, eds. Advances in epileptology. New York: Raven Press, 1987; 611-614.

Trenerry MR, Jack CR Jr, Cascino GD, Sharabrough FW, Ivnik RJ. Gender differences in post-temporal lobectomy verbal memory and relationships between MRI hippocampal volumes and preoperative verbal memory. *Epilepsy Res.* 1995; 20:69-76.

Tucha O, Smely C, Preier M, Lange KW. Cognitive deficits before treatment among patients with brain tumors. *Neurosurgery* 2000; 47:324–333.

Upton D, Thompson PJ. General neuropsychological characteristics of frontal lobe epilepsy. *Epilepsy Research* 1996; 23:169–177.

Vecchio ND, Liporace J, Nei M, Sperling M, Tracy J. A dissociation between implicit and explicit verbal memory in left temporal lobe epilepsy. *Epilepsia* 2004; 45:1124-1133.

Vermeulen J, Aldenkamp AP, Alpherts WCJ. Memory complaints in epilepsy: correlation with cognitive performance and neuroticism. *Epilepsy Res.* 1993; 15:157-170.

Vickrey BG, Hays RD, Hermann BP, Bladin PF, Batzel LW. Outcomes with respects to quality of life. In: Engel J Jr. Surgical treatment of epilepsies. 2nd ed. New York: Raven Press Ltd, 1993 a; 623–635.

Vickrey BG, Perrine KR, Hays RD, Hermann B, Cramer J.A, Gordon J, Meador K, Devinski, O. Quality of Life in Epilepsy. QOLIE-89 (version 1.0). Scoring Manual and Patient Inventory. Santa Monica: RAND 1993 b.

Vingerhoets G, Deblaere K, Backes WH, Achten E, Boon P, Boon PJ, Hofman P, Vermeueln J, Vonck K, Wilmink J, Aldenkamp AP. Lessons for neuropsychology from functional MRI in patients with epilepsy. *Epilepsy and Behavior,* 2004; 1(Suppl 5):S81–S89.

Volicer L, Smith S, Volicer BJ. Effect of seizures on progression of dementia of the Alzheimer type. *Dementia* 1995; 6:258–263.

Wada J, Rasmussen TB. Intracarotid injection of sodium amobarbital for the lateralization of cerebral speech dominance: experimental and clinical observations. *J. Neurosurg.* 1960; 17: 266–282.

Wagner JL, Smith G. Psychosocial intervention in pediatric epilepsy: A critique of the literature. *Epilepsy and Behavior* 2006; 8:39-49.

Wagner JL, Smith G. Psychosocial services in pediatric epilepsy clinic: Referral patterns and feasibility. *Epilepsy and Behavior.* 2007; 10:129-133.

Weintraub D, Buchsbaum R, Resor SR Jr, Hirsch LJ. Psychiatric and behavioral side effects of the newer antiepileptic drugs in adults with epilepsy. *Epilepsy and Behavior* 2007; 10:105-110.

Wheelock I, Peterson C, Buchtel HA. Pre-surgery expectations, post-surgery satisfaction, and psychosocial adjustment after epilepsy surgery. *Epilepsia* 1998; 39:487–494.

Whitman S, Dell J, Legion V, Eibhlyn A, Statsinger J. Progressive relaxation for seizure reduction. *Journal of Epilepsy* 1990; 3:17–22.

Wiebe S, Blume WT, Girvin JP. A randomized, controlled trial of surgery for temporal-lobe epilepsy. *N. Engl. J. Med.* 2001; 345:311-318.

Wiebe S, Matijevic S, Eliasziw M, Derry PA. Clinically important change in quality of life in epilepsy. *J. Neurol. Neurosurg. Psychiatry* 2002; 73:116–120.

Wilson BA. Memory rehabilitation. In: Squire LR, Schachter DL, eds. Neuropsychology of memory. 3rd ed. New York: The Guilford Press, 2002; 263–272.

Wilson SJ, Bladin PF, Saling MM. Paradoxical results in the cure of chronic illness: the "burden of normality" as exemplified following seizure surgery. *Epilepsy and Behavior* 2004; 5:13-21.

Wilson SJ, Bladin PF, Saling MM, McIntosh AM, Lawrence JA. The longitudinal course of adjustment after seizure surgery. *Seizure* 2001; 10:165–172.

Wohlrab GCh, Rinnert S, Bettendorf U, Fischbach H, Heinen G, Klein P, Kluger G, Jacob K, Kahn D, Winter R, Pfäfflin M. famoses: A modular educational program for children with epilepsy and their parents. *Epilepsy and Behavior* 2007; 10: 44-48.

Wyllie E, Naugle R, Chelune G, Luders G, Morris H, Skibinski C. Intracarotid amobarbital procedure: II. Lateralizing value in evaluation for temporal lobectomy. *Epilepsia* 1991; 32:865-869.

Zatorre RJ. Perceptual asymmetry on the dichotic fused words test and cerebral speech lateralization determined by the carotid sodium amytal test. *Neuropsychologia* 1989; 27: 1207–1219.

In: Cognitive Deficit in Mental and Neurological Disorders ISBN: 978-1-60741-957-0
Editors: H. Kucerova, M. Preiss

Chapter X

Huntington's Disease

Jan Roth and Jiri Klempir

Abstract

Huntington's disease (HD) is an autosomal dominantly inherited neurodegenerative disease caused by gene mutation on a short arm of the 4th chromosome, with incidence of about 1: 10-15,000. The mutation consists in expansion of CAG triplet with critical limit of about 40 repeats. HD is manifested by combination of motor symptoms (especially, the choreatic dyskinesias are characteristic), neuropsychiatric disorders (depression, anxiety, irritability or apathy, obsession and compulsion, psychotic symptoms) and progressing dementia. Typically, HD begins between the 35th and 50th year of age, however, juvenile and late forms also exist.

The progression of HD cannot be substantially therapeutically influenced, but some of the symptoms may be at least temporarily effectively confronted using pharmacological and psychosocial interventions. However, the course of HD leads unevitably to the total dependency on the neighbourhood and patients die in uncontrollable marasmus.

The diagnosis of HD is confirmed by a genetic test. In persons at risk (the offspring of the ill or positively tested person) who want to know their genetic state, presymptomatic DNA testing is performed using a specific protocol. Prenatal testing is also possible.

1. Introduction into the Issue

Huntington's disease (HD) is an autosomal dominantly inherited, progressive neurodegenerative disease. The first compact description was made by George Huntington in 1872 (Huntington, 1872).

The prevalence of HD in European and North American countries is estimated to about 5 to 10/100 thousand inhabitants (Harper, 1992; Kremer, 1994; Al-Jader, 2001). HD is relatively more frequent in all countries in which the emigration from Europe was historically directed (USA, Canada or Australia). However, Europe may not be the only source of the HD gene mutation. There is indirect evidence that another source of mutation may also be in Africa (Harper, 1992). In Japan and other Far East countries, its prevalence is rarer (Harper, 1992).

The best-known epidemiological study in Europe is a study of South Wales (Walker, 1981; Quarrell, 1988) and, in the U.S.A., that of Maryland (Folstein, 1987). The epidemiological studies on HD are available on the website http://uwcmml1s.uwcm.ac.uk /uwcm/mg/fidd/data/143100.html.

A discovery of a source of HD in Venezuela, located in an isolated community near the Maracaibo Lake, where about 10 thousand persons with more than 100 HD-afflicted persons are living, was of extreme importance for the research of HD (Penney, 1990).

Localization of the mutation of the 4th chromosome was found in 1983 (Gusella, 1983); in 1993, the character of the mutation conditioning HD was explained - multiplication of trinucleotide (triplet) CAG exceeding 39 repeats (Huntington's Disease Collaborative Research Group, 1993). In HD, an inverse relationship between the CAG triplet repeats and the age-at-onset of clinical manifestations was shown (the more triplets, the sooner the disease flares up) (Andrew, 1993; Snell, 1993).

A product of the mutation is an aberrant protein called huntingtin. The substance of the pathogenetic activity of huntingtin is not clear yet; its influence on a series of neurotrophic factors, induction of apoptosis or changes of ubiquitin-proteasome system are discussed (Paulson, 2000, Valera 2005).

The principal incipient neuropathological change in HD consists in a loss of GABA-ergic, so-called medium-size spiny neurons in the striatum (Perry, 1973; Spokes, 1980). Further progression manifests with atrophic changes of pallidum, degenerative changes in the cortex, and afterward, general atrophy of the brain (Vonsattel, 1985).

In a typical case, HD is manifested with a clinical triad: motor, cognitive and neuropsychiatric symptoms. There are three forms of the disease, for which age at the onset of HD is primarily decisive.

Classical form of HD (90% of all patients) with the onset of clinical manifestation between the 35th and 50th years of age is by far the most frequent. The first signs of the disease are usually unspecific neuro-psychiatric (behavioural and affective symptoms) and cognitive changes. However, they do not provide for correct diagnosing. The right diagnosis is often determined only after the manifestation of motor symptoms, especially choreatic dyskinesias (involuntary rapid movements, accidentally occurring at various parts of the body, which may be compared with occasional dancing-like movements) which are typical for HD. Gradually, other neurological symptoms occur: dysarthria and dysphagia, eye movement disorders, symptoms of cerebellar or pyramidal tracts lesions, gait disorders, incontinence and, later also cachexia. In advanced stages, the involuntary movements often decline or change from the original choreatic ones to dystonic ones. Further progression brings atypical parkinsonian syndrome. The patient becomes fully dependent on his/her neighbourhood and dies in uncontrollable marasmus, mostly of infections and secondary complications, approximately after 15 to 20 years. The cognitive deficit is also progressing during the course of the disease; continuous disintegration of the personality and severe progressing dementia occur.

The juvenile form of HD (onset of the disease before the 20th year of age) develops in about 5% of all cases. The first symptoms are usually mental changes. The behavioral abnormalities quickly progress, and the psychotic conditions are relatively often manifested.

Dementia is concomitantly developed. From the point of view of movements, a progressing parkinsonian syndrome occurs; in about 30% of affected persons epileptic paroxysms are manifested. The choreatic dyskinesias are very rare in the juvenile form. The progression is quick and the survival time is shorter (8 to 10 years) than in case of the classic form (Ribaï, 2007).

The HD form with late onset is manifested in persons over 60. Again, this represents about 5% of all cases. Such a form of the disease shows relatively benign course and most of the patients live to the average age of the healthy population. The principal and incipient symptom is chorea, whose distribution and character do not differ from the classical form of the disease, but they are less intensive and progress more slowly. Cognitive dysfunctions and other mental abnormities are usually not conspicuous and dementia does not usually develop. However, isolated cognitive deficits may be present.

HD is usually diagnosed on the basis of a typical clinical picture and result of a genetic test. The genetic test itself, however, only confirms the presence of mutation - the positivity of test with the absence of symptoms only means the presence of a genetic propensity of the disease (which flares up if the mutation bearer lives for a sufficient period).

The test can be (on condition of the presence of the specific procedure) carried out in so far healthy persons who are at risk of HD (the so-called predictive presymptomatic and prenatal test).

The progression of HD is insusceptible to any treatment. However, some of the symptoms may be effectively confronted using pharmacological and psychosocial interventions.

Pathophysiological Background of Development of Mental Disorders in HD

The area of the basal ganglia regulates and readjusts motor abilities as far as inborn, automatic and learned patterns are concerned. Other basic function of the basal ganglia consists in the regulation of motivation, affective and cognitive functions and behaviour. Therefore, in case of impairment within the basal ganglia region, a combination of motor (parkinsonian syndrome, dyskinetic syndromes) and mental (neuro-psychiatric and cognitive symptoms) changes is often apparent.

The complexity of basal ganglia is functionally connected by links that form parallel working circuits (Alexander, 1986). These circuits are linked to the systems and functional units that are further connected to structures located outside basal ganglia (thalamus, frontal lobes and limbic system).

At present, the striatum, a nucleus that is in case of HD dominantly damaged already in the incipient stages of HD, is considered to be the principal input into the system of basal ganglia (Albin, 1989; Alexander, 1990).

Striatum can be divided into three parts: dorsal, medial and ventral (Flaherty, 1994):

Dorsal striatum (most of putamen, dorsal part of caudate nucleus) is connected especially in motor circuits;

Medial striatum (most of caudate nucleus, ventral part of putamen) is primarily connected to the structures of so-called associative cortex - thus its function is already a modulation of cognitive functions and behaviour;

Ventral striatum (ventral caudate nucleus, incl. accumbens, tuberculum olfactorium) is primarily connected to the limbic system, including the amygdala and hippocampus. This part plays an important role for regulation of the motivation/affective functions; in addition, it takes part in creation of the memory traces.

One of the dominant areas determining the character of development of psychopathologic symptoms in HD and other conditions of basal ganglia consists, according to the present knowledge, in changes of three functional circuits of the striatum (especially the ventral part) connected with certain areas of the frontal lobes (Cummings, 1993; Tekin, 2002, Bonelli, 2008):

Dorsolateral circuit, whose affection is primarily manifested by executive dysfunction;

Orbitofrontal circuit, whose affection is primarily manifested by changes of personality, disinhibition, disorder of the attention, motivation, initiative, emotional instability, inadequate euphoria and irritability;

Anterior cingulate circuit, whose affection is primarily manifested by signs like immobility, incontinence, apathy, abulia, loss of communication, food-intake, up to the so-called akinetic mutism.

The extent of affection of the respective circuits and combination of the symptoms gives rise to an individual demonstration of patient's psychic dysfunction.

However, the neuropsychological changes, present in diseases of basal ganglia, thus also in HD, may originate in areas outside such striatofrontal circuits. Actually, transmitter dysbalances in the ascendant brain stem tracts practically always occur. Such dysbalances play an important role in regulation of the mental symptoms (serotonin – nuclei raphe – depression, aggression, anxiety; noradrenalin – locus coeruleus – wake/sleep, attention, dopamin – substantia nigra – mesolimbic system and mesocortical system – cognitive, affective, motivation function, behaviour) (Graybiel, 1990).

2. Principal Domains of the Affected Psychic Functions

The mental disorders (neuropsychiatric and cognitive ones) are an integral part of HD and often belong to the most frequent symptoms of the disease and precede manifestation of the movement symptoms by several years. Also, for most of the patients and their families, they form the most serious symptoms affecting the quality of life.

The publications of the 1980s and 1990s usually studied a lower number of patients and did not use unified diagnostic instruments. Only recently, thanks to research organizations such as e.g., Huntington Study Group v USA (www.huntington-study-group.org) and European Huntington's Disease Network (www.euro-HD.net), the number of the observational studies carried out on big multi-centric groups of uniformly examined patients (e.g., study of the frequency of depression in the study of Paulsen et al., 2005, predictors of the HD diagnosis in the study of Langbehn et al., 2007 or obsessive - compulsive disorders in the study of Beglinger et al., 2007) has increased.

The multi-centric groups also enable the analysis of larger groups of persons at risk of HD in the "preclinical" phase (e.g., Julien et al., 2007).

Table No. 1. The main psychopathological symptoms of the Huntington's disease

Personality changes and behaviour disorders,
Affective disorders,
Anxiety disorders (anxiety, obsession, compulsion),
Psychotic symptoms,
Cognitive deficits and dementia.

Table No. 2. Frequency of respective psychiatric symptoms of the classical form of HD

Irritability	over 50%	(Thompson, 2002)
Apathy	70%	(Craufurd, 2001)
Anxiety	over 50%	(Paulsen, 2001)
Depression	over 40%	(Mendez, 1994)
Suicidal behaviour	12.7%	(Schoenfeld, 1984)
Bipolar affective disorder	10%	(Folstein, 1987)
Obsession, compulsion	20 to 30%	(Marder, 2000)
Delusions, hallucinations	1 to 5%	(Marder, 2000)

(Naarding et al., 2001, modified)

2.1. Personality and Behavioural Disorders

The personality changes and behavioural disorders are usually the first signs of development of pathological changes, and it seems that they may precede any manifestations of typical motor symptoms even by many years (Di Maio et al., 1993. Shiwach et al., 1994).

An HD person changes continuously, especially in the sense of an increased interest in his/her own person and needs that are in contrast, however, to a lack of interest in work, his/her own appearance and needs of other persons (Paulsen, 2001; Mendez, 1994). In the early stages of the HD, changes of sexual appetency in the sense of hypersexuality, possibly related aggressivity, promiscuity or sexually provocative behaviour are rare. A much more frequent problem of the HD persons consists in loss of libido or impotence, developing in the course of HD (Fedoroff, 1994).

In the very beginning of HD, petty criminality/offences may also occur (e.g., thefts, recklessness while driving, drunk driving, vandalism) (Jensen, 1998); more rarely, it is alcohol abuse (King, 1985). The neighbourhood perceives such events as "unscrupulous" demonstrations, however, they already result from pathological changes.

A frequent symptom is a *loss of insight (*especially when the patient wants to carry on the activities that he/she cannot cope with - driving, finance management, etc.). It is usually a source of frequent conflicts with his/her family. Insufficient or completely lacking insight of the disease may be interpreted as a defence mechanism - "denial" However, it may also be based on the cognitive deficit.

Increased *irritability* occurs in nearly 50% of patients, at least in a certain period (Paulsen, 2001; Mendez, 1994; Folstein, 1987; Thompson, 2002); it does not correlate with their mood and often also not with their manifestation of aggressivity. The increased irritability is provoked by circumstances that would not have induced such response of the patient in the past. Also, the intensity and duration of such responses are not proportional to circumstances. According to some important studies, irritability or apathy (see below) seem to be the main and characteristic features of the behavioural disorders in persons suffering from HD, and correlate neither with the duration of the disease nor with the severity of the motor and cognitive signs (Craufurd, 2001; Thompson, 2002).

Aggressivity (both verbal and brachial) is more frequently manifested in such patients who have had tendency to it in all their lives. Very often, it is only directed towards the closest family members, but usually, it is not demonstrated in the public/hospital environment. The predisposing factors are as follows: abuse of psychoactive substances, anxiety, depressive/psychotic symptoms, obsessive-compulsive disorder, delirious conditions and, last but not least, psychosocial stress induced by an assignment of more tasks within a short period, problems with common tasks or conflict with authorities etc. (Burns, 1990).

The problems of *apathy* should be mentioned separately. For HD, the apathy is the characteristic and frequent symptom. Apathy significantly influences the quality of life and, in the research of HD, has to be dealt with separately.

The apathy may be defined as a reduction of the emotional reactivity linked with internal feelings of indifference to one's own personality and to the environment, with loss of energy/drive. It can occur as an independent psychopathological phenomenon (Levy, 1998, Kingma, 2008) or accompany depressive symptoms and physical/psychical exhaustion. It has a tendency to run deep, along with the cognitive deterioration. Apathy may be induced or potentiated by overloading the patient with excessive requirements. Apathy negatively influences cognitive performance (Thompson, 2002) and occurs in nearly 70% of all patients with HD (Craufurd, 2001). Diagnostically, it is often mistaken for depression.

2.2. Affective Disorders

Depression accompanies HD patients in nearly 40% of cases (Mendez, 1994; Folstein, 1987; Shiwach, 1994; Paulsen, 200), while about 20% of those patients suffer from more serious forms of depression. In up to 30% of patients, depression manifests several years before the first motor symptoms, and it is also manifested in persons who are not aware of their risk. There are families with a high prevalence of depression and families with a low prevalence. With gradual progression of the disease, the number of depressive conditions decreases (Folstein, 1983; Paulsen 2005). In about 10% of patients, we identify a picture of bipolar affective disorder (Folstein, 1987; Mendez, 2000).

Suicide is a serious problem. Patients commit suicide four to six times more frequently than the healthy population; more than 2% of all patients suffering from HD commit suicide (Farrer, 1986; Di Maio, 1993; Rosenblatt, 2000). Some data indicate the prevalence of suicidal behaviour reaching more than 10% in this group of patients (Schoenfeld, 1984; Paulsen 2005). It should be stressed that the suicidal behaviour is a threat in any HD stage, even in case when the disease has not yet been diagnosed.

2.3. Anxiety Disorders

At least 30% of patients complain about anxiety verging on panic (Paulsen, 2001). Due to their anxiety, they are often unable to solve previously banal tasks. Family members can, for instance, note a disquieted reaction of the patient to common and unimportant events - late arrival home; decision as to what to put on; decision as to whether to accept an invitation and so on. The anxiety in patients suffering from HD often and persistently manifests with somatoform signs (headaches, back pain, gastrointestinal disorders), which patients very often refer to as dominant problems.

Obsessions (persistent, obtrusive ideas, thoughts, concepts) are present relatively often (in up to 24% of patients) and in up to 12% of patients, *compulsions* (compulsive behaviour) and possibly *perseverations* (adherence to certain ideas, but more frequently persistent repetition of words, gestures or movements) occur. The incidence of obsessions and compulsions increases with the period of HD (Marder, 2000; Anderson, 2001; Beglinger 2007).

2.4. Psychotic Symptoms

The incidence of psychotic complications in the course of HD is reported in 3.4 to 12% of the patients (Mendez, 1994; Folstein, 1987; Rosenblatt, 2000). However, in some later studies, the incidence of psychotic manifestations is reported only rarely (Marder, 2000). Patients with earlier onset of HD show higher risk of development of psychotic symptoms (Rosenblatt, 2000).

The so-called negative symptoms are more striking: loss of initiative, inability to keep personal relationships. Another possible dominating feature in psychotic patients is a generalized paranoid attitude or even delusions connected with irritability and aggressive behaviour. This paranoid attitude is especially obvious towards family members, not the medical staff. Patients are hostile, mistrustful, "arrayed" and do not want to be examined. Hallucinations are much rarer. Psychotic signs may develop at the beginning of HD or at some point during its course.

The psychotic symptoms are often unidentified - many physicians and non-psychiatrists cannot identify or address them. Without contacts with caregivers, even a psychiatrist or neuropsychologist may not reveal them. This may explain a low detection of psychotic complications in the studies.

2.5. Isolated Cognitive Deficits and Dementia

There is a series of studies aimed at cognitive deficit in HD (Folstein, 1983; Bylsma, 1992; Butters, 1978, 1985; Lawrence, 1996, Verny, 2007). The results of these works indicate that even before the clinical manifestation of motor symptoms, slight changes very often occur in the area of cognitive functions (Verny, 2007).

Hahn-Barma et al. (1998) examined 91 persons at risk of HD during the testing protocol, prior to the genetic analysis. A genetic mutation for HD was subsequently shown in 42 persons. In those subjects, a positive correlation between the increased number of the CAG triplets and performance in tests of executive functions (Symbol Digit Modalities Test - SDMT, Stroop's Test) and impaired learning of pair associations in Wechsler Memory Scale (WMS) were observed. However, Snowden et al. (2000) did not show any relationship between the number of the CAG triplets and speed of the cognitive deterioration on a group of 87 patients suffering from HD.

Lawrence et al. (1998) tested 22 persons with HD but without obvious clinical symptoms using a battery of the CANTAB cognitive tests (Cambridge Neuropsychological Test Automated Battery) and compared them with a group of 32 persons without mutation. They found a decreased performance in tests of divided attention and semantic verbal fluency.

The reduction of cognitive functions in HD is neither global nor gradually progressing. In a study of Snowden et al. (2000), it was the psychomotor speed and verbal fluency that were impaired most and at a most rapid speed. On the contrary, the executive functions (Wisconsin Card Sorting Test–WCST) and spatial (extra-personal) functions (the so-called Road Map Test) did not change even three years later.

Ho et al. (2003) used for the identification of cognitive changes in 61 persons in initial stages of HD a battery of neuropsychological tests of the CAPIT-HD protocol and the CANTAB electronic battery. The patients showed progressive disorder of their attention, short-term memory, executive functions and deceleration of the psychomotor speed. On the contrary, the semantic memory and remote recall were relatively well preserved. The general cognitive performance was not noticeably reduced.

Lemiere et al. (2004) prospectively compared cognitive functions in the group of persons with HD, persons at risk of HD and in a control group. In the group with HD, they observed a significant decrease in tests of executive functions (SDMT, Stroop's Test, Trail Making Test B - TMT-B) and visuospatial functions (Object and Space Perception test). When comparing the persons at risk of HD with the control group, they observed a reduced performance in tests of the working memory (SDMT, repetition of numbers backwards from WAIS III, spatial extent backwards from WAIS III), in tests of verbal learning and remote recall (Hopkins Verbal Learning test) and also in conditional associative learning (Conditional Associative Learning Test). Lemiere et al., among others, dealt with the interpretation of results of the so-called time-limited tests (SDMT, Stroop's Test, TMT) and concluded that the performance in these tests is more influenced by the total deceleration of the information processing than by patient's own cognitive deterioration. Lemiere et al. consider SDMT a very sensitive test that is suitable for longitudinal monitoring of cognitive changes.

Thompson et al. (2002), of the Manchester Group, studied the influence of behavioural disorders (apathy, depression, irritability) on independence and cognitive performance in patients suffering from HD. They assess the behavioural disorders in the same way as Craufurd, using the Problem Behaviour Assessment Scale for Huntington's disease (PBA-HD). According to the results of this study, the presence of apathy negatively affects cognitive (designation of objects, test of verbal fluency, Stroop's Test) and motor performances.

Therefore, in early stages of HD, the isolated cognitive deficits, e.g., attention, learning process and memory disorders, dominate. Step-by-step, dysexecutive syndrome develops. The psychomotor speed also changes during the course of the disease. Sooner or later, the patient reaches the level of dementia, largely of a subcortical type. The cognitive deterioration in HD has a progressive character but its speed is individual. Sometimes even a long-term stationary character may be observed. The rate of cognitive deterioration need not be directly proportional to behavioural or neurological symptoms.

Attention, Learning and Memory Disorders

One of the first cognitive symptoms of HD is an *attention disorder.* Both simple and divided attention are reduced. Typically, the persistence is low and the concentration is bad. The decreased attention and memory disorders often belong to the first troubles that are perceived by the patient and his/her neighbourhood (e.g., in the family, at workplace).

Attention disorders negatively affect the learning process and memory. Already in the initial stages of the disease, disorders of learning new information and its recollection occur. The learning curve varies and increases only very slowly. In patients with HD, Lundervold et al. (Lundervold, 1994) observed a decreased ability to remember, tendency to passive method of learning new information, but normal ability of acquired knowledge *retention.* During acquisition and learning new information, *the interference effect* functions very easily. The disorders in shifting attention from one task to another are caused by perseverance of the previous, already learned information.

The most severely, and first of all, affected is the *working memory,* which is significantly utilized for the solution of topical problems and new situations. The capacity of working memory is significantly reduced with HD.

In patients not just with HD but with any cause of the frontal dysfunction, *the prospective memory* is damaged (Baddeley, 1987). The patient does not remember what to do in the right moment, how to apply the previous decision (he/she forgets about a check-up with the physician or to pick up a child from school). The recall of the information after its reminder is typical for the prospective memory disorder. The disorder of prospective memory is the result of impaired explicit memory and executive dysfunction.

The patients most often complain about the disorder of a free recall of information (new names and events, time data) -the impairment of the *explicit (declarative, intentional) memory,* which acts for retention of memories in time and space (episodic memory) and knowledge of the surrounding world and events (semantic memory). However, *the semantic memory*, whose disorders are predominantly linked with the temporal cortex, is usually preserved for a long time in HD. Sometimes, a patient suffering from HD surprises his/her neighbourhood with his/her knowledge watching a TV knowledge contest. On the other hand, his/her performance in tests of the semantic memory (e.g., designation of pictures) may be paradoxically reduced (Hodges, 1990).

The HD patient's inability to select and classify a higher amount of acquired pieces of information also significantly contributes to the disorder in remembering and recalling of important information.

The recognition is, however, surprisingly good in HD when compared with *free recall* (Butters, 1985). *Cuing* (cue reproduction) or *creation of associations* helps with the organization of memory and facilitates the recall of necessary information from the memory. According to Jacobs et al. (1990), the patients also more frequently confabulate.

The weakened *verbal memory* limits the patient in conversation, watching the TV program or reading of a continuous text.

In case of HD, the *procedural memory* (i.e. learning of motor skills) is also significantly affected. The disorders of procedural memory are typical for the impairment of basal ganglia, especially the striatum. In practice, any dysfunction of the procedural memory is manifested by disorder of acquiring and maintenance of learned motor formulas (e.g., driving, dancing, playing a musical instrument). Performance of such operations needs an increased concentration of attention, leads to exhaustion, failure and subsequently to loss of motivation and mood/behavioural disorders. In advanced stages of the disease, also the malfunction of basic motor operations appears (skill necessary to walking, dressing and eating).

The long-lasting memory is well preserved, even in advanced stages of the disease. Patients remember many events but have problems with their arrangement in time (they remember the first signs of the disease, but they do not know when the disease started or how long it has been lasting, when he/she quit his/her employment and so forth).

The disorders of attention, learning and memory are supported by prompt fatigue, anxiety, disinhibition, executive dysfunction, dyskinetic syndromes and the treatment.

Disorders of Visual Perception and Visuospatial Functions

The visual perception deficit is obvious when comparing and distinguishing figures and objects (Brouwers, 1984; Lawrence, 1996). Patients have difficulties in percepting the emotional content of faces (expression), especially in case of negative emotions (anger, disgust, fear, sadness) (Jacobs, 1995; Sprenglemeyer, 1996, Johnson et al., 2007). The recognition of negative emotions gets worse with increasing cognitive deterioration and motor affection (Johnson et al., 2007). The ability of patients with HD to recognize disgust correlates with atrophy of the anteroventral insula and the recognition of joy correlates with the volume of the amygdala (Kipps, 2007).

The visuospatial memory for the arrangement of outer space (*alocentric memory*) in patients with HD is affected from the early stages of the disease. Unlike the alocentric memory, the visuospatial memory for the position of the own body (*egocentric memory*) is only affected in the advanced stages of cognitive deterioration (Davis, 2003).

The limited spatial memory often leads to disorders of orientation, especially in a new environment (shopping centres, hospitals). The patients with HD show a deficit of *intrapersonal orientation*. It is manifested, for instance, when the patient follows a premarked route on the map, which is divided in square fields, and the position of the map towards the subject is concomitantly changed (Brouwers, 1984; Bylsma, 1992). *Extrapersonal orientation* in space is, on the contrary, well preserved - the patients suffering from HD do not have bigger problems with localising objects in their neighbourhood as is the problem of patients suffering from dementia of the Alzheimer's type. They can also localise their position in relation to the environment (Potegal, 1971).

Visuo-constructional deficit is manifested especially in tests requiring planning and organization, for instance in a WAIS-R subtest (Bamford, 1989). Apraxia, typical for cortical affection, is a very rare phenomenon in HD (Derix, 1994).

The patients often err in tracing geometric figures. *The deficit of mental rotation* with three-dimensional objects was similarly described (Mohr, 1991, 1997). Already in the initial stages, HD patients reproduce movements of the examining person despite repeated notices and training and mostly do not realize it.

The perception disorders may also be affected by *oculomotor dysfunction* (pursuit and saccadic movements), even in the initial stages of the disease (Leigh, 1983; Folstein, 1986). The initiation and smoothness of ocular movements is disturbed. The speed of the ocular movements is reduced, and the patients are not often able to suppress concomitant head movements. The patients are not able to suppress reflex saccadic movements to a visual stimulus despite understanding of the instruction (Lasker, 1987).

Language and Speech

In HD, language is relatively preserved in comparison to speech. Vocabulary, grammar and syntax are usually preserved up to advanced stages of dementia (Bayles, 1988). The ability of understanding the speech is retained even though patient's own speech expression is not possible any longer. The patients predominantly express themselves in short, uncomplicated sentences and have a tendency to semantic errors (Folstein, 1990). In common conversation, they do not have any problems with using proper terms and no paraphrasia occurs. With the progression of the disease, they often seek proper words; and although their vocabulary is maintained, the free recall stagnates (explicit memory). Change of the speed of speech is typical (acceleration or deceleration). The patients have problems in initiating conversation and sticking to the theme. In addition, the verbal expression is negatively affected by reduced ability of the concentration. Echolalia and perseverance of words and phrases is common, sometimes even in inadequate situations. From the point of view of the content, the executive dysfunction participates in the organization of the speech expression. In advanced stages, a disconnection of the speech program and motor sequences, the so-called *verbal apraxia,* occurs. It is not a aphasia, as it is confirmed by results of the Aachen Aphasia Test (Wallesch, 1988).

One of the first symptoms of the cognitive deterioration consists in decreased *verbal fluency* (Bayles, 1985), which is considered one of the most sensitive tests of executive functions. It is thus not primarily a linguistic problem. Better preserved semantic verbal fluency (e.g., animals, fruits) is typical for HD, although it does not reach the standard (Randolph, 1993).

The speech expression in HD is complicated as early as in the initial stages by *articulation and prosody disorder (hyperkinetic dysarthria)* (timbre and pitch of voice, loudness, pauses, melody, speed and accent) (Gordon, 1987). In advanced stages, the verbal expression is also impaired by cognitive deficit and dyskinesias of the orofacial, lingual, pharyngeal and expiratory muscles (Folstein, 1989). The speech of patients suffering from HD reminds one of the speech of a drunken man. In advanced stages, the speech is disjointed or even completely incomprehensible.

The speech perception, especially prosody, is also damaged. The inability to understand the rhythm and changes of intonation may cause conflicting situations and lead to social isolation (Speedie, 1990). If the patient is overloaded with information extent, he/she may have problems with understanding the speech even in the initial stages.

Dysexecutive Syndrome

The words *executive function* describes a subset of cognitive functions that helps to create and execute plans, respect the rules of social conduct, solve problems, adapt to unexpected changes of circumstances, carry out several activities at a time, place events in time and space, store, process and retrieve information from memory. The dysexecutive syndrome is manifested in case of damage of the frontal lobes and frontostriatal circuits, especially the dorsolateral prefrontal circuit (Duffy 1994).

The expression of executive dysfunction in HD is especially the inability to create a concept, plan and maintain mental setting, unaltered activity and repetitive operations. The control of the course of a specific performance and its time structure is disrupted. The ability of a quick change of the current activity in a specific situation is also reduced (Lawrence, 1996). Folstein et al. (1992) found a correlation between atrophy of the caudate nucleus and attention deficit and retention of thoughts. The quality of the executive functions influences the activity of the working memory and free recall. The patients with HD themselves can often see deterioration of their short-term memory and performance in trivial arithmetic operations (shopping, home budget). The executive functions also participate in the creation and implementation of the motor programs for locomotion and fine movements including articulation. The loss of mental flexibility then leads to the loss of employment and later to failures in common daily routines and self-sufficiency.

Dementia

The progressive cognitive deterioration is for the patient subjectively often a more serious problem than the behavioural and motor expressions of HD.

As for HD, *dementi*a of the so-called *subcortical* type, in which disorders of attention and executive functions, deceleration of the psychomotor speed, behaviour disorders (irritability, apathy, obsessive-compulsive expressions, etc.), depression and anxiety dominate. Unlike dementia of the cortical type (Alzheimer's type), phatic, practical and gnostic functions are relatively maintained up to the advanced stages of HD. However, cortical functions are markedly affected with further progression of the cognitive deterioration.

According to recent studies, the disorders of cognitive functions precede the development of motor affection (Hahn-Barma, 1998; Farrow, 2006; Stout, 2007; Verny, 2007). Slight deficits of deceleration of the psychomotor speed and weakening of attention, executive and memory functions were observed in otherwise asymptomatic carriers of HD mutation (Verny, 2007). The macrostructural atrophic changes are visible at least 10 years before the clinical onset (Aylward, 2007). Therefore, there is the question when, actually, HD begins.

In addition to the number of the CAG triplets, the start of the disease will also be influenced by other genetic factors (Metzger, 2006) but also by the premorbid capacity of the central nervous system. The isolated cognitive deficits commonly appear as early as at the clinical onset of the disease; gradually, they deepen and are joined by other ones (Paulsen, 2001; Mendez, 1994; Jason, 1997; Snowden, 2001). The disorders of attention, memory and mental flexibility belong to the first cognitive expressions of deterioration, which are often perceived by the patient him/herself or by his/her neighbourhood. In the early stages, the patients also show some disorders of attention, executive functions and short-term memory, and show reduced performance in time-limited, psychomotor-oriented tests.

On the contrary, the general abilities are maintained including remote recall and semantic memory. However, more discrete changes remain unrevealed in the initial stages of the disease and may only be detected during a careful psychological examination. The early stages of HD are characteristic of maintenance of normal performance in the tests aimed at global cognitive abilities (Mini Mental State Examination - MMSE, Mattis Dementia Rating Scale - MDRS).

The dementia of the subcortical type is usually *accompanied by motor impairment and change of the psychomotor speed*. In the initial stages, the psychomotor speed may be accelerated, but it continuously decelerates during the course of the disease.

It is common for the subcortical type of cognitive deterioration that the patient maintains at least partial insight of his/her own abilities, which is strikingly different from the dementia of the cortical type (e.g., dementia of Alzheimer's type). In the patients with HD, the insight is disrupted mostly quantitatively in the sense of an estimate of the degree of the cognitive deficit, behavioural disorders and functional capacity (Hoth, 2007). In the patients with Alzheimer's disease, it is more or less qualitative disorder of the insight that relates to full loss of information in the memory and has a tendency to fill the vacant positions in the memory by confabulations.

The patients with HD often spontaneously admit disorders of attention, learning and memory. Due to them, the patients often feel frustrated and depressive. However, some of them paradoxically do not draw any conclusions from their failures and want to continue driving, working activity, independent financial management and so forth.

On the contrary, the motor problems are often belittled or even not realized by the patients (Snowden, 1998). The question as to which symptoms are the most bothering ones is usually answered by the patient in such a way that mostly even in case of a significant motor deficit, the patient enumerates other ones. A particular question whether he/she has some involuntary movements is by most of the patients with the dyskinetic syndromes usually answered affirmatively. Some patients spontaneously mention motor impairment. According to Snowden et al. (2001), some patients do not spontaneously realize the extent of the motor deficit, but if they have an opportunity to watch themselves on a video recording, they are often very surprised. An insight of the motor deficit cannot be interpreted only as a result of cognitive deterioration or as a defence mechanism. Anosognosia in the neurological sense is quite rare in HD.

However, the HD patients often show a quite incorrect insight of their behavioural disorders (Hoth, 2007). In some patients, a correct insight of their health state was observed, but they recurrently refused a genetic confirmation of HD - the definitive and confirming verdict.

3. Measurement

3.1. Measurement of Behavioural Disorders

Cummings et al. (1994) published a structured interview for detection and quantification of behavioural disorders, the so-called *Neuropsychiatric Inventory* (NPI). The NPI consists of ten areas aimed at the presence of delusions, hallucinations, depression and dysphoria, anxiety, agitation and aggression, euphoria, disinhibition, apathy, irritability and aberrant motor behaviour. In order to increase validity, it is suitable to carry out assessment in cooperation with the person who cares for the patient.

For both clinic and experimental purposes, the so-called *Unified Huntington's Disease Rating Scale, UHDRS*, has been created (Huntington Study Group, 1996). The UHDRS has been formed with the aim to comprehensively chart the neurological, behavioural and cognitive deficits. The UHDRS also contains questionnaires targeted at dealing with daily activities and needs of care for other persons. The UHDRS screening of the behavioural disorders (*UHDRS Behavioural Assessment*) is more concise than the NPI.

The Core Assessment Program for Intracerebral Transplantation in Huntington's Disease - *CAPIT-HD* protocol (Quinn, 1996) - contains a battery of tests and scales aimed at behavioural expressions: Beck's depression scale, Spielberg's questionnaire for assessment of anxiety and distress and computer-controlled structured interview (Computerised Diagnostic Interview, CIDI-Auto).

Craufurd et al. (2001) dealt with utilization of a semi-structured interview (Problem Behaviour Assessment for Huntington's disease - *PBA-HD*) with the patient, possibly also with the caregiver, in order to identify symptoms related to disorders of the insight, mood, somatic symptoms, apathy, irritability, obsessive-compulsive and psychotic symptoms.

The questionnaire was compiled according to the list of symptoms of behavioural changes detected by patients and their caregivers during the clinical meetings in Manchester. In addition, literature data and theoretical knowledge of cognitive impairment in general and that of specific patterns of the frontal lobes syndromes were taken into account. Forty items were created, each of them assessed from zero to four points, with seriousness and frequency separated. Using the factor analysis of data obtained on a set of 134 persons with HD, Craufurd found three principal domains of the behavioural changes: apathy, irritability and depression.

3.2. Measurement of Cognitive Functions

Quinn at al. (1996) published an extensive battery of tests aimed at selection of suitable candidates with HD for intracerebral transplantation therapy (Core Assessment Program for Intracerebral Transplantation in Huntington's Disease**,** *CAPIT-HD*).

The battery includes motor, cognitive, behavioural and electrophysiologic testing. CAPIT-HD also covers examination by magnetic resonance and positron emission tomography. The battery of neuropsychological tests is aimed at the whole spectrum of cognitive functions affected in HD. This battery is very exacting for patients, and therefore, an abridged version is used for consecutive testing.

The battery of the cognitive tests in the UHDRS consists of three tests: Verbal Fluency, Symbol Digit Modalities Test and Stroop's Test. The battery is short but highly sensitive to cognitive deficits, even in the initial stages of HD.

In the study of Ho et al. (2003), the computer battery of neuropsychological tests -. Cambridge Neuropsychological Test Automated Battery (CANTAB) - was also used for testing of persons in early stages of HD in addition to the CAPIT-HD battery. **CANTAB** (Sahakian, 1988) consists of an extensive flexible battery of standard tests, transferred into an electronic form. As stated by its authors, the advantage of this battery consists in the minimization of the influence of the motor performance on cognitive tasks. The battery is suitable to testing of both cortical and subcortical cognitive deficits.

In clinical practice, a series of cognitive tests in various modifications is used to test cognitive deficits of HD. The batteries of such tests are aimed especially at the psychomotor speed, attention, learning, memory, visually spatial functions and executive functions. A list of the most frequently used tests is given in Table No. 4.

4. The Course of Neuropsychological Affection

The progression of HD is inevitable; nevertheless, in many patients, also long-term plateau phases may be observed during the disease; however, they are usually followed by devastating acceleration of motor and cognitive symptoms. In some patients, we may also find a long-term stationary condition in the advanced phase of HD, when the patient is not self-sufficient anymore and needs a continuous care of his/her neighbourhood. This is connected with an extreme load on the caregiver; however, the stationary course and survival several years in this condition are not only due to the good quality of the care. Individual symptom complexes, i.e., motor, cognitive and psychiatric ones, very often do not show mutual interconnections in clinical practice.

Particularly psychiatric expressions such as irritability, depression, etc. are often reduced during the course of the disease; other symptoms appear, but always within an individual pattern. However, according to some studies, patients with apathy and without concomitant depression symptoms show much worse cognitive performance and voluntary motor impairment than patients with HD without apathy (Thompson, 2002; Baudic, 2006). Surprisingly, depression does not negatively affect motor/cognitive performance (Thompson, 2002; Baudic, 2006). In patients with obsessive-compulsive symptoms, a worse cognitive performance was observed than in patients without those symptoms (Anderson, 2001). The cooperation with the patient is usually complicated due to his/her overlooking of symptoms, anosognosia and perseverance, stubbornness and repulsion to cooperate.

There are not many studies dealing with the dynamics of development of mental changes in HD (Marder, 2000; Mahant, 2003; Andrich, 2007). For such purpose, long-term prospective studies on many patients are necessary. Among other things, that is why multicentric groups of experts were established - the Huntington Study Group in the U.S.A. and the Huntington's Disease Network in Europe.

5. The Proposal of a Standardized Neuropsychological Examination

Table No.3. Behavioural tests

Domain	Test
Global screening	Symptom Checklist 90—Revised (SCL-90-R) (Derogatis, 1975) Neuropsychiatric Inventory (NPI) (Cummings, 1994) Behavioral Assessment Scale (part of UHDRS) Problem Behavior Assessment
Depression	Beck's Depression Scale (BDI-II) Zung's Depression Scale Hamilton's Depression Scale (HDS) Montgomery and Asberg Depression Rating Scale (MADRS)

Table No.3. (Continued)

Domain	Test
Anxiety	Hamilton's Anxiety Scale (HAS) Beck's Anxiety Scale (BAI)
Aggressivity	Overt Aggression Scale (Yudofsky, 1986)
Apathy	Lille Apathy Rating Scale (Dujardin, 2008)
Obsession, compulsion	Yale-Brown Obsessive Compulsive Scale (YBOCS) (Goodmann, 1989)
Psychotic expressions	Positive and Negative Syndrome Scale (PANNS) (Kay, 1987) Brief Psychiatric Rating Scale (BPRS) (Overall, 1962)

Table No. 4. Cognitive tests

Domain	Tests
Global screening	Mini Mental State Examination (MMSE) Mattis Dementia Rating Scale (MDRS)
Working memory	Digit Span (subtest WAIS-R) Corsi Blocks (Milner, 1971)
Memory	Rivermead Behavioural Memory Test (RBMT) (Wilson, 1985) Hopkins Verbal Learning Test (HVLT) (Brandt, 1991) Auditory Verbal Learning Test (AVLT) California Verbal Learning Test (CVLT)
Language	Boston Naming Test (BNT, abridged version) (Kaplan, 1978) Token Test (abridged version) (De Renzi, 1978)
Visually-spatial functions	Object and Space Perception Battery (Warrington, 1991) Rey-Osterrieth's Complex Figure /copy (ROCF) Block Design (subtest of WAIS) Benton Visual Retention Test Money Road Map Test Clock Test
Executive functions and attention	Test of Verbal Fluency Stroop's Test (modified) (Huntington Study Group, 1996) Wisconsin Card Sorting Test (modified) (Nelson, 1976) Digit Symbol Modalities Test (DSMT) or Symbol Digit Modalities Test (SDMT) Frontal Assessment Battery (FAB) (Dubois, 2000) Trail Making Test

6. Rehabilitation and Psychotherapy of Cognitive Deficit

A slowly developing cognitive deficit from the very beginning of the disease, progressing up to the stage of severe dementia of subcortical type, leading to the loss of self-sufficiency and full dependence on the care of other persons is typical for HD. In HD, it is possible to temporarily alleviate pharmacologically some motor and behavioural symptoms; however, we have not yet succeeded to influence the loss of cognitive functions. The efficacy of state-of–the-art drugs - inhibitors of acetylcholinesterase - is disputable (Cubo, 2006).

On the basis of such information, an incorrect impression may appear that any intervention in the area of cognitive processes in HD is worthless and unreasonable. The cognitive deterioration in HD shows a progressive character, however, the mental processes are not globally affected (for details, see Isolated Cognitive Deficits in HD). In HD, the beginning deficit is primarily manifested by disorders of attention, learning of new knowledge and skills. Primarily, the short-term memory is disrupted and the free recall stagnates, but the retention and recognition of acquired information is maintained. For instance, the semantic memory is preserved up to the advanced stages. The deficits of visually-perceptive functions, especially orientation (of the person in the neighbourhood) in space, are also typical for HD. Dysarthria manifests relatively early after the onset of the disease; in the advanced stages, the patient is not able to orally express him/herself, despite the fact that he/she understands verbal instructions. Motor deficit also often contributes to the decrease of cognitive performance. The overall mental and motor performance is negatively affected by the growing executive dysfunction.

The knowledge about maintained and affected cognitive skills may be sensibly utilized to the benefit of the patient and his/her neighbourhood. A prerequisite of successful cognitive rehabilitation is its appropriate selection and the method corresponding to patient's abilities. The cognitive rehabilitation has several important aspects. The first objective is to keep the patient in such a good mental condition that his/her dependence on other persons' help be as low as possible. The rehabilitation should start in the period when the patient is still able to learn new strategies. They can be then applied (already prepared and routinized) in advanced stages of the disease. The training is focused especially on communication skills, spatial orientation, decision-making and solution of new situations and self-attendance.

The method of rehabilitation is quite individual; it is necessary to respect needs and interests of the patient. People suffering from HD easily get tired and lose interest. The training must be regular and eventful ("learning by play"). However, if a balanced and sufficiently attractive rehabilitation programme is found, not only independence will increase, but also behavioural expressions will be adjusted and positive emotions will be evoked.

In cognitive rehabilitation, both specialists (psychologist, speech therapist, music therapist, art therapist, physiotherapist and ergotherapist) and family members or volunteers can take part.

Communication with the Patient

When communicating with the patient, it is necessary to express clearly and concisely, not to use long and complicated sentences. When transferring an exacting message from the viewpoint of content, it is necessary to select and logically arrange essential pieces of information. It is good to use non-verbal, emotionally loaded means (to show pictures, photos, objects and to use gestures). The patient must have enough time to process and evaluate every new piece of information, because he/she is not able to concomitantly perceive additional verbal/nonverbal impulses. After communicating a whole set of information, it is necessary to summarize substantial information and to make certain that the patient has understood the message.

The persons with HD typically display disorders of speech initiation and long intervals between words and sentences; they use short, uncomplicated and often-set phrases. The patients have problems with prompt recall of adequate words and information. Even if the patient understands well, he/she answers with a long, latent period and often leaves an impression that he/she does not understand. The conversation is then prematurely stopped or its theme is changed. The patient is not only confused and frustrated, but he/she is also unjustifiably considered incompetent. Therefore, the patient must be provided a sufficient space in the conversation to express him/herself, and the caregiver should have enough patience to listen to him/her. The speech is also limited due to deteriorating articulation.. The communication with the patient can be made more effective when using short sentences with the possibility of answering yes or no or selecting from two alternatives. Another useful aid consists in a prompt of suitable words.

In the advanced stages, when the patient is not able to articulate comprehensibly, various external aids (table with the alphabet or basic sentences for the most frequent needs of the patient, albums with pictures of important objects, photographs of persons) may come in handy. Only rarely, some patients are able to communicate in writing (even if their motor deficit is severe) by means of specially adjusted electronic equipment (e.g., a computer keyboard with buttons providing for a single push of a button or notebooks with a display and word reproduction).

7. Problems of Persons at Risk

7.1. Impacts of the Pre-Symptomatic Test

Since HD is an autosomal dominant hereditary disease with full penetration, all direct offspring and siblings of an ill or positively tested person show 50% probability of the mutated gene transfer.

Since 1993, there has been an opportunity for a genetic test. This opportunity has led to a very complicated situation - the detection of possible presence of mutation does not currently allow for any therapeutical strategy improving the prognosis; the persons at risk may finally loose their hope for a healthy life, etc.

About 60% of all persons at risk who learn about the possibility of genetic testing want immediately to have their tests done (the principal reasons are usually as follows: to know for sure the facts, to plan the future, to inform the descendants, and so on). The course of the protocol procedure (International Huntington Association and the World Federation of Neurology Research Group on Huntington's Chorea, 1994) will significantly reduce this percentage. The final acceptance of the testing is between 9 to 20% of all original applicants (their principle reasons being possible loss of hope in case of capture of the mutation, fear of self-monitoring and searching for the first symptoms etc.) (Tibben, 2007).

The persons who were tested show less depressive and distressing expressions than the persons at risk who have not undergone the testing. The highest risk of depression applies to childless persons who are at the age approaching the usual time of manifestation of HD who have not undergone the genetic testing.

7.2. Preclinical Neuropsychological Markers of Mutation Carriers

Quite a different type of problems consists in the investigation whether or not the carriers of the mutation bear subtle changes even before the clinical manifestation of typical symptoms of HD.

According to some studies (Lawrence, 1998; Kirkwood, 2000), some noticeable cognitive and motor symptoms precede the clear manifestation of HD. In the study of Kirkwood, five basic components were defined: oculomotor changes, movements speed, petty disorders of voluntary movements, cognitive functions and reaction times.

An interesting finding also consists in a specific inability to recognize facial expressions, especially negative emotions not only in patients with HD but also in carriers of mutation of HD (Sprengelmeyer, 1996; Gray, 1997; Johnson, 2007).

The period during which the above-mentioned symptoms may be observed, may last during the several years that precede the manifestation and diagnosing of HD (Marshall, 2007; Duff, 2007).

Similar results have been identified in the study with functional magnetic resonance in persons at a risk of HD (Zimbelman, 2007), when the changes were obvious even before the clinical manifestation of HD.

8. Problems of the Caregivers

The partner of the patient must solve a series of problems: lower socio-economic status, loss of free time, loss of safe background, the role of a caregiver that takes practically all the time, etc. Other important problems are represented by the risk of transfer of HD to descendants (feelings of guilt for mutation transfer, inability to tell children about their endangerment, etc.) and the character of symptoms of the disease itself, which usually seriously disrupt the mind of the partner (Kessler, 1993). The patients change their behaviour and personality; sometimes, they use violence against their partners (pathological jealousy, sexually motivated violent behaviour) or their children. In addition, the children in families with HD cannot fully understand the situation with all its consequences (why their parent is so aggressive, behaves differently, etc.). The impacts of such long-term problems on children's enlightenment cannot be generalized, however, there is surely some additional impact on the functioning of the whole family.

In most of the partners, severe depression, distressing conditions up to panic disorders, negativistic behaviour, bursts of aggressivity against the patient, etc. may develop during the course of common life with the patient due to the impact of the stressing situation. Some cases of alcoholism and suicidal attempts of the partners have been described. The theme of HD in the family is often taboo and can be discussed neither in public nor within the broader family. The partners, similar to the persons at risk, describe their condition as "permanent sadness."

Supportive patients societies offer considerable help to both risk groups.

Conclusion

HD is a fatal nervous disease, with yet unexplained pathogenesis. The pathophysiological background of the development and progression of individual symptoms of the disease are supported by structural neurodegenerative changes, especially in the area of basal ganglia and then in other cortical-subcortical areas. However, specific functionally-morphologic connections have not been investigated in detail yet. HD is a typical neuropsychiatric disease with the impact on the whole family of the affected person (psycho-socio-economic impacts of the devastating disease with its onset in the productive age, autosomally dominant type of heredity with full penetration). For high-quality care of patients with HD, it is necessary to form multidisciplinary teams embracing the possibilities of medical, psychological, rehabilitation, consulting and social intervention. An important role is also played by supportive societies, e.g., International Huntington Association (www.huntington-assoc.com).

Scientific organizations take a significant part in the research of HD: in the U.S.A., it is the Huntington Study Group (www.huntington-study-group.org), and in Europe the European Huntington's disease Network (www.euro-HD.net).

References

Albin, R. L., Young, A. B., Penney, J. B.: The functional anatomy of basal ganglia. *Trends Neurosci*. 1989;12:366–375.

Alexander, G. E., Crutcher, M. D.: Functional architecture of basal ganglia circuits: neuronal substrates of parallel processing. *Trend Neurosci.* 1990;13:266–271.

Alexander, G. E., DeLong, M. R., Strick, P. L.: Parallel organization of functionally segregated circuits linking basal ganglia and cortex. *Annu. Rev. Neurosci.* 1986;9:357–81.

Al-Jader, L. N., Harper, P. S., Krawczak, M., Palmer, SR.: The frequency of inherited disorders database: prevalence of Huntington disease. *Community Genet*. 2001;4 (3):148–57.

Anderson, K. E., Louis, E. D., Stern, Y., Marder, K. S.: Cognitive correlates of obsessive and compulsive symptoms in Huntington's disease. *Am J Psychiatry*. 2001;158:799–801.

Andrew, S. E., Goldberg, Y. P., Kremer, B., et al.: The relationship between trinucleotide (CAG) repeat length and clinical features of Huntington's disease. *Nature Genet.* 1993;4:398–403.

Andrich, J, Saft, C, Ostholt N, Muller T. Complex motor behaviour and progression of Huntington´s disease. *Neurosci. Lett.* 2007;416(3):272-4.

Aylward, EH. Change in MRI striatal volumes as a biomarker in preclinical Huntington's disease. *Brain Res. Bull.* 2007 Apr 30;72(2-3):152-8.

Baddeley, A., Harris, J., Sunderland, A., et al.: Closed head injury and memory. In: Levin HS, Grafman J and Eisenberg HM eds. Neurobehavioral recovery from head injury. New York, Oxford University Press 1987.

Bamford, K. A., Caine, E. D., Kido, D. K., Plassche, W. M., Shoulson, I.: Clinical-pathologic correlation in Huntington's disease: a neuropsychological and computed tomography study. *Neurology.* 1989;39(6):796–801.

Baudic, S., Maison, P., Dolbeau, G., Boissé, M.F., Bartolomeo, P., Dalla Barba, G., Traykov, L., Bachoud-Lévi, A.C.. Cognitive impairment related to apathy in early Huntington's disease. *Dement. Geriatr. Cogn. Disord.* 2006;21(5-6):316-21.

Bayles, K. A., Tomoeda, C. K., Kaszniak, A. W., Stern, L. Z., Eagans, K. K.: Verbal perseveration of dementia patients. *Brain Lang.* 1985;25 (1):102–16.

Bayles, K. A.: Dementia: The clinical perspective. Seminars in Speech and Language, 1988, 9, 149–165.

Beglinger, L.J., Langbehn, D.R., Duff, K., Stierman, L., Black, D.W., Nehl, C., Anderson, K., Penziner, E., Paulsen, J.S.; Huntington Study Group Investigators. Probability of obsessive and compulsive symptoms in Huntington's disease. *Biol. Psychiatry.* 2007 Feb 1;61(3):415-8.

Bonelli, R.M., Cummings, J.L.. Frontal-Subcortical Dementias. *Neurologist.* 2008 Mar;14(2):100-107.

Brandt, J.: The Hopkins Verbal Learning Test: Development of a new memory test with six equivalent forms. *The Clinical Neuropsychologist.* 1991;5:125–142.

Brouwers, P., Cox, C., Martin, A., Chase, T., Fedio, P.: Differential perceptual-spatial impairment in Huntington's and Alzheimer's dementias. *Arch. Neurol.* 1984;41(10):1073–6.

Brown, R. G., Marsden, C. D.: "Subcortical dementia": the neuropsychological evidence. *Neuroscience.* 1988;25(2):363–87.

Burns, A., Folstein, S., Brandt, J., Folstein, M.: Clinical assessment of irritability, aggression, and apathy in Huntington and Alzheimer disease. *J. Nerv. Ment. Dis.* 1990;178:20–26.

Butters, N., Sax, D., Montgomery, K., Tarlow, S.: Comparison of neuropsychological deficits associated with early and advanced Huntington's disease. *Archives of Neurology.* 1978;35:585–589.

Butters, N., Wolfe, J., Martone, M., Granholm, E., Cermak, L. S.: Memory disorders associated with Huntington's disease: verbal recall, verbal recognition and procedural memory. *Neuropsychologia.* 1985;23:729–743.

Bylsma, F. W., Brandt, J., Strauss, M. E.: Personal and extrapersonal orientation in Huntington's disease patients and those at risk. *Cortex* 1992;28(1):113–22.

Craufurd, D., Thompson, J. C., Snowden, J. S.: Behavioral changes in Huntington´s disease. *Neuropsychiatry, neuropsychology and behavioral Neurology.*, 2001;4:219–226.

Cubo, E., Shannon, K.M., Tracy, D., Jaglin, J.A., Bernard, B.A., Wuu, J., Leurgans, S.E. Effect of donepezil on motor and cognitive function in Huntington disease. *Neurology.* 2006;67:1268-1271.

Cummings, J. L., Mega, M., Gray, K., Rosenberg-Thompson, S., Carusi, D. A., Gornbein, J.: The Neuropsychiatric Inventory: comprehensive assessment of psychopathology in dementia. *Neurology.* 1994;44:2308–2314.

Cummings, J. L.: Frontal-subcortical circuits and human behavior. *Arch Neurol.* 1993; 50:873–880.

Davis, J.D., Filoteo, J.V., Kesner, R.P., Roberts, J.W.. Recognition memory for hand positions and spatial locations in patients with Huntington's disease: differential visuospatial memory impairment? *Cortex.* 2003 Apr;39(2):239-53.

De Renzi, E., Faglioni, P.: normative data and screening power of a shortened version of the Token Test. *Cortex.* 1978;14:41–49.

Derix, M. M. A.: Neuropsychological differentiation of dementing syndromes. Lisse, The Netherlands: Swets and Zeitlinger, 1994.

Derogatis, LR. Symptom Checklist-90-R (SCL-90-R), NCS Assessments, Minneapolis, MN (1975).

Di Maio, L., Squitieri, F., napolitano, G., Campanella, G., Trofatter, J. A., Conneally, P. M.: Onset symptoms in 510 patients with Huntington´s disease. *J. Med. Genet.* 1993;30:289–92.

Di Maio, L., Squitieri, F., Napolitano, G., Campanella, G., Trofatter, J. A., Conneally, P. M.: Suicide risk in Huntington's disease *J. Med. Genet.* 1993; 30(4):293–5.

Dubois, B., Slachevsky, A., Litvan, I., Pillon, B.: The FAB: a Frontal Assessment Battery at bedside. *Neurology.,* 2000;55(11):1621–6.

Duff, K., Paulsen, J.S., Beglinger, L.J., Langbehn, D.R., Stout, J.C.; Predict-HD Investigators of the Huntington Study Group. Psychiatric symptoms in Huntington's disease before diagnosis: the predict-HD study. *Biol. Psychiatry.* 2007 Dec 15;62(12):1341-6.

Duffy, J.D. and Campbell, J.J.. The regional prefrontal syndromes: theoretical and clinical overview. *J. Neuropsychiatry Clin. Neurosci.* 6 (1994), 379–387.

Dujardin, K., Sockeel, P., Delliaux, M., Destée, A., Defebvre, L.. The Lille Apathy Rating Scale: Validation of a caregiver-based version. *Mov Disord.* 2008 Feb 28; [Epub ahead of print]

Farrer, L. A.: Suicide and attempted suicide in Huntington´s disease: implications for preclinical testing of persons at risk. *Am. J. Med. Genet.* 1986;24(2):305–11.

Farrow, M., Chua, P., Churchyard, A., Bradshaw, J.L., Chiu, E., Georgiou-Karistianis, N.. Proximity to clinical onset influences motor and cognitive performance in presymptomatic Huntington disease gene carriers. *Cogn. Behav. Neurol.* 2006 Dec;19(4):208-16.

Fedoroff, J. P., Peyser, C., Franz, M. L., Folstein, S. E.: Sexual disorders in Huntington's disease. *J. Neuropsychiatry Clin. Neurosci.* 1994; 6(2):147–53.

Flaherty, A. W., Graybiel, A. M.: Anatomy of the basal ganglia. In: *Movement Disorders* 3, eds Marsden CD, Fahn S. Butterworth-Heinemann, 1994, 3–27.

Folstein, M. F., Brandt, J. Starkstein, S.: Cognition in Huntington´s disease: characteristics and correlates. In: Function and dysfunction in the basal ganglia. Franks, A. J, Ironside, J. W., Mindham, R. H. S., Smith, R. J., Spokes, E. G. S. and Winlow, W. eds. Oxford, Pergamon 1992, 218–223.

Folstein, S. E., Abbott, M. H., Chase, G. A., et al.: The association of affective disorder with Huntington´s disease in a case series and in families. *Psychological Medicine.* 1983;13:537–542.

Folstein, S. E., Brandt, J., Folstein, M. F.: Huntington's disease. In JL Cummings (Ed.) Subcortical dementia. New York, Oxford University Press 1990.

Folstein, S. E., Chase, G. A., Wahl, W. E., et al.: Huntington's disease in Maryland: Clinical aspects of racial variation. *Am. J. Hum. Genet.* 1987;41:168–79.

Folstein, S. E., Leigh, R. J., Parhad, I. M., Folstein, M. F.: The diagnosis of Huntington's disease. *Neurology*. 1986;36(10):1279–83.

Folstein, S. E.: The emotional disorder. In: Huntington's disease. A disorder of families. Foroud, T., Gray, J., Ivashing, J. and Conneally, P. M. eds. Baltimore, John Hopkins University Press 1989, 49–64.

Goodman, W.K., Price, L.H., Rasmussen, S.A., Mazure, C., Fleischmann, R.L., Hill, C.L., Heninger, G.R., Charney, D.S.. The Yale-Brown Obsessive Compulsive Scale. I. Development, use, and reliability. *Arch. Gen. Psychiatry*. 1989 Nov;46(11):1006-11.

Gordon, W. P., Illes, J.: Neurolinguistic characteristics of language production in Huntington's disease: a preliminary report. *Brain Lang*.1987;31 (1):1–10.

Gray, J. M., Young, A. W., Barker, W. A., Curtis, A., Gibson, D.: Impaired recognition of disgust in Huntington's disease gene carriers. *Brain*. 1997;120:2029–38.

Graybiel, A. M.: Neurotransmitters and neuromodulators in the basal ganglia. *Trends Neurosci*. 1990;13:244–254.

Gusella, J. F., Wexler, N. S., Conneally, P. M., et al.: A polymorphic DNA marker genetically linked to Huntington´s disease. *Nature*. 1983;306:234–238.

Hahn-Barma, V., Deweer, B., Durr, A., Dode, C., Feingold, J., Pillon, B., Agid, Y, Brice, A., Dubois, B.: Are cognitive changes the first symptoms of Huntington's disease? A study of gene carriers. *J. Neurol. Neurosurg. Psychiatry*. 1998;64(2):172–7.

Harper, P S.: The epidemiology of Huntington's disease. *Hum Genet*. 1992;89:365-376.

Ho, A. K., Sahakian, B. J., Brown, R. G., Barker, R. A., Hodges, J. R., Ane, M. N., Snowden, J,. Thompson, J., Esmonde, T., Gentry, R., Moore, J. W., Bodner, T.: NEST-HD Consortium. Profile of cognitive progression in early Huntington's disease. *Neurology*. 2003;61(12):1702–6.

Hodges, J. R., Salmon, D. P., Butters, N.: Differential impairment of semantic and episodic memory in Alzheimer's and Huntington's diseases: a controlled prospective study. *J. Neurol. Neurosurg .Psychiatry*.1990;53(12):1089–95.

Hoth, K.F., Paulsen, J.S., Moser, D.J., Tranel, D., Clark, L.A., Bechara, A.. Patients with Huntington's disease have impaired awareness of cognitive, emotional, and functional abilities. *J. Clin. Exp. Neuropsychol.* 2007 May;29(4):365-76.

Huntington Study Group: Unified Huntington's Disease Rating Scale: reliability and consistency. *Mov. Disord.* 1996;11(2):136–42.

Huntington, G.: On chorea. Med. *Surg. Reporter*. 1872;26:317–321.

Huntington's Disease Collaborative Research Group: A novel gene containing a trinucleotide repeat that is expanded and unstable on Huntington's disease chromosomes. *Cell*. 1993;72:971–983.

International Huntington Association and the World Federation of Neurology Research Group on Huntington's Chorea: Guidelines for the molecular genetics predictive test in Huntington's disease. *J. Med. Genet*. 1994;31(7):555–9.

Jacobs, D. H., Shuren, J., Heilman, K. M.: Impaired perception of facial identity and facial affect in Huntington's disease. *Neurology*. 1995;45(6):1217–8.

Jacobs, D., Tröster, A. I., Butters, N. et al.: Intrusion errors on the Visual Reproduction Test of the Wechsler memory Scale and the Wechsler Memory Scale-Revised: An analysis of demented and amnestic patients. *The Clinical Neuropsychologist*. 1990;4:177–191.

Jason, G. W., Suchowersky, O., Pajurkova, E. M.: Cognitive manifestations of Huntington´s disease in relation to genetic structure and clinical onset. *Arch. Neurol.* 1997;54(9):1081–8.

Jensen, P., Fenger, K., Bolwig, T., Sørensen, S. A.: Crime in Huntington´s disease: a study of registered offences among patients, relatives, and controls. *J. Neurol. Neurosurg. Psychiatry*. 1998;65:467–471.

Johnson, S.A., Stout, J.C., Solomon, A.C., Langbehn, D.R., Aylward, E.H., Cruce, C.B., Ross, C.A., Nance, M., Kayson, E., Julian-Baros, E., Hayden, M.R., Kieburtz, K., Guttman, M., Oakes, D., Shoulson, I., Beglinger, L., Duff, K., Penziner, E., Paulsen, J.S.; Predict-HD Investigators of the Huntington Study Group. Beyond disgust: impaired recognition of negative emotions prior to diagnosis in Huntington's disease. *Brain.* 2007 Jul;130(Pt 7):1732-44.

Julien, C.L., Thompson, J.C., Wild, S., Yardumian, P., Snowden, J.S., Turner, G., Craufurd, D.. Psychiatric disorders in preclinical Huntington's disease. *J. Neurol. Neurosurg. Psychiatry*. 2007 Sep;78(9):939-43.

Kaplan, E. F., Goodglass, H., Weintraub, S.: The Boston naming test. Boston, Kaplan and Goodglass 1978.

Kay, S.R., Fiszbein, A. and Opler, L.A. 1987. The Positive and Negative Syndrome Scale (PANNS) for schizophrenia. *Schizophr. Bull.* 1987;13(2):261–276.

Kessler, S.: Forgotten person in the Huntington disease family. *Am. J. Med. Genet.* 1993;48(3):145–50.

King, M.: Alcohol abuse in Huntington´s disease. *Psychol Med*. 1985;15:815–819.

Kingma, E.M., van Duijn, E., Timman, R., van der Mast, R.C., Roos, R.A.. Behavioural problems in Huntington's disease using the Problem Behaviour Assessment. *Gen. Hosp. Psychiatry.* 2008 Mar-Apr;30(2):155-61.

Kipps, C.M., Duggins, A.J., McCusker, E.A., Calder, A.J.. Disgust and happiness recognition correlate with anteroventral insula and amygdala volume respectively in preclinical Huntington's disease. *J. Cogn. Neurosci.* 2007 Jul;19(7):1206-17.

Kirkwood, S. C., Siemers, E., Hodes, M. E., Conneally, P. M., Christian, J. C., Foroud, T.: Subtle changes among presymptomatic carriers of the Huntington's disease gene. *J. Neurol. Neurosurg. Psychiatry* 2000;69:773–9.

Kremer, B., Goldberg, P., Andrew, S. E. et al.: A worldwide study of the Huntington's disease mutation: the sensitivity and specificity of measuring CAG repeats. *New Eng. J. Med.* 1994;330:1401–6.

Langbehn, D.R., Paulsen, J.S.; Huntington Study Group. Predictors of diagnosis in Huntington disease. *Neurology.* 2007 May 15;68(20):1710-7.

Lasker, A. G., Zee, D. S., Hain, T. C., Folstein, S. E., Singer, H. S.: Saccades in Huntington's disease: initiation defects and distractibility. *Neurology.* 1987;37(3):364–70.

Lawrence, A. D., Sahakian, B. J., Hodges, J. R., Rosser, A. E., Lange, K. W., Robbins, T. W.: Executive and mnemonic functions in early Huntington´s disease. *Brain.* 1996;19(Pt 5):1633–45.

Lawrence, A. D., Weeks, R. A., Brooks, D. J., Andrews, T. C., Watkins, L. H., Harding, A. E., Robbins, T. W., Sahakian, B. J.: The relationship between striatal dopamine receptor binding and cognitive performance in Huntington's disease. *Brain.* 1998;121(Pt 7):1343–55.

Leigh, R. J., Newman, S. A., Folstein, S. E., Lasker, A. G., Jensen, B. A.: Abnormal ocular motor control in Huntington´s disease. *Neurology*. 1983;33(10):1268–75.

Lemiere, J., Decruyenaere, M., Evers-Kiebooms, G., Vandenbussche, E., Dom, R.: Cognitive changes in patients with Huntington's disease (HD) and asymptomatic carriers of HD mutation—a longitudinal follow-up study. *J. Neurol.* 2004;251(8):935–42.

Levy, M. L., Cummings, J. L., Fairbanks, L. A., Masterman, D, Miller, B. L, Craig, A. H., Paulsen, J. S., Litvan, I.: Apathy is not depression. *J. Neuropsychiatry Clin. Neurosci.* 1998;10 (3):314–9.

Lundervold, A. J., Reinvang, I., Lundervold, A.: Characteristic patterns of verbal memory function in patients with Huntington's disease. *Scand. J. Psychol.* 1994;35(1):38–47.

Mahant, N., McCusker, E. A., Byth, K., Graham, S., Huntington Study Group.: Huntington´s disease. Clinical correlates of disability and progression. *Neurology*. 2003;61:1085–92.

Marder, K., Zhao, H., Myers, R. H., Cudkowicz, M., Kayson, E., Kieburtz, K., Orme, C., Paulsen, J., Penney, J. B., Jr, Siemers, E., Shoulson, I.: Rate of functional decline in Huntington's disease. Huntington Study Group. *Neurology*. 2000;54(2):452–8.

Marshall, J., White, K., Weaver, M., Flury Wetherill, L., Hui, S., Stout, J.C., Johnson, S.A., Beristain, X., Gray, J., Wojcieszek, J., Foroud, T..: Specific psychiatric manifestations among preclinical Huntington disease mutation carriers. *Arch. Neurol.* 2007 Jan;64(1):116-21.

Mendez, M. F.: Huntington´s disease: Update and review of neuropsychiatric aspects. I*nt J. Psychiatry Med.* 1994;24(3):189–208.

Mendez, M. F.: Mania in neurologic disorders. *Curr. Psychiatry Rep.* 2000;2(5):440–5.

Metzger, S., Bauer, P., Tomiuk, J., Laccone, F., Didonato, S., Gellera, C., Mariotti, C., Lange, H.W., Weirich-Schwaiger, H., Wenning, G.K., Seppi, K., Melegh, B., Havasi, V., Balikó, L., Wieczorek, S., Zaremba, J., Hoffman-Zacharska, D., Sulek, A., Basak, A.N., Soydan, E., Zidovska, J., Kebrdlova, V., Pandolfo, M., Ribaï, P., Kadasi, L., Kvasnicova, M., Weber, B.H., Kreuz, F., Dose, M., Stuhrmann, M., Riess, O.: Genetic analysis of candidate genes modifying the age-at-onset in Huntington's disease. *Hum Genet.* 2006 Sep;120(2):285-92.

Milner, B.: Interhemispheric differences in the localization of psychological processes in men. *Br. Med. Bull.* 1971;27:272–7.

Mohr, E., Brouwers, P., Claus, J. J., Mann, U. M., Fedio, P., and Chase, T. N.: Visuospatial cognition in Huntington's disease. *Mov. Disord.* 1991;6:127–132.

Mohr, E., Claus, J. J., Brouwers, P.: Basal ganglia disease and visuospatial cognition: are there disease specific impairments? *Behavioral Neurology*. 1997;10:67–75.

Naarding, P., Kremer, H. P. H., Zitman, F. G.: Huntington´s disease: a review of the literature on prevalence and treatment of neuropsychiatric phenomena. *European psychiatry*. 2001;8:439–445.

Nelson, H. E.: A modified card sorting test sensitive to frontal lobe defects. *Cortex*. 1976;12:313–324.

Overall, J. E., Gorham, D. R.: The Brief Psychiatric Rating Scale. *Psychological Reports*.1962;10:790 –812.

Paulsen, J. S., Ready, R. E., Hamilton, J. M., et al.: Neuropsychiatic aspects of Huntington's disease. *J. Neurol. Neurosurg. Psychiatry*. 2001;71:310–14.

Paulsen, J. S., Zhao, H., Stout, J. C., Brinkman, R. R., Guttman, M., Ross, C. A., Como, P., Manning, C., Hayden, M. R., Shoulson, I: Huntington Study Group. Clinical markers of early disease in persons near onset of Huntington's disease. *Neurology.* 2001;57(4):658–62.

Paulsen, J.S., Hoth, K.F., Nehl, C., Stierman, L.. Critical periods of suicide risk in Huntington's disease. *Am. J. Psychiatry.* 2005 Apr;162(4):725-31.

Paulsen, J.S., Nehl, C., Hoth, K.F., Kanz, J.E., Benjamin, M., Conybeare, R., McDowell, B., Turner, B.. Depression and stages of Huntington's disease. *J. Neuropsychiatry Clin. Neurosci.* 2005 Fall;17(4):496-502

Paulson, H. L., Bonini, N. M., Roth, K. A.: Polyglutamine disease and neuronal cell death. *Proc. Nat. Acad. Sci.,* 2000;97:12957–12958.

Penney, J. B. Jr., Young, A. B., Shoulson, I., Starosta-Rubenstein, S., Snodgrass, S. R., Sanchez-Ramos, J., Ramos-Arroyo, M., Gomez, F., Penchaszadeh, G., Alvir, J., et al.: Huntington's disease in Venezuela: 7 years of follow-up on symptomatic and asymptomatic individuals. *Mov. Disord.* 1990;5 (2):93–9.

Perry, T. L., Hansen, S., Kloster, M.: Huntington´s chorea: deficiency of gamma-aminobutyric acid in brain. *New Engl. J. Med.* 1973;288:337–342.

Potegal, M.: A note on spatial-motor deficits in patients with Huntington's disease: a test of a hypothesis. *Neuropsychologia.* 1971;9(2):233–5.

Quarrell, O. W., Tyler, A., Jones, M. P., Nordin, M., Harper, P. S.: Population studies of Huntington disease in Wales. *Clin. Genet.* 1988;33(3):189–195.

Quinn, N., Brown, R., Crauford, D., et al.: Core Assessment Program for Intracerebral Transplantation in Huntington´s disease (CAPIT-HD). *Mov. Disord.* 1996;2:143–150.

Randolph, C., Mohr, E., Chase, T. N.: Assessment of intellectual function in dementing disorders: validity of WAIS-R short forms for patients with Alzheimer's, Huntington's, and Parkinson's disease. *J. Clin. Exp. Neuropsychol.* 1993;15(5):743–53.

Ribaï, P., Nguyen, K., Hahn-Barma, V., Gourfinkel-An, I., Vidailhet, M., Legout, A., Dodé, C., Brice, A., Dürr, A.: Psychiatric and cognitive difficulties as indicators of juvenile Huntington's disease onset in 29 patients. *Arch. Neurol.* 2007 Jun;64(6):813-9.

Rosenblatt, A., Leroi, I.: Neuropsychiatry of Huntington's disease and other basal ganglia disorders. *Psychosomatics.* 2000;41:24–30.

Sahakian, B. J., Morris, R. G., Evenden, J. L., Heald, A., Levy, R., Philpot, M., Robbins, T. W.: A comparative study of visuospatial memory and learning in Alzheimer-type dementia and Parkinson's disease. *Brain.* 1988;111(Pt 3):695–718.

Schoenfeld, M., Myers, R. H., Cupples, L. A., et al.: Increased risk of suicide among patients with Huntington's disease. *J Neurol Neurosurg Psychiatry.* 1984;47:1283–7.

Shiwach, R.: Psychopathology in Huntington's disease patients. *Acta Psychiatr Scand.,* 1994;90(4):241–6.

Snell, R. G., MacMillan, J. C., Cheadle, J. P., Fenton, I., Lazarou, L. P., Davies, P., MacDonald, M. E., Gusella, J. F., Harper, P. S., Shaw, D. J.: Relationship between trinucleotide repeat expansion and phenotypic variation in Huntington´s disease. *Nat. Genet.* 1993;4:393–7.

Snowden, J.S., Craufurd, D., Griffiths, H.L., Neary, D.: Awareness of involuntary movements in Huntington disease. *Arch. Neurol.* 1998 Jun;55(6):801-5.

Snowden, J., Craufurd, D., Griffiths, H., Thompson, J. and Neary, D.: Longitudinal evaluation of cognitive disorder in Huntington´s disease. *Journal of International Neuropsychological Society.* 2000;6:33–44.

Snowden, J., Craufurd, D., Griffiths, H., Thompson, J., Neary, D.: Longitudinal evaluation of cognitive disorder in Huntington´s disease. *J. Int. Neuropsychol .Soc.* 2001;7(1):33–44.

Speedie, L. J., Brake, N., Folstein, S. E., et al.: Comprehension of prosody in Huntington's disease. *J. Neurol. Neurosurg. Psychiatry.* 1990;53:607–610.

Spokes, E. G. S.: Neurochemical alterations in Huntington's Chorea. A study of post-mortem brain tissue. *Brain.* 1980;103:179–210.

Sprengelmeyer, R., Young, A. W., Calder, A. J., Karnat, A., Lange, H., Hömberg, V., et al.: Loss of disgust. Perception of faces and emotions in Huntington's disease. *Brain.* 1996;119:1647–65.

Stout, J.C., Weaver, M., Solomon, A.C., Queller, S., Hui, S., Johnson, S.A., Gray, J., Beristain, X., Wojcieszek, J., Foroud, T.: Are cognitive changes progressive in prediagnostic HD? *Cogn. Behav. Neurol.* 2007 Dec;20(4):212-8.

Tekin, S., Cummings, J. L.: Frontal-subcortical neuronal circuits and clinical neuropsychiatry: an update. *J. Psychosom. Res.* 2002;53(2):647–54.

Thompson, J. C., Snowden, J., Craufurd, D., Neary, D.: Behavior in Huntington´s disease: Dissociating cognition-based and mood-based changes. *Journal of Neuropsychiatry and Clinical Neuroscience*s. 2002;1:37–44.

Tibben, A.. Predictive testing for Huntington's disease. Brain Res *Bull.* 2007 Apr 30;72(2-3):165-71.

Valera, A.G., Díaz-Hernández, M., Hernández, F., Ortega, Z., Lucas, J.J.. The ubiquitin-proteasome system in Huntington's disease. *Neuroscientist.* 2005 Dec;11(6):583-94.

Verny, C., Allain, P., Prudean, A., Malinge, M.C., Gohier, B., Scherer, C., Bonneau, D., Dubas, F., Le Gall, D.: Cognitive changes in asymptomatic carriers of the Huntington disease mutation gene. *Eur. J .Neurol.* 2007 Dec;14(12):1344-50. Epub 2007 Oct 17.

Vonsattel, J. P., Meyers, R. H., Stevens, T. J., et al.: Neuropathological classification of Huntington´s disease. *J. Neuropathol. and Exp. Neurol.* 1985;44:559–77.

Walker, D. A., Harper, P. S., Wells, C. E. C., Tyler, A., Davies, K., Newcombe, R. G.: Huntington's chorea in South Wales: a genetic and epidemiological study. *Clin. Genet.* 1981;19:213–221.

Wallesch, C. W., Fehrenbach, R. A.: On the neurolinguistic nature of language abnormalities in Huntington's disease. *J. Neurol .Neurosurg. Psychiatry.* 1988;51(3):367–73.

Warrington, E. K., James, M.: Visual Object and Space perception Battery. Bury St. Edmunds: Thames Valley Test Co., 1991.

Wilson, B., Cockburn, J., Baddeley, A.: The Rivermead Behavioural Memory Test. Bury St. Edmunds: Thames Valley Test Co., 1985.

Yudofsky, S.C., Silver, J.M., Jackson, W., Endicott, J., Williams, D.. The Overt Aggression Scale for the objective rating of verbal and physical aggression. *Am. J. Psychiatry.* 1986 Jan;143(1):35-9

Zimbelman, J.L., Paulsen, J.S., Mikos, A., Reynolds, N.C., Hoffmann, R.G., Rao, S.M.. fMRI detection of early neural dysfunction in preclinical Huntington's disease. *J. Int. Neuropsychol. Soc.* 2007 Sep;13(5):758-69.

The study was supported from the Czech Ministry of Education (research program MSM 0021620849)

In: Cognitive Deficit in Mental and Neurological Disorders ISBN: 978-1-60741-957-0
Editors: H. Kucerova, M. Preiss

Chapter XI

Hydrocephalus

Marketa Mohaplova

Abstract

Normal Pressure Hydrocephalus (NPH) in adults is a disease with varied etiology. In typical examples, it is manifested by a triad of symptoms—gait disorders, incontinence and cognitive functions disorders or even dementia. It develops most often with an, as yet, unexplained etiology (idiopathic hydrocephalus, iNPH) or less often as a result of another disease or injury. Normal pressure hydrocephalus occurs in all age groups, but most cases occur in the over those over 60. Both forms of NPH—Normal Pressure Hydrocephalus— cause 3 to 6% of all dementia and may be very effectively treated by shunting. In cases with a timely diagnosis, the cognitive abilities may be restored to premorbid levels—it is an extraordinary form of reversible dementia. Other forms of hydrocephalus occurring in the adulthood include diagnoses of slowly developing obstruction hydrocephalus and atrophic hydrocephalus. Within differential diagnostics, neuropsychology primarily deals with NPH. A significant problem in NPH involves making the correct diagnosis in patients over 60. A suspicion of NPH can be confirmed using imaging methods such as CT and MRI.

The loss of cognitive functions is especially related to memory, attention and executive functions. The cognitive deficit develops concomitantly with gait disorders and is not apparent to those around them, since no changes in personality or behavior occur. Left untreated, progression of the NPH will begin to affect cognitive abilities; manifesting as orientation disorders and significant memory/attention disorders, additionally qualitative consciousness disorders also begin to appear. These stages are accompanied by a loss of mobility and self-reliance. However, in cases with an early NPH diagnosis, coupled with timely surgery, improvement or even full recovery can occur or, at the very least, the progression of the clinical symptoms can be stopped.

1. Introduction

Hydrocephalus is defined as "an abnormal build-up of cerebrospinal fluid (liquor) in the intracranial space due to an imbalance in its production, flow or reabsorption" (Sameš, 2002, p.6). Cerebrospinal fluid accumulates in the ventricles and, sometimes, even in the subarachnoid spaces of the brain; this accumulation occurs at the expense of cerebral tissue. The ventricles are extended (ventriculomegaly), and this is usually linked to intracranial hypertension. The pathophysiological mechanisms are multifarious and, therefore, an occurrence of hydrocephalus is considered a pathological condition and not a specific disease or etiopathogenetic unit (Hebb et al., 2001).

Note 1, Related to the History

The name hydrocephalus comes from Greek: hydro = water, kephale = head. Up to the sixteenth century, there were disputes over the localization of the liquid—whether it was under the skin, under the cranial bone, under the dura mater or whether it was dispersed in the cerebral tissue. Most physicians believed that the liquor was accumulated under the skin; only Vesalius, in the sixteenth century, observed that hydrocephalus in children led to an increase in head volume, while in adults head volume was not altered. The disease had been observed in antiquity, but it was only at the beginning of the last century that attempts to find an effective treatment were successful. No pharmacological treatment exists; the only functional procedures involve surgery. The first operations occurred at the end of the nineteenth and at the beginning of the twentieth century. At present, a ventriculo-peritoneal shunt, which carries the liquor away from the cerebral ventricles through a one-way valve into the abdominal cavity is most frequently used. The principal objective of the therapy consists in optimization of the functions and decrease, preferably normalization, of intracranial pressure; having the ventricles return to their original size is not necessary.

Anatomic and Physiologic Circumstances

Under physiological conditions, cerebrospinal fluid is primarily produced by the chorioid plexi of the lateral ventricles with additional small amounts produced by plexi of the third and fourth ventricles. From the lateral ventricles, the fluid penetrates into the third and fourth ventricles through foramen Monroi and the aqueduct of Sylvius, respectively; from here, it flows out into the basal cisterns and ultimately to the surface of the hemispheres where it is absorbed into the vascular bed. Flow between the sites of production and sites of reabsorption are supported by pulsation of blood in the arteries and changes in venous volume during the breathing cycle. Total volume of the cerebrospinal fluid in the ventricles and subarachnoid spaces in adults is about 150 ml, and the daily production of the fluid averages about 500 ml per 24 hours.

Pathology

A CSF flow disorder may develop at any point—if flow disruption is caused by an obstacle it is called *obstructive hydrocephalus*. The underlying cause of *normal pressure hydrocephalus* lies in decreased reabsorption. The speed of development and seriousness of the disease depends on the ratio between CSF production, the degree of obstruction and maintenance of a compensatory reabsorption. Other factors influencing onset and seriousness of hydrocephalus include: the duration period of the obstruction or insufficient reabsorption, possibility of extension of CSF routes as partial compensation, the possibility of cranial extension (especially in cases of a hydrocephalus developing in infants) and the original volume and compliance of cerebral tissue.

Hydrocephalus may be inborn or acquired. From the psychological point of view, monitoring of cognitive functions in cases of both hydrocephalus types are within the competence of developmental psychologists. On the basis of clinical classification in adults, the following diagnoses are met in practice (according to MKN-10):

- • obstructive hydrocephalus—an obstacle found in the ventricular system,
- • normal pressure hydrocephalus—a reabsorption disorder,
- • atrophic hydrocephalus—a condition developed after cerebral tissue atrophy occurs with normal intracranial pressure and extension of the ventricles (in the case of Alzheimer's disease).

Obstructive hydrocephalus usually develops quickly; patients present with persistent headache, nausea, consciousness disorders, and even episodes of loss of consciousness. Thus it is a quantitative consciousness disorder within the scope of neurologists. From the psychological point of view, acute hydrocephalus, which over time becomes compensated hydrocephalus, does not result in any sequelae.

Normal Pressure Hydrocephalus

The typical neuropsychological practice can expect to encounter patients suffering from slowly developing hydrocephalus, due to either obstructive (although exceptional and most often associated with slowly growing tumors) or NPH. In cases of NPH, the most important issue is a proper diagnosis.

Note 2. Related to the History

Normal pressure hydrocephalus, as a clinical entity, was first described by Hakim and Adams (Hakim, 1965) in 1965; the authors were the first to link patients having the symptom triad—dementia, balance disorders, and incontinence and a finding of communicating hydrocephalus (through imaging).

Patients with the diagnosed NPH can be divided into two basic subgroups from an etiological point of view:

1. In patients of the first subgroup, no reason for NPH development can be found—this is called *idiopathic NPH.* From a clinical point of view, the only evidence of a correct diagnosis comes from improvement of clinical symptoms after shunt surgery. This form is present in 45 to 50% of the diagnosed cases (Dunn, 2002). A neuropsychological examination may contribute, in the diagnostics stage, to a definite determination of the disease and, in the postoperative period, to an unambiguous assessment of NPH sequelae and changes in cognitive functions after surgery.
2. NPH can develop *as a consequence of a primary disease that leads to* CSF malabsorption. The most frequent causes are subarachnoid bleeding, infectious meningitis, cranio-cerebral injury, tumors, and intracranial surgery. In secondarily developing NPH, it may be very difficult to distinguish the affects of the primary disease from those of hydrocephalus during a neuropsychological examination.

In normal pressure hydrocephalus, an extension of the cerebral ventricles at the expense of cerebral tissue occurs. The cerebral tissue becomes, especially in older ages, more pliable and recedes in reaction to the pressure of expanding ventricles. With the extension of the ventricular system, reduced blood flow to periventricular structures and association routes in local white matter occurs. However, if shunt surgery is carried out in a timely fashion, there can be a full recovery.

According to statistical data, NPH incidence in Great Britain averages seven to ten cases per 100,000 inhabitants. In Sweden four to five cases per 100,000 inhabitants are successfully resolved every year (Dunn, 2002).

Clinical Picture of NPH

NPH is characterized by a triad of symptoms—gait disorder, dementia, and incontinence.

The gait disorder is the most conspicuous symptom—the patient moves with small steps and a wide base, the impairment is most noticeable when the patient must overcome a small obstacle—entering an elevator, stepping over an object on the floor; the patient may also present with apraxia (magnetic phenomenon).

The urinary incontinence is manifested in later stages of the disease.

Diagnostics

Morphological examinations (CT, MRI) show an extension of the ventricular system, especially in the area of the frontal corners of the lateral ventricles; in clearly expressed hydrocephalus, an erasure of the subarachnoid space over the hemispheres and transependymal transfer of cerebrospinal fluid into the periventricular white matter is observed.

Functional Examination

- *Tap test*—repeated lumbar punctures with discharge of large volumes of cerebrospinal fluid leads to an improvement of the clinical symptoms in communicating hydrocephalus.
- *Lumbar drainage*—excessive cerebrospinal fluid is drained, using a catheter, from the area of lumbar spine to an exterior reservoir—if the condition improves, similar effects can also be expected after shunt surgery.
- *Lumbar infusion test*—using a needle inserted into the area of the lumbar spine, a specific amount of a liquid, which exceeds the normal production of cerebrospinal fluid, is introduced, and dependence between the amount of the supplied liquid and pressure increase in the CSF routes is monitored; should values exceed physiological values, it may indicate a reabsorption disorder.

Therapy

Shunt surgery—involves drainage of the cerebrospinal fluid from ventricular routes into other bodily cavities, most often into the abdominal cavity, where reabsorption can occur.

After the introduction of a drain, a favorable prognosis for NPH patients who had the complete triad of symptoms and known etiology is 60 to 75% (Prigatano, 2000). In idiopathic NPH, improvement is only visible in 10 to 40 % of cases. It appears that the longer the patient experiences the symptoms, the lower the probability of successful treatment.

Although shunt surgery is relatively undemanding, the percentage of patients who experience post-operative complications is high. Prigatano (Prigatano, 2000) found that the percentage of complications presented in the literature was as high as 38%; 22% of patients needed a shunt revision (second surgery), and in 6% of patients, serious neurological complications or death occurred.

2. Principal Domains of Measured Cognitive Functions

The described changes of cognitive functions primarily relate to patients with idiopathic NPH or patients with secondary NPH, in whom the primary disease did not cause any sequelae (which is only a theoretical assumption).

Although, in connection with hydrocephalus, dementia is regularly described as one of the symptom of the triad, however, the *complex diagnostic criteria for dementia is only fulfilled in more developed disease stages.* In patients who benefit from surgery and have a real hope of recovery of their cognitive performance, impairment of cognitive performance is generally limited to the area of memory, attention and executive functions. In NPH, some monitored functions, in which deterioration with frequent dementia occurs, are maintained for a long period—episodic memory component; also, neither qualities of personality nor behavioral expressions change—social competence persists. In the following text, we will try to describe a profile of the cognitive deficit in NPH in the sense of positive symptoms and missing typical symptoms of the respective dementia types in more detail.

Considering the current classification, cognitive deficit in NPH comes close to the so-called *subcortical type* of dementia with slowed psychomotor pace (Lezak, 1995) and a disorder of frontal functions. Localization of anatomical changes in cases of extended cerebral ventricles corresponds to such a type of defect. The extension of the temporal corners of the lateral ventricles causes hippocampal dysfunctions and, therefore, disrupts an important part of the cortical-subcortical circuit, which is important for execution of cognitive functions. Another theory directly mentions a defect of the frontal lobes (and not only a similarity to the frontal dementia). The reason is reduced blood flow associated with a defect of the anterior cerebral arteries that pass over the corpus callosum (Todd, 2003).

In Table 1, expressions of the cortical/subcortical dementia and sequelae of hydrocephalus are presented.

Table 1. Comparison of symptoms of cortical/subcortical dementia

According to Vašina and Diamant (1994)

	Cortical dementia	*Subcortical dementia*
Speech	normal	abnormal, motor dysarthria, dysphonia
Language	Aphasia	no disorders
Memory	Amnesia	forgetfulness
Cognition	disorders of judgment and abstraction	abnormal, slow and deteriorating
Numerical operations	Acalculia	disrupted due to deceleration of mental processes
Visual perception	Abnormal	normal
Spatial orientation	Abnormal	normal
Mood	Indifference, apathy	disinhibition, depression

The most important difference seen in NPH involves the *absence of speech disorders;* in addition, in NPH, spatial orientation disorder occurs; mood disorders are not common, even if depressive temper/experience often occurs.

Orientation disorder is associated with developed stages of the disease. According to our clinical experience, time disorientation primarily occurs (from day to century confusion); on the other hand, we have never seen location disorientation in communicating patients. Total cognitive affection continues with confusion and decelerating psychomotor pace; however, in those cases, physical symptoms are clearly visible and the patient is not capable of independent movement (gait is characterized with short ataxic steps, marked balance and incontinence disorders also develop, completing the symptom triad, which should lead to a suspicion of NPH, even without a neuropsychological examination). General deterioration of cognitive abilities may lead to qualitative changes in consciousness and total inability to communicate.

The neuropsychological examination under the terms of differential diagnostics of dementia will primarily be focused on testing of memory, attention, and executive functions; other possible deficits have been included in a survey of possible defects presented in Table 2.

Table 2. Survey of disrupted cognitive functions and form of the defect

	Type of disorder/reduced ability
Memory	semantic, short- and long-term one
Attention	planning, problem-solving, flexibility
Executive functions	planning, problem-solving, flexibility
Visuo-spatial abilities	movement in an unknown environment (hospital)
Orientation	in time
Confusion	confusion of events/persons
Consciousness	quantitative disorders/loss of consciousness

Memory

The memory may be briefly defined as *the ability to notice, keep, and recall* information. For a description of the development of memory disorders in normal pressure hydrocephalus, Tulving's classification is suitable (in Kulišťák, 2003):

- *The episodic memory* notices and keeps specific events connected with the respective context. The experienced event is linked with the time, place, feelings etc. which accompanied the event;
- *The semantic memory* arranges remembering and maintenance of knowledge about the surrounding world.

In NPH, the episodic memory is maintained; if a defect in early stages of hydrocephalus occurs, it is related to time designation. In practice, problems accompanying anamnesis detection often occur: the patient is unable to determine the respective years of important events. The non-declarative (implicit) memory for unintentional processes, e.g., learned skills, adaptation reactions, are preserved for extended periods without any decline. Cognitive reduction relates to *semantic memory,* the ability to reproduce verbal information without a logical sequence being especially badly affected (we can observe substandard performance on the AVLT). Other limitations of semantic memory may be observed in lexical verbal fluency (recalling words beginning with a specific letter). The result of this combination of the memory affection is a "social unobtrusiveness." NPH patients are well aware of their diminished ability and often they try to conceal the deficit in normal contact.

Reduction of memory abilities is mentioned by all authors, without exception, who have dealt with normal pressure hydrocephalus (Hakim, Adams, 1965; Iddon et al, 2004; Hebb, 2001, etc). Due to extensive variability of classification of memory, its disorders and description, the given characteristics of cognitive deficits slightly differ from each other. Lezak (1995, s. 251) quotes: "Typical endangered functions are represented by memory and learning, of both visual and verbal content, even if memory of new and remote events probably remain intact." The same, in other words, is given by Luciano (2001, s. 675): "Episodic memory remains intact while an impairment may at first be observed in learning and recalling of visual/verbal inputs; later more profound weakening of the memory may be seen."

Attention

Attention is one of the principal conditions of cognitive functioning; any attention disorder may significantly reduce cognitive performance. In NPH, a decrease in concentration after a short time period and inability to divide attention occurs. Along with executive function disorders, it causes an inability to shift attention among multiple inputs, e.g., failure in the B-version of the Trail Making Test.

More serious attention disruptions may also cause orientation disorders. In the early stages of the disease, low performance on instant recall tests—short-term memory and learning—may indicate confusion and reduced attention rather than memory disorders (Lezak, 2003).

Executive Functions

In patients with NPH, some executive functions disorders that are, despite some uncertainties, still localizationally classified to prefrontal structures, may be found and frontal lobe damage should be expected. The processes in question are of "higher order" like planning, problem-solving, cognitive flexibility, and the rate of information processing (Luciano, 2001; Devito, 2005). Normal pressure hydrocephalus causes quick deterioration of the aforementioned items. Patients may have more difficulties coping with this deficit than simple memory disorders and, especially in less elderly patients, it is the main reason for seeking medical help (see Caser report No. 1).

Case report No. 1:

A woman (41) sought a neurological examination due to deteriorating memory and "becoming stupid." In the previous four months, she had observed forgetfulness and the inability to solve common problems, both at work and at home, with the same decisiveness as before. She was university-educated (economics) and is employed as a chief accountant in a large insurance company. She repeatedly forgot what she had already done/solved, the last incident being her inability to close a common monthly accounting balance. One month ago, she had been able to cope with work problems. She believed that nobody had observed her decrease in cognitive abilities (at least, nobody had drawn her attention to it); at home, her husband and daughter noted some minor hesitations but did not assign any importance to it. She was tested with the following: Orientation of WMS, AVLT, Rey-Osterrieth figure, Trail Making Test version A and B for adults. The results of the neuropsychological tests showed average performance, only AVLT (30-40 percent) and Trail Making Test, version B (19-28 percent), were substandard. In the tests, no failures were recorded; however, with respect to education and vocabulary, the results clearly indicated a decrease in performance. The physical symptoms were limited to minor gait impairment, which had not caused her any significant problems. Following shunt surgery, she spent five months on sick leave. During this period, she actively trained her memory—she recapitulated read texts and TV news, revised her German language, disposed of administrative/tax matters and revised accountancy. The tests were repeated six month later, at which time the patient achieved maximum performance on the AVLT and Trail Making Test, version A; other results exceeding 90 percent.

The executive functions also include abilities of cognitive estimates; however, this is probably not affected, at all, in patients in the initial stages of hydrocephalus. In a pilot study, we verified that the results of the Cognitive Estimate Test did not correlate with results of other tests (Mohaplová, 2004). Even in patients with substandard performance on memory tests, the cognitive estimate was normal or even above average. This fact may be explained by an opportunity to deduce answers on the basis of previous knowledge and experience, which is only lost in NPH patients in stages of general advanced deterioration of their abilities and the accompanying confusion.

Psychic Disorders

In patients suffering from NPH, depressive episodes are not uncommon; these episodes are not a consequence of development of hydrocephalus, but are triggered, in predisposed patients, by circumstances accompanying the loss of cognitive abilities and self-reliance. The presence of depressive episodes is often seen from the very beginning of the disease; if the condition is not treated, apathy, anxiety, and paranoid fantasies may also occur (Luciano, 2001). An assessment of current mood should be a part of every examination in patients suspected of having hydrocephalus, because depression can significantly decrease cognitive performance and decelerate rehabilitation and recovery after surgery.

The delay in diagnosing may lead to deteriorating symptoms of neurological/psychiatric affection. We have recorded the development of a panic disorder in a 30-year-old patient who had observed a decrease in cognitive abilities without any explanation. After NPH surgery, there was a remission of the panic disorder, but full recovery of original abilities did not take place.

Case report No. 2

In a 30-year-old woman, normal pressure hydrocephalus of unknown etiology was diagnosed. The first signs, which she described as increased tediousness, forgetfulness of normal daily things (e.g., what she had wanted to buy), distraction and loss of attentiveness, had prompted her, several times, to see a doctor. Initially, these symptoms were attributed to her pregnancy, then to post-delivery exhaustion and changes associated with recovery from her pregnancy (at the time of diagnosis, she was 20 months on her maternity leave). After the above-mentioned symptoms had been ignored by a general practitioner, gynecologist, and neurologist, she sought a healer and expert in homeopathy. Despite subjective complaints of continued impairment of, primarily, memory and attention, nothing was "objectively" found, and the patient began to believe she was ill with malign disease. She was referred to a psychiatric department where she was treated for manic disorder—her worries regarding her "malign disease" induced several panic attacks. Eventually, she underwent magnetic resonance examination with a finding of a developed normal pressure hydrocephalus. In response to the diagnosis, she discontinued her psychiatric medication and both the panic attacks and symptoms of depression returned, despite immediate surgery. Immediately after being released from the hospital, she went to see a psychiatrist; with pharmacological treatment (anxiolytic drugs), her condition improved. In spite of a statistically insignificant improvement in cognitive functions, three months after surgery, she indicated a significant subjective improvement. She went back to work as a bank clerk-teller, which is a rather demanding job. She is able to better manage her panic disorder and takes medication prior to anticipated stressful situations; oddly, the attacks do not occur on weekends, despite not taking any medication during these days.

3. Measurement, Tests, Methods

The selection of testing methods suitable for examination of a patient with normal pressure hydrocephalus should be considered from two principal points of view:

1. Etiology of the disease:

- *Idiopathic NPH*—when preparing the test battery, we should expect disorders mentioned in the previous chapter and choose from methods that check the level of memory, attention, and executive functions.
- *Secondary NPH,* which develops as a result of a primary disease, mostly an injury, bleeding, tumor, and operation—it is necessary to individually consider the sequelae of the primary disease and judge whether it is possible to obtain valid results through testing.

2. Examination purpose. We will focus on the two most frequent objectives:

- Examination within differential diagnostics; a neuropsychologist cannot diagnose but "only" pronounce a suspicion of NPH, which should be verified by imaging and lumbar infusion tests. An assessment of total (even physical) condition of the patient, especially of his/her gait, may present a significant indication. Distinguishing between dementia types is generally demanding, the profile of cognitive function in NPH differs from other irreversible dementias in only a few details.
- Reassessment of cognitive function level with clear diagnosis—there may be progression monitoring, assessment of the condition before/after surgery, assessment of rehabilitation benefits (the recommended battery of tests for those purposes is given in the next chapter).

Table 3 - Selected testing methods suitable for administration to NPH patients

Function	Method
Memory	Wechsler memory scale-III AVLT, RAVLT California verbal learning test Rey Osterrieth Complex Figure Test – reproduction Rey Auditory-Verbal Learning Test Repetition of numbers WAIS III (WAIS-R)
Executive functions	Trail Making Test, A, B Stroop Test Verbal Fluency Tests Wisconsin Card Sorting Test

In Table 3, the Wechsler Memory Scale III is given as a complete unit—an administration of all subtests would require additional meetings because increased tediousness and decreased concentration ability often limit patients to single-hour testing. However, it is possible to use the respective WMS subtests. If there is an opportunity to meet the patient on more occasions, the Wechsler memory scale is a very useful method for assessing hydrocephalus, especially because of the possibility of a detailed assessment of the post-operative changes and determination of rehabilitation procedures. The same time limitation applies to the WAIS-R (WAIS III), the subtests of which are regularly part of neuropsychological batteries (Lezak, 1995; Boon et al., 1999; Burtscher et al., 2003 and others). If the administration of the entire test is not possible, the Numbers Repetition (assessment of the working memory level), Calculations (ability to concentrate and cognitive flexibility), and Dices (visual-spatial abilities and ability of analysis/synthesis) subtests seem to be especially useful.

Very often, the Mini Mental State Examination (MMSE), which is especially popular with physicians and neuropsychologists carrying out research studies, is used and is assessed as an introductory orientation method. Undoubtedly, the test may be used for a primary differential appraisal, if the patient actually suffers from dementia. A problem with this method relates to the fact that in patients in the fully reversible stage of the disease, a decrease in performance is not noticed—so-called ceiling effect. A lower score is only reached by patients having moderate dementia (Pettersen, 2001). Within the differential diagnostics of hydrocephalus, use of the Mini Mental State Examination appears to be an informative method that does not, from the neuropsychological point of view, contribute to a final diagnosis. However, due to easy administration and evaluation, frequency of utilization of the test is quite high.

Structures of testing batteries in published studies are alike; in most research cases, their administration does not exceed one hour, and tests of memory, attention and executive functions are submitted (many tests, in fact, unify all monitored areas). The most extensive research is represented by a Dutch study_(Boon et al., 1999). It included 101 patients who underwent a pre-surgery and, within half of a year, a post-surgery neuropsychological examination. The authors' drew up a so-called Dementia scale consisting of four psychological tests: Digit span forward and backward (repetition of numbers), 10-word test, Trail Making Test and the Finger Tapping Test.

There are two interesting studies that focused on differential diagnostics. The first was published by Iddon et al. (1996): they compared cognitive functions in patients with normal pressure hydrocephalus and Alzheimer's disease. In all cases, the administration was carried out both prior to the surgery and then six months after the surgery. The battery of tests included a subtest of attention from the CANTAB battery—Cambridge Neuropsychological Test Automated Battery, NART—The National Adult Reading Test (to assess the level of pre-morbid intellect), Test of executive functions, Test of verbal fluency, and the Kendric object learning test (KOLT). The second study (Helstrom et al, 2007) documents the influence of other somatic factors on cognitive performance in NPH. A group of patients with iNPH was compared with a group of patients with iNPH and a significant vascular risk with expected concurrence of hydrocephalus and vascular dementia.

Methods mapping the current state of experience should be a necessary part of the test battery, because the incidence of mood disorders up to depressive experience is common in patients with hydrocephalus (Lezak, 2004). In order to assess depression, short questionnaires are suitable, e.g., a common test is the Beck Depression Inventory (BDI); other self-assessment methods include: the HAMA (Hamilton Anxiety Scale) and Geriatric Depression Scale for older patients.

In patients in an advanced stage of the disease, who may not be able cooperate in the administration of the test battery; it is reasonable to monitor self-reliance and functional abilities using CDR (Clinical Dementia Rating).

4. Course of the Cognitive Deficit

Normal pressure hydrocephalus is clinically manifested by Hakim's triad. Due to the difficulties regarding differential diagnostics of dementia, we believe it is important to become acquainted with a general picture of the disease. Gait disorders, specifically, may be a significant clue in making the right diagnosis:

1. Balance/gait disorders . The picture and seriousness of gait problems change over time—ranging from slight clumsiness to the inability to stand or walk. The gait usually has a wide-base, with small steps; shambling may make the gait resemble that of Parkinson's disease. To turn, the patient will use a large number of very short steps, for an "about-face" perhaps as many as 12 to 15 steps (Todd, 2003). The disorder is amplified when small obstacles have to be overcome—a small step, getting on an elevator. Often there are problems with gait initiation; they feel to be glued to the ground—so-called magnetic phenomenon (Lucianno, 2001). The gait disorders are among the first and most common symptoms seen in normal pressure hydrocephalus. The extending ventricles damage more white matter than gray; therefore, motor functions are affected more and sooner, as axon collaterals are compressed.

2. Incontinence. Full incontinence is rare; in most cases, only increased frequency of urination occurs. In the first stage, the patients indicate imperative micturition—with the first feeling of the urge to urinate, they must proceed for the toilet. Only later does incontinence in its full sense occur (Lucianno, 2001). However, some patients do not have any sphincter problems. Like other clinical symptoms, the diagnosis is aggravated by the incidence of age-related incontinence disorders.
3. Deterioration of the cognitive functions, up to dementia. In typical cases, cognitive problems appear concomitantly with development balance/gait disorders or soon afterwards. Cognitive deterioration is creeping and inconspicuous; especially in patients over 60, the symptoms are often ascribed to the aging process. First symptoms involve a loss of interest for existing activities, a decline in organizational abilities, and short-term blackouts. With further development of hydrocephalus, confusion and orientation disorders begin to appear, the extent of attention decreases and memory problems, which also involve long-term memory traces, increase. Self-image and self-assessment ability is, more or less, preserved, and patients are aware of their impaired conditions. Therefore, very often depression, anxious experiences (see Case report No. 2), and sometimes even paranoid symptoms occur.

Should hydrocephalus develop secondarily on the basis of a primary condition (injury, bleeding, or tumor), the onset of symptoms may be obscured with health problems caused by the primary condition.

In the case of normal pressure hydrocephalus development, cognitive performance decrease starts immediately at the beginning of the disease. It develops concomitantly or immediately after the onset of the gait/balance disorder. The start is slow and creeping, and the first symptoms may easily be mistaken for other problems. Above all, loss of interests and tiny memory blackouts occur; which is, especially in elderly persons, too often ascribed to aging. With the development of the disease, memory disorders worsen, attention and the ability to concentrate fluctuate, and confusion or even disorientation appears. However, even people who suffer from an extensive cognitive disorder usually visit the doctor because of their deteriorating gait and loss of balance. An exception is younger patients, particularly those involved in business; they tend to seek medical care because cognitive blackouts prevent them from managing everyday activities (see Case report No. 1).

Later stages of the disease are characterized by Luciano (2001) in the following way: "In advanced stages, emotional and psychiatric symptoms—agitation, anxiety, depression, and paranoid thoughts may occur." As NPH progresses, memory is unevenly affected; typically, learning and recognition of both visual and verbal content deteriorate first, while episodic memory remains intact. Also, disorders linked with dysfunction of the frontal lobe, related with verbal fluency, cognitive flexibility, and attention are also frequently seen.

In untreated cases, orientation progressively worsens up to full confusion and dependency. The course and rate of cognitive function decline is highly individual.

Differential Diagnostics

In normal pressure hydrocephalus, there is a principle that the sooner the surgery, the smaller the damage to nervous structures and the greater the chance of a full recovery of cognitive performance. Definitely, it is not appropriate to only look for diffuse cognitive disorders, which do not fulfill the criteria for dementia determination. The biggest problem is the differential diagnosis in patients over 60; this is because all three clinical symptoms are often generally associated with the aging process. The elderly often expect and accept that they must live with age-related problems and adapt to them. Subtle symptoms may have been present months or even years before the patient seeks medical help. The symptoms progress with time, and often the elderly are forced to seek medical attention because of continued deterioration of their gait and balance. Cognitive changes are unpleasant for most of the seniors, however; because of simplified daily routines, they are often more limited by their physical (gait-related) problems. It is family members who often draw their attention to their forgetfulness. Since neurosurgery may improve or at least stop the progression of the disease, we should think of normal pressure hydrocephalus as a counterweight of other types of irreversible dementias.

To return the patient to normal life as completely and quickly as possible, it is not only important to make the correct diagnosis of the disease but also proceed with surgery in a timely fashion.

In the following text, some diagnostic clues are given that may help in making the proper differential diagnosis.

Dementia

As in dementia, memory problems and other cognitive functions may be seen in hydrocephalus. The dementia criteria, according to MKN-10—*decrease in emotional control, motivation, and changes of social behavior*—do not show up in the initial phases of the NPH. Those changes only occur in advanced stages of the disease, along with severe deterioration of cognitive functions; at this stage, even a shunt operation does not offer any real chance of improvement.

When taking into account the other symptoms supporting dementia diagnosing, in NPH patients sometimes *confabulations* occur, however, unlike demented persons, *NPH patients are aware of them* even if they are not able to reproduce them. *Aphasia, apraxia, agnosia and other cortical disorders have only been recorded where another serious disease/injury preceded the discovery of hydrocephalus* (e.g., cerebral vascular event, aneurysm, injury). With deepening dementia, difficulties finding proper words gets more frequent, but, as Prigatano states (BNI, s. 11), it is not aphasia.

Dementia in Alzheimer's Disease

A differential diagnosis, especially at the beginning of the disease, is very difficult. Even in theory, the difference between the initial and moderate stages of Alzheimer's disease and normal pressure hydrocephalus is only small, and, in practice, in a normal examination, nearly undistinguishable. One of the principal clues could be *the absence of so-called magnetic gait with wide base in Alzheimer's dementia,* which is, on the contrary, typical for NPH. Other differences, e.g., personality changes, agnosia, apraxia, aphasia and other speech disorders, as well as motivation changes, are variable and individual. In differential diagnosis consideration, physicians and psychologists should also take accounts of *family members* and close personal contacts before they recommend further examination. In his extensive research, Lucianno (2001) monitored differences in cooperation while examining that may help improve the diagnostic process.

A patient with normal pressure hydrocephalus does not answer the questions of the examiner immediately *(akinetic mutism)* but, if the examiner repeats the question and insists on an answer, the patient answers, and answers are mostly correct. Patients with Alzheimer's disease usually answer immediately but incorrectly. Patients with NPH *tend to stay without movement and speak softly*. If there is an opportunity to speak with the patient over the phone, the answers to questions are prompter and louder (so-called *phone phenomenon*). The mental changes in NPH may differ from patient to patient. A decrease in intellectual initiative, spontaneity, and communication is usual. Volitive movements are delayed and decelerated. The answers may decrease down to an abulia stage. *NPH offers an important characteristics that may significantly help in diagnosing, namely variation of symptoms intensity from one day to another*. The patient's gait is sometimes better, he/she can go to the toilet, and his/her memory may be improved to such extent that he/she may take part in conversation without any noticeable problems. This information may only be available from family members, since no long-term observation is possible. However, physicians should ask pointed questions because such possible variability is seldom spontaneously referred to by relatives. This phenomenon does not appear in Alzheimer's disease or other organic dementias, for which a slow continuous progression of the condition without any improvement is typical; only occasional stagnation in the decrease but no improvement, however temporary, occurs.

Attention should also be drawn to the beginning of the disease, even if it is difficult to obtain quality information several months or years later. In *Alzheimer's disease, dementia precedes the gait disorders* while *in NPH both the disorders occur concomitantly* or the cognitive disorders are only observed after gait problems appear.

Vascular Dementia

The differential diagnosis of vascular dementia and normal pressure hydrocephalus is difficult. The only really reliable and objective method is magnetic resonance because even tiny ischemic changes following the ictus are visible. For the appraisal, a clue could be taken by presence of neurological syndromes exceeding the gait disorders and also phatic and gnostic disorders in multi-infarction dementia.

Another type of the vascular dementia, often mentioned within the differential diagnosis of NPH, is Biswanger's disease. It develops on the basis of vascular affection of the subcortical structures, and it is then a subcortical dementia. Clinical expressions are very similar to those of NPH and, in addition, and unlike in Alzheimer's disease, some cortical disorders of phatic and practical functions do not appear as they do in cases of NPH.

Since vascular changes are very a frequent finding in people over 60, a concurrence of cerebrovascular disease and normal pressure hydrocephalus may occur. In such case, "the shunt surgery may only have a minimal effect or may have no effect at all" (Boon, 1999).

Depression

In patients with NPH, depressive experiences are often recorded. If a patient scores on a depression test, which should always be part of the battery, a psychiatrist should be consulted. The symptoms of depression can give the impression of dementia and differential diagnosis could be difficult. Depression causes cognitive inhibition, attention and memory reduction and, on the other hand, cognitive deficit, is accompanied by depressive experience. Despite that, some important differences may be found:

- Depression shows a prompt onset compared to slow progress in NPH;
- Depression is accompanied by vegetative problems, e.g., alteration of appetite, digestion problems and sleeping disorders;
- Patients with depression do not try to hide their conditions, they not only admit the memory disorders but also often aggrandize them; patients with dementia try to "mask" the problems, they answer aptly but incorrectly;
- In depression, reduction of short- and long-term memory is visible;
- The depressive patients are fully oriented and quite seldom confused.

Scoring on depression tests may be significantly influenced, especially in seniors in advanced phases of the NPH, by fears of the future and uncertainty about the future course of life. After their existential uncertainty had been resolved, subjectively referred gait/cognitive deficit improvement was often reported, even if the only statistically significant changes occurred on the depression scale (see the Case report No. 3).

Case Report No. 3

An old woman (80) whose daughter had been upset by the rapidly progressing gait disorder and loss of balance of her mother, was examined. When asked pointed questions, the daughter also confirmed marked forgetfulness and total loss of cognitive flexibility, which had been, however, assigned to aging. The patient is frequently weepy and speaks about her fears of the future. So far she lives alone in a family house in different part of the village from her daughter, who helps her often with her household duties. She visits the family on weekends and is delighted with her two-year-old great-grandson. She assesses herself as "quite self-reliant;" she can dress herself, heat up her meals, can do simple chores. Objectively a significant reduction of monitored cognitive functions occurred, she is not time-oriented, in tests of verbal/visuomotor memory, verbal fluency, and in attention she scores under the fifth percentile; she completely failed the Trail Making Test and showed moderate depression on the BDI (she refused an offer of psychiatric care). Six months after the surgery, the gait and balance improved, but she always uses a cane and moves slowly; the results of the cognitive tests have not statistically improved, although objectively a small improvement has been recorded. However, on the BDI questionnaire, the gross score is 3,—without depression, shown marked improvement. Subjectively, the patient describes improvement in all respects, is in a good mood, smiling, and fully cooperates. As the first information, she says she is living with her daughter who moved her during the period of the first hospitalization to her home; from the hospital, she directly went to her home (at the time of the first testing she had not known about that; her daughter wanted to surprise her). She is satisfied with her life and future expectations as well as with the result of the operation. She spends her days in the presence of her great-grandson who, as she states, "looks after her and orders her about on walks."

Other

Of the diseases that come under the psychiatric diagnoses, also delirium, schizophrenia and mental retardation are worthy of consideration within the frame of the differential diagnostics.

Other diseases whose symptoms may be mistaken for the beginning of dementia are slowly growing cerebral tumors, infection of the central nervous system and metabolic disorders.

As expected, however, the second biggest group (after dementias) of non-diagnosed patients with normal pressure hydrocephalus is formed by people in whom the clinical triad symptoms are mistaken for common aging problems. Smolík (1996, p. 68) defines forgetfulness in normal course of aging as follows: "The memory disorders caused by aging are only slight and do not significantly disturb the daily activities. Dementia is not synonymous with aging."

5. Proposal for Standardized Examination

A selected test battery has been proposed for common practical use within differential diagnostics and also for comparison before and after surgery, and possibly for comparison of rehabilitation success rates. Currently, the test battery is used in a contemporary research carried out in order to assess changes of the cognitive abilities prior/after normal pressure hydrocephalus. The time required for administration is about 45 to 60 minutes (including the introductory discussion), and a more specific anamnesis should be completed, in most of the patients, by discussion with family members. *Conversation with close contacts is considered necessary for any differential diagnostic appraisal*; it may bring valuable detailed information that cannot be reported by the patient (dating of the first symptoms, concurrence of individual symptoms, rate of their development and variability and so on).

As it was mentioned in the previous chapter, complex administration of WMS and WAIS III maps the complex profile of cognitive abilities, offers data on development of the intellectual powers and allows assessing performance smoothness, psychomotor rate and level of attention. However, such tests are time-consuming and stressful for NPH patients; therefore, in most patients, any administration involving all tests should be divided into at least two visits. Their use may be considered in cases of motivated patients after individual rehabilitation program has been drawn.

The selection of methods corresponds to the monitored domains of measured cognitive functions—memory, attention and executive functions. At the end, BDI-II is included in order to assess the current condition of experience.

Table 4. Proposed examination algorithm

Test	Monitored function
Orientation from WMS	
Rey AVLT	verbal memory, learning
Rey Osterrieth Complex Figure	visuo-construction abilities, attention
Rey Osterrieth Figure – reproduction	memory
Trail Making Test A,B	attention, flexibility, psychomotor rate
Verbal Fluency Test	verbal recall
Rey AVLT–remote recall	verbal memory
BDI	level of depression

For the first test, we propose a subtest Information and Orientation of *the Wechsler Memory Scale* (WMS-III, 1999). Its principal advantage consists in its potential to reveal deeper damage in a very short period, and thus it is an input for possible change of the test battery with respect to the current state. The Information and Orientation subtest is the first of 13 parts of Wechsler's memory scale. It includes 18 questions, of which 14 are to be assessed (the last four questions relate to health restrictions). The test informs about basic orientation in person, time, and place. It only picks up severe disorders. While processing, gross scores are used—each correct answer means one point. Should inaccurate orientation in time or even an information error be found, an alternative of Trail Making Test version B for children is adequate, however, failure should also be expected. In that case, the available standards cannot be used, but we can have a notion of the level of the cognitive flexibility (most of the patients can cope with an internship with prompts) and especially monitor a post-operation improvement.

Note—Even patients with full failure in the children's version B of the Trail Making Test may be inconspicuous in normal contacts for their environment, especially if they had above-average intellect prior to the disease and they are socially competent.

The next battery method is *AVLT.* It was selected because of its sensitivity to tiny damages of memory, focused on verbal contents. It allows both short-term (experiments I-V) and remote (experiment VII) recalls. The time for administration is, with respect to the extent of obtained information, adequate to include the test into a more extensive battery without exhausting the patient. Also, the number of repetitions of identical words in a single experiment, distortion, and confabulation are monitored. The test also offers alternative retest sets of words, so it is possible to objectively assess the postoperative and rehabilitation changes. The available standards for this test are also suitable; in higher age groups up to 87, the standards are well differentiated according to Ivnik et al., 1999. If WAIS-R was administered, we can also use a standard of IQ stratification according to Wiens et al, 1988. An alternative may consist in the use of the extended California Verbal Learning Test.

The next is *Rey-Osterrieth Complex Figure,* an alternative form of the Taylor Figure; other alternatives are also offered —by Lezak, 2003. The method allows a possibility to pick up disorders of constructional/psychomotor abilities by tracing a copy; and, as a useful method, it is utilized in the assessment of memory for non-verbal content while drawing a reproduction (Lezak, 1995; Preiss, 1997; Kulišťák, 2003). As for the assessment, we propose a milder scoring system according to Osterrieth. Due to a non-uniform procedure of assessment, any comparison to healthy populations is more-or-less informative because the scoring system used may, because if its benevolence, show quite diverse results depending on the evaluator. The advantage of the test consists in both its qualitative and quantitative assessment. NPH patients have below-average scores; in tracing a copy often a visuo-construction ability disorder may be seen, the picture is drawn without any frame, just piling up details. While making a reproduction, a memory disorder for content without logical sequence is visible.

The *Trail Making Test* is a relatively difficult test for patients with hydrocephalus. As for the A-version for the adults, most patients are below average; in the B-version for the adults, total failure is very frequent. The level of attention and cognitive flexibility do not allow patients to complete the test even if there is support. In order to map the seriousness, part B for children is used—but even here some patients totally fail. Despite that, the test is considered useful since after a successful operation, significant improvement of the monitored abilities may be recorded. The standards according to Ivnik et al., 1996, again differentiate well in higher age groups, up to 80.

In order to assess the disorders of the frontal lobe functions, the *Test of verbal fluency* has been included. This quick method assesses verbal fluency and long-term memory. NPH patients perform below average prior to surgery. Higher age groups standards were prepared by Tombaugh et al. (1999).

6. Rehabilitation and Psychotherapy

Rehabilitation of hydrocephalus cognitive disorders is always part of complex rehabilitation, which also includes a movement part. It is necessary to individually select methods taking into account many variables:

- Total physical and psychological condition related to age/fitness;
- Etiology of hydrocephalus and possible further defects of cerebral structures and nervous functions due to the primary disease (e.g., effects of bleeding, injury and so on);
- Depth of the total cognitive deficit (from a mild form without disruption of the daily routine, up to confusion and disorientation);
- Depth of disruption of individual functions (e.g., serious disorder of the verbal memory while maintaining the ability to keep attention);
- Physical restrictions resulting from previous diseases and pre-surgery condition (e.g., partial loss of motility, muscular contractures);
- Current psychical condition dependent on associated psychological disorders, primarily taking into account presence and depth of depressive experiences;
- Motivation of the patient and his/her ambitions;
- Familial environment and potential cooperation with family members.

The form of rehabilitation of cognitive functions is also bound to subsequent postoperative care. Some patients remain in the hospital or rehabilitation facility, some come to complex rehabilitation in the outpatients' department, some "only" pursue an improvement of physical problems, and some are released home without any follow-up professional care.

The range of cognitive rehabilitation is very wide and includes an entire spectrum of procedures ranging from specialized narrow-profile programs to common daily activities carried out without professional supervision. They may be divided into three groups:

1. Neuro-rehabilitation carried out under professional supervision focused on specific deficits of memory, attention, and executive functions disorders. This form is especially suitable for motivated patients who struggle to return to work.
2. Training of general cognitive performance without closer specialization within other rehabilitation activities. This method is especially used in patients with continuing hospitalization and patients assigned to motion rehabilitation. The ergotherapeutic procedures, but also cooperation in practice of physical activities, regular attendance, and active contact with rehabilitation workers and co-patients, especially belong to this group.
3. Practicing in a form of common daily routine without any professional supervision. We recommend activities that are in connection with the patient's interest or return to previous hobbies. This will assure a smooth and long-term continuation of practice. At the beginning, at least, support of the family in monitoring of daily activities, control and encouragement is helpful. Some examples of the recommended activities are given in the next table:

Note: In practice, determination of former patient's interests (even in youth) as soon as during the dialogue and their recommendation as a suitable form of rehabilitation has been again and again proven useful. A positive emotional animation significantly enhances not only common routine repetition of an activity but, above all, its development in the extension of the interest and increase in demands. Our most successful case is a man (62) who returned, after a lapse of several decades, to aero modeling—at first with the intent to peruse his old materials and find out new information; and ultimately, he actively started to assemble models, subscribed to a special magazine, and engaged himself in club activities.

Even if we work with a group of patients with a view toward improvement, it is necessary to reduce unrealistic expectations that follow from a quick onset of gait adjustment—there is, without exception, an objectively recognizable improvement in gait within several hours of introduction of preoperative lumbar drainage. An improvement in cognitive deficit should be expected over weeks or months. According to clinical experience, in cases of hydrocephalus with idiopathic etiology, an improvement of cognitive disorder is the least and the slowest when compared with the other triad symptoms (Luciano, 2001). In this sense family members, who, in good faith, relatively often overtax the patient with difficult and excessive tasks, should also be educated regarding recovery times.

The assessment of the neuro-rehabilitation benefit is very difficult because after a successful surgery, a spontaneous improvement of cognitive abilities to a large extent occurs. Nevertheless, it is clear that nearly any actively pursued activity contributes to a quick recovery or, at least, to maintenance of cognitive abilities; therefore, patients should be supported in their interests.

Table 5. Recommended activities carried out within rehabilitation without any professional supervision

Memory	summary of daily program (in written or oral form)
	crosswords (puzzles)
	recapitulation of a read text (own selection)
	recall of previous series episode
	revision of a foreign language
	information about leisure activity
	shopping without prompts
Executive functions	planning of the daily program
	Sudoku
	brain teasers
	little errands
	cinema/theatre, including selection and ticket-booking
	planning and implementation of an excursion, meeting of family/friends

Psychotherapy in patients with hydrocephalus is an absolutely individual matter. Depression is a recurring reason for starting treatment in NPH patients. In the Beck Depression Inventory (a questionnaire), patients most frequently score on the parts referring to their own failure and, above all, to worries about the future. Rather exceptionally, other psychological disorders associate; however, they are exceptional events. We recommend dealing with persisting psychological problems through individual meetings since a preparation of a group of patients with NPH is unrealistic due to the number of operations and entry into a group of patients suffering from dementia is not appropriate. The primary reason lies in the expected inverse development of cognitive abilities (in NPH an improvement, in dementias a reduction) and an entry to such group could be demotivating and worrying for all people concerned.

Another area of a possible therapeutic intervention is paired/family therapy, primarily focused on changes in the patient's position within the family and on demands associated with cohabitation with a family member with a cognitive disorder.

Conclusion

Hydrocephalus is a disease known and described from antiquity; however, it is has only been effectively surgically treated since the half of the twentieth century. At present, the most frequent surgical method consists of an introduction of a ventriculo-peritoneal shunt that conducts superfluous cerebrospinal fluid away from the ventricular system to the abdominal cavity. The clinical symptomatology comprises three principal areas: gait/balance disorders, incontinence and disorders of the cognitive functions. The affected cognitive functions include decrease in the short-term memory and later, disorders of attention, cognitive flexibility, verbal fluency, and rate of information processing. Often, associated psychological disorders such as depression, apathy, anxiety, and paranoid thoughts appear in patients. If the disease is correctly and quickly diagnosed and surgery is carried out in a timely fashion, full recovery to premorbid conditions in all spheres of the clinical triad is possible. The restoration of cognitive performance is partly spontaneous; however, full recovery should be supported by rehabilitation.

The clinical symptoms of NPH are relatively easily mistaken with a series of other diseases, especially irreversible forms of dementia, depression, infections of CNS and slowly growing tumors. Often gait disorders, the beginnings of incontinence and memory impairment are ascribed to aging. A suspicion of normal pressure hydrocephalus can only be confirmed by imaging examinations (CT, magnetic resonance).

References

Beck AT, et al.: Beckova sebeposuzovací škála depresivity pro dospělé. Bratislava, Psychodiagnostika a.s. 1999.

Boon AJ, Tans JT, Delwel EJ, et al.: Dutch normal-pressure hydrocephalus study: How to select patient for shunting. *Surg. Neurol*: 201–207, 2000.

Boon AJ, Tans JT, Delwel EJ, et al.: Dutch normal-pressure hydrocephalus study: The role of cerebrovascular disease. *J. Neurosurg*: 221–226, 1996.

Bret J, Guyotat J, Chazal J: Is normal pressure hydrocephalus a valid concept in 2002? A reappraisal in five questions and proposal for a new designation. *J. Neurol. Neurosurg. Psychiatry*: 9–12, 2002.

Burtscher J, Bartha L, Twerdy K, Eisner W: Effect of endoscopic third ventriculostomy on neuropsychological outcome in late onset idiopathic aqueductus stenosis. *J. Neurolog. Neurosurg. Psychiatry:* 222–225, 2005.

Cross JJ, Griffiths PD, Czosnyka M, et al.: Specific patterns of cognitive impairment in patients with idiopathic normal pressure hydrocephalus and Alzheimer's disease: a pilot study. *J. Neurol. Neurosurg .Psychiatry:* 723–32, 1999.

Černý I: Normotensní hydrocefalus. *Neurologie pro praxi*: 83–84, 2003.

DesRosiers G.: Depressive pseudodementia. In: *Memory disorders in psychiatric practice*. Cambridge University Press 2000, 268-277.

DeVito EE, Pickard JD, Salmond CH: The neuropsychology of Normal Pressure Hydrocephalus (NPH). *British Journal of Neurosurgery 19(3)*:217-224, 2005.

Dunn L: "Normal pressure hydrocephalus": what's in a name? *J. Neurol. Neurosurg. Psychiatry*: 8–9, 2002.

Fillit HM, et al.: Achieving and maintaining cognitive vitality with aging. M*ayo Clinics Proceedings*: 681–690, 2002.

Friedman MA, Meyers Ch, Sawaya R: Neuropsychological effects of third ventricle tumor surgery. *Neurosurgery*: 791–798, 2003.

Goodman M, Meyer W: Dementia Reversal in Post-Shunt Normal Pressure

Hydrocephalus Predicted by Neuropsychological Assessment. *Clinical Neuropsychology*: 323–330, 1988.

Fuld PA: Guaranted stimulus processing in the evaluation of memory and learning. *Cortex:* 255–272, 1980.

Hakim S, Adams RD: The special clinical problem of symptomatic hydrocephalus with normal cerebrospinal fluid pressure. Observation on cerebrospinal fluid hydrodynamics. *J. Neurol.* Sci: 307–327, 1965.

Hejl A, Hoegh P, et al.: Potentially reversible conditions in memory clinic patients—A prospective study. *J. Neurol. Neurosurg. Psychiatry:* 390–399, 2002.

Hebb AO, Cusimano MD: Idiopathic normal pressure hydrocephalus: a systematic review of diagnosis and outcome. *Neurosurgery*: 1166–1184, 2001.

Hellstrom P, Edsbagge M, Archer T, et al.: The Neuropsychology of Patients with Clinically Diagnosed Idiopathic Normal Pressure Hydrocephalus. *Neurosurgery 6*: 1219-1228, 2007.

Iddon J, Morgan D, Loveday C, Sahakian B: Neuropsychological profile of young adults with spina bifida with or without hydrocephalus. *J. Neurolog. Neurosurg. Psychiatry*: 1112–1118, 2004.

Jakubec J: Doporučené postupy pro praktické lékaře – hydrocefalus. Závěrečná zpráva grantu IGA MZ ČR 5390-3, 2000.

Jirák R, a kol.: Demence. Praha, MAXDORF 1999.

Koukolík F: Lidský mozek, Funkční systémy, Norma a poruchy. Praha, Portál 2000.

Kulišťák P*: Neuropsychologie.* Praha, Portál 2003.

Leonard A, Cantraine F, Desmyttere F: Cognitive recovery in idiopathic normal pressure hydrocephalus: A Prospective Study. *Neurosurgery*: 397–405, 1994.

Lezak M: Neuropsychological Assessment, 3rd. ed. New York, Oxford University Press, 1995.

Lezak M: Neuropsychological Asseeement, 4. ed. New York: Oxford University Press, 2003.

Luciano MG: Neurosurgery Clinics of North America. Hydrocephalus. Philadelphia: A Harcourt Health Sciences Company, 2001.

Mohapl M.: Hydrocefalus jako následek subarachnoidálního krvácení – vliv modality léčby aneuryzmatu. Závěrečná zpráva grantu IGA MZ ČR 6616-3, 2003.

Petersen RC, Stevens JC, Ganguli M, et al.: Practice parameter: early detection of dementia: mild cognitive impairment (an evidence-based review). Report of the Quality Standards Subcommittee of the American Academy of Neurology. *Neurology* 56:33-1142, 2001.

Preiss M, a kol.: Klinická neuropsychologie. Praha, Grada 1998.

Preiss M, Laing H, Rodriguez M: Neuropsychologická baterie Psychiatrického centra Praha. Praha, PCP, 2002.

Prigatano GP, Palencia B: Halstead Impairment Index, Wechsler IQ, and the BNI Screen for Higher Cerebral Functions. *BNI Quarterly*: 22–27, 2000.

Rey A, Osterrieth PA: Rey-Osterriethova komplexní figura. Úprava Novák, J., Košč, M. Bratislava, Psychodiagnostika s.r.o., 1997.

Sameš M, Vaněk P: Lumbální infusní test a transkraniální doppler v diagnostice normotensního hydrocefalu. Závěrečná zpráva grantu IGA MZ ČR 6072-3, 2002.

Silverberg GD, Bloch D, Levinthal E: Effects of chronic CSF drainage on cognition and concentration of bichemical markers on Alzheimer disease. Proceedings of 11th international symposium on intracranial pressure and brain monitoring. Cambridge, 2000.

Smolík P: Duševní a behaviorální poruchy. Praha, MAXDORF, 1996.

Svoboda M: Psychologická diagnostika dospělých. Praha, Portál, s.r.o., 1999.

Todd RA, Karis P: Normal pressure hydrocephalus: Diagnostic imaging and prognostic assessment. *BNI Quarterly*: 16–22, 2003.

Topinková E, Jirák R: Kognitivní poruchy ve vyšším věku – diferenciální diagnostika. Závěrečná zpráva grantu IGA MZ ČR 5390-3, 2001.

Supported by the grant IGA MZ ČR NR 9436-3.

In: Cognitive Deficit in Mental and Neurological Disorders ISBN: 978-1-60741-957-0
Editors: H. Kucerova, M. Preiss

Chapter XII

Parkinson's Disease

Evzen Ruzicka, Olga Klempirova and Natasa Spackova

Abstract

Parkinson's disease (PD) is a serious neurodegenerative disease affecting one to two persons out of every 1,000 in the general population. In addition to being a movement disorder characterized by progressive hypokinesia, rigidity, tremor at rest, and stance/gait disorders, PD is also often associated with mental changes. Cognitive disorders, especially executive dysfunction, affect up to 90% of patients. Subcortical-type dementia develops in at least 20% of these patients. Over the course of the disease, at least 50% of patients experience depression, which is often combined with anxiety. Psychotic complications of drug therapy affect relatively few patients, although patients with cognitive defects are at an increased risk.

In addition to the crucial deficit of dopamine, disturbances in other neurotransmitters that participate in basal ganglia circuits and ascending pathways constitute the neurobiological background of the mental symptoms associated with PD. Consequently, not all of these disorders can be managed pharmacologically through dopamine replacement therapy.

Neuropsychological examinations help in the diagnosis and determination of the severity of various components of mental problems associated with PD. The recommended tests help in evaluation and long-term monitoring of global cognitive deficits, cognitive disorders (especially executive dysfunction), and depression.

Keywords

Parkinsonian syndrome (Parkinsonism): motor impairment with hypokinesia, rigidity, tremor at rest, stance, and gait disorders. The most common cause is Parkinson's disease.

Parkinson's disease: a disease manifested by Parkinsonian syndrome and due to the degeneration of neurons in the substantia nigra of the midbrain, which leads to depletion of the neurotransmitter, dopamine.

Hypokinesia: limitation, reduction of extent, slowed movements, impaired initiation of movement.

Rigidity: plastic muscle hypertonus, which is manifested in both active and passive movements.

Dopamine: neurotransmitter that modulates the function of the striatum; its depletion causes the symptoms associated with Parkinson's disease.

Striatum: part of the basal ganglia consisting of the putamen and the caudate nucleus.

Basal ganglia: paired masses of gray matter, deep within the cerebral hemispheres. They are part of the functional circuits controlling motor and cognitive functions, affectivity, and behavior.

Executive dysfunction: impairment of functions associated with planning and performance of goal-oriented activities.

Subcortical dementia: dementia with predominant executive dysfunction, with cortical functions remaining largely intact.

1. Introduction

Parkinson's disease (PD) is one of the most common chronic neurodegenerative diseases in adults. It affects one to two persons per 1,000 and up to 1 in 100 people over the age of 60.

The main manifestations of PD are hypokinesia and rigidity. Other characteristic symptoms of PD include tremor at rest, mainly in the hands, and postural abnormalities (flexed posture, instability while standing, and gait disorders). These motor symptoms of PD are mainly caused by a deficit of the neurotransmitter dopamine acting on the striatum. Dopamine is produced by neurons in the substantia nigra of the midbrain and is transported via cell projections to the nuclei of the striatum (i.e., caudate nucleus and putamen). In PD, a gradual degeneration of the substantia nigra, with an accompanying decline in dopamine in the striatum, occurs without any clear cause, although genetic and endo- and exotoxic mechanisms are thought to play a role. Causal therapy of PD is currently not available. Symptomatic therapy (suppression of motor symptoms) consists mainly of dopamine replacement therapy with levodopa or dopamine agonists. Levodopa, also known as L-DOPA (L-3,4-dihydroxyphenylalanine), is metabolized into dopamine while dopamine agonists (e.g., pramipexol, ropinirole, etc.) act directly on dopamine receptors in the brain. PD is typically a slowly progressive disease. Initially, mild and non-specific motor dysfunctions gradually deteriorate, eventually progressing to a point that requires pharmacotherapy. Further progression of the disease is characterized by late motor complications (so-called wearing-off i.e., reduced duration of levodopa dose effect, response fluctuations (on/off phenomena), and involuntary movements linked to pharmacotherapy).

Mental disorders, as symptoms of PD, were not mentioned in early studies, and the condition was considered to be purely motor (J. Parkinson, 1817: "Senses and intellect remain unaffected"). Studies that described the occurrence and characteristics of mental changes in PD appeared more frequently after 1970. Introduction of therapy with levodopa significantly improved the prognosis for the disease and suppressed motor impairment, making differentiation of other components of the disease possible. Undoubtedly, extended survival and prolonged progression of cerebral changes played a role. Indeed, recent pathological studies have found that the pathological process also affects regions outside the brain stem, including cortical and subcortical areas (Braak, 2008). Awareness of mental disorders associated with PD may also be attributed to greater interest among neurologists in the mental functions of patients and an extension of neuropsychological testing methods. In the last three decades, the existence of cognitive, behavioral, and affective disorders in PD has been fully confirmed, and the number of studies describing these issues continues to grow. Research on cognitive functions in PD has become a significant source of information about the mechanism of action of the basal ganglia and the functionally associated subcortical-cortical circuits of the central nervous system.

2. Mental Changes and their Mechanisms in PD

2.1. Executive Functions

Executive functions enable a person to adaptively respond to new situations and are the basis for cognitive, emotional, and social skills. Executive functions consist of four components: intention, planning, purposeful behavior, and effective performance.

Deficits of executive functions are considered to be the most common cognitive problems in PD. Because executive functions are part of most neuropsychological tests, a reduction in performance will appear across a broad scale of cognitive domains, especially with regard to working memory and visuospatial functions. Instrumental functions, practice, and speech are not commonly impaired in PD. It is still not completely clear if cognitive changes at the beginning of the disease are isolated deficits or if they indicate dementia in PD (Levin, 2005).

2.2. Memory and Learning

Memory disorders can be found in patients in early stages of PD, independent of dementia. Newly diagnosed patients with PD have consistently lower performance during recall of a semantically sorted list of words (California Verbal Learning Test, CVLT), where the strategy for word sorting is based on categorization. They are also more sensitive to distractions during the process of verbal learning. This deficit in recall is apparently due to reduced planning capabilities, which are caused by executive dysfunction. According to Marié et al. (2007), patients with PD have somewhat reduced short-term recall, but markedly reduced delayed recall compared to healthy subjects. A pronounced activation of prefrontal and parietal regions, which are associated with attention demanding roles, has been found in PD patients. These results indicate effective compensatory mechanisms, within the framework of short-term memory, in patients with PD. They also found a correlation between perfusion, in the inferior parietal cortex bilaterally, and short-term recall performance.

2.3. Visuospatial Functions

Proctor et al. (1964) described, for the first time, isolated **visuospatial deficits** in PD. This field includes all tasks that use visual perception including recognition of faces, visual analysis and synthesis, visual differentiation, visual recall, spatial memory, perception of personal space, spatial planning, visuomotor integration, visual vigilance, and orientation.

2.4. Speech and Language

Language abilities remain well preserved in PD (Borod, 1980; Freedman, 1984). In a study evaluating spontaneous speech, Hanson and Iritani (1987) found that patients with PD composed longer sentences since they paused more frequently during their speech, however *verbal fluency* disorders are typical for PD patients. PD patients without dementia have *reduced content of spontaneous speech and reduced comprehension of complex instructions* (Grossmann, 2002). Furthermore, patients with PD have problems expressing their emotions through speech (prosody).

2.5. Dementia

Dementia in PD is clinically characterized by a slowly progressive reduction of cognitive abilities with prevailing dysexecutive syndrome, which is associated with various behavioral disorders such as depression, anxiety, psychotic disorders, and excessive daily sleepiness. Dementia in PD probably occurs due to subcortical and cortical pathological structural changes of the Lewy-type and associated structural changes of the Alzheimer-type (Caballol, 2007).

2.6. Other Psychical Symptoms in PD

2.6.1. Patients' Personality

Classical conceptions about the premorbid personality in PD have not been completely confirmed or disproved (Menza, 2000). Based on older studies, PD patients, prior to the first symptoms of the disease, were described as markedly introverted with quiet conformist behaviors, unassertive, and rarely expressed emotions (Lit, 1968; Poewe, 1983). In addition, it is not clear whether the observed behavioral patterns or characteristics are related to etiological factors of the disease or if they are simply prodromal symptoms of PD (Paulson, 1991).

However, based on clinical experience and studies, there are certain common characteristics that fit most patients with PD. Except for common symptoms of depression and anxiety, various specific characteristics have been described in patients, these include: closeness, propensity toward rigid thinking, pedantry, perfectionism, and conformism. Occurrence of the described personality characteristics is more common in PD compared to the general population and even more common than in other chronic diseases that limit mobility (e.g., rheumatism and orthopedic disorders). These personal characteristics may be one possible explanation for the high percentage of non-smokers among PD patients (Jimenez-Mimenez, 1992). However, it has not been confirmed that the described personal characteristics are specific for PD or useful as early indicators of the disease.

A possible relationship between dopaminergic activity in the central nervous system and personal characteristics of patients with PD has been discussed. Consistent with previous descriptions of PD, Menza et al. (1993) found that there were significantly lower values for the temperament dimension of "novelty seeking" (Cloninger, 1994) in PD patients compared to the norm, which correlates with the following personality characteristics: rigid, thoughtful, quiet, slow, mannered, and steadfast. However, the anticipated association between low scores on the temperament dimension and reduced dopaminergic activity in the ascendant mesocorticolimbic system has not been convincingly demonstrated.

2.6.2. Depression

At least 50% of PD patients experience depression over the course of the disease. Therefore, depression is the most common psychiatric symptom in PD. Although the possibility of a reactive component for depression related to severe functional impairment of basic motor function cannot be ruled out, there is no biological basis for a neuromediator imbalance related to depression in PD; especially since the lack of dopamine and its derivates (catecholamines) and serotonin are arguably associated with depression (Schrag, 2004).

Depression in PD is frequently associated with cognitive deficits and dementia (Schrag, 2004). Apparently, this coincidence is associated with a broader affection of ascendant neuromediator systems and frontal cortico-subcortical circuits (see further).

2.6.3. Anxiety

Anxiety is often found in association with depression in PD, but it develops separately. Anxiety is generally a symptom that accompanies any serious chronic disease. However, an imbalance in catecholamine levels within the underlying pathological mechanism may contribute to depression in PD as well.

Anxious mood and nosophobia are most often found in patients with PD. Acute episodic anxiety, which disappears with motor improvement (i.e., after drug dose), develops in some cases when there is a serious fluctuation in mobility associated with the hypodopaminergic "off" condition. Acute anxiety, associated with motor unrest, may develop into a panic attack. These conditions may be related to the transient lack of dopamine and other neuromediators in the patient's brain.

2.6.4. Post-Drug Psychotic Symptoms and Delirium

While the above stated disorders (cognitive disorders, changes in personality, depression, anxiety) may appear in both treated and non-treated PD, treatment of PD is usually associated with development of psychotic symptoms.

Mechanisms of psychotic symptoms are associated with excessive stimulation of extrastriatal dopamine receptors, especially in the limbic system and frontal cortex. With regard to psychotic symptoms, drugs with indirect dopaminergic effects (e.g., selegiline), amantadine, and anticholinergic agents are equally or more hazardous than dopaminergic medication, especially if administered in combinations. Patients with PD onset at older ages and patients with underlying cognitive disorders, dementia, or depression, are at increased risk of psychotic symptoms.

3. Prevalence of Cognitive Dysfunction in PD

With the use of suitable neuropsychological tests, cognitive disorders can be seen in a considerable percentage of non-demented patients with PD, even in the earliest stages of the disease (Lees, 1983; Taylor, 1990). Estimations of the prevalence of cognitive disorders in

PD vary depending on test methods used and the patients selected (in some studies exceeding 90% (Pirozzollo, 1982)). Isolated impairment of executive functions are mostly concerned or associated with specific memory disorders, impairment of visuospatial functions, speech, etc. Global cognitive deficits that reach the level of dementia are rare; and if it develops, it occurs in the late stages of PD or in patients with a concomitant underlying dementia causing disease. The prevalence of dementia in PD is most often reported to range between 15 and 20% (Mayeux, 1988). However, the actual incidence may be higher since the data is probably biased by shortened survival of demented patients with PD (Dubois, 1991; Bosboom, 2004).

4. Principal Domains of the Cognitive Functions and their Measurements

4.1. Executive Functions

Cognitive disorders found in PD are associated with affection of single functional components of the executive domain that are involved in targeted behaviors leading to specific mental or motor performances (formulation of the target of the activity, creation and performance of the activity, adjustment of the performance to external conditions and completion of the activity according to plan). Executive functions are often affected in frontal lobes convexity lesions, especially in the dorsolateral cortical area. It appears that in PD, similar disorders may also occur in cases of impairment of other functional components of the frontal system that consist of the frontal cortex and subcortical structures, especially the basal ganglia. They can be detected by examination using tests focused on cognitive flexibility and internally controlled behavior in problem-solving tasks (see Table 1).

The *Wisconsin Card Sorting Test, WCST* appears to be the most sensitive task for demonstrating executive dysfunction, and in some studies, the pathological findings on the WCST were the only symptoms of a cognitive disorder in patients with PD (Dubois, 1991). In PD, the WCST demonstrates, particularly well, impaired conceptualization of solutions (lower number of achieved categories) and reduced ability to change and maintain a mental set (perseveration and non-perseveration errors) (Bowen, 1975; Brown, 1988).

The *Trail Making Test, Stroop test* and other tasks confirm impaired ability to change a mental set in PD (Pirozzolo, 1982; Taylor, 1986). These findings indicate reduced cognitive flexibility in PD patients from the earliest stages of the disease (Hietanen, 1986), which may support views regarding specific premorbid personality in PD. Inability to change a mental set, according to task requirements, may also explain characteristic problems that patients with PD have in concomitant performance of two or more competitive activities. As results from *verbal fluency* testing and other tasks show, in addition to WCST, the ability to maintain a mental set is impaired in PD. A recent metanalysis of results from verbal fluency studies, somewhat surprisingly, showed that semantic fluency was more markedly reduced, whereas phonemic (lexical) fluency was relatively less affected (Henry, 2004). The *"tower" tests,* which monitor problem-solving abilities and planning a succession of actions, document prolongation of the task-solving time; which is partly related to general cognitive deceleration, but also specifically reflects a disorder of activity planning. Compared to healthy individuals, patients with PD needed more moves to complete the task, which may also indicate a specific disorder in procedural learning (Saint-Cyr, 1988).

Table 1. Tasks used for testing executive functions in Parkinson's disease

Tested functional components	Tasks
Creation of a concept of the solution, finding the rules	Wisconsin Card Sorting Test, WCST Delayed Response Tasks
Mental set change (set-shifting)	Trail Making Test Odd Man Out Test WCST Stroop test
Mental set maintenance	verbal fluency tests WCST Stroop test Odd Man Out Test
Systematic problem-solving	The "tower" tests (Tower of London, Tower of Hanoi, Tower of Toronto Test, etc.)

Therefore, executive dysfunction is a nearly universal finding in patients with PD. The ability to conceptualize a behavior, plan, maintain a mental set, sustain and complete an activity, and task repetition are typically impaired. Control of specific performance and its time structure is impaired, and the ability to perform rapid changes in the actual activity, according to external needs, is also reduced. Despite different severities of the disorder and extents of affection of single components of executive functions in single patients, it appears that cognitive disorders in PD develop due to certain basic dysfunctions comprising several elements: we can assume that *the impairment of regulation of behavior* is the basis for problems involving change and maintenance of a mental set; problems with problem-solving are caused by *impairment of internal plan creation;* and inability to solve more complex multistep tasks is due to a *reduction of attention* and *lack of internal sources of processing* (Brown, 1988). Similar basic features of dysfunction can be found in focal lesions of the frontal lobes and also in structural or functional impairment of the basal ganglia; however, they do differ in some aspects. For example, neither patients with PD nor those with frontal lobe impairment are able to attain a satisfactory number of categories on the WCST, however perseveration errors are more common in frontal lesions, i.e., patients are easily distracted from the original mental set, whereas patients with PD also make non-perseveration errors, since they have problems maintaining the actual mental set (Owen, 1993; Partiot, 1996). This may be related to the functional impairment of the striatum in maintaining a mental set (Taylor, 1986) and in sensory integration in which the striatum ensures focusing of attention on a particular event, while suppressing other perceptions (Hassler, 1978).

4.2. Visuospatial Functions

Visuospatial disorders may be easily overlooked in patients with PD. They are much less prominent compared to memory affections or dementia, although they constitute a serious limitation to the everyday life of the patient. The disorders affect the ability to evaluate positions and mutual relationships between objects and stimuli in the environment, including objects in the continual spatial framework and performance of spatial intellectual operations.

Numerous experimental studies on animals have documented the affect on visuospatial functions of lesions of the basal ganglia or substantia nigra (e.g., Mura, 2003). Disruption of these functions (impairment of spatial orientation, reproduction of spatial relations, inability of spatial structuring, drawing, etc.) has been repeatedly found in patients with PD through the use of visual perception tests with minimal motor components—e.g., the discrimination *line orientation test* (Boller, 1984) and the *Benton visual retention test* (BVRT) with multiple choice answers (Ransmayer, 1987). Therefore, impairment in visuospatial relations is assumed in PD, which causes incorrect spatial images. It appears that the affection is most markedly seen in complex visuospatial tests that require the creation of a plan and the selection of successive steps needed for solving a task (Richards, 1993). Hence, executive visuomotor mechanisms located in the frontal lobes are also involved, beside the affection of primary information processing.

4.3. Memory

Memory impairment is generally considered to be the main symptom of dementia. However, memory disorders can also be found in non-demented patients with PD, while some memory qualities may be preserved in PD patients with dementia .

If disorders of *primary memory* (short-term or working memory) are found in patients with PD, they reflect attentional deficits rather than involvement of the respective memory mechanisms (Cooper, 1993). Problems imprinting new information occur, especially, when the patient is anxious, depressed or if there are other reasons for decreased concentration of *attention*.

Among *secondary (long-term) memory* components, both *explicit (declarative) memory*—which includes facts and data acquired by learning and accessible to conscious recall—and *implicit memory*—which includes automatic memory processes *(nondeclarative, procedural memory)* with a low proportion of conscious control—are impaired in PD.

A more detailed analysis reveals that a more passive form of declarative memory—*recognition*—is normal for verbal and visuospatial information in PD, but *recall,* which requires effort and some cognitive capacity, is affected (Pillon, 1993). If a patient receives categorical help, they are able to use it. Clues function as keys to information stored in memory. Therefore, it appears that the ability to notice verbal or visuospatial information is preserved in patients with PD, but the ability to use the memory record created this way is impaired (Pillon, 1996). Impairment of insertion of past events into a timeline has also been observed (Cooper, 1993).

Procedural memory disorders are found in patients with PD, and the capacity for procedural learning is also affected. (Procedural learning is the basis for the ability to acquire perceptive and motor routines and skills during a specific, repeated activity, without the acquired successful strategy being accessible to conscious recall; and it is manifested by accelerated and improved task completion.) Therefore, patients loose both the ability to perform previously learned automated tasks and the ability to learn new skills. This condition may be associated with the fact that the striatum (especially nucleus caudatus) plays an important role in the mechanisms of procedural memory (Sarazin, 2002). A significant differential diagnostic fact is that procedural memory is often preserved in amnesias of various origin and in Alzheimer's disease.

4.4. Speech

In very advanced cases of PD, which were observed especially often before the era of L-DOPA, speech loss may have been observed as a severe motor deficit (aphonia—loss of the ability to create vocal sounds, anarthria—loss of articulation). Limitation of speech functions, which may partly consist of the impairment of mainly neuromechanical processes of articulation and partly impairment of higher communication mechanisms, is often seen in milder cases of PD.

The most common symptoms of PD include *hypophonia* (silent speech, soundless voice) and *dysprosody* (reduction of the ability to modulate loudness and melody of speech). The later is closely related to *hypokinetic dysarthria* and to inaccurate and blurred articulation, sometimes associated with an accelerated speech pace *(tachyphemia)* and compulsive repetition of syllables, words, or whole sentences *(palilalia)*. These symptoms are caused by muscle rigidity and reduced mobility of respiratory and articular muscles (i.e., the symptoms of Parkinson's rigidity and bradykinesis) but also impairment of the speech plan (i.e., speech control mechanisms) as well. On the contrary (and in contrast to speech impairment in Alzheimer's disease), aphasia is not a typical symptom of PD. However, patients with PD can show reduced naming ability and verbal fluency, which are rather related to involvement of executive functions (see above).

4.5. Dementia in PD

The clinical picture of dementia in PD is, in some aspects, different from the classic picture of Alzheimer's-type cortical dementia. In contrast to Alzheimer's disease, reduction of performance scores on psychometric scales is more marked comparing to reduction in verbal scores (Aarsland, 2003). Executive functions are typically more affected and memory is less affected in PD. Demented patients with PD have impaired learning of new information, show affection on the WMS scale and in tasks involving learning of a list of words, but the deficit is not as marked as it is in Alzheimer's disease. Although demented patients with PD have reduced ability of free verbal recall, the recall of words is significantly improved if they receive semantic help, as with the Grober and Buschke test (Pillon, 1993). This means that the processes of information reception and storage remain relatively preserved, but recall of memory tracks is impaired. Speech functions usually remain preserved except for verbal fluency. Executive dysfunction is the common denominator for specific involvements of speech and memory. Due to the fact that similar picture of dementia occurs typically when frontal cortex or associated subcortical structures are affected, the terms of "frontal-type dementia" or "subcortical dementia" are commonly used withe regard to dementia in PD (Cummings and Benson, 1984). The clinical picture of subcortical dementia includes:

- cognitive slowing,

- difficulties in processing new information,
- impairment of planning and abstract reasoning,
- changes in personality and mood,
- absence of aphasia, apraxia and agnosia.

The diagnosis of dementia is based on the DSM-IV criteria, which assume cognitive impairment to be so serious that it impairs social and professional life. However, the usefulness of these criteria in patients with PD is reduced due to underlying motor impairment that limitsby itself the activity of the patient. In addition, most of the test batteries used do not include executive function tests, which are crucial in PD—not only for finding cognitive deficits and monitoring progression but also for differentiation of Parkinsonian dementia from dementia caused by another neurodegenerative disease (e.g., concomitant Alzheimer's disease).

8. Neuropsychological Examination in Parkinson's Disease

8.1. Objectives of Examination

Neuropsychological examination is not a basic procedure in the *diagnosis of PD.* However, neuropsychological findings can help differentiate between PD and other diseases characterised by hypokinetic-rigid syndrome associated with concomitant disorders of cognitive functions, affectivity, and behavior. Examples include rare neurodegenerative diseases from the Parkinson plus group, e.g., progressive supranuclear palsy (Steele-Richardson-Olszewski disease), corticobasal ganglional degeneration, dementia with Lewy bodies, or Alzheimer's disease with associated motor impairment. In most cases of those, the main differential diagnostic sign is a very early occurrence of dementia, which is generally not present in early stages of PD, and a different profile of cognitive deficits (e.g., amnesia and aphasia in Alzheimer's disease, and apraxia in corticobasal degeneration). Last, but not least, the neuropsychological examination of patients with PD is a significant tool for clinical research into *functions of the basal ganglia* regarding control of movement, cognitive functions, and behavior.

Requirements for the clinical neuropsychological examination in patients with PD come up most often when there is a *suspicion of cognitive deficit or dementia.* Detection of the deficit, determination of its severity and assessment of whether the limit for dementia has been exceeded are mainly concerned. Monitoring changes over time is important for therapy management and evaluation of therapeutic effects.

The current trend in neuropsychological diagnostics is toward flexible batteries, which are combinations of quantitative approaches involving fixed batteries and qualitative interpretation of neuropsychological functions (Sweet, 2000). This diagnostic approach is very suitable for examination of cognitive functions in PD. It enables both intra- and interindividual psychometric comparison of cognitive performance and captures qualitative changes in performance and behavior. Information about the extent and type of the neuropsychological deficit can be used in preparation of a treatment strategy and implementation of measures, in the patient's home setting, to minimize the impact of the clinical and psychosocial affection as much as possible. Performance on neuropsychological tests may be significantly affected by *depression and anxiety,* which are among the most common mental disorders in PD. Symptoms of depression and anxiety must be monitored in the course of contact with the patient during the examination.

8.2. Examination of Global Cognitive Deficit

Determination of the presence and evaluation of the severity of a global cognitive deficit in PD (Tab. 2) are important for selection of therapeutic approaches and adjustment of the patient's environment.

Screening scales, which comprise tests of the basic areas of cognitive functioning, are most often used for the first quantitative analysis of a global cognitive deficit. In the clinical setting, the most commonly used scale is *the Mini-Mental State Examination (MMSE),* an effective diagnostic tool, especially for recognition of moderate and severe Alzheimer's dementia. The MMSE scale can also provide early information that may raise suspicion of initial dementia, but without differentiation of type. The MMSE scale is not suitable for diagnosis of mild dementia in PD since its single tests do not correspond to the profile of cognitive deficits in PD. Impairments of executive functions that may already interfere with daily-life activities may not be reflected on the MMSE scale or are inadequately reflected. It is also important to observe behavioral impairments—depression, apathy, or psychotic symptoms. Mild stages of dementia in PD can be difficult to distinguish from depression, anxiety and other behavioral complications. Therefore, if there is suspicion of depression, it is important to perform a neuropsychological examination that includes a battery of tests specific for the range of cognitive deficits in PD and methods of examination for depression and other mental impairments. The degree of motor impairment, which negatively interferes with cognitive performance, must always be considered in the evaluation of the severity of cognitive deficits in PD.

The *Mattis Dementia Rating Scale (MDRS)* is the most suitable scale for a more precise estimation of severity and type of dementia in PD (Dujardin, 2006). The MDRS scale is divided into five basic subscales—attention, initiation, construction, conceptualization, and memory. Deficits that correspond mainly to subcortical-type (frontal) impairment in PD particularly affect attention, initiation, and free recall of memory. Deficits in construction, conceptualization and memory retention indicate impairments in the cortical functions, e.g., in Alzheimer's-type dementia.

In patients with PD, it is suitable to add a screening examination of frontal (executive) functions that help to further specify the type of cognitive deficit relative to a diagnosis of dementia, such as the Frontal Assessment Battery (FAB, Dubois, 2000, Paviour, 2005) or the Behavior Dyscontrol Scale (BDS, Grigsby, 1992). The short form of the Neuropsychiatric inventory, NPI-Q, can help evaluate initial depressive and anxiety symptoms, apathy, and psychotic symptoms (Kauter, 2000).

Table 2. Tests for evaluation of global cognitive deficit in PD

Test	Followed function
Mini-Mental State Examination (MMSE)	Global deficit/dementia
Matis dementia scale (DRS)	Global deficit/ differentiation of dementia attention initiation conceptualization construction memory
Frontal Assessment Battery (FAB)	set of short tests for frontal/executive functions
Neuropsychiatric Inventory (NPI-Q)	depression, apathy, psychotic symptoms

8.3. Symptoms and Evaluation of Depression and Anxiety

Depression can manifest directly during the initial interview or in patient symptoms such as communicating depressive thoughts during the examination. The depressive patient is often less communicative and, therefore, their indirect verbal insinuations and non-verbal symptoms must be observed.

The patient can easily tire and become less motivated to perform. In contrast to patients with purely cognitive deficits, depressive patients try less and tend to end tasks early. Their cognitive performance is inhibited by reduced self-confidence. Depressive patients with PD often say that they are not able to cope with the task even before they get it. Transient attention impairments, which affect performance in all other cognitive domains, are typical of depressive patients; depressive mood can also be seen in the face of patients. However, motor impairment of the mimic muscles is typical for patients with PD, and, therefore, a blunt or rigid face may be misleading and may be wrongly assumed to be depressive.

Subjective scales, such as the Beck Depression Inventory, BDI-II, and objective evaluation scales, e.g., the *Montgomery and Asberg Depression Rating Scale, and the MADRS* can be used to evaluate depression.

Depression and apathy can be easily treated in dementia patients with PD. In contrast to depression, depressive thoughts are missing in apathy. Apathy is manifested as a loss of interest in oneself and one's environment. In contrast to a depressive patient, patients with apathy do not express dissatisfaction when asked about their situations; however physical and cognitive activity and emotional expression are reduced (Pluck, 2002). Recent studies have shown an association between apathy and executive dysfunction (Zgaljardic 2007, Czernecki, 2008).

Anxiety is often closely related to depression in PD. As with depression, anxiety negatively affects cognitive performance. Some patients do not talk about anxiety, either because they do not recognize it or they are trying to mask it. The *STAI* Anxiety *Questionnaire* (STAI) measures both actual levels of anxiety as a characteristic personality feature. *The Beck anxiety scale (BAI)* includes more somatic symptoms that, however, often overlap with symptoms of PD.

8.4. Examination of Focal Cognitive Deficits in PD

8.4.1. Memory and Learning

Auditory subtests of the WMS-III that, except for immediate and delayed recall, also test learning on the first attempt, learning trend, retention and recall from memory are suitable for examination of verbal memory and learning. Impaired ability to create a learning strategy is most often seen in the verbal paired association subtest. To find the effect of interference during the verbal learning process, the Auditory verbal learning test (AVLT) is often used, in which the transfer of attention to the second series of words causes problems in the subsequent recall of the first series of words in patients with greater deficits.

The visual subtests of the WMS-III are suitable for detection of deficits in visuospatial memory. Patients have difficulties in the free recall of the whole scene in the subtest of family pictures because they retain the visual information in their memory less effectively. They do not form a spatial plan of the picture. The *Benton visual retention test (BVRT)* can be used for testing short-term visual memory, which in addition to distortions frequently shows perseveration errors that are typical for subcortical-type deficits. The *working memory subtests (WMS-III)*, involving an arrangement of numbers and letters, and spatial span, can be used for the examination of working memory.

8.4.2. Attention and Executive Functions

Reduced psychomotor pace in PD is manifested by slowed processing of new information. The deficit is more apparent in more complex attention tasks that require more self-motivation. They especially include tasks involving divided or selective attention in which executive functions are applied. The problem with a change of mental set is manifested by an increase in time and mistakes on the *Trail making test B (TMT-B)* or by perseveration mistakes on the Wisconsin card sorting test (WCST). Problems with maintaining a mental set are manifested in situations that require sticking to one type of answer, e.g., within one category of the WCST test. Selective attention can be evaluated by means of the *Stroop test,* in which reduced ability to suppress undesirable stimuli and to focus attention on a certain stimulus may be manifested in PD. In more complex executive functions tasks, such as the Tower tests and WCST, deficits are also manifested in the ability to plan, problem-solve, and create concepts. Fluency tests are suitable methods for detecting impairments of initiation that require activation of cognitive resources, which is necessary for initiation of any activity. Patients with PD have problems in *verbal fluency* tests, not only at the beginning of the task but also during word production that may be interrupted by arrests.

Table 3. Complex examination of the cognitive functions in PD

Test	Followed function
Tapping test	psychomotor pace
Trail making test (TMT)	attention Executive functions (changes of the mental set)
Verbal fluency tests (category: animals; lexical: words starting on N-K-P)	speech executive functions (initiation and maintaining of the mental set)

Table 3. (Continued)

Test	Followed function
Stroop test	attention executive functions (resistance against a distractor)
WMS-III Arrangement of numbers and letters Spatial range	 work auditory memory work visual memory
WMS-III Logic memory Verbal paired associations	 immediate verbal memory verbal learning
Wisconsin card sorting test	executive functions (conceptualizations, changes and maintenance of the mental set)
London tower	Executive function (planning, problem-solving)
WMS-III Logic memory Verbal paired associations Recognition	 delayed verbal memory Recognition
BDI-II (or MADRS)	Depression
STAI	Anxiety
Additional tests for evaluation of memory	
Auditory verbal learning test (AVLT)	verbal memory and learning, interference effect
Benton visual retention test	short-term visual memory
Questionnaires for evaluation of personality	
Multiple Minnesota Personality Inventory (MMPI-II)	diagnosis of psychopathological symptoms
Cloninger's temperament and character inventory (TCI)	diagnosis of basic structure of a personality

8.5. Particulars and Pitfalls of the Neuropsychological Examination in PD

Performance in patients with PD is significantly affected by motor impairment. The speed and dexterity of movements are reduced and require still more effortas the disease progresses. Patients must exert a disproportionate amount of energy for many common activities. They tire quickly and their endurance, during neuropsychological testing, is very limited. Motor impairment especially affects performance on all tests that include motor activities. Therefore, this must be taken into account; complete testing, including the interview, should not take longer than 90 minutes. Patients with more marked motor or cognitive deficits tire even more quickly. In such cases, it may be necessary to reduce the examination time by using alternative shorter tests (AVLT and BVRT instead of the WMS-III) and to omit some of the more difficult tests (London tower). Not only it is important to take into account the influence of motor impairment but also the effects of depression and anxiety on cognitive performance when making final interpretations.

The level of motor impairment and performances on neuropsychological tests can be different, depending on which phase of response to therapy the patient is in. The patient's condition usually deteriorates after the effect of the drug dose disappears (the "off" condition)—motor slowing, muscle rigidity, and tremor significantly worsen motor performance components of the tests. In addition, the "off" condition can be associated with increased anxiety, depression, pain, and other problems that can further reduce the patient's performance. On the other hand, the patient's movements are markedly better in the "on" state after administration of therapy, and the performance on neuropsychological tests can improve. However, the "on" condition may be complicated by dyskinesias, which can also impair performance on tests. Therefore, when planning the examination, it is necessary to take into account oscillation of the patient's condition and that a satisfactory testing period may be only a few tens of minutes between drug doses and thus the examination must be divided into several phases. The key prerequisite for a reliable comparison of results of repeated examinations is to perform the examinations while the patient is in the same motor condition.

9. Prevention, Rehabilitation and Psychotherapy of Mental Disorders in PD

Cognitive disorders in PD represent both medical and social problems. The patient's family and caregivers should know the situations in which the patients will generally have difficulties and should help them in coping with these situations. From the therapeutic point of view, there is no strategy available that can prevent cognitive deficits or reduce their progression. Possibilities for cognitive rehabilitation are limited, and they are generally not used in PD. Speech therapy, which might somewhat improve speech comprehension, may be partially successful in PD patients with more severe dysphonia, dysarthria, and other speech impairments.

The affective disorders must be recognized and adequately treated as soon as possible however; pharmacological approaches clearly dominate over psychotherapy treatment because of the biological origin of depression in PD.

In patients with hallucinations, delusions, delirium and other psychiatric complications associated with PD and its therapy, procedures that are known to increase the risk of psychotic complications must be avoided (e.g., administration of anticholinergic drugs and other high-risk substances in elderly patients or in cases of preexisting cognitive deficits).

10. Ability to Work and Disability in PD

Primary motor impairment is generally the leading factor that determines the ability to work and places limitations on patients with PD. More significant cognitive deficits, which would interfere with work assignments, generally occur only in the later stages of the disease, and mainly in elderly patients. Depression, which can occur in PD since the early stages, is a significant risk factor that limits the ability to work.

From the psychosocial point of view, it is best that patients, especially younger ones, be maintained in their work environments if they can cope with their jobs and if it does not cause undue exhaustion and stress; however, clearly this may require reduction of performance standards expected of the patient. Similarly, it is also desirable to maintain household activities and other daily life activities of the patient, whenever possible.

Conclusion

Subcortical-type dementia, focal cognitive deficits, depression and/or anxiety and specific personality traits represent the broad spectrum of possible mental symptoms of PD. Although typical motor impairment remains the primary focus and target for neurological care in PD, careful attention needs to be paid to the mental component of the disease, which is now generally recognized as significant. The role of the clinical neuropsychological examination is irreplaceable. An adequate assessment of the severity of cognitive deficits and evaluation of depression are necessary prerequisites for adequate therapy and monitoring of its effects during the relentless progression of the disease.

Grant support: IGA MZ CR NR 9220-3, MSM 0021620849.

References

Aarsland, D., Litvan, I., Salmon, D. et al.: Performance on the dementia rating scale in Parkinson's disease with dementia and dementia with Lewy bodies: Comparison with progressive supranuclear palsy and Alzheimer's disease. *J. Neurol. Neurosurg. Psychiatry*, 2003, 74, s. 1215-1220.

Benton AL, Sivan AB, Hausher K et al. Contributions to neuropsychological assessment. A clinical manual (2nd ed.). New York: Oxford University Press. 1994

Boller, F., Passafiume, D., Keefe, N. C., Rogers, K., Morrow, L., Kim, Y.: Visuospatial impairment in Parkinson's disease. Role of perceptual and motor factors. *Arch. Neurol.,* 1984, 41, s. 485-490.

Borod, J. C., Goodglass, H., Kaplan, E.: Normative data on the Boston Diagnostic Aphasia Examination, Parietal Lobe Battery, and the Boston Naming Test. *J. Clin. Neuropsychol.*, 1980, 2, s. 209–215.

Bowen, F. P., Kamienny, R. S., Burns, M. M., Yahr, M.: Parkinsonism: effects of levodopa treatment on concept formation. *Neurology*, 1975, 25, s. 701-704.

Braak H, Del Tredici K. Invited Article: Nervous system pathology in sporadic Parkinson's disease. *Neurology*. 2008 May 13;70(20):1916-25.

Brown, R. G., Marsden, *C. D.:* Internal versus external cues and the control of attention in Parkinson's disease. *Brain*, 1988, 111, s. 323-345.

Caballol N, Martí MJ, Tolosa E. Cognitive dysfunction and dementia in Parkinson's disease. *Mov. Disord.* 2007;22(Suppl. 17):S358-S366

Cloninger, C. R.: Temperament and Personality. *Curr Opin Neurobiol*, 1994, 4, s. 266-273.

Cooper, J. A., Sagar, H. J., Sullivan, E. V.: Short-term memory and temporal ordering in early Parkinson's disease: effects of disease chronicity and medication. *Neuropsychologia*, 1993, 31, s. 933-949.

Cummings, J. L., Benson, D. F.: Subcortical dementia. *Arch. Neurol.*, 1984, 41, s. 874-879.

Czernecki V, Schüpbach M, Yaici S, Lévy R, Bardinet E, Yelnik J, Dubois B, Agid Y. Apathy following subthalamic stimulation in Parkinson's disease: A dopamine responsive symptom. *Mov. Disord.* 2008 Apr 8 [Epub ahead of print]

Dubois, B., Boller, F., Pillon, B., Agid, Y.: Cognitive deficits in Parkinson's disease. In: Boller F, Grafman J, eds. *Handbook of Neuropsychology,* Vol. 5, Elsevier, Amsterdam, 1991, s. 195-239.

Dubois, B., Slachevsky, A., Litvan, I., Pillon, B.: The FAB: a Frontal Assessment Battery at bedside. *Neurology*, 2000, 55, s. 1621-1626.

Dujardin K, Devos D, Duhem S, Destée A, Marié RM, Durif F, Lacomblez L, Touchon J, Pollak P, Péré JJ. Utility of the Mattis dementia rating scale to assess the efficacy of rivastigmine in dementia associated with Parkinson's disease. *J. Neurol.* 2006 Sep;253(9):1154-9.

Freedman, M., Rivoira, P., Butters, N., Sax, D. S., Feldman, R. G.: Retrograde amnesia in Parkinson's disease. *Can. J. Neurol. Sci.,* 1984, 11, s. 297-301.

Grigsby, J., Kaye, K., Robbins, L. J.: Reliabilities, norms and factor structure of the Behavioral Dyscontrol Scale. *Percept Mot Skills*, 1992, 74, s. 883-892.

Grossman M, Lee C, Morris J, Stern MB, Hurtig HI. Assessing resource demands during sentence processing in Parkinson's disease. *Brain. Lang.* 2002 Mar;80(3):603-16.

Hassler, R.: Striatal control of locomotion, intentional actions and of integrating and perceptive activity. *J. Neurol. Sci.*, 1978, 36, s. 187-224.

Hietanen, M., Teravainen, H.: Cognitive performance in early Parkinson's disease. *Acta Neurol. Scand,* 1986, 73, s. 151-159.

Jimenez-Jimenez, F. J., Mateo, D., Gimenez-Roldan, S.: Premorbid smoking, alcohol consumption, and coffee-drinking habits in Parkinson's disease: a case-control study. *Mov Disord*, 1992, 7, s. 339-44.

Lees, A. J., Smith, E.: Cognitive deficits in the early stages of Parkinson's disease. *Brain,* 1983, 106, s. 257-270.

Levin BE, Katzen HL. Early cognitive changes and nondementing behavioral abnormalities in Parkinson's disease. *Adv. Neurol.* 2005;96:84-94

Lit, A. C.: Man behind a mask. An analysis of the psychomotor phenomena of Parkinson´s disease. *Acta Neurol. Belg*., 1968, 68, s. 863-874.

Marié RM, Lozza C, Chavoix C, Defer GL, Baron JC. Functional imaging of working memory in Parkinson's disease: compensations and deficits. *J. Neuroimaging.* 2007 Oct;17(4):277-85.

Mayeux, R., Stern, Y., Rosenstein, R. et al.: An estimate of the prevalence of dementia in idiopathic Parkinson's disease. *Arch. Neurol,* 1988, 45, s. 260-252.

Menza, M. A., Golbe, L. I., Cody, R. A., Forman, N. E.: Dopamine-related personality traits in Parkinson´s disease. *Neurology,* 1993, 43, s. 505–508

Menza, M.: The personality associated with Parkinson's disease. *Curr. Psychiatry Rep.*, 2000, 2, s. 421-426.

Mura, A., Feldon, J.: Spatial learning in rats is impaired after degeneration of the nigrostriatal dopaminergic system. *Mov. Disord.,* 2003, 18, s. 860-871.

Owen, A. M., Beksinska, M., James, M., et al.: Visuospatial memory deficits at different stages of Parkinson's disease. *Neuropsychologia,* 1993, 31, s. 627-644.

Partiot, A., Verin, M., Pillon, B., Teixeira-Ferreira, C., Agid, Y., Dubois, B.: Delayed response tasks in basal ganglia lesions in man: further evidence for a striato-frontal cooperation in behavioural adaptation. *Neuropsychologia*, 1996, 34, s. 709-721.

Paviour DC, Winterburn D, Simmonds S, Burgess G, Wilkinson L, Fox NC, Lees AJ, Jahanshahi M. Can the frontal assessment battery (FAB) differentiate bradykinetic rigid syndromes? Relation of the FAB to formal neuropsychological testing. *Neurocase.* 2005 Aug;11(4):274-82.

Pillon, B., Deweer, B., Agid, Y., Dubois, B.: Explicit memory in Alzheimer's, Huntington's, and Parkinson's diseases. *Arch. Neurol.,* 1993, 50, s. 374-379.

Pillon, B., Dubois, B., Agid, Y.: Testing cognition may contribute to the diagnosis of movement disorders. *Neurology*, 1996, 46, s. 329-334.

Pillon, B., Ertle, S., Deweer, B., Sarazin, M., Agid, Y., Dubois, B.: Memory for spatial location is affected in Parkinson's disease. *Neuropsychologia*, 1996, 34, s. 77-85.

Pirozzolo, F. J., Hansch, E. C., Mortimer, J. A., Webster, D. D., Kuskowski, M. A.: Dementia in Parkinson disease: a neuropsychological analysis. *Brain Cogn.*, 1982, 1, s. 71-83.

Pluck, G. C., Brown, R. G.: Apathy in Parkinson disease. *J Neurol Neurosurg Psychiatry,* 2002, 73, s. 636-642.

Richards, M., Cote, L. J., Stern, *Y.:* The relationship between visuospatial ability and perceptual motor function in Parkinson's disease. *J. Neurol. Neurosurg. Psychiatry,* 1993, 56, s. 400-406.

Saint-Cyr, J. A., Taylor, A. E., Lang, A. E.: Procedural learning and neostriatal dysfunction in man. *Brain*, 1988, 111, s. 941-959.

Sarazin, M., Deweer, B., Merkl, A., von Poser, N., Pillon, B., Dubois, B.: Procedural learning and striatofrontal dysfunction in Parkinson's disease. *Mov. Disord.,* 2002, 17, s. 265-273.

Schrag, A.: Psychiatric aspects of Parkinson's disease - an update. *J. Neurol.* 2004, 251, s. 795-804.

Sweet, J. J., Moberg, P. J., Suchy, Y.: Ten-year follow-up survey of clinical neuropsychologists:part I. Practice and beliefs. *Clin. Neuropsychologist.*, 2000, 14, s. 18-37.

Taylor AE, Saint-Cyr JA, Lang AE. Memory and learning in early Parkinson´s disease. *Brain Cogn.* 1990;2:211-232.

Taylor, A. E., Saint-Cyr, J. A., Lang, A. E.: Frontal lobe dysfunction in Parkinson's disease. The cortical focus of neostriatal outflow. *Brain*, 1986, 109, s. 845-883.

Zgaljardic DJ, Borod JC, Foldi NS, Rocco M, Mattis PJ, Gordon MF, Feigin AS, Eidelberg D. Relationship between self-reported apathy and executive dysfunction in nondemented patients with Parkinson disease. *Cogn. Behav. Neurol.* 2007 Sep;20(3):184-92.

In: Cognitive Deficit in Mental and Neurological Disorders ISBN: 978-1-60741-957-0
Editors: H. Kucerova, M. Preiss

Chapter XIII

Subarachnoid Hemorrhage from Intracranial Aneurysms

Lenka Kramska

Abstract

Subarachnoid hemorrhage (SAH) from aneurysms of the cerebral arteries (AN) is a medical term referring to the bleeding in the subarachnoid space. The bleeding mostly occurs in the region of the basal cisterns, which is in close relation to the arterial circle of Willis. The occurrence of SAH is 6 to 12 cases/100.000 inhabitants every year. SAH is often fatal and represents a significant cause of invalidity in a young and otherwise healthy population. The natural course leads to death in 25 to 30% of cases within a 24-hour period. Without treatment, another 30% of patients die within the next four weeks.

The aetiology of the aneurysm formation is a defect of elastic tissues, genetically based and specifically evolved during embryonal development. The exact pathophysiology is not certain. There are several risk factors for rupture, such as hypertension, alcohol abuse, smoking and physical/psychical stress. The signs of the rupture include headache, nausea, vomiting and loss of consciousness.

During the acute phase, the patient is endangered by increased intracranial pressure and a limited amount of oxygen blood to the brain. SAH can be diagnosed by a lumbar tap (bloody cerebrospinal fluid); the next step is a CT scan of the brain, showing characteristic blood clots in the area of the basal cisterns. Further investigations depict the exact location, size and shape of the aneurysm—a CT angiography or digital subtraction angiography are used.

The choice of adequate treatment is based on the results of a radiological examination and the condition of the patient. A surgical solution is traditional and uses clips to exclude the aneurysm from the circulation (clipping). A more modern method is the endovascular solution by filling of the aneurysm with platinum coils (coiling).

It is impossible to influence the acute phase of the SAH. The solution of the primary source of the SAH is chosen and performed. Even after successful treatment, there are still delayed and very serious complications of SAH. Most often seen are cerebral vasospasms, mineral metabolism disbalances and a development of hydrocephalus. The management of these complications is challenging, since they often produce delayed cerebral ischemia with subsequent neuropsychological impairments. The most often are disorders of speech, movement, memory, and there are also emotional and social disturbances, personality changes, or drop in IQ.

Personality changes and cognitive changes, if present, have a significant influence to everyday life of the patients. Patients after SAH thus require not only rehabilitation of motor and speech deficits, but also extensive and systematic neuropsychological care. Postoperative cognitive rehabilitation as well as crisis interventions (if needed) should start as soon as possible, and the patients should be followed in long-term aspect. The role of the neuropsychologist is of major importance in both diagnostics and postoperative care.

Introduction

Aneurysms of the cerebral vessels (AN) represent one of the most problematic and complex diseases that are faced by the field of neurosurgery and neuroscience. Although benign in terms of cellular biology, these lesions can cause intracranial bleeding with disastrous and often fatal effects. In the past, neurosurgeons were happy for every patient to simply survive, and they did not tend to investigate a further postoperative status. With certain improvements of diagnostics and treatment modalities, neurological deficits came into scope and a good result was claimed when the patient was "walking and talking" (Adams et al., 1976; Testa, et al., 1985).

However, it is not always the neurologic deficit that represents the crucial limitation in the patient's life. Several studies have showed that neuropsychological impairments are not as apparent as "true neurological deficits," but they can be even more important. It has been elucidated that an otherwise healthy person confined to a wheelchair can have a much better quality of life compared to a "walking and talking" person (Glasgow Outcome Scale I. i.e., neurologically excellent result) with severe memory, intelligence or personality disorder (Ogden et al., 1993; Samra et al., 2007).

The interest of neuropsychologists in neurobehavioral aspects of SAH is a matter of the last several decades. There were studies dealing with memory and personality changes published in the 50s, but focussed mostly on correlation with the organic site of the brain injury and type of the disorder. Contemporary studies concentrate not only on the origin of the impairment, but also on preventive measures and the treatment options.

Contemporary results show no correlation between neuropsychological deficits and the site or size of the aneurysm, not even a focal injury apparent on the CT. The most important factor predictive of quality of life is a severity of the initial bleeding and secondary brain injury (Hütter 2000; Ogden 1994; Vilkki 1989, 1990). However, the question remains which type of secondary brain damage can be attributed to neurobehavioral consequences. One way of understanding this relations lies in the functional anatomy of frontobasal and midline structures that are often affected by SAH and that are well known (and widely investigated) for an intimate relation to emotional and cognitive functions. A second important aspect is an understanding of SAH pathophysiology, the way it can influence these structures, and the treatment modalities available to alleviate its undesirable effects.

In accordance with Sanchez et al. (2007) we ask: 1) What modalities should be measured or scored for an effective evaluation of the patients after SAH and other cerebrovascular diseases? 2) What are the proper diagnostic tools in patients with cerebrovascular disorders and what is their relation to the medical treatment modalities? 3) What are contemporary trends in the evaluation of cerebrovascular disorders? 4) What should be the priorities of future studies?

A description and understanding of SAH from the neuropsychological point of view should form a base for psychosocial care and rehabilitation of individual patients. It is an interdisciplinary approach that is the key for understanding of the various contexts of this disease, including social relations, working opportunities, etc. Apart from lowering of mortality and neurological morbidity, the focus of contemporary treatment also lies in the minimalization of neuropsychological impairment and its effects on a patient's everyday life. The ultimate target of these efforts should be a clear description of neuropsychological influences and the development of adequate therapeutical and rehabilitation programs.

1. Anatomy and epidemiology of SAH

Cerebral aneurysm (AN) is a medical term for a fairly specific bulge in the wall of the major vessels of the brain. It consists of the bulging part called the "fundus" or the "dome" and a connecting part close to the parent vessel called the "neck." Aneurysms can be sorted according to size as small (<15mm), big (>15 mm) and giant (>25 mm). The majority of aneurysms are 4 to 15 mm in diameter. Around 80 to 90% of aneurysms are located in the anterior part of the Willis Circle; the remaining 20% are located in the vertebro-basilar (posterior) part (Kassell et al., 1990). They usually arise at the bifurcation of the arteries, in regions with defective architecture of the vessel wall. The aetiology of these defects and pathophysiology of the aneurysm formation is not certain; however, two major theories speak of an inherited lesions and a progressive, degenerative development. The impairment of the vessel wall seems to be of a more systemic nature since there is a double risk of mortality of cerebrovascular or cardiac origin in patients after successful treatment of SAH within the first 12 months after the insult (Ronkainen et al., 2001).

Once the aneurysm ruptures, the blood flows between the surface of the brain and arachnoid membrane. This situation is called a "subarachnoid haemorrhage" (SAH). There are also other causes of SAH, but aneurysmal ruptures represent the majority (around 50 to 90%) of non-traumatic cases. Apart from SAH, AN rupture can also lead to intracerebral haemorrhage, subdural haemorrhage and intraventricular haemorrhage.

According to a large series of autopsies, the prevalence of AN is surprisingly large and varies between 0.2 and 8% (Taylor 1995, 1996). It is the rupture, or to put it properly SAH, that makes these lesions so dangerous. The incidence of SAH itself is much lower—roughly 6 to 10 new bleedings per 100,000 people every year. In absolute terms, especially as compared to the numbers of cerebral ischemia, that does not seem to be a very high number. However, the severity of this disease lies in its natural course and the population affected. The incidence does not spare young and otherwise healthy patients, and it rises linearly from the age of 20 peaking between 40 to 60 years. Women slightly predominate (55 to 65%), mainly in younger age groups. Risk factors include smoking, arterial hypertension and a consumption of more than 150g of alcohol/week (Teunissen et al., 1996). The risk of a rupture is increased with heavy physical activity and physiological rise of systemic of intracranial pressure, typically lifting heavy objects, defecation, sexual activities, emotional stress (Ogden et al., 1993).

Several external factors have been identified, such as time of the year, weather changes, etc. (Chyatte et al., 1994).

In around 15% of cases, aneurysms are multiple, and it is very rare to see more than six aneurysms in one patient. Around half of multiple aneurysms occur on internal carotid artery, one-third on middle cerebral artery and 15% on anterior communicating artery (Yasagril, 1984). After negative screening, a new aneurysm develops in less than 1% of cases. (Marchel et al., 1991). The probability of the rupture of an intact intracranial aneurysm is 1 to 2% per year and it depends on size—the probability is higher in aneurysms larger than 6 to 7 mm.

No matter how much the neuroscience advanced in the past time, the mortality rate remains over 50% (Bamford et al, 1990; Kassell et al., 1990), which is much more in comparison with ischemic brain disease (10%—Bamford et al., 1990). Another 25% of victims end up with a permanent neurological disability. All of the survivors, including the remaining "otherwise healthy" cases, can suffer less apparent insults leading to various neuropsychological disorders.

There are 14,000 survivors of SAH in the USA every year. This is an enormous socioeconomic influence not only on patients, but on all society. According to Kassel (Kassel, 1990), the situation in Europe is comparable to the USA in all major aspects.

2. Pathophysiology of SAH

There can be very complex, unusual and surprising findings in the profile of the patients that have recovered from SAH. The origin of these findings lies in an equally complex pathophysiology. We present basic information and preferably aspects that are relevant to neurobehavioral consequences.

There are three major components inside the patient's skull: brain tissue, blood in the vessels, and approximately 150mL of cerebrospinal fluid (CSF). The human skull provides a constant amount of space for these elements. The Monroe-Kelly doctrine points out that these elements are not compressible, and in the case of the expansion of one, another must exit the intracranial space, keeping constant volume.

In the region of the skull base, subarachnoid space is widened and the space is divided by septa into interconnected compartments called cisterns. The space is filled with CSF, and it harbours major arteries, too.

The rupture of the aneurysm wall is produced by a wave of arterial pressure as it exceeds the mechanical limits of the aneurysm wall (Kim et al., 1992). In the case of a haemorrhage to the subarachnoid space, pulsating blood replaces the CSF, pushes it away from the cistern surrounding the site of the rupture. As intracranial and local pressure increases, the pressure gradient between blood and CSF decreases, bleeding slows down until the conditions reach a point where a clot can (and is) formed and bleeding stops.

Sudden increase of the intracranial pressure (ICP) causes severe headaches and usually a rapid loss of consciousness; decreased blood flow in cerebral vessels results in hypo-perfusion and neuronal ischemia. After approximately five minutes, the acute phase ends and complex sub-acute changes develop. At this stage (5 to 20 minutes), ICP decreases, and it is the overall cerebral metabolic activity of the brain that is most predictive for outcome.

Once ICP decreases, there is a high risk of repeated rupture. Each repeated rupture is associated with and a 30% increase in mortality risk.

Up to this moment, it is usually impossible to influence the disease, and the data comes mostly from experimental works. Subsequent chronic changes matter the most in clinical medicine. Blood in the subarachnoid space leads to a complex biological cascade with vascular irritation and contractures of arterial walls. This phenomenon is called vasospasms. If the patient survives the acute phase of the bleeding, it is vasospasms that have the utmost influence on outcome and morbidity/mortality rates. Within an onset approximately 72 hours after the bleeding, the spasm of the arterial wall decreases the amount of blood entering brain and causes another wave of cerebral ischemia. This time, it lasts for several days, and it involves slow changes. The severity of the cerebral vasospasm can be measured by transcranial Doppler ultrasonography (TCD). As specific vessels supply specific territories of the brain and different areas of the brain have different resistance to ischemia, resulting ischemic changes can lead to a very variable impact on the patient's outcome and final neuropsychological status (Bornstein et al., 1987; De Luca, 1992).

In a case of severe ischemia, cerebral oedema can develop with further increase of ICP and subsequent loss of perfusion (Hornyak et al., 1991) forming a classical example of "circulus vitiosus."

The second most common delayed complication of SAH is hydrocephalus. This condition develops in approximately 20% of patients, and it is caused by disrupted blood elements that block natural sites of CSF resorbtion. The production of the CSF continues, and this time, it is the CSF itself that causes an increase of intracranial pressure and subsequent neurologic symptomatology. Hydrocephalus needs to be recognized. In contrast to the vasospasms, it can be treated much more effectively. The solution is usually a ventriculo-peritoneal shunt—CSF is derived from the brain via a system of tubes and pressure valves into the abdominal cavity, where it resorbs.

There are further complications, namely infection, electrolyte and water imbalances such as cerebral salt wasting (CSW), syndrome of inappropriate adiuretin secretion (SIADH), or diabetes insipidus. These factors can significantly contribute to the outcome in terms of both neurologic and neuropsychological morbidity.

From the standpoint of neuropsychology, it is important to mention associated haemorrhages. Bleeding from the aneurysm can extend intraventriculary (intraventricular haemorrhage—IVH) and intraparenchymally (intracerebral haemorrhage—ICH). IVH seems to play a significant role in neuropsychological consequences of SAH (Hütter, 1999; Le Roux, 1996). Mechanisms involved in cerebral damage are thought to be obstruction of CSF pathways and a compression of periventricular structures. (Shapiro et al., 1994).

Intraventricular haemorrhage is usually present in middle cerebral artery aneurysms. Patients with ICH have worse clinical status on admission. All types of haemorrhage have a significant role in the prognosis and outcome (morbidity, mortality).

According to Hütter (2000), one of the promising directions in neuropsychological research is a detailed neuro-anatomical topographic analysis of the subarachnoid space affected by SAH. It seems that there can be differences in cognitive deficits at least partially correspondent to the anatomical location blood clots in cisterns.

Table 1. Basal cisterns and surrounding neural structures (Hütter, 2000)

Basal cistern	Related neuro-anatomical structure
C. carotis	Parts of the orbital frontal lobe Parts of the medial temporal lobe Uncus
C. laminae terminalis	Rostrum corpus callosi Gyrus rectus Commissura anterior
C. olfactorii	Parts of the orbital frontal lobe Gyrus rectus
C. fossa sylvii	Parts of the orbital frontal lobe Parts of the baso-medial temporal lobe Limen insulae
C. cruralis(interpeduncularis)	Parahippocampal gyrus
C. ambiens	Lateral sections of the tegmentum Cerebral peduncles Parts of the medial temporal lobe Uncus Velum interpositum Pulvinar thalami
C. vena magna Galeni	Dorsal sections of the tegmentum Splenium corporis callosi
C. velum interpositum	Splenium corporis callosi Fornix Pulvinar thalami
C. corpus callosi	Rostrum corpus callosi Cingulate gyrus Corpus callosum
C. interpeduncularis	Tegmentum Substantia perforata rostralis Mamillary bodies Parts of the medial temporal lobe
C. praepontina	Pons
C. medullaris anterior	Pons Medulla oblongata
C. cerebellopontina	Pons
C. cerebellomedullaris lateralis	Medulla oblongata
C. magna	Medulla oblongata

3. Clinical Findings in SAH

Diagnosis of SAH includes clinical findings, laboratory findings and radiological findings. Patients with SAH usually experience a sudden, extremely strong and sharp headache. Even if they do not loose consciousness, there can be multiple neurological impairments; typically seen is nausea, vomiting, diplopia, and photophobia. Nuchal rigidity develops, causing positive meningeal signs (inability to flex head for reflexive neck muscle spasms). Typical symptoms are summarized in Table 2.

Table 2. Symptoms of aneurysmal SAH

Symptoms	%
Meningeal irritation	
earlier warning leaks (headache)	30 to 50
severe headache	more 85
nausea and/or vomiting	more than 50
meningism (after 12 to 24 hours)	70
Neurological/neuropsychological deficits	30
visual fields defects	
oculomotor palsy	
hemiparesis	
aphasia	
disorientation/agitation	
Epileptic seizures	4 to 26
Clouding of consciousness/coma	40
Sudden death	15

According to Smith and Miller (1990), in Hütter (2000).

Diagnostics of SAH

The process of diagnostics involves three basic steps: 1. proof of SAH, 2. localizing the source of the SAH, 3. proof of the complication closely related to SAH (hydrocephalus, vasospasm, ICH, SDH). If SAH is suspected, the modality of first choice is a CT scan. In case of unavailability of the CT, a lumbar puncture is the second option.

After SAH confirmation, there is a need to confirm or to rule out any underlying vascular pathology. These are the three major diagnostic tools: magnetic resonance angiography (MR-AG), computer tomography–based angiography (CT-AG) and digital subtraction angiography (DSA). MR-AG and CT-AG are non-invasive methods, with MR-AG having less sensitivity as it can detect only larger aneurysms over 3mm in diameter (Gilsbach, Poeck, Piscol, 1993). DSA, on the other hand, is performed invasively, using access through patient´s femoral artery. A catheter is placed in the patient´s aorta and a contrast agent is injected into the arteries with subsequent X-ray evaluation. As compensation for the invasiveness, there is a possibility to treat some of the diagnosed vascular lesions right away, using endovascular techniques. DSA is considered and unmatched "golden standard," as it has highest sensitivity.

In some cases, no source of SAH can be found. There are two main reasons: 1) the source is too small to be detected (mild SAH, usually) 2) the source has been obliterated by blood clot and cannot be detected on initial examination. Some of the obliterated sources can spontaneously re-open in time. It is, therefore, necessary to perform additional examinations, usually one week and two months after the bleeding. Despite advanced technologies involved, in more than 20 to 30% of AG and CT-verified cases of SAH, no underlying pathology is detected (Rinkel, van Gijn, Vijdicks, 1993).

4. Evaluation and Scaling of SAH

The Most Commonly Used Tools and Scales to Evaluate Patients with SAH:

A proper initial evaluation of patients with SAH remains essential as it has direct implications in the prognosis and treatment options. The evaluation and classification according to consistent methodology also allows a comparison between the clinical centres and ensures consistency in the cooperation of research. It also provides a platform of unbiased communication between specialties involved in the treatment of a particular patient.

There are scales evaluating levels of consciousness, severity of SAH according to various criteria and neurological and psychosocial impact of SAH.

The most commonly used is a five-grade scale according to Hunt and Hess (Cavanagh, 1968; Vickie, 2002), sorting the initial status of the patient according to cutoffs in prognosis. It is also a leading argument in the decision of involving early treatment (Hütter et al., 1999).

Table 3. Hunt and Hess Scale

Grade 1	Mild headache and/or neck stiffness
Grade 2	Severe headache and/or pronounced neck stiffness and/or cranial nerve deficits, photophobia
Grade 3	Drowsiness and/or mild disorientation and/or slight pareses and/or dysphasia
Grade 4	Stupor or sopor and/or fair to severe hemiparesis and/or dysphasia
Grade 5	Coma, decerebrate rigidity, acute middle-brain syndrome

Table 4. Botterell Scale et al. (1956)

Grade I	Patient presents with clear consciousness
Grade II	Patient is tired/drowsy but has no neurological deficits
Grade III	Patient is tired/drowsy but presents with neurological deficit (s)
Grade IV	Patient presents with severe neurological deficit (s) and clinical deterioration
Grade V	Moribund or nearly moribund

Another similar scale is the World Federation of Neurological Surgeons (WFNS SAH scale, 1988).

Table 5. Classification according to WFNS SAH scale (1988)

Grade	GCS (Jennet et al. 1981)	Motor deficit
I	15	none
II	14 to 13	none
III	14 to 13	present
IV	12 to 7	present or not present
V	6 to 3	present or not present

After the introduction of the CT, Fischer, Kistler a Davis (1980) developed a "Fischer-scale," which divides SAH into categories according to its appearance on CT scans.

Table 6. Fischer-scale: grading system for quantification of the severity of SAH

Grade 0	No blood can be detected on the CT scan
Grade 1	Diffuse distribution or thin, localized layer of blood in all vertical layers (inter-hemispheric fissure, insular cistern, ambient cistern) less than 1 mm of thickness
Grade 2	Localized clots of blood and/or vertical layers of blood more than 1 mm of thickness
Grade 3	Diffuse or no subarachnoid blood; but intracerebral or intraventricular blood

Jennett and Bond published the Glasgow outcome Scale in 1975, as a quantification tool for and outcome after cerebral injury (in general).

Table 7. Glasgow Outcome Scale

Result	Definition
GOS I	no/minimal impairment
GOS II	modest impairment (needs no help for daily life)
GOS III	severely impaired (needs help for daily life)
GOS IV	persistent vegetative state
GOS V	patient is dead

Mhoney and Barthel developed the Barthel Index (BI) in 1965. The index evaluates coping with tasks of everyday life. Although developed for patients after ischemic ictus, it is widely used for evaluation in other groups of neurologic disorders. It consists of 10 functions or abilities significant for everyday routines, and there are points corresponding to the (in)ability of the patients to perform the tasks by themselves, or with help of someone else. The result can be anything from 0 (unable for independent life) to 100 (fully independent).

5. Clinical Course and Therapy of SAH

After a single, mild spontaneous SAH with no sign of vascular pathology on the initial angiography and with repeatedly negative angiographic (AG-negative) follow-ups (one week and approx. two months after bleeding), the prognosis is generally good, and a risk of severe SAH in the future is small. Patients with mild SAH generally experience less severe clinical signs, such as headache, nausea, photophobia, stiffness of the neck, and these typically last for several days, rarely weeks. However, the risk of recurrence in this group (low) must be clearly distinguished from the risk of SAH-associated complications, as these can develop even in the case of a small and AG-negative SAH. It is necessary to provide full monitoring, and the stay in the hospital is usually up to two weeks.

In the case of severe SAH, the clinical course gets worse as a risk of vasospasm and other complications rises. The first goal of the diagnostics is to detect the source. It is possible, but less probable, to see AG-negative cases with severe bleeding. In most of the patients with severe SAH, the source is located and it is usually necessary to treat it as soon as possible. The risk of re-rupture is quite high, especially in the early hours and days after the first rupture (Inagawa, 1994). Furthermore, mortality of the second and further ruptures steeply rises. Severe forms of bleeding and especially intraventricular bleedings tend to progress into acute hydrocephalus. This condition cannot be treated by a VP shunt, since blood degradation products would obliterate the tubing and delicate pressure valves. For a limited period of time, an external ventricular drainage is applied. A catheter is inserted in one of the cerebral ventricles and extends out of the patient´s head. CSF stained with blood is drained into a reservoir and disposed. After CSF clears, the catheter system can be transformed into VP shunt if necessary.

It takes about 72 hours for the blood clot degradation cascade to cause vasospasms, and it is desirable to exclude the aneurysm from the blood circulation before this happens. Once vasospasms occur, the arteries become very thin and the brain becomes very vulnerable. It is dangerous to perform surgery under these circumstances and usually impossible to perform endovascular treatment as well. Once the early period is missed, the causal treatment of the aneurysms must be postponed until vasospasms cease, which is typically two weeks after bleeding. Considering purely the risks of re-rupture, patients treated early are clearly at an advantage. There are other beneficial implications of the early treatment (mainly the possibility to keep the arterial pressure high and provide sufficient brain perfusion). The main drawback of an early surgical approach is clear: the amount of blood in the cisterns around the aneurysm, brain oedema and its metabolic changes make surgery more difficult and risky. Delayed surgery (after the CFS clears and vasospasms cease) is less difficult to perform, but the patient has to be exposed to the risk of either re-rupture or brain perfusion decompensation. There is no consensus whether to operate right away or to wait, but early surgery seems to be preferred by the majority of neurosurgeons.

As mentioned before, there two main possibilities of the treatment. Surgery requires opening of the head and treats the aneurysm by applying a clip (clipping), and endovascular treatment uses catheters introduced to the arteries and treats aneurysms by platinum coils (coiling).

Surgery is the traditional approach, with very well-defined techniques, approaches and a definitive treatment at the moment of a precise clip application. It requires a head opening (craniotomy). The aneurysm has to be located, clearly distinguished from other vessels and the surrounding structures. Then, a clip can be applied to its neck and thus it is instantly excluded from the circulation. Clipping of the aneurysm ensures a 98% certainty of no further bleeding.

Another option has emerged quite recently. It is an endovascular solution, where the interventional radiologist advances a catheter through the femoral artery, far into the arteries of the brain, finds the aneurysm and places platinum strands (coils) into it using a micro-catheter. This is controlled by an advanced X-Ray. The aneurysm is filled by foreign material "from inside" and thromboses in time. This modality does not exclude the aneurysm right away, it is very expensive, but it has comparable short-term results as surgery and requires no head opening.

It seems that certain groups of patients will clearly benefit from the endovascular approach, and certain groups will remain in the domain of surgery with quite broad field remaining, where both methods would be possible. As of now, the experience of the physician with the method used is essential in the decision of which modality to choose.

There are ongoing clinical trials evaluating all aspects of both methods (Wermer et al., 2007), but long-term results are not conclusive yet. According to Frazer et al. (2007), both modalities possess approximately the same risk of morbidity. Neuropsychological evaluation has showed that it is the site and severity of the bleeding, plus several other initial parameters, that are relevant to the cognitive outcome. The choice of treatment influences the outcome far less (Hütter et al, 1999).

The results of available studies are often controversial. The International Subarachnoid Aneurysm Trial (ISAT) shows a better mortality ratio in patients after coiling, but this advantage lasts only up to seven years. There are more re-bleedings compared to the clipping (Molyneux et al., 2005). The patients were presented with the same deficit in verbal and visual memory (Bellebaum et al., 2004). Patients with the clipping show a little more compromise in the affective area and self-evaluation executive functions. Frazer et al. (2007) concludes that there are no differences in the cognitive outcome in the long-term period. Endovascular treatment provides slightly better results at the beginning, but this difference has been assigned to the necessity of opening the head in a surgery group. Subsequently, all the difference disappears. Another study of Solheim et al. (2006) followed 73 patients with un-ruptured aneurysms after clipping and coiling and did not find any major differences in the quality parameters of their lives. The study of Koivisto at al. (2000) comparing endovascular and the surgical approach found no significant difference in neuropsychological status on a one-year follow-up.

5.1. Historical Developments of the Treatment and Psychological Evaluation of the Patients with Intracranial Aneurysms

Compared to the other types of intracranial bleedings, SAH has been clouded in mystery for a long time. The first description is from Morgagni (1762), but it was Sir Charles Symonds who introduced SAH as a diagnostic category. The first reminiscence of aneurysm treatment is a ligature of artery in the region of the knee for a popliteal aneurysm, and it comes from Hunter (1784). Sir Victor Horsley ligated a carotid artery for an intracranial aneurysm in 1885. These methods are called trapping (achieved by ligature of the feeding artery) and have enormous complications and mortality rates due to ischemic "collateral damage." More advanced surgical solutions of intracranial aneurysms came to life with the invention of angiography by Egas Monitz in 1927. The first intended surgery for intracranial aneurysms was performed by Normann Dott in 1931, as he operated on an acutely bleeding aneurysm. Despite serious bleeding he succeeded with bands of muscles wrapped around the aneurysmal dome. Wrapping, however, is not a perfect treatment in the majority of cases. It was Walter Dandy, a true neurosurgical genius, who used a silver McKenzie clip for the first time (1937). Several authors (Olivecrona, Schvartz, Mayfield, Scovill) developed various clip modifications and there were substantial developments in operative techniques. Nonetheless, results of aneurysm treatment remained very poor with a very high mortality rate. From the point of neuropsychology, there is a very important study of Webster from this era. In 1960 he evaluated neuropsychological effects of the anterior cerebral artery occlusion. This condition can occur with aneurysmal rupture and sometimes effectively results from a severe vasospasm of the artery. Observations included anxiety, loss of initiative, worsening of intellectual powers and other defects—all in the absence of a marked neurologic deficit.

Further progress in diagnostics was bound to the invention of a CT scanner in 1971 and especially an operating microscope (1964). At the end of the 1970s and the beginning of the 1980s, advances in pathophysiology of SAH, vasospasm and recognition of risks of re-bleeding (Mizukami et al., 1982) improved an otherwise very poor prognosis of the patients. Together, these major improvements led to a renaissance of aneurysm surgery.

Modern techniques utilize aneurysm clips made of non-ferromagnetic alloys allowing postoperative examinations in MRI scanners. Apart from simple clipping, there are several advanced microsurgical possibilities such as trapping using bypass, complex vascular reconstructions etc.

The treatment of the aneurysm itself evolved, but there was another evolution in the treatment of the effects of SAH. After the aneurysm is clipped or coiled, the "battlefield" moves from the operating theatre to the intensive care unit (ICU). A better understanding of vasospasm, hemodynamic therapy, antagonist of calcium, use of nimodipin and other pharmacological substances—all of this forms the cornerstone of modern treatment, which has decreased the mortality rate substantially (Baker, 1996).

6. Neuropsychological Impacts of SAH

Initial studies dealing with the neuropsychological impacts of SAH were not very systematic. There were mostly case studies, random descriptions of symptoms and summaries of medical records. The outcomes and recommendations of such studies did not match the reality, and there were many misunderstandings (Hütter, 2000).

The first description of the neuropsychological effect of SAH is connected with Hamilton Roe (1851). He described a case of a 21-year old woman treated for a loss of memory and a loss of vision in one eye at the Westminster hospital. After her death, the autopsy revealed a thrombosed aneurysm as a cause of the symptoms. In 1866, Herman Lebert emphasized an importance of the aneurysm localization in relation to the neurological and mental deficit. He also speculated about the possibility to localize the aneurysm according to the clinical symptomatology.

The interest in the neuropsychological effects of SAH rose in the 1920s (Hütter, 2000). Author interested in neuropsychological aspects of SAH is Dott (1933); however his works did not include enough details about objective findings and test results. Many of the psychological peculiarities were misdiagnosed as a Korsakow psychosis. The most common symptoms include anterograde and retrograde amnesia. Disorientation and confabulations were common in the first days and weeks after SAH, whereas memory disturbances, emotional changes and mood impairments lasted much longer. Walton (1953) describes as some of the patients improved and reached their premorbid "self" in various periods of time, however, some never reached their personality profile again.

The first systematic follow-up of the effects of SAH dates back to the 1960s. In 1964, Norlen described 14 patients after AcoA aneurysm rupture. Korsakow syndrome was diagnosed in nine of them.

The most often cited classical work is a case report of Talland et al. (1967) following two patients for four years. After the intervention, both patients were cooperative, neuropsychological test showed normal memory, however, there was a persistent confusion, confabulations and anterograde amnesia. One of the patients returned to work (not to his previous job), and there were significant personality changes in both (in Hütter, 2000).

Despite many studies dealing with cognitive, emotional and motivation abnormalities, the main interest was focused on memory disturbances with respect to the Korsakow syndrome (Hütter, 2000). The first group study included a neuropsychological follow-up and was performed by Linquist and Norlen in 1966. There were 33 patients after the rupture of the AcoA aneurysm. Storey (1970) published a psychiatric study of 261 patients evaluated six months to six years after the rupture of aneurysm (ACoA, MCA, PCoA). In psychiatric terms, 45% of patients were within the norm. He depicted a decrease of initiative, irritability and anxiety in 55% and mild to severe psychiatric disturbances in 21% of patients. There was no correlation between the specific psychiatric disorder and a localization of the aneurysm, but some of the symptoms (depression, emotional lability and anxiety) occurred predominantly in patients with MCA aneurysm on the right side. Logue et al. (1968) followed a group of 79 patients between 7 and 101 months after the rupture of the aneurysm. Memory disturbances were found in 29% of the patients; the average IQ did not differ from the normal population using WAIS-R. There was a marked decrease of initiative in 60.7% and an emotional control disturbance in 30% of the patients.

Lurias systematic neuropsychological testing of two patients after the rupture of AcoA (1976) aneurysm performed nearly daily showed an increase of absent-mindedness and pathological sensitivity. As compared to the patients with deep structural lesions or tumors, they did not express a global consciousness and lucidity impairment.

Sengupta, Chinu and Brierley (1975) found significant correlations between personality changes, lack of initiative, loss of will and severity of bleeding, initial clinical status and severity of vasospasms. Vilkki et al. (1989) studied a relation between CT findings and cognitive deficits. Patients with an ischemia on the left side suffered from verbal performance deficiency, memory loss and the ability to classify. The right sided ischaemias expressed visuomotor disturbances and visuoconstruction impairments.

There are many studies dealing with the results of SAH. Contrary to mainstream Penrose and Storey (1970) investigated, if and how the emotional disturbances can cause SAH. In patients without an apparent source of SAH on angiography, an increase of psychiatric care for emotional problems was observed prior to SAH. Another study by Ogden (1993b) showed increased emotional stress before SAH. Although there are signs of the role of emotional stress in facilitating aneurysmal rupture; no longitudinal epidemiologic study is available to prove such an assumption.

In the clinical settings, we can see premorbid emotional stress, social or interpersonal problems, increased work load, which are both of long and short (peak) character. There is also a question of possible personality structures and specific patterns that predispose for SAH (as it is proven in cardiovascular diseases).

Table 8. Neuropsychology, Anatomic division and blood supply. According to Synder, Nussbaum (2003)

Function	Impairment	Brain structure	Blood supply
Sensorimotor	paralysis of contralateral	primary motor area	middle cerebral artery
	face, arm and leg	precentral gyrus anterior	cerebral artery
	sensory impairment over	primary sensory area	middle cerebral artery
	face, arm and leg	postccentral gyrus	anterior cerebral artery
Language	Broca´s aphasia	inferior frontal gyrus in dominant hemisphere	middle cerebral artery
	Wernicke´s aphasia	superior temporal gyrus in dominant hemisphere	middle cerebral artery
Visual Perception	homonymous hemianopia	optic radiation deep in temporal convolution	middle cerebral artery posterior cerebral artery
	visual integration, spatial neglect, visual agnosia	parietal-occipital lobe, nondominant hemisphere	middle cerebral artery
	constructional appraxia, dressing apraxia	parietal lobe, nondominant hemisphere	middle cerebral artery
	Gerstmann´s syndrome	angular gyrus of the dominant	middle cerebral artery
	(agraphia,)		
	acalculia, alexia, finger agnosia, right-left confusion	hemisphere	
Movement	ideomotor and ideational Apraxia	left temporal, parietal and occipital area	middle cerebral artery posterior cerebral artery
Memory	short-term and long-term	hippocampus, medial temporal	medial cerebral
	memory impairment	lobes, frontal lobes, basal forebrain, medial thalamus	posterior cerebral anterior choroidal Posterior communicating artery
	working memory impairment	dorsolateral frontal lobes	anterior cerebral artery
Frontal-executive	impairment in set maintenance, problem solving, planning, self-evaluation, ability to modify behaviour	dorsolateral frontal	middle cerebral artery
	impairment in inhibition, emotional regulation	orbital frontal	anterior cerebral artery
	akinesia, bradykinesia,	basal ganglia, putamen, globus	anterior choroidal artery
	dyskinesia	pallidus, caudate nucleus, amygdaloid	middle cerebral artery

6.1. No Neurological Deficit and Neuropsychological Disorders

A neuropsychologist often faces a patient without apparent neurological deficit who on the other hand expresses signs of severe neuropsychological disturbances.

Significant alteration of a specific performance is considered as 2 standard deviations below the average score of normal test results (Lezak, 2004). The most often used outcome scale in neurology is quite simply the Glasgow Outcome Score (GOS). However, this scale is focused on a level of physical function only (Egge et al., 2005).

There are many studies proving a top GOS score with severe alterations in cognitive capacity, emotional balance and other areas leading to a significant drop in quality of life. (Sonesson, 1987; Bornstein et al., 1987; Desantis, 1989; Hütter, 1998; Kim et al., 2005).

The most often explored disorders in good neurological outcome cover verbal and nonverbal capacity, short- and long-term memory, abstract thinking, flexibility, concentration and accuracy of perception (blood supply and neuropsychological functioning, see Table 8).

Hütter and Gilsbach (1993) followed 31 patients (GOS=1) one to five years after the SAH. The deficit was most often found in the following areas: complex reaction time (Wiener Determinationsgerat) 28 to 62% of patients, figural short-term memory (Benton test) 53% of patients, long-term memory 21%, concentration and alertness 7 to 16%, fatic lesion (Token Test) 10%. Only 20% presented with no signs of cognitive deficit. Over 54% of patients with good neurological deficit (GOS I) showed a disturbance in cognitive capacity in three main cognitive domains.

Despite apparent differences in patient populations, surgical and endovascular indications, ICU care, testing methods, it can be concluded that most often, SAH related effects are short memory disturbances, overall psychomotor deceleration and a decreased ability to concentrate. Good neurological outcome (GOS I) does not warrant the absence of neuropsychological impairments (Hütter 2000; Ropper et al., 1984; Vilkki et al., 1990). The cognitive level can be much different from the neurological.

The above-mentioned facts call for a practical use of a more complex evaluation. Including neuropsychological tests in outcome measures is the only way for a real insight into patient´s everyday life, emotional status and overall quality of life.

7. Basic Principles of Neuropsychological Diagnostics in Patients after SAH

The complex evaluation of brain functions includes five main areas:

1. neurologic deficit
2. cognitive performance
3. emotional status
4. activities in daily living
5. health-related quality of life

A neuropsychological evaluation should not be reduced to a simple evaluation of a cognitive performance of the patient, but it should include the emotional status and other aspects (family, profession). Only such an approach allows a transfer from pure diagnostics to the therapy.

Diagnostics of the effects of SAH faces complex pathophysiology and a possibility of diverse pathology with no specific anatomical site. Also, most of the neuropsychological changes have no detectable correlation using radiologic evaluations. Another problem is a marked heterogeneity of population effected, but this is a known limit of nearly all neuropsychological studies (Mesulam 1986; Hütter 2000; Sanchez 2007). Moreover, neuropsychological research is often based on presumptions and concepts that were validated on brain injuries of other aetiology, and the validity of the results can be questionable.

For a true insight into patient´s functional status, there is a need for a systematic and rigorous methodology. The spectrum of instruments available today is very broad though, and it is often up to the personal preferences of the researcher which method is to be used. However, it should be a method standardized for SAH-patients and not formal administrative method designed for general psychiatric use.

Interestingly, it is not practical to compare average scores in SAH patients with a population norm. The average usually corresponds with the expected value, even though some of the patients show substantial cognitive deficits in separate scales (Hütter, 2000).

The basics of a neuropsychological battery should include short- and long-term memory tests, tests of concentration and screening tests for aphasia. In an acute stage of the disease, the bedside evaluation should be adjusted according to the patient´s physical health status.

Further investigations, especially after dismission, should include personality psychopathology, quality of life evaluation and assessment of patient´s adaptation from the viewpoint of the relatives.

Table 9. The most common neuropsychological disorders after acquired brain injury (Hütter, 2000)

1) Visual field defects
2) Neglect
3) Defects of visuo-spatial constructive capacities
4) Distortion of face and object recognition
5) Memory disorders
6) Language disturbances (aphasias)
7) Deficits in problem-solving
8) Impairments of motor fine coordination
9) Impairments of complex sensory-motor coordination
10) Apraxias
11) Attention deficits
12) Mental rigidity
13) Dementia
14) Deficits of concentration capacity
15) Personality changes/emotional disorders
16) Behavioral disorders

7.1. Diagnostics of Attention Disorders

Disorders of attention are described in 80% of patients with brain damage. Attention is a process providing the reaction to specific sources, selected according to specific criteria, where other criteria are suppressed. It is a readiness for a quick and adequate reaction on selected input (Broadbent, 1958; Posner, 1987, 2007).

There are many more definitions of attention, such as major topics of cognitive psychology. Modalities evaluated within this term include a pure reaction time, vigilance, selectness/tendency towards perseveration, attention capacity, divided attention, etc. Modern understanding of attention is connected with Posner (2007), who discriminates three major aspects: selectivity, capacity and controlled processing. There are specific disorders matching these categories.

Table 10. Measurement of attention

Auditory attention	Wechsler Adult Intelligence Scale –Revised: Digit Span	Wechsler, 1994, 1955, 1981
	Paced Auditory Serial Addition Test	Gronwell, 1977
	Verbal and Nonverbal Cancellation	Mesulam, 1988
	Continuous Performance Test of Attention	Cicerone, 1997
Visual attention and spatial neglect		
	Line Bisection Test	Smith, 1982
	Symbol Digit Modalities Test	
	Trail Making test	Reitan, 1958

Another test of selective reactivity is a Go/NoGo test. The principle is to react only to specific signals and ignore all others, no matter how similar they are. The tendency to perseverations is also evaluated (inability to stop automatic flow of reactions). This test can be considered as an indicator of performance capacity of frontal-cortical regions. (Hütter, 1997 b).

7.2. Diagnostics of Memory and Learning Disorders

The most often used are partial subtests of complex tests of intelligence (WAIS-R/WAIS-III) of complex psychological methods such as Wechsler Memory Scale–III. Mnestic functions are often tested by specific neuropsychological methods (see Tab. 11), as they provide a higher sensitivity for the differentiation of specific memory deficits. The Wechsler Memory Scale is an example of test transfer influence: the test is originally part of an intelligence test—and it correlates much better with general intelligence. Moreover, the results are dependent on the level of education and linguistic performance, so it is no longer considered optimal for pure memory deficit evaluation.

Benton´s test (Benton, 1981) is very often used for the evaluation of short-term visual memory and is suitable for patients after SAH. The test includes ten simple geometric figures that are shown for ten seconds, and the proband reproduces the figures on a blank sheet of paper. The results are formed by two scores: first includes the amount of mistakes and the second, the number of correct reproductions. Benton´s test is very precise for cases of diffuse brain injury (as it can happen in SAH).

Table 11. Methods focused on the memory and learning (Lezak, 2004)

Short-term, long-term, working memory	
Wechsler memory scale – III	Wechsler, 1945, 1987, 1997
California Verbal Learning Test	Delis, Kramer, Kaplan, Ober, 1987, 2000
Buschke Selective Reminding Test	Buschke, Fuld, 1974
Hopkins Verbal Learning Test	Brandt, 1991; Benedict, Schretlen, et al., 1998
Rey Auditory Verbal Learning Test	Rey, 1964; Taylor, 1959; Schmidt, 1996
Rey-Osterreith Complex Figure	Osterreith, 1944
Benton Visual Retention Test	Benton, 1974; Sivan, 1992
Corsi Block Tapping Test	Milner, 1971
Serial digit learning	Benton, Sivan, Hamsher et al., 1994
Interference Learning Test	Schmidt, Coolidge, 1999
Memory Assessment Scales	Williams, 1991

7.3. Visual Perception, Sensimotor Coordination, Concentration Capacity and Visuoconstructive Capacity

Concentration capacity, visual sensation, accuracy and speed of work can be evaluated by a D2 test with a prognostic validity for a patient's return to work. It is actually a modification of Bourdon Wiersma Dot Cancellation test (Brickenkamp, 1978). The proband is given a pencil and a paper, and he or she is to mark all D2 signs. This test includes four parameters—the amount of correctly marked signs, percentage of mistakes, the overall results without mistakes and a continuity of the performance. There are several modifications of this test.

7.4. Diagnostics of Verbal Disorders

Aphasia is an impairment of the ability to express by means of spoken language and/or impairment of understanding of spoken language, both due to damage to the brain.

It is one of the most frequent areas of neuropsychological diagnostics as well as therapy. This is mainly because of the importance of the spoken language in human life.

Table 12. Visual sensation and visuoconstructional capabilities

Vizual perception		
Homonymous hemianopia	Double Simultaneous Stimulation Test	Walsh, 1987
Visual organization and Integration	Hooper Visual Organization Test	Hooper Organization Test Manual, 1983
	Visual Object and Space Perception Battery	Warrington, 1983 James,1991
Visual motor construction	WAIS-R: Block Design Object Assembly	Wechsler, 1994
	Complex Figure Test	Corwin, Bylsma, 1993
Visual recognition	Visual Form Discrimination Test	Benton, Hamsher, 1983, 1994
Face recognition	Test of Face recognition	

Table 13. Tests of aphasia (Snydder, Nussbaum, 2003)

Function or impairment	Test	References
Broca´s aphasia Wernicke´s aphasia	Boston Diagnostic Aphasia Examination	Goodglass, Kaplan, 1983 Benton, Hamsher, 1989
Transcortical motor aphasia Global aphasia	Multilingual Aphasia Examination	Kertesz, 1979
Transcortical sensory aphasia, Conduction aphasia	Western Aphasia Battery	
Comprehension	Token Test	Boller, Vignolo, 1966
Naming	Boston Naming Test	Kaplan,Goodglass, Weintraub, 1983, 2001
Vocabulary	Peabody Picture Vocabulary Test	Dunn, Dunn, 1981, 1997
Verbal fluency	Controlled Oral Word Association Test	Benton, Hamsher, 1989 Spreen, Strauss 1991
Reading	National Adult Reading Test	Nelson, 1978, 1991
	Wide Range Achievement Test: Reading	Wilkinson, 1993
Writing	Boston Diagnostic Aphasia Examination: Cookie Theft Picture	Goodglass, Kaplan, 1983

7.5. Thinking and intelligence

It is possible to use Wechsler intelligence scales WAIS-R and WAIS-III, or their respective abbreviated versions. These tests are too demanding for patients early after SAH, and it is, therefore, advised to choose only one of the subtests and to postpone a complex evaluation after patient's sufficient recovery. The variety of Wechslers tests are usually administered between 6 and 84 months after SAH (Stenhouse et al., 1991).

Table 14. Tests of thinking

Concept formation	California Proverb Test	Delis, Kaplan, Kramer, 2001
Verbal	WAIS: Similarities	Wechsler, 1955,1981,1997
Concept formation	Category Test	Halstead, 1947; Reitan, Wolfson, 1993
Visual	Raven Progressive Matrices	Raven, 1996
Sort and shift	Sorting Test	Delis, Kaplan, Kramer, 2001
	Wisconsin Card Sorting Test	Berg, 1948
Reasoning	WAIS: Comprehension	Wechsler, 1955,1981,1997
Verbal Reasoning	WAIS: Picture Completion, Picture Arrangement	Corsini, Renck, 1992 Wechsler, 1955,1981,1997

7.6. Premorbid Intelligence

From the knowledge of pathophysiology of SAH and its sudden onset, it is clear that there are no means to test patients before SAH occurs, and thus there can be no comparison between premorbid results and the status after the recovery. The only information available is data and feedback from the family and relatives. The only areas with a possibility of pre-op/post-op testing are accidental findings of aneurysms and selective operations (patients with and intact aneurysm, no SAH, and a scheduled operation). In this setting, we can evaluate the influence of the operation, but not of the SAH (there is no bleeding).

These are methods usually used for evaluation of premorbid intelect (Snyder, Nussbaum, 2003):

I) Life history approaches
1) Indicators of socioeconomic status
a) Academic evolution Evaluates achieved education, problems at school, average grades.
b) Indicators of employment

Highest rank achieved at work, changes in effectivity at work

2) Medical history
a) Birth and early development;
Abnormalities in early development, Apgar score, perinatal trauma if present
b) Comorbidity;

diseases with relation to cognitive development, pervasive developmental disorders, phenylketonuria, childhood injuries to the head.

3) Other demographic entries:

Age, sex, race, education, residence.

4) Other sources:
   Records of standardized tests (school, army, etc.)

II) Methods of estimation

1) Information/Vocabulary scatter

Based on a variance of the results of other Wechsler subtests with respect to Vocabulary and Information.

2) Methods of best performance based on the comparison of different markers (test methods, anamnesis, and observation). We get the best performance of all tasks, and we set this performance as the marker of the premorbid status. This method has its obvious limitations, but it also has advantages (Lezak, 2004). It belongs to the most simple, but it is not really possible to use this method in healthy subjects.

III) Approaches working with actual capabilities

1) National Adult Reading Test

NART is, by origin, a British test of reading and pronunciation, which consists of 50 simple and phonematically irregular words. Previous exposure and active knowledge of the word is necessary for proper pronunciation. This test is supposed to show premorbid (mostly education-based) intellect performance.

The test was developed based on observations of patients with dementia, where the ability to read suffers much less than lexical knowledge. We prepare the Czech version of the NART (Kramska, 2007, 2009).

1. National Adult Reading Test—Revised (NART-R) Modification by Blair and Spreen (1989) with North American pronunciation.
2. Wide Range Achievement Test—Revised (WRAT-R, Jastak, Wilkinson, 1984)

The test consists of words that both follow general rules of pronunciation and do not. Reading subtest score can be transformed to a standard score (average 100, SD 15).

IV) Combination of life history and today´s approaches

1) Combination of NART and variables of life history. Uses the results of NART and a system of regression equations for demographic variables such as sex, social group, education (Crawford et al., 1989).
2) Combination of American NART version (AMNART) and a variables of life history (Grober, Sliwinski, 1991)

Demographic parameters for an estimation of premorbid capabilities are based on regression equations with known data such as age, race, sex, education, job, etc. These are very specific to a particular culture. On the left side of the equation, we can find IQ, on the right side, demographic parameters. Modern standardization of the tests of intelligence count with demographic influences, and the data is gained from test persons. The method is used on a research basis rather than clinically.

7.7. Neuropsychological Evaluation of the Executive Functions (Frontal Lobe Functions)

This is very important in SAH population. Many aneurysms involve anterior circulation and a feeding artery for the major part of the frontal lobes (a cerebri anterior). The ischemic injury can be caused by occlusion of severe and prolonged vasospasm of the vessel. Methods included should be sensitive to frontal-cortical dysfunctions. It is still unclear which method is the best. The most often used are tests of fluency (Benton, 1968), Labyrints (1950), Go/NoGo tasks (Drewe, 1975) and Wisconsin Card Sorting Test (Heaton et al., 1993).

Table 15. Neuropsychological diagnostics of frontal lobe functions (Hütter, 2000)

Standardized	Non-standardized
Wisconsin Card Sorting Test (WCST)	Tower of Hanoi task
Heaton et al., 1993)	Anzai, Simon (1979), Shallice (1982)
Go/NoGo test	Mental rotation tasks
Drewe (1975)	Shepard, Metzler (1971)
Halstead Categories test	Clinical interwievs, proxy ratings
Halstead (1947)	Lezak (1982), Hutter, Gilsbach (1995, a,b)
Porteus Labyrinth test	Labyrinth tasks
Porteus (1950)	Walsh (1987), Karnath, Zimmermann, Wallesch (1991)
Benton Word Fluency test	Estimaton tasks
Benton (1968)	Smith, Milner (1984)
Stroop test (FWIT)	Behavioral observation
Bäumler (1985), Jensen, Hohwer (1966)	Luria (1970), Goldberg, Costa (1986)
Tower of London	
Culbertson, Zillmer, (2001)	
Design Fluency Test	
Delis, Kaplan, Kramer (2001)	
Frontal Assessment Battery	
Dubois, Slachevsky, (2000)	

The Word fluency Test (WFT) shows the highest sensitivity for organic damage to frontal lobes of the brain (Crockett et al., 1986; Benton, 1968).

7.8. Personality and Emotivity Disorders in Patients after SAH

This area was not in the scope of neuropsychology until recently (Prigatano, 1986, 1999). The studies focused more on psychiatric symptoms and not specific neuropsychological disorders (Storey, 1967; Okawa et al., 1980). Nearly all psychodiagnostic methods are developed for patients without organic damage to the brain.

The major target is the mapping of emotional adaptation, behavior, personal experience and personality characteristics. SAH represents a very strong existential experience. The emotional status can be altered not only by organic causes but purely by psychological trauma with fears of another bleeding and then death.

The sudden onset of bleeding without any signs of prior warning symptoms can produce signs similar to the post-traumatic stress disorder (McMillan, 1996).

Most often seen psychopathological signs are apathy, organic personality changes, mood and emotional disbalances (can be organically based), affective lability, psychosocial maladjustments, aggression, loss of initiative (King et al., 2005).

These changes are most often connected with damage to frontal lobes with apathy and emotional indifference being prominent symptoms.

Blumer and Benson (1975) distinguish two types of brain damage based on which part of frontal lobes is affected.

1. dorsolateral area—apathy, loss of initiative, inability of long-term planning, loss of emotional robustness. Authors speak of pseudo-depression.
2. frontal-orbital region—egoistic, careless behavior, aggressive, combined with sexually explicit humor. The authors call this type of behavior as pseudo-psychopathic.

In the study of Hütter and Gilsbach (1995a), patients after SAH and with an infarct to the frontal lobe presented a significantly lower rate of depression and cared less about their health, and they even considered themselves as equally affected as other patients.

Table 16. Methods focused on personality psychopathology and emotions

Depression Scales	Beck Depression Inventory	Beck, Steer, Brown, 1996
	Geriatric Depression Scale	Yesavage et al., 1983
Psychiatric Scales	Minnesota Multiphasic	Butcher et al., 1989
	Personality Inventory	Graham, 1990
	Sickness Impact Profile	Bergner et al., 1981
	Symptom Check List-90-R	Derogatis, 1994

8. Quality of Life (QOL) in Patients after SAH

As neuropsychological diagnostics evolve, there are emerging areas suitable for neuropsychological therapy as well. All of the patients are seen and treated by neurologists who have no means (and no interest) to answer areas outside their scope. However, changes in emotivity, moods and cognitive performance have a major influence on the family, partners and general social relations. It is clear that proper care by a specialist can influence these interactions dramatically. Analysis and proper evaluation of a patient's final status has an important role for nursing persons, families and, last but not least, taxpayers.

In the studies available, the major neuropsychological effects of SAH are described in surprising detail. However, the implications of neuropsychological diagnoses on the patient´s quality of life (WHO 1980) are still clouded. Psychological follow-up of the patient is closely linked to QOL. By its nature, this area inevitably falls into the scope of a neuropsychologist. However, proper evaluation of QOL brings many additional variables into play, making neuropsychologists' work (and related research) even more complex.

Very few studies include instruments for QOL evaluation, the tests are diverse and include anything between semi-structurized dialogues and standardized tests. The timing of the evaluation also varies widely (two weeks to one year).

Buchanan et al. (2000) tried to follow studies evaluating personality changes, psychological distress and family dispositions. The main target of the research was to 1) evaluate the origin and extent of personality changes from the viewpoint of the patient himself and close relatives, too; 2) to capture patient's psychosocial functions again from the viewpoint of the patient and the relatives; 3) to evaluate a degree of overall psychosocial distress in patient's close relatives; 4) to measure a degree of family dispositions 5) to compare future perspectives to actual psychological results.

Hellawell et al. (1999) used a self-evaluating scale HISC (Head Injury Symptom Checklist), commonly used in patients after traumatic brain injury (TBI), assuming patients with SAH have the same problems. They also used Relative's Questionnaire (RQ) to evaluate everyday situations with respect to the premorbid lifestyle and work stress, and finally evaluation of the stress felt by the relatives. It was a stress presented among the relatives of patients after TBI presented, and a significant factor with close relations to the changes of behavior and psychological functions. In their follow-up of 193 patients and 18 relatives treated by coil, Raaymakers et al. (2000) evaluated a negative effect of the neurological evaluation itself, handicap and invalidity by Rankin Scale and Barthel index, QOL by Sickness Impact Profile (SIP) and SF-36. Hop et al. (2001) followed 64 patients after SAH with an average mean time of examination of 18 months (modified Rankin Scale–mRS) in 48 patients and 35 nursing personnel, they evaluated QOL by SF-36, Sickness Impact Profile (SIP) and Visual Analog Scale. These results were compared with measurements after four months. There was an improvement of subjectively experienced QOL between 4 and 18 months after SAH.

Barthel index and Rankin scale are reliable and valid methods usually used in neurology. SIP is a test of 136 issues focusing on QOL in 12 domains—sleep/rest, emotional behavior, body care and sport, coping with household, motoric abilities, social interactions, communication, ability to walk, agility and behavior, work, recreation time, food intake. SIP describes the quality of life in terms of behavior and reflects changes in time.

Medical outcomes study short form 36 (SF-36) is 36-item self-evaluation scale focused on the subjective view of health. It involves eight areas—physical and social functions, limited functions due to physical problems, limited functions due to psychical problems, psychical health, vitality, pain and an overall view of health.

In contemporary research, QOL scales include Quality of Well-Being; Self-Administered SF-12 is a 12-item downscale of SF 36, which is considered reliable and valid for SAH patients (King et al, 2005). Study of Hütter et al. (1995), based on the model of Flanagan (Flanagan 1975, 1982), utilized a systematic psychometric evaluation of QOL and cognitive capacity. They used an 11-item scale parallel for patients and family members as a control of the patients (Mc Glynn, Schacter, 1989). The results show a reduced quality of life in several aspects: feeling of uncertainty in social relations (39%), limitations of free-time activities (52%), limitations of psychical capacity (47%), concentration of attention (70%), reduction of interest in everyday problems and their solutions (47%), loss of motivation (50%), problems in coordination and delicate motor tasks (25%), sleep disorders (47%), feeling of lack of information about the disease, headaches (77%) and body problems.

Methods focused on HRQOL (Hütter, 2000)

Medical Outcome Study (MOS) Short Form 36 (SF-36)	Anderson et al., 1996
Quality of Well-Being, Self-Administered SF-12	
EORTC Euro Quol (QLCQ -30)	Dorman et al., 1996
Nottingham Health Profile	Ebrahim et al. (1986)
Aachen Life Quality Inventory for Aphasic (ALQI-A)	Hütter et al. (1995)
Subjective Quality of Life Analysis	Zannotti, 1995
Sickness Impact Profile (SIP)	Visser et al. (1996)

9. Rehabilitation of Patients after SAH

Bahavioral assessment is concerned with identifying and measuring problem behaviors encountered in the everyday lives of those, who have suffered injury to the brain. Assessment is conducted in order to answer specific question, the nature of the question posed in any particular case will determine the assessment tool or procedure adopted (Wilson et al., 2003). Neuropsychological assessment answers different questions, which are required in rehabilitation:

a) Is this person intellectually impaired?
b) What is the predicted level of premorbid functioning?
c) What kind of language, reading, perceptual and memory disorder does this person have?
d) Which cognitive skills remain intact or appear less damaged?
e) How does this person compare with others of the same age and/or others with the same diagnosis?
f) Is the score in a particular test in the abnormal range?
g) Is failure on a particular test due to a disorder of comprehension, recognition, planning or memory?
h) Is the person faking or exaggerating problems?

One of the main neuropsychological questions in patients with SAH is whether there is an improvement in the early diagnosed neuropsychological deficits and, if yes, whether these can be resolved completely in time. The subsequent question is whether there are any specific characteristics of SAH-induced neuropathology.

There is a large amount of studies showing that there can be persistent residual neuropsychological deficits, but there is still chance of improvement over more than two to three years after the insult.

In series of 93 patients with aphasia (either treated or not treated by a logopedist), there was also a subgroup of patients after SAH. This subgroup showed several specifics, mainly great variability in the course of the therapy and overall satisfactory results as compared to the traumatic brain injury group. Severe and persistent aphasias were associated with left MCA aneurysm ruptures (Kertesz, McCabe, 1977).

According to Busch (1987), the prognosis of rehabilitation in patients with cerebrovascular disorders remains worse in comparison with a tumor and TBI cases. In the series of 171 patients receiving rehabilitation after SAH, over 24% were presented with fatic disorder and 38% with organic psycho-syndrome. The results of the study are not fully coherent due to inclusion of patients after the rupture of the aneurysm, but they provide a source for the indication of rehabilitation: Bush found out the improvement of aphasia in 36%, improvement of cognitive functions in 49% and resolution of organic psycho-syndrome during a seven-week rehabilitation in 36% of cases (Bush, 1987). Only 11% of patients regained their working capabilities. However, at the same time, only 11% of patients recovered to their full working capacity. These results only cover cases with mild cognitive deficit. Although there is a clear effect of cognitive rehabilitation, it is seldom effective enough to allow the patients to re-enter their previous positions at work.

Another study of Hampl et al. (1990) advocates a use of an intensive cognitive rehabilitation, as it has an important influence on final outcome; however, the results show no influence on the rate of return to work—47% with rehabilitation vs. 48%.

All of the studies are usually focused on three main areas: physical damage, psychological disorders and impairments of everyday life and social functions. The rehabilitation of patients after SAH should consider all of these areas, and it should start as soon as possible.

Neuropsychologists dealing with acute phase at the departments of neurosurgery should consider bed-sided assessment and interventions for following disorders:

Speech impairment: once diagnosed, a logopedist should be involved as soon as patient's status allows. The neuropsychologist can make further differential diagnostics of the disorder and help to target the rehabilitation accordingly.

Memory impairments: early diagnostics of memory disturbance should be focused on further specification of the problem (instilment or evocation area), which compound of the memory is affected the most (semantic, explicit, implicit, auditive or visual). Based on these results, it is possible to design training and compensation strategies.

Executive functions disorders: mostly concerns planning, ability to organize and to analyze the results of one's efforts and to gain experience. This area is crucial for emotional and social adaptation (Sohlberg, 1989), and it is a cornerstone of overall cognitive performance profile.

Targets of rehabilitation (Hütter, 2000):

1) restoration of impaired functions
2) optimalization of residual functions
3) acquisition of new strategies for compensation of persistent impairments
4) improvement of persistence
5) acquisition of coping strategies
6) encouragement of coping with illness
7) information about causes and consequences of the illness
8) acquisition of adaptive illness behavior

9) adjustment to the affordance of work and daily life in relation to the functional capacities of the patient
10) support of professional reintegration

Both somatic and cognitive rehabilitations should start in the early postoperative period, as soon as the patient's status allows. All steps of rehabilitation should be followed for a feedback and a possibility to form general conclusions. The target of the somatic and cognitive efforts is the same: restitution of patient's previous social and occupational level. The problem is, according to Wilson (2003), that standardized neuropsychological tests cannot answer questions such as the following: How is the person with brain injury and the family affected by the cognitive or neuropsychological problems identified? Can the patient return home or continue with schooling? What treatment methods should be employed? How should be efficacy or treatment be measured?

The best option seems to be rehabilitation on outpatient basis, which allows immersion of the patient into a well-known home environment, and it activates all the relatives and brings them into the rehabilitation process. The ultimate goal of cognitive rehabilitation is not an isolated improvement of a specific cognitive scale measurement, but facilitation of the wide re-integration of the patient into his/her natural environment.

Conclusion

Developments in medical care and management of patients with SAH have substantially improved the prognosis of this severe disease. This fact brings new research areas on one side and the influence on everyday family life on the other.

The purpose of the text is to map the problems of SAH, aetiology, pathogenesis, history, general course of the disease, possibilities of treatment, methods of neuropsychological assessment, prognosis and influence of the disease on a patient and his/her relatives and families. Even though we deal with a single medical entity, we face a very diverse pool of patients, with very different results and fates.

It is clear that it is not only a neurological status of the patient that matters. There is a whole other world of neuropsychological and psychosocial issues with a surprisingly strong influence on a patient´s life. Around one-third to half of the patients after SAH present with cognitive deficits in many areas, predominantly in memory and attention. Concerning emotional evaluation, there is a question of proper tests and the influence of the awareness of the insult, and some studies show similarities with post-traumatic stress disorder (PTSD). However, diagnostics cannot be restricted only to the area of raw intelligence. It is not only the pure brain hemorrhage or ischemia that produces problems, and some of the major issues can extend beyond a hospital stay, into patient's social relations, working and financial opportunities, and form a complex sphere of the quality of life.

Some of the results suggest that there is no difference in cognitive deficits between the two main treatment modalities, and others suggest the opposite; the results are not definitive yet. However, it is clear that there is a very strong influence of the initial condition of the patient and a severity of complications, especially vasospasms (Hütter 2000; Ogden et al., 1997).

Despite all the inventions of contemporary medicine, the damaged areas of the brain cannot be routinely displayed, and it is the function (with neuropsychological methods as diagnostic tools) that matters the most.

Early neuropsychological diagnostics and systematic longitudinal follow-ups, availability of consultations and focused cognitive and social rehabilitation should become standard in the complex care of this group of patients.

Study is supported by Czech Science Foundation GAČR 406/07/1444

References

Adams CBT, Loach AB, O´Laire S. Intracranial aneurysm: analysis of results of microneurosurgery. *Brit. Med. J.* 1976; 2: 607-609.

Bamford JM, Sandercock P., Jones L., Warlow C. The natural history of lacunar infarction: The Oxfordshire Community Stroke Project Stroke 1987;18:545-551.

Barbarotto R., De Santis A., Laiacona M., Basso A., Spagnoli D., Capitani E. Neuropsychological follow-up of patients operated for aneurysm of the middle cerebral artery and posterior communicating artery. *Cortex* 1989; 25: 275-288.

Bellebaum, C., Schäfers, L., Schoch, B., Wanke, I., Stolke, D., Forsting, M. and Daum, I. Clipping vs. Coiling: Neuropsychological follow-up after aneurysmal subarachnoid hemorrhage (SAH). *Journal of Clinical and Experimental Neuropsychology,* 2004; 26, 1081-1092.

Benson and D. Blumer, eds. Psychiatric Aspects of Neurologic Disease. New York: Grune and Stratton, 1975.

Berry E., Jones RAC, West CGH, Brown JDK. Outcome of subarchnoid hemorrhage. An analysis of surgical variables, cognitive and emotional sequale related to SPECT scanning. *Br. J. Neurosurgery* 1997;115:378–387.

Bornstein RA, Weir BKA, Petruk KC, Disney LB. Neuropsychological function in patients after subarachnoid hemorrhage. *Neurosurgery* 1987; 21:651–654.

Brickenkamp R. Test d2 Aufmerksamkeits-Belastungs-Test. Göttingen: Hogreve, 1978.

Brinker T., Seifert V., Dietz H. Cerebral blood flow and intracranial pressure during experimental subarachnoid hemorrhage. *Acta Neurochir.* (Wien) 1992;115:47-52.

Broadbent D E. Perception and communication. London: Pergamon Press, 1958.

Buchanan KM, Elias LJ, Doplen GB. Differing perspectives on outcome after subarachnoid hemorrhage: The patient, the relative, the neurosurgeon. *Neurosurgery* 2000; 46: 831-838.

Carter BS, Buckley D., Ferraro R. Factors associated with reintegration to normal living after subarachnoid hemorrhage. *Neurosurgery* 2000;46:1326–1334.

Cavanagh SJ, Vickie LG. Grading Scales in the Management of Aneurysmal Subarachnoid Hemorrhage: A critical Review. *Journal of Neuroscience Nursing* 2002; 34: 288-295

De Luca J. Cognitive dysfunction after aneurysm of the anterior communicating artery. *J. Clin. Neuropsychol.* 1992; 14: 924-934.

De Santis A., Laiacona M., Barbarotto R. et al. Neuropsychological outcome of patients operated upon for an intracranial aneurysm. *J. Neurol. Neurosurg. Psychiatry* 1989: 52: 1135-40.

Dombovy ML, Drew-Cates J., Serdans R. Recovery and rehabilitation following subarachnoid hemorrhage: part II long-term follow up. *Brain Injury* 1998;12:887–894.

Dott NM, Intracranial aneurysms: cerebral arterio-radiography: surgical treatment. *Edinburgh Med. J.* 1933; 40:219-234.

Egge A., Waterloo K., Sjoholm H., Ingebrigsten T., Forsdahl S., Jacobsen EA, Romner B. Outcome one year after aneurysmal subarachnoid hemorrhage: relation between cognitive performance and neuroimaging. *Acta Neurol. Scand.* 2005; 112: 76-80.

Fisher CM, Kistler JP, Davis JM. Relation of cerebral vasospasm to subarachnoid hemorrhage visualized by computerized tomographic scanning. *Neurosurgery* 1980;6:l-9.

Flanagan JC. Measurement of quality of life: current state of the art. *Arch. Phys. Med. Rehab.* 1982; 63: 173-5.

Flanagan JC. The concept of quality of life for American community members. *Social Indicators* 1975; 63:56-9.

Frazer D., Ahuja A., Watkins L., Cipolotti L. Coiling versus clipping for the treatment of aneurysmal subarachnoid hemorrhage: a longitudinal investigation into cognitive outcome *Neurosurgery* 2007; 60(3):434-41.

Gade A. Amnesia after operations on aneurysms of the anterior communicating artery. *Surg. Neurol.* 1982; 18: 46-49.

Hamburger C., Schönberger J., Lange M. Management and prognosis of intracranial giant aneurysms. A report on 58 cases. *Neurosurg .Rev.* 15:97-103, 1992.

Hellawell D., Taylor R., Pentland B. Persisting symptoms and carer's, views of outcome after subarachnoid hemorrhage. *Clin. Rehab.* 1999;13:333–340.

Hop JV, Rinkel GJE, Algra A, Gin J. Changes in functional outcome and quality of life in patients and caregivers after aneurysmal subarachnoid hemorrhage, *J. Neurosurg.* 2001; 95: 957-963.

Hornyak M., Gilsbach J., Harders A. Clinical significance of computed tomography in early aneurysm surgery. *Neurochirurgia (Stuttg).* 1991 Sep;34(5):135-40.

Hütter B., Gilsbach J. Which neuropsychological deficits are hidden behind a good outcome (Glasgow=I) after aneurysmal subarachnoid hemorrhage? *Neuropsychology.* 1993; 7: 273–295.

Hütter BO, Gilsbach JM, Kreitschmann I. Quality of life and cognitive deficits after subarchnoid hemorrhage. *Brit. J. Neurosur.* 1995; 9: 465-475.

Hütter BO, Gilsbach JM. Early neuropsychological sequelae of aneurysm surgery and subarachnoid hemorrhage. Acta Neurochir (Wien). 1996;138(12):1370-8; discussion 1378-9.

Hütter BO, Kreitschmann-Andermahr I., Gilsbach JM. Cognitive deficits in the acute stage after subarachnoid hemorrhage. *Neurosurgery* 1998;43:1054–1064.

Hütter BO, Kreitschmann-Andermahr I., Mayfrank L., Rohde V., Spetzger U., Gilsbach JM. Functional outcome after aneurysmal subarachnoid hemorrhage. *Acta Neurochir. Suppl.* 1999;72:157-74.

Chan, A. S., Ho, S., Poon, W. S. Neuropsychological sequelae of patients treated with microsurgical clipping or endovascular embolization for anterior communicating artery aneurysm. *Eur .Neurol.* 2002;47:37-44.

Chyatte D., Chen TL, Bronstein K., Brass LM. Seasonal fluctuation in the incidence of intracranial aneurysm rupture and its relationship to changing climatic conditions. *J. Neurosurg.* 1994; 81:525-530.

Jennett B., Bond M. Assessment of outcome after severe brain damage. *Lancet* 1975; 1: 480-484.

Jennett, B.., Snoek J., et al. Disability after severe head injury: observations on the use of the Glasgow Outcome Scale. *J. Neurol. Neurosurg. Psychiatry* 1981; 44(4): 285-93.

Kassell NF, Torner JC, Haley EC Jr, Adams HP. The international cooperative study on the timing of aneurysm surgery. Part 2 : Surgical results. *J. Neurosurg.* 1990; 73 : 37-47. a.

Kassell NF, Torner JC, Haley EC Jr. The international cooperative study on the timing of aneurysm surgery. Part 1 : Overall management results. J Neurosurg 1990; 73 : 18-36. b.

Kim C., Cervos-Navarro J., Patzold C., Tokuriki Y., Takebe Y., Hori K. In vivo study of flow pattern at human carotid artery bifurcation with regard to aneurysm development. *Acta Neurochir.* (Wien) 1992;115:112–117.

Kim DH, Haney CL, Ginhoven GV. Utility of outcome measures after treatment for intracranial aneurysms: a prospective trial involving 520 patients. *Stroke.* 2005; Apr;36(4):792-6.

Kim JM, Kang SD. Benefits of antifibrinolytic therapy before early aneurysm surgery. *J. Korean Neurosurg. Soc.* 2001; 30 : 729-732.

King JT, Horowitz MB, Kassam AB, Yonas H., Roberts MS. The Short Form-12 and the measurement of health status in patients with cerebral aneurysms: performance, validity and reliability. *J. Neurosurg.* 2005; 102: 489-494.

Koivisto T., Vanninen R., Hurskainen H., Saari T., Hernesniemi J., Vapalahti M. Outcomes of early endovascular versus surgical treatment of ruptured cerebral aneurysms. A prospective randomized study. *Stroke.* 2000 Oct;31(10):2369-77.

Kramska, L. The possibilities of evaluation of premorbid intellect in patients after subarrachnoid hemorrhage. Design of Czech version of the NART. Dissertation thesis. FF UK Prague, 2009.

Krámská L. Preiss M. Evaluation of premorbid status—word reading test. *Psychiatrie* 2007; 11: 4-8.

Le Roux PD, Elliot JP, Newell DW, Grady MS, Winn HR. The incidence of surgical complications is similar in good and poor grade patients undergoing repair of ruptured anterior circulation aneurysms: a retrospective review of 355 patients. *Neurosurgery.* 1996 May;38(5):887-93; discussion 893-5.

Lee KC, Joo JY, Huh SG, Lee KS. Surgical experience of 1,000 cases of intracranial aneurysm. *J. Korean Neurosurg. Soc.* 1992; 12 : 1599-1606.

Lindqvist G., Norlen G. Korsakoff's syndrome after operation on ruptured aneurysm of anterior communicating artery. *Acta psychiat. scand.* 1966; 42, 24-34.

Linn FH, Rinkel GJ, Algra A., et al. Incidence of subarachnoid hemorrhage: role of region, year, and rate of computed tomography: A meta-analysis *Stroke* 1996;27:625-629

Ljunggren B., Sonesson B., Saveland H., Brandt L. Cognitive impairment and adjustment in patients without neurological deficits. *J. Neurosurg.* 1985;62:673–679.

Logue V., Durward M., Pratt RT, Piercy M., Nixon WL. The quality of survival after rupture of an anterior cerebral aneurysm. *Br. J. Psychiatry* 1968; 114: 137–60.

Luria, A. R. (1976). The neuropsychology of memory. Washington D. C.: V. H. Winston and Sons, 1976.

Mahoney FI, Barthel D. "Functional evaluation: The Barthel Index." *Maryland State Medical Journal* 1965;14:56-61.

Marchel A., Bidzinski J., Bojarski P. Formation of new aneurysms: report of five cases. *Acta Neurochirugia* (Wien) 1991;112:96–99.

Mavaddat N., Kirkpatrick PJ, Rogers RD. Deficits in decision-making in patients with aneurysm at the anterior communicating artery. *Brain* 2000;123:2109–2117.

Mc Glynn SM, Schacter DL. Unawareness of deficits in neuropsychological syndromes. *J. Clin. Exper. Neuropsychol.* 1989; 11: 143-205.

McCormick WF. Pathology of closed head injury. In: Wilkins RH, Rengachary SS (eds) Neurosurgery. 1985; McGraw-Hill, New York, pp 1544-1570.

McKenna P., Willison JR, Phil B., Lowe D., Neil-Dwyer G. Cognitive outcome and quality of life one year after subarachnoid hemorrhage. *Neurosurgery* 1989;24:361–367.

McMillan TM. Post-traumatic stress disorder following minor and severe closed head injury: 10 single cases. *Brain Injury* 1996; 10:749-758.

Mesulam, M. Frontal cortex and behavior. *Ann. Neurol.* 1986; 19 (4), 320-325.

Mizukami M., Kawase T., Usami I., Tazawa T. Prevention of vasospasm by early operation with removal of subarachnoid blood. *Neurosurgery* 1982;10:301—307.

Norlen, C., Lindqvist, C. The anatomy of memory. Lancet, 1964; 1, 335.

Ogden JA, Mee EW, Henning M. A prospective study of impairment of cognition and memory and recovery after subarachnoid hemorrhage. Neurosurgery 1993;33:572–587.a.

Ogden JA, Mee EW, Henning M. A prospective study of psychosocial adaptation following subarachnoid hemorrhage. *Neuropsychological Rehab. 1*994, 4: 7–30.

Ogden JA, Utley T., Mee EW. Neurological and psychosocial outcome 4 to 5 years after subarachnoid hemorrhage. *Neurosurgery* 1997; 41: 25-34.

Ogden, JA, Mee EW, Henning M. "Life-Events Stress: A Significant Precursor to subarachnoid hemorrhage. *Neuropsychiatry Neuropsychol. Behav. Neurol.* 1993; 6: 219-228.b.

Okawa M., Maeda S., Nukui H., Kawafuchi J. Psychiatric symptoms in ruptured anterior communicating aneurysms: social prognosis Acta Psychiatrica Scandinavica 1980; 61 (4) 306–312.

Okawa M., Maeda S., Nukui H, Kawafuchi J. Psychiatric symptoms in ruptured anterior communicating aneurysms: social prognosis. Acta Psychiatr Scand 1980; 61: 306–12.

Penrose R., Storey P. Emotional disturbance and subarachnoid hemorrhage. *Psychother. Psychosom.* 1970;18:321-325.

Posner MI, Rothbart MK. Research on attention networks as a model for the integration of psychological science. *Annu. Rev. Psychol.* 2007; Vol. 58: 1-23.

Prigatano GP, Fordyce DJ, Zeiwer HK, et al. Neuropsychological Rehabilitation After Brain Injury. Baltimore, Md: Johns Hopkins University Press; 1986.

Prigatano GP. Principles of Neuropsychological Rehabilitation. New York: Oxford University Press; 1999.

Raaymakers TWM, MARS study group. Functional outcome and quality of life after angiography and operation for unruptured intracranial aneurysm. *J. Neurol. Neurosur. Psychiatry.* 2000; 68: 571-576.

Richardson JTE. Cognitive performance following rupture and repair of intracranial aneurysm. *Acta Neurol. Scand.* 1991;83:110–122.

Rinkel GJ, van Gijn J., Wijdicks EF. Subarachnoid hemorrhage without detectable aneurysm. A review of the causes. *Stroke* 1993; 24: 1403–9.

Ronkainen A., Niskanen M., Rinne J., Koivisto, T., Hernesniemi J., Vapalahti M. Evidence for excess long-term mortality after treated subarachnoid hemorrhage. *Stroke* 2001;32:2850-3.

Ropper AH, Zervas NT. Outcome one year after SAH from cerebral aneurysm: management morbidity, mortality and functional status in 112 consecutive good-risk patients. *J. Neurosurg.* 1984; 60: 909-915.

Samra, Satwant K., Giordani B., Caveney AF, Clarke WR, Scott PA, Anderson S., Thompson BG, Todd MM. Recovery of Cognitive Function After Surgery for Aneurysmal Subarachnoid Hemorrhage. *Stroke* 2007; 38(6):1864-1872.

Sanchez CE, Oglivy CS, Carter BS. Outcomes studies in cerebrovascular neurosurgery. *Neurosurg. Focus* 2007; 22 (3):E11.

Sengupta RP, Chiu JSP, Brierley H. Quality of survival. following direct surgery for anterior communicating artery aneurysms. *J. Neurosurg.* 1975; 43:58-66.

Shapiro SA, Campbell RL, Scully T. Hemorrhagic dilation of fourth ventricle. *J. Neurosurg.* 1994; 80:805-809.

Solheim O., Eloqayli H., Muller TB., Unsgaard G. Quality of life after treatment for incidental, unruptured intracranial aneurysms. *Acta Neurochir.* 2006; 148: 821-830.

Sonesson B., Ljunggren B., Saveland H. Cognition and adjustment and early operation for ruptured aneurysm. *Neurosurgery* 1987;21:279–287.

Sonesson B., Säveland H., Ljunggren B., Brandt L. Cognitive functioning after subrachnoid hemorrhage of unknown origin. *Acta Neurol. Scand.* 1989;80:400-410.

Stenhouse LM, Knight RG, Longmore BE, Bishara SN. Long-term cognitive deficits in patients after surgery on aneurysms of the anterior communicating artery. *J. Neurol. Neurosurg. Psychiatry* 1991; 54:909—914.

Storey PB. Psychiatric sequelae of subarchnoid hemorrhage. *Brit. Med. J.* 1967;3:261–266.

Stuss DT, Alexander MP, Lieberman A., Levine H. An extraordinary form of confabulation. *Neurology*, 1978; 28: 116-172.

Talland GA, Sweet WH, Ballantine HT. Amnestic syndrome with anterior communicating artery aneurysm. *J. Nerv. Ment. Dis.* 1967;114:137-160.

Taylor CL, Selman WR, Kiefer SP, Ratcheson RA: Temporary vessel occlusion during intracranial aneurysm repair. *Neurosurgery* 1996; 39:893-906.

Taylor CL, Yuan Z., Selman WR, Ratcheson RA, Rimm AA: Cerebral arterial aneurysm formation and rupture in 20,767 elderly patients: hypertension and other risk factors. *J. Neurosurg.* 1995; 83:812-819.

Testa C., Andreoli A., Arista A., Limoni P., Tognetti F. Overall results in 304 consecutive patients with acute spontaneous subarachnoid hemorrhage. *Surg. Neurol.* 1985; 24: 377-385.

Teunissen LL, Rinkel GJE, Algra A., van Gijn J. Risk factors for subarachnoid hemorrhage: a systematic review. *Stroke* 1996; 27: 544-9.

Vilkki J., Holst P., Ohman J. et al. Cognitive deficits related to computed tomographic findings after surgery for a ruptured intracranial aneurysm. *J. Neurol. Neurosurg. Psychiatry* 1989;52:1135-1140

Vilkki J., Holst P., Ohman J., Servo A., Heiskanen O. Social outcome related to cognitive performance and computed tomographic findings after surgery for a ruptured intracranial aneurysm. *Neurosurgery* 1990;26:579–585.

Walton. The Korsakov syndrome in spontaneous subarachnoid hemorrhage. *J. Ment. Sci.* 1953; 99, 521.

Wermer MJ, Kool H., Albrecht KW et al; Subarachnoid hemorrhage treated with clipping: long-term effects on employment, relationships, personality, and mood. *Neurosurgery.* 2007; Jan;60(1):91-7.

Wilson B., Herbert C.M., Shiel A. Behavioural Approaches in Neuropsychological Rehabilitation. New York: Psychology Press; 2003.

World Health Organization. International classification of impairments, disabilities and handicaps. A manual of classification relating to the consequences of disease. Geneva: WHO, 1980.

Yasargil MG (ed): Microneurosurgery. New York, G. Thieme, 1984, vol I, pp 72-96.

In: Cognitive Deficit in Mental and Neurological Disorders ISBN: 978-1-60741-957-0
Editors: H. Kucerova, M. Preiss

Chapter XIV

Traumatic Brain Impairment

Petr Kulistak

1.1. Abstract

Cognitive functions impairment as a consequence of a head/brain injury represents a wide-ranging and heterogeneous spectrum of disorders. Seriousness of such disorders, as well as their duration and extent of recovery, depend on both the severity of the trauma itself (i.e., on a primary process) and consequent events inside the skull (i.e., on a secondary impact). In general taxonomy, severe, moderate, and mild forms of traumatic impairment are described. The severe head injuries have their structural correlates visible on CT (Computed Tomography) or MRI (Magnetic Resonance Imaging) – —it is an impaired parenchyma. The moderate and mild forms, as well as a so-called diffuse axonal impairment (DAI), do not need to have a structural finding. They can be thus even more dangerous, since such sufferers are only rarely neuropsychologically explored. Moreover, they are often not medically examined at all or they are considered as healthy and without any damage when leaving a medical institution. Incidence of mild brain injuries is ever more frequent as a result of increasing popularity of sports activities of all kinds (especially of the adrenaline ones preferred by the young generation, in which the health hazard is even higher), as well as of strong pressure of media, which emphasize that sport contributes to health maintenance. Neuropsychological evaluation of a person with a head/brain traumatic impairment usually finds deficiencies in the following areas: attention/concentration, memory/learning, and executive functions. Furthermore, also cognitive domains, such as thinking, language, visuospatial abilities, mathematics, etc., may be affected. Additional problems in emotional living and behavior (irritability, impulsiveness, apathy, loss of motivation, lack of interest in the others) can even lead tdo psychotic disorders (mania, touchiness, delusions) in some cases. Depressions and suicidal thoughts are not rare. The neuropsychological examination itself begins with a detailed interview – —with a patient, their relatives or a partner, or with their friends – — and should lead to a "holistically integrated neuropsychological evaluation" (Klonoff, Dawson, 2004). Collection of such an amount of data is necessary especially in mild forms of head and brain impairments, since a relevant medical resource may be absolutely absent (actually, from a medical point of view, the person in question does not have any damage). Subsequently, the data collection leads to a choice of diagnostic tools and a plan of neurocognitive retraining (see chapter on neuropsychological rehabilitation). Since the supply of neuropsychological tests is extensive, their selection is based mainly on the previously defined areas of cognitive functions, emotions, behavior, and personality. Responsibility for a proper diagnosis of a mild form of head impairment tends to be emphasized, for instance, in forensic proceedings regarding injury consequences, compensation of treatment expenses, etc. The examination of a person in question must be carried out by an experienced neuropsychologist, who is familiar with the subject, since a sole clinically psychological examination is only rarely sufficient and its later revision is usually very problematic. However, this domain does not tend to be properly regulated in the forensic practice.

1.2. History

Neuropsychology itself does not have a „"significant"" history yet,; it is rather linked mainly to neurotraumatology, as Smrčka et al. (2001) note. It tends to be connected with basic skull operations, trephinations, which were carried out in primeval times perhaps on every continent. The authors (Smrčka et al., 2001, p. 15) also report that first mentions of trephinations carried out in Bohemia date back to 5,000 years BC. Hippocrates (460 – 377 BC) wrote a book called *„On head injuries,"* and he made a link between head injuries and paralysis of the opposite limbs. He also specified a fact that sinistral brain impairments might cause a loss of speech (apropos, it is interesting that thereafter, all research regarding human body and thus human „"soul,"" too, was repressed by the church for long years – —and it was not sooner than in the year 1861, when Paul-Pierre Broca, a professor of external surgery, found expressive aphasia in his patient „"Tan-tan"—" – however, this was a result of stroke).

1.3. Role of Neuropsychology in the Treatment of Brain Impairment

In comparison with the rest of the world (see e.g. e.g.Cooper, Cooper et al., 1982, 1993), where all essential publications on brain impairments contain at least one comprehensive chapter devoted to its neuropsychological consequences, diagnostics and treatment, there is no reference to neuropsychology in connection with craniocerebral trauma in Czech publications (Nebudová, 1998; Smrčka et al., 2001), and the psychic consequences tend to be very briefly mentioned on only one page or not at all. It is even more striking when we realize that approximately 20 years have already passed since publication of the mentioned books by Cooper et al. (1982, 1993). Moreover, with regard to "mild brain impairment" (see classification below), neuropsychological perspective highly dominates in the world, since neurosurgery, neurotraumatology, and neurology deal with this diagnostic unit only marginally, if ever (see e.g. e.g., Varney, Roberts et al., 1999; Podell, 2004). Based on our own experiences, as well as on several of Podell's (2004) observations, the neuropsychological examination is especially crucial in these "medically unattractive" head and brain injuries. The reason is that the related medical disciplines do not have sufficiently sensitive tools that would be able to reveal consequences of the events on cognitive systems.

1.4. Epidemiology of Brain Traumas

National Institutes of Health consider and call the realm of traumatic brain injuries (TBI) as a „"quiet epidemic"" (i.e., similarly to dementias in elderly age).

In our country, this category is studied independently under the cluster of head injuries as „"intracranial injuries"" (dg. S 06, according to ICD 10). When considering brain injuries within all affections of central nervous system, Smrcka et al. (2001) report that they are the second most frequent events – —having 149.6 cases/100,000 inhabitants. While vascular brain diseases in the first place (180.1 cases) are followed by schizophrenic disorders (85.2) and epilepsy (37.0), malignant tumors take the ninth place (12.1). The question of classification of traumatic brain injuries is linked also to their frequent common incidence with an extracranialextra cranial injury – —which averages 36% % (with a high variance in particular countries: e.g. e.g., Sweden 24% %%, Benelux 56% %) according to a European multi-centric study with 67 neurocentres involved (Murray et al., 1999). Therefore, we usually speak about a polytrauma, in which a head – —and possibly a brain – —is one of the impaired parts of the body. The research (Murray et al., 1999) has also shown that average age of the injured persons was 38 years, 74% %% out of them were males, and 51% %% of all injuries were caused by traffic accidents. On reception of patients to a hospital, 58% %% of the impairments were labelledlabeled as severe ones, 17% %% as moderate ones and 19% %% as having a transitional character.

The latest statistics published by Institute of Health Information and Statistics of the Czech Rrepublic (2007) show that number of hospitalized patients with the mentioned diagnosis of intracranial injury is as follows (for Diagram 1, see Appendix):

Year	2003	2004	2005	2006
Males	25,241	24,384	23,272	21,152
Females	12,643	12,021	11,916	11,142
Total	37,884	36,405	35,188	32,294
Prevalence (cases/100,000 inhabitants)	371.4	356.7	343.8	342.7

In comparison with the statistics reported by Smrčka et al. (2001, p. 21), which present data applicable to the period before the year 1997, figures of the period between the years 2003 and 2007 are slightly higher. For age distribution of intracranial injuries occurred between 2004 and 2007, see Diagram 2 in the Appendix.

From the neuropsychological point of view, information about deaths caused by brain traumas (year 1997, as reported by Smrčka et al., 2001) is very interesting: a diagnosis of diffuse impairment + contusion highly dominates (323 cases) and is followed by subdural haematoma (67 cases) and epidural haematoma (15 cases). In the Czech Republic, approximately 1,750 patients die every year after an injury in which a craniocerebral lesion is one of the stated diagnoses. The nNumber of the deadsdead (percentage distribution in males and females) are shown in Diagram 3 in the Appendix.

1.5. Classification of Brain Impairments

The basic classification is shown in Table 1 (Savage, Wolcott, 1994).

Table. 1. Classification of brain impairments

Acquired brain traumas		
Not caused by injury	Caused by injury	
	Open	Closed
1. Anoxia		
2. Infection	Penetrating	Internal pressure and ruptures
3. Stroke	1. Hits	1. Hits
4. Tumors	2. Falls	2. Falls
5. Metabolic disorders	3. Accidents	3. Accidents
4. Physical abuse	4. Physical abuse	
	5. Surgery	

In terms of pathophysiology, the impairments (e.g. e.g., Pang, 1989) are classified as follows:

- primary and secondary;
- focal and diffuse.

Primary impairment (brain tissue lesion, which results from an injury):
focal – —brain contusion and acute haematoma occurring within the brain;
diffuse – —e.g. e.g., commotion and diffuse axonal impairment.

Secondary impairment resulting from:

a system process (i.e., not directly connected with brain) – —hypoxia (e.g. e.g., caused by obstruction), hypotension (e.g. e.g., caused by visceral wounds bleeding), hypercapnia (increased amount of carbon dioxide in blood), anemia (caused by loss of blood), hyperthermy, hyponatraemia (secondary water retention in the body caused by, for instance, inadequate secretion of antidiuretic hormone) and hypoglycaemia;

intracranial pathological events – —oedemaedema (vasogenic, cytotoxic, ischemic and hydrocephalus), vasospasm and also hernia caused by deformation, shift and consequent nip (due to a stoppage of breath caused by direct pressure on the medulla oblongata, a patient is at risk of death).

Aa „"classic"" classification of brain injuries (Angerova, 1999) is as follows:

a) injury on cranial extracerebral soft tissue,
b) concussion (commotio cerebri) – —a reversible malfunction without a morphological correlate;,
c) brain contusion (contusio cerebri) – —a morphological lesion with initial blackout;

d) brain rupture (dilaceratio cerebri) – —a morphological brain impairment caused by a trauma, usually combined with a skull fracture;,
e) post-traumatic complications.

Severity of Brain Impairments

Generally, head injuries may be divided into severe, moderate and mild ones (see below). Naturally, many factors must be taken into account when evaluating a patient's condition after a head injury from a neurosurgical (neurotraumatological) and neurological perspectives. There are also dozens of scales used for state of consciousness evaluation (a vertical point of view). Glasgow Coma Scale (GCS) by Teasdale and Jennett (1974) is the most common in the world. In the Czech Republic, there are also other modified versions—, for instance, those by neurosurgeons Benes senior (1981; disturbances of consciousness scheme) and Benes junior (1984; fundamental symptoms scheme). According to GCS, head injuries can be also classified as follows:

- mild head injury GCS > 13
- moderate head injury GCS = 9 to 12
- severe head injury GCS ≤ 8

For description of the severity of the patient's condition after a head injury, a parameter of duration of post-traumatic amnesia (PTA; Jennett and Teasdale, 1981) is also monitored. PTA is defined as the time period between the injury and retrieval of anterograde memory. However, in the Czech rRepublic, this criterion is rarely employed in practice and, for instance, Smrčka et al. (2001) do not mention it at all (maybe, the reason is that currently used modern treatment methods do not enable us to accurately monitor the time period).

However, from the neuropsychological point of view, the information about PTA duration is very important and applicable in primary diagnostics, as well as in formulation of prognosis and in selection of appropriate forms of cognitive functions rehabilitation.

Table 2. Posttraumatic amnesia: correlation with severity of patient's condition after head injury

Duration	Severity
less than 5 minutes	very mild
less than 1 hour	mild
1 to 24 hours	moderate
1 to 7 days	severe
more than 7 days	very severe
more than 4 weeks	extremely severe

When cognitive condition in an acute or subacute stage of a cranio-cerebral trauma must be neuropsychologically evaluated, "Rancho Los Amigos scale of cognitive functioning"

(Hagen, Malkmus, Durham, 1972) is excellently applicable. It is not yet known in the Czech Republic and it has eight8 qualitative – —based on patient's reactions – —anchored points:

1. no response,
2. generalized response,
3. localized response,
4. confused-agitated,
5. confused, inappropriate, non-agitated,
6. confused-appropriate,
7. automatic-appropriate,
8. purposeful and appropriate.

1.6. Short Overview of Several Researches

There are numerous resources on evaluation of neuropsychological consequences of traumatic brain injury, and their quantity currently grows mainly in connection with the mentioned mild forms of the injury (Podell, 2004). Authors of the overviews tend to emphasize the finding that patients with a brain injury have cognitive, as well as emotional and behavioral, problems, and that their extent may vary in severity and length of time interval since the injury. Brooks (1990) reports that following impairments may be observed:

1) impairment in the so-called core domains: attention/concentration, memory/learning, executive functions; and
2) in other cognitive domains: those including visuo-spatial abilities and the language.

Prigatano, Fordyce (1986) found out that an injury leads directly to disorders of the following:

1) learning and memory
2) complex processing of information (speed of information reception, planning, etc.)
3) perception and communication.

In a meta-analytic research (Binder, Rohling, and Larrabee, 1997) of eight published neuropsychological studies on patients with mild head injuries, general impairments of various cognitive areas were found out. The areas included attention/concentration, memory, hand laterality, performance abilities, cognitive flexibility and abstraction, and verbal abilities. The most substantial difference between patients and a control group was observed in the attention/concentration area.

In addition to the cognitive functions, all performed researches have studied emotional and personality (i.e. i.e., in terms of personality disorders) changes. In a large examined population of Massachusetts (Mangione et al., 1988), approximately 50 %% of persons had a post-traumatic depression (which had not been present in antecedent anamnesis), and in 33 %%, some kind of psychiatric disorder (which, again, had not been present premorbidly) was found out. Moreover, between 10 and 15 %% of the sample manifested suicidal signs and between 6 and 7 %six and seven percent began to misuse drugs or alcohol. In another large sample from the same state (Kamen et al., 1988), approximately 20 – to 30 %% of patients with head and brain injury had subsequent interpersonal problems, such as inability to identify the impact of their own behavior on others, unconsidered behavior without anticipation of potential consequences, misunderstanding or not admitting one's their own problems, difficulties in finding friends, situationally inadequate conversations, and consequent feelings of – —or even real – —social isolation and loneliness, and suffering from such situation.

Similar findings are reported also by, for instance, Wood, 1984; Prigatano, 1986; Lezak, 1989, and they are summarized in Table 1.4.

Table 1.4 Major symptoms following traumatic brain injury (Morse, Montgomery, 1992, p. 86)

Cognitive areas

a) Attention-concentration
b) Memory-learning
c) Executive functions: problem identification, goal formulation
d) Other cognitive areas: reasoning, intelligence, language, visuo-spatial, mathematics

Emotional-behavioral areas

A. Depression, suicidal ideation
B. Apathy, lack of initiation (motivation)
C. Changes in emotional regulation (emotional lability, irritability, aggressive outbursts)
D. Impulsivity, disinhibition, (sexual disturbances, inappropriateness)
E. Unawareness of problems (loss of insight, denial)
F. Insensitivity, unconcern for others
G. Other emotional/behavioral problems (anxiety, mania/hypomania, paranoid /psychotic ideation, child-like behavior)

1.7. Issue of Inaccurate Diagnosis in Mild Brain Impairments

Since the scale of cognitive and emotional/personality disorders tends to be wide-ranging in persons after a head injury, their symptoms – —and especially in case of a mild brain impairment – —may be initially evaluated in terms of a psychiatric diagnosis (the situation is interpreted in such terms by the patient's family or by the patient themselves). Therefore, it is necessary to consider a head injury as a differential or an additional diagnosis in psychiatric patients in general – —in depressive or anxious individuals, in those with signs of impaired interpersonal/social abilities (personality disorders), with drugs or alcohol abuse (e.g. e.g., in case of alcohol related falls), sexually abused ones (often combined with physical violence and head wounds), and possibly also in individuals with orthopedic or spinal-cord-afflicting injuries, in which the patient could have hitted their his/her head (if this alternative is not examined).

In the neurological field, a differential diagnosis must be stated in case of a head injury, especially when elder and old populations is are evaluated (falls, dementias) and in individuals with a paroxysmal disease (various etiologies).

1.8. Neuropsychological Evaluation of a Patient with Brain Impairment

In connection with the already mentioned, ever -increasing number of head (and thus usually also brain) injuries, as well as with limitations that medical disciplines (neurotraumatology, neurosurgery, neurology, psychiatry) have when diagnosing especially the "mild impairments,", significance of the neuropsychological diagnostics rises. This situation has triggered changes in the attitude towards evaluation – —or towards neglect – — of some factors and has resulted in a "holistically integrated neuropsychological evaluation" (Klonoff, Dawson, 2004), which includes following variables:

Demographics

- age,
- gender,
- date and place of birth,
- educational history (grade/degree completed and academic status, including prior history of learning problems),
- marital status (current and past) and current family composition,
- occupational history (current and past, including major job fields, job transiency, problems on the jobs),
- residence (e.g. e.g., with family, independent, group home).

Social History

- pre-injury and current alcohol and drug use,
- pre-injury psychiatric diagnosis and treatment,
- pre-injury financial status,
- pre-injury legal problems (e.g.,e.g., arrest),
- pre-injury hobbies and interests,
- family history (including medical and psychiatric health of parents and siblings),
- childhood experiences.

Medical History

- developmental history (prenatal or postnatal complications; gestational age and weight; developmental delays in walking, talking, etc.),
- previous brain injury or disease (e.g.,e.g., loss of consciousness, seizures, high fever),
- general medical history (systemic illness; comorbid disease),
- medications.

Injury-Related Data

- circumastancecircumstance of injury (date, location, and surrounding events; mechanism of injury; presence/absence of paramedics and/or hospitalizaionhospitalization/surgery),
- absence or presence of loss of consciousness and lenghtlength of tiemtime,
- estimated period of post-traumatic amnesia,
- Glasgow Coma Scale score,
- radiographic findings (CT and/or MRI),
- hospitalization records.

Subjective Report of Post-Injury Status

- perception of injury-related information (relative to factual information),
- perception of current status: cognitive, physical, emotional status with detailed description of problem areas with specific examples and severity levels,
- perception of course of recovery; improvement versus deterioration,
- sleep, appetite and libido,
- driving status,
- work status (with performance evaluations, if working),
- perception of work capacity (if not working),
- living situation and activities of daily living with level of independence,
- degree of unsupervised time,
- hobbies, interests, and socialization,
- use of strategies or compensation (e.g.,e.g., datebookdate book, pillbox),
- presence or absence of litigation or financial disincentives,
- goals and aspirations for the future.

Current Medical Treatment

- rehabilitation (prior and perception of proposed need),

- medical management (other medical services/practitioners involved),
- medications, including psychotrophics,
- medical complications (e.g.,e.g., pain, seizures).

Collateral Data

- relative's assessment of patient's functioning,
- objective data in the form performance evaluation and academic records.

Observational Data by Clinician

- affect,
- hygiene,
- pragmatics of communication (eye contact, openness to questions),
- behavior (impulsivity, frustration tolerance),
- emotional status,
- route finding in vicinity of office,
- observed recall of salient information versus subjective report of memory problems,
- consistency of effort and test performance,
- consistencye of self-report, and behavioral manifestations,
- level of satisfaction with health care professionals.
- *Since TBI is an acquired disorder, a thorough history is essential in:*
- establishing the patient's premorbid level,
- documenting changes in function following a head injury relative to premorbid level,
- identifying the contribution of other premorbid, pre-existing conditions (e.g.,e.g., neurological, psychiatric, learning/emotional disorders, substance abuse) which that may complicate the assessment of the sequelae of a TBI,
- generating hypothetical areas for formal evaluation.

In cases of mild head injuries, a combination of anamnesis and a high-quality evaluation of behavior (and of performance) is even more important. The main reason is that results of a formal testing may be minimal (or none) in such cases. A neuropsychologist's conclusion regarding the impairment must be thus based on exact anamnestic data and on their his/her own observations.

Pieces of *information provided by the patient's family* play an extremely important role in gathering anamnestic data. They often represent the sole resource of facts that enable us to form an image of the patient's common work, sports, etc., performance – —with regard to both its physical and mental aspects. Sometimes, they also provide data on the injury itself and/or on the patient's antecedent behavior. Moreover, the relatives often look after the patient in the subsequent acute stage. It is favorable to obtain the information before initiation of formal testing, because they this may lead to formulation of main hypotheses, as well as to constitution of the neuropsychological examination's design. Furthermore, the data are essential for subsequent considerations of post-traumatic rehabilitation of cognitive functions (we will not get into difficulties, because we will not attempt to get the patient to a better performance level than was the premorbid one). The cooperation with the patient's relatives or friends will be mentioned also in the chapter on neuropsychological rehabilitation. Nevertheless, it is beneficial to establish positive contacts with the family members already at „"the beginning of the story"" – —when recording the patient's anamnesis – —and to cultivate the contacts gradually during the patient's hospitalization or their his/her stay in various rehabilitation institutions, and so to create appropriate conditions for the period after moving home.

Furthermore, it is important not to forget to obtain results of any previous psychological or neuropsychological examinations (carried out, for instance, when entering the school, or even in the pre-school age, then when dealing with educational problems in various advisory centrescenters or in connection with transfer to a selective school, later when entering a job – —in which psychological testing is almost a standard nowadays; and possibly also in connection with forensic investigations or with execution of sentence).

A patient's complete medical documentation should be always and unconditionally available for a neuropsychologist, which means records regarding the patient's acute hospital/emergency care and postacutepost-acute hospitalization should be obtainable, as well as data on their his/her stay in other rehabilitation institutions, all stated diagnoses when both entering and leaving an institution, all executed therapies/operations, all laboratory findings (including e.g. e.g., EEG[8], CT[9], MRI[10], SPECT[11], PET[12] images and their descriptions), evidence of loss of consciousness, and data on duration of the patient's coma (preferably the GCS or a similar scale and information on PTA). For the sake of the neuropsychological evaluation itself, it is useful to make a summary of the examination data and neurosurgical, neurological, psychiatric, psychological or logopedic, occupational therapy, and physiotherapeutic findings, as well as of information about the patient's ability to perform everyday activities (self-attendance and similar ones, which tend to be recorded by nurses or other hospital staff).

1.8.1. Interview with a Patient

The structure of an interview with a patient corresponds with the mentioned structure of anamnesis. The data obtained from the patient after accidental head and brain injury may differ substantially from the facts obtained „"objectively"." The exploration itself is a time-consuming, but highly important part of a formal neuropsychological examination. In addition, in case of a mild head injury, one has to always bear in mind that the patient's symptoms/complaints often last much longer than the (decreased) performance in standard tests shows.

The interview should be carried out – —with respect to the patient's capacity of attention/concentration – —during their his/her "best" time of the day and only for a short

[8] Electro-encephalography
[9] Computed Tomography
[10] Magnetic Resonance Imaging
[11] Single Photon Emission Computed Tomography
[12] Positron Emission Tomography

time, especially when the patient tends to get tired quickly. For easily distracted patients, a calm and quiet environment is preferable (and also without excessive amount of visual stimuli). Some people can be "distracted" even by their own thinking, which is a highly demanding situation for the examiner. Furthermore, the patient may become overloaded by information (the patients after head injuries tend to have a deteriorated ability to process information – —which are the author's own findings based on his work with KAI test – — Kurztest für allgemeine Basisgrössen der Informationsverarbeitung). Therefore, simple, short, and concise questions should be asked, and breaks between different topics should be done. Retrieval from memory is another problematic area when interviewing the patient, which is manifested either by incorrect information recall, their inaccurate time-localization, or by confabulations present in the answers. In such a case, a confrontation of the data obtained from the patient with those obtained from other resources is necessary. Impairment of executive functions may be manifested during the interview with the patient by a considerably slow change in their his/her focus of attention, which worsens the ability to understand a question and may be potentially demonstrated by either lingering on a previous topic (perseveration) or by blending two lines of thought together. Parts of a response to a preceding question may freely continue in the following topic. This characteristic must be distinguished from the confabulated responses. The area of speech, or, to be more specific, its disturbances, will probably have the most substantial impact on the communication during the interview. On one hand, patients with various types of aphasias may be present – —with global, expressive, or perceptional one – —on the other hand, patients that we will not be able to speak with may also be present. We often deal with patients having auditory problems, which is essential to know before initiation of the interview (for example, in case of unilateral impairment, one can appropriately arrange the position of the patient and the examiner). Cases of deteriorated central auditory discrimination may also be present, which requires a slowdown of the neuropsychologist's speech, clear articulation, and sometimes also decrease in number of questions. When dealing with a patient who suffers from a combination of the mentioned memory difficulties and anomic (an amnestic) aphasia, their extensive answers – —thanks to their circumlocution – —may become a rebus for us, and the situation will be a mental burden for the both sides – —the examinant and the examiner. Patients with frontal lobe impairment often have problems with use of language when regulating their own behavior. They may have difficulties in controlling their own verbal reactions, as well as in awareness of or insight into their own problems. In such cases, the examinatorexaminer should try to structure the topics of the conversation, as well as to narrow their focus. A state of "disconnection" of the patient's speech from their his/her behavior may become an extremely important element in observation of their his/her expressions (for example, although the patient claims: "I don't like my neuropsychotherapist, because I don't have any mental problems,", they arehe/she never late in arrival to the psychotherapist). With regard to the emotional/behavioral aspect, the interview itself may be complicated by the fact that only a few patients with head injuries (especially in case of its mild form) have had an opportunity to speak about their problems before the neuropsychological consultation. Such a situation often results in a too long interview, in which the examiner has to respond to the patient's states of tearfulness, their suicidal ruminations, and general emotional lability. The situation thus requires to sensitively "balance" among support, continuous direction of questions towards the main theme, and thinking about topics that are not related to the interview itself. Furthermore, another group of patients may manifest a significant disinhibition of their emotional/social expressions; they behave in a socially inappropriate manners – —for example, in an excessively familiar or lax way; they often make indecent proposals or they want to touch the examiner; some of them are verbally or even physically aggressive.

We try to prevent such situations by means of appropriate arrangement of environment, in which the interview is conducted, as well as by elimination of ambiguous or unstructured questions, which may cause the patients to "link them with their emotions.". In such cases, we must always bear in mind that regulation of cognition tends to be based rather on "lower" levels of brain and the disinhibition occurs quickly and (in terms of the controlled cognition) unpredictably. We can repeatedly remind the main points of the interview in a calm, but consistent way, so as to keep it under control. The interview should be as short as possible, or divided into tangible performance tasks, which should help to prevent the mentioned problems. Again, the absence of insight in "frontal" patients may lead to expressions of resistenceresistance/irritability towards the questions being asked. They often do not understand why they are talked to or they change meaning of the questions (such as "What do my problems in school and the accident have in common?").

Another different group is comprisesd of patients with mild head injuries whose composition of complaints develops during a very short time period. While at the beginning, they complain mainly about somatic changes (predominantly headaches, fatigue, nausea, diplopia, etc.), the complaints about poor concentration, memory, difficulties in suitable words finding, which tend to disrupt work and leisure activities, join the list of symptoms later (Dikmen et al., 1989). Such a moment is especially noticeable in persons who were highly active (in work, sports, etc.) before the injury. After somatic symptoms of the mild injury subside, they expect a quick return to their activities and premorbid performance levels, which is, however, complicated by the mentioned set of cognitive difficulties.

A short case study: A 28-year-old man spontaneously comes for a neuropsychological consultation. Basically, he is a professional athlete – —a pole vaulter – —who has already took part in Olympiad with an average result. He had an injury two years ago – —he landed partly outside the landing area – —and he had mild wound in the area of his shoulder. At that time, the head injury was evaluated as a mild commotion. His somatic consequences subsided very quickly, but in a period of 6 six following months, many "pseudoneurasthenic" symptoms (using the words of his sports doctor) were developed. They gradually decreased the vaulter's performance to such extent that he began to seriously consider termination of his sports career. His current weak performance was associated mainly with his average result in the Olympiad, high competitiveness among top athletes, a need to get back among the Olympic contestants, etc. Unfortunately, in these "stressful" hypotheses, he was supported also by sports and clinical psychologists, who recommended him to undertake psychotherapy. A neuropsychological examination shows deficiencies in attention, memory and partially in executive functions. The finding is confirmed also by a functional image of blood flow in the brain done by the SPECT method. The man's state was evaluated as consequences of mild brain injury.

1.8.2. Formal Testing

As mentioned above, the consequences of head and brain injuries may be very heterogeneous in their expressions, and thus one must choose between a fixed and a flexible test approach – —out of which the latter one seems to be more rational. However, if we have experiences rather with a fixed neuropsychological battery, we may use it and resolve uncertainties with the help of other techniques. Obviously, the examination is different in the case of a patient with severe impairment – —its duration ranges between 15 minutes and 1 hour, maximally. On the contrary, patients with mild injuries are normally able to finish the examination in its almost necessary length, i.e. i.e., several hours (with breaks for rest, of course).

In severe/moderate cases, short screening tools are recommended, such as Neurobehavioral Cognitive Status Examination – Cognistat (Kiernan, Mueller, Langston, 1995; translation into English and modification of experimental form of examination done by Kulišťák, 1996), which provide us with a quick overview of a patient's orientation, attention, memory, speech, visuospatial and constructional abilities, inference, arithmetic abilities, and fine motor skills. Alternatively, one may also employ several screening items from frequently used tests (basic information about orientation – —in person, time, place; Trail Making Test A or B; CLOX – —clock face drawing; picture copying – —a house, bicycle, cube; selected items from Boston Naming Test – —or alternatively, Pictorially-Lexical Test (Kondáš, 1970); in the Czech Rrepublic;, selected items from the Comprehension subtest in WAIS[13]; memorizing a short list of words, as well as current events). On the basis of the "screening,", a structure of cognitive functions rehabilitation is planned, as well as a subsequent comprehensive examination of "problematic" cognitive domains.

On the contrary, patients with mild head injuries require more extensive testing (usually WAIS and WMS[14], which inform us about strengths and weaknesses in the patient's cognitive performance; patients with a sole frontal impairment are an exception – —in these cases, the testing sets usually provide us with insufficient or even misleading information – —see below). In these patients, we have to devote a lot of time to testing various "types" of memory (e.g. e.g., RAVLT[15], CVLT[16], ROCFT[17]), as well as attention (e.g. e.g., PASAT[18], CPT[19], Capacity of Attention Test) and executive functions (WCST[20], Trail making A and B, COWA/FAS[21], Stroop Test, Porteus Maze Test, TOL[22], TOH[23], BDS[24]).

The selection of tests for a particular patient will often depend on the following issues (Morse, Montgomery, 1992):

- the importance of results that are quantitative in nature with appropriately referenced normative samples,
- the importance of information about the underlying processes (e.g.,e.g., learning processes) involved in cognition, and

[13] Wechsler Adult Intelligence Scale
[14] Wechsler Memory Scale
[15] Rey Auditory Verbal Learning Test
[16] California Verbal Learning Test
[17] Rey Osterrieth Complex Figure Test
[18] Paced Auditory Serial Addition Test
[19] Conner's Continuous Performance Test
[20] Wisconsin Card Sorting Test
[21] Controlled Oral Word Association, i.e., Word Fluency
[22] Tower of London
[23] Tower of Hanoi
[24] Behavioral Dyscontrol Scale

- the importance of briefly covering a broad range of assessment areas vs. fewer areas in depth.

1.8.3. Diagnostic Contribution of Tests in Mild Head and Brain Impairment

In terms of differential diagnostic use of test methods, a meta-analytic research (Zakzanis, Leach, and Kaplan, 1999), in which 12 studies published between the years 1980 and 1997 were included, is considerably interesting. Overall, results of neuropsychological testing obtained from 952 patients with mild head impairment and 495 healthy persons (control group) were analyzed. The findings show the function of cognitive flexibility and abstraction was the most sensitive when detecting consequences of mild head injuries; and methods focused on delayed memory recall, information learning (verbal learning and memorizing), attention/concentration, and verbal skills did not differ much when speaking about their contribution to diagnosis stating. Techniques that examined performance and manual skills had only a minimal contribution. Zakzanis, Leach a Kaplan (1999) also present every test method used in the mentioned cognitive areas. The best technique for detecting insufficiencies in *cognitive flexibility and abstraction* domain was the measurement of phonemic fluency in COWA/FAS test, and similar success was achieved by semantic fluency parameter. Its nonverbal counterpart – —fluency in shapes (designs) formation – —was not as contributory and distinguished approximately 50 %% of patients with an impairment from the healthy control population. In the WCST technique, criteriumcriteria of perseveration errors predicted the impairment more reliably than number of categories criteriumcriteria. Both WCST categories were more sensitive than the Trail making Making B and interference parameter in the Stroop test. The Tower of Hanoi, the last diagnostic technique in the field, did not prove to be much contributory for stating a differential diagnosis in mild brain impairments. In the area of *delayed memory recall*, which was the second most sensitive for this type of patients, subtests *Logical Memory* and *Paired Associates Learning* from WMS-R were the best predictors, and they were followed by RAVLT. As to the nonverbal techniques, while the ROCFT was the most sensitive, delayed memory recall of WMS-R subtest *Visual Reproduction* was not so contributory. Memory recall similar to WAIS subtest *Information* did not prove to be as predictory as monitoring of recently retained information (e.g. e.g., RAVLT or CVLT). Furthermore, another nonsensitive technique was monitoring loss of amount of information in Bushke test, when comparing results of 30-minute and 4-hour delay. Similarly, examination of recognition aspect of memory (one of the parameters in CVLT) did not prove to be contributory. The *memorizing and learning* domain was predominantly also impaired and memory recall of material with a short-term delay in the RAVLT method, as well as immediate reproduction of stories in *Logical Memory* subtest and of *Paired Associates* subtest from WMS-R, were shown to be sensitive. On the contrary, performance in *Digit Span* subtest (WAIS) was not deteriorated in any way, as well as performance in *Visual Reproduction* – —immediate recall – —subtest (focus on operating with nonverbal material) in WMS-R. Similar results were obtained also in "completion of lexical stem" (priming), which suggests system of implicit memory in people with mild brain impairment is usually very well preserved. The meta-analytical study has brought significant findings also for *attention/concentration* domain, which is usually considered to be the most impaired in patients with accidental head and brain injuries. However, in the study, the attention/concentration domain was shown to be less sensitive than the mentioned *flexibility and abstraction* and *memory*. The area was evaluated by *interference* parameter of the Stroop test, and the same result was found out by Seashore Rhythm Test and PASAT. The authors remark that although Trail making MakingMaking Test A does not serve for a pure evaluation of attention and concentration, in the research, it proved to be the most sensitive in assessing this area. As already mentioned above, measurements in the area of *verbal skills* were the most sensitive indicators of mild brain impairment (phonemic and semantic fluency); the *Vocabulary* subtest of WAIS was not shown to be so contributory, as well as the overall verbal score of the scale, which distinguished patients from control persons even less (also in comparison with the performance score of WAIS).

Skills in working with visual material, measured as visuo-spatial and visuo-constructional skills, were the second most sensitive in evaluating patients with mild head impairments. The most contributory was copying of ROCF; on the contrary, results of the highly promoted *Block Design* subtest of WAIS were almost the same in patients and healthy persons (!). As was already mentioned above, the overall performance score in WAIS was more contributory (in terms of differential diagnosis stating) than the overall verbal score in the same method (they were able to distinguish 30 %% and 20% % of patients, respectively). The *manual skills* domain was shown to be hardly significant for evaluation of mild traumatic impairments. This area was represented in the research by Finger Tap Test, and not even a lateral asymmetric deficit was found. In addition, the authors of the meta-analytic study (Zakzanis, Leach, and Kaplan, 1999) included two scales focused on emotional aspects – —Beck Depression Inventory and *Detecting Sources of Anxiety* questionnaire; results obtained from the patients with mild brain impairment were elevated in both scales. The anxiety increase was interpreted rather as a reaction to the injury than as a premorbid personality trait.

In conclusion, Zakzanis, Leac, and Kaplan (1999) state that in patients with mild head and brain injury, the neuropsychological deterioration is present in many cognitive tasks and variables of the tests. This appears to them as a syndrome of „"frontal dysfunction,"" as defined by Stuss and Gow (1992). Unfortunately, at this point, a possibility of diffuse brain impairment interferes, which may result in insufficient performance in executive tests. In some cases, secondary deficits are definitely in question, in which diffuse axonal impairment lies in the background (sometimes confused with mild head and brain impairment – —which is, however, a very severe condition). For the sake of differential diagnosis, we must then employ measurement of delayed memory recall and memorizing (learning).

Based on our own findings (Matěcha, Kulišťák, Roubíčková et al., 1997), as well as on generally presented information about impairments of cognitive systems (e.g. e.g., Binder, Rohling, and Larrabee, 1997), attention is usually the most impacted cognitive area.

A short case study: A young man sustained a head injury in a sports accident, when riding his mountain bike. After a fall on a root of tree, he suffered a blackout (GCS data are not available) and was transferred to an emergency neurosurgical ambulance. When no finding on CT was shown, the hospitalization was terminated the following day. His mother came to pick him up and at home, she found out her son did not recognize the environment in which he had lived for 24 years;, he identified neither photographs from his youth nor things he had brought home from his mountain hiking abroad. During the following days, his state "continued": he regarded his girlfriend (with whom he had been in a relationship already for for 4four years) as a stranger and similarly, he did not recognize his friends and colleagues from school. When he mentioned his problems to his doctor, to whom he payedpaid a visit because of a medical check-up, the problems were dismissed as impossible ("it is not possible, he makes up everything for sure"). The young man accidentally found out there was an opportunity to be neuropsychologically examined. In the neuropsychological evaluation, an extensive damage in autobiographic memory was detected, as well as impairment of executive functions, attention, and several milder deficiencies in other cognitive domains. After two years of outpatient neuropsychological rehabilitation, he managed to finish his university studies, but a mild memory and executive insufficiency still continues to be present.

1.8.4. Course of Cognitive Deficit In Head and Brain Impairment

The point of turnabout, i.e. i.e., the period of coming around from coma, is not immediate,; it is rather a stage in which lucid intervals lengthen and self-awareness, as well as awareness of environment gradually increase. This stage is followed by the mentioned post-traumatic amnesia (PTA – —see the Appendix). Similarly, the process of approaching to stability of memory is also periodic and at this point – —when the medically studied functions are more or less stable – —the cognitive functioning of a patient after a brain injury represents 40 to -60 %% of their premorbid level. Therefore, a neuropsychological examination is especially important at this stage, since an overall level of functioning is being evaluated and main areas of weakness (as well as of well preserved functions) are being searched for. An accurate and thorough evaluation will be helpful in the process of clarification of the emerged problems to the patient and their relatives, as well as in the preparation of a corresponding and effective rehabilitation plan. A patient and other involved persons are often interested in the question of duration of problems that are connected with the brain damage (cognitive impairment). It is very difficult to answer such question, since it embraces numerous factors, which that can never be totally grasped. Moreover, other psychosocial phenomena may emerge during the recovery process, which may impede a successful development in spite of an optimally led complex, and especially neuro-psychological rehabilitation.

A short case study: A young clinical psychologist informed wife and parents of a young, 32-year-old man suffering from severe brain lesion that the actual state of his intellectual functions corresponded to performance of a 1.5-year-old child, and that such situation was probably permanent and presumably, it would never be changed. Subsequently, the man's wife, together with their daughter left the family, and property problems arose (the wife took a car, computer, etc., which will have to be solved by legal proceedings). In addition to the severe state of their son, the wife's reaction upset the man's parents and all care about him, participation in the rehabilitation, etc., had to be done by themselves. Optimal conditions for the process of a long period of recovery were spoiled already in its beginnings. Our neuropsychological examination found well -preserved – —though temporarily weakened – —functions in almost all cognitive areas. The biggest problems were present in the attention domain, the ability of "full" concentration ranged in an interval of a few minutes. Maybe this was the reason of the clinical psychologist's conclusion and the patient thus did not have any chance to apply his other (less- impaired) cognitive functions.

1.8.5. Utilization of Imaging Methods

Introduction of Computed Tomography (CT) to diagnostics and therapy of patients with head injuries meant a real revolution in the 1970's (until then, X-ray examination and angiography had been used). Arrival of Magnetic Resonance Imaging (MRI), which is able to depict structure of brain parenchyma, did not represent such leap any more, but it enabled higher resolution of tissues and thus contributed to, for instance, diagnosing of diffuse axonal impairment. Further progress brought techniques depicting functional modalities – —blood flow, metabolism, and oxygenation – —such as Single Photon Emission Computed Tomography (SPECT), Positron Emission Tomography (PET), and Functional Magnetic Resonance Imaging (fMRI). In case of brain traumas, SPECT is the most widely used, because it is financially undemanding, as well as diagnostically contributory.

1.8.6. Proposal of Neuropsychological Examination of Patients after Accidental Brain Injury

The Czech repertoire of neuropsychological diagnostic tools corresponds with the report by Morse and Montgomery (1992, p. 118), with the only exception of less frequent use of WAIS. The reason is that WAIS tends to distort results of patients with craniocerebral traumas, in which the injury affects mainly the frontal lobe of brain. In this area, the potential of Wechsler's examination of intelligence is considerably limited – —speaking about both global score and scores obtained in individual subtests (maybe this is also due to the fact that the scale was not created with this aim – —see the following case study).

A short case study: A 38-year-old man, after a heavy car accident, suffered from a predominant frontally sinistral impairment, mainly orbitally and laterally (in neuro-traumatologic terms described as a fracture of base of anterior cranial pit – —frontally bilaterally – —and of facial skeleton). The so-called intelligence was repeatedly examined by the WAIS-R method, and always an average result was found (overall score 97, 99, 101; verbal score 106, 111, 108; performance score 86, 86, 94; almost a flat profile of subtests). Consequently, the man was recommended – —not by us – —to return to his job. He came to contact with us after a total failure in work – —the main problem had been his inability to anticipate consequences of his own behavior. Since examination of "intelligence" was requested again, we used Intelligence Structure Test (1965), which excellently discriminated impaired and non-impaired functions. Moreover, the overall result in the test (77; considerable elevations and falls) led to certification of the man's full disability.

If we proceed in accordance with the intentions of the proposed schema of neuropsychological tools (applicable to patients after accidental head and brain injury), we may recommend the following:

Attention/concentration:

- observation
- Continuous Performance Test (CPT),
- Reaction Time (FePsy – computer test battery "The Iron Psychologist"),
- Vigilance Test (FePsy),

- Attentional Capacity Test (d2 – computer test battery “Neurop2”),
- Cancellation Test,
- Trail -mMaking Test (version A and B),
- Paced Auditory Serial Addition Test (PASAT),
- digit span (test battery KAI – Germany test of information processing),
- visual span (WMS-III),
- mental control (WMS-III),
- Stroop (short Victoria-version),
- Wisconsin Card Sorting Test (WCST),
- arithmetic (WAIS-III),
- digit symbol (WAIS-III),
- Behavioral Inattention Test (BIT).

Memory/Learning:

- California Verbal Learning Test (CVLT-9 word version),
- Rey-Auditory Verbal Learning Test (RAVLT),
- Buschke Selective Reminding Test,
- Luria Memory Learning Test (LMLT – words and numbers),
- Serial and simultaneous recognition of words and shapes (FePsy),
- Wechsler Memory Scale (WMS-III; as exeptionexception, haven’t ecological validity)
- Rivermead Behavioral Memory Test (RBMT; better ecological validity),
- Reyova-Osterrieth Complex Figure Test (ROCFT; copy, immediate and delayed reproduction),
- Warringtonové Recognition Memory Test (RMT – words, faces),
- Rey 15-items Memory Test (2 versions),
- Graham-Kendall Memory Test (shapes),
- Bentonův Visual Recogniton Test (BVRT),
- Peterson Interference Task,
- Famous Faces (private version),
- WCST.

Executive Function:

- Frontal Assessment Battery (FAB),
- Verbal Fluency (phonemic, semantic),
- Design Fluency („“five dots test“),
- WCST,
- Stroop,
- Go/No-Go (computer battery ANT 2.0 – Amsterdam Neuropsychological Tasks),
- Trail-m Making Test (A and B),

- Tower of London (computer test battery “Neurop2”),
- Tower of Hanoi (computer test battery “Neurop2”),
- Tower of Toronto (computer test battery “Neurop2”),
- Porteus Mazes,
- Behavioral Dyscontrol Scale (BDS),
- Behavioral Assessment of Dysexecutive Syndrom (BADS),
- Hayling and Brixton Test,
- Executive Interview (EXIT25).

Language:

- Token-Test,
- Picture-Vocabulary Test (OSS-Czech version),
- Boston Naming Test,
- Spontaneous speech,
- Wepman-Halsteadt Screening Aphasia Test,
- Western Aphasia Battery (WAB),
- Luria Assessment of Expression and Perception of Language,
- Prague Aphasia Battery (PAB),
- Dichotic Listening Task.

Visuospatial Abilities:

- ROCFT (copy),
- Corsi Blocs (FePsy),
- Visual Searching Test (CVST; FePsy),
- Line Bisection Test,
- Copy of Cube,
- Hooper Test of Visual Organization,
- Cancellation Test,
- Benton Judgment of Line Orientation Test,
- Benton Shapes Discrimination Test,
- Benton Constructional Test (Photo, Design, Model),
- Visual Object and Space Perception Battery (VOSP).

Motor:

- Behavioral Dyscontrol Scale (BDS— - Luria and Head tasks),
- Finger Tapping (FePsy),
- Grip Strength,
- Grooved Pegboard,

- Florida Screening Test of Apraxia (FAST).

Emotion/Behavior/Personality:

- observation,
- Perception of Emotion (ANT2),
- Self-evaluation Inventory (BDI, SDS, etc.),
- Minnesota Multiphasic Personality Inventory 100 (Czech short version),
- Drawing (tree, house, Figural Drawing Test).

Other:

- Tactual Perception (Benton),
- Finger Localization (Benton),
- KAI— – Germany test of information -processing.

Battery:

- Cognistat,
- Luria-Nebraska Neuropsychological Battery,
- FePsy (Computer Test Battery with EEG),
- Neurop-2 (Computer Test Battery— – Czech version).

From the mentioned overview of neuropsychological tools follows that a neuropsychologist definitely does not suffer from lack of tests. However, issue of norms may be problematic sometimes. Nevertheless, the norms often do not play the leading role in "clinical practice,", which we have noted after consultations with foreign colleagues, and which was also confirmed by cross-cultural studies of healthy population (in the USA, Germany, Mexico, Denmark, Slovakia, Russia). With regard to patients with severe accidental brain injuries, this is certainly a minor issue. Sometimes, difficulties may arise when evaluating persons with mild or moderate cranio-cerebral traumas, as well as in forensic assessment of such people.

1.9. Psychosocial Consequences of Traumatic Head Injuries (Disability)

A long-term monitoring of individuals after TBI has not been yet carried out systematically in the Czech rRepublic and available are only partial data obtained in the year 2003 (only within the dg S06 category – —according to ICD 10 – intracranial lesion) – — they are presented in the Diagrams 4 and 5 in the Appendix.

Conclusion

Based on our own practical findings about neuropsychological evaluation of impaired cognitive functions in cases of brain injuries of various severity (which, basically, correspond with the opinions of other authors – —e.g. e.g., those of Morse and Montgomery, 1992, p. 164), we may conclude the following:

- consequences of craniocerebral traumas represent a considerably heterogeneous spectrum of cognitive functions impairments;
- the resultant image of a cognitive functions impairment comprises of severity of the trauma – —mild, moderate, or severe one— –, as well as of extent of “primary” and consequent “secondary” events;
- the primary consequences are caused by mechanisms of a lesion— – i.e. i.e., by type of impact and of possible “counterimpactcounter impact” (whiplash), torsional movement (inertial movement of brain against the direction of skull movement), diffuse axonal impairment (emerging mainly during accelerated forward movement of head);
- the secondary consequences reflect many changes in brain tissue (swelling, infection, hypoxia, regulation of vital somatic functions in case of lesion on stem structures, etc.);
- since localization of lesions in traumatic brain impairments highly varies, we may search for general changes (attention, memory, and learning) – —which are present in almost all cases— - in the area of cognitive functions, as well as for the specific ones (perception, speech, reading, writing, arithmetic, visuospatial abilities, and executive functions) — – i.e. i.e., those relating to a place of the most severe impairment of brain parenchyma; insufficiencies in the mentioned areas are then reflected in overall behavior and in functionality in everyday life;
- individual differences of people before a head and brain injury may affect their personality structures after the event, or the change may even be so profound that a “new” personality is being formed in the process of rehabilitation (however, the process is a matter of long-lasting neuropsychotherapy);
- the post-injurial development of emotional living is similarly complicated. Predominant problems in the area of emotions and behavior include difficulties in regulation of affective expressions (irritability or even aggression), loss of activity initiation caused by depression (motivation), impulsiveness and disinhibition, unawareness (denial) of own problems, insensitivity, and lack of interest in the others. In addition to anxiety, also psychotic symptoms (mania, paranoia, delusions) may be temporarily present;.
- many patients after a head injury are not neuropsychologically diagnosed at all (especially those without a positive structural imaging finding); furthermore, in a standard examination carried out by a clinical psychologist (which includes, for example, intelligence tests and tests of the so-called organicity), the patient’s main problems tend to stay unrevealed; moreover, problems in various cognitive domains do not necessarily need to be accompanied by symptoms that could be considered as “organic” ones; the similar situation prevails in the emotional and behavioral area; a

comprehensive interview with the patient should play an essential role in the examination, and a further analysis with help of appropriately selected test methods should lead to a "holistically integrated evaluation" (see above);.

- Every head and brain impairment – —which means also a mild one – —deserves, firstly, a subsequent rehabilitation (together with instruction of the patient) of cognitive functions (neurocognitive training), which has to be organized and planned in accordance with the patient's condition, and secondly, psychological counsellingcounseling, a short-term neuropsychotherapy, or a crisis psychotherapeutic intervention (in case of emotional and behavioral problems); thirdly, supportive groups are also favorable for this type of patients, since a standard group therapy is usually not contributory with regard to the patient's specificities (which are, most importantly, continuing cognitive and sensory limitations).

Appendix

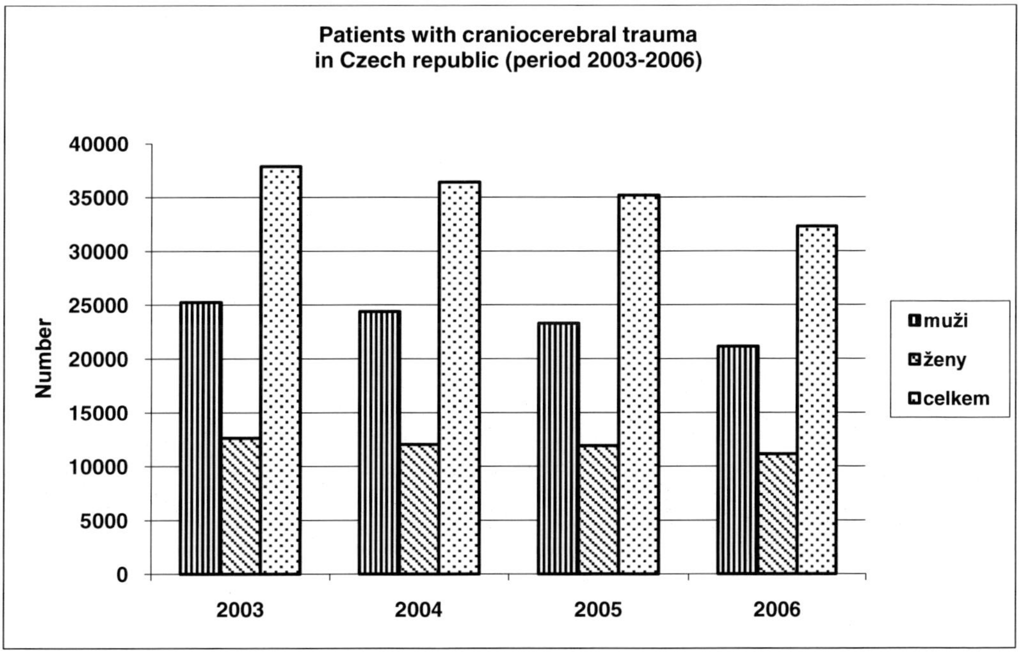

Diagram 1.

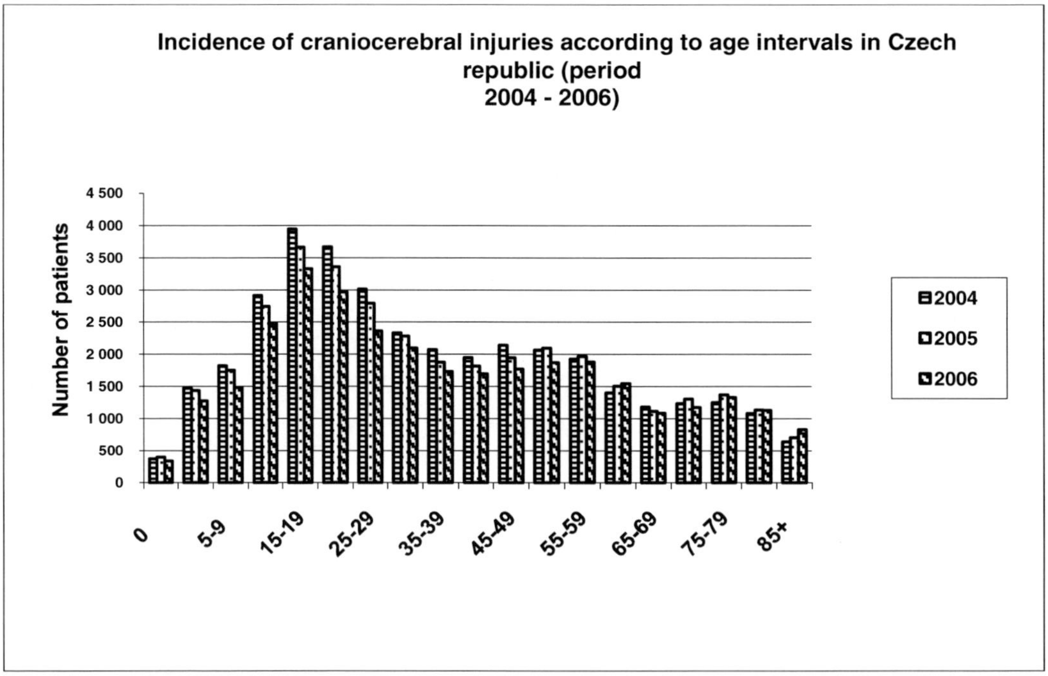

Diagram 2.

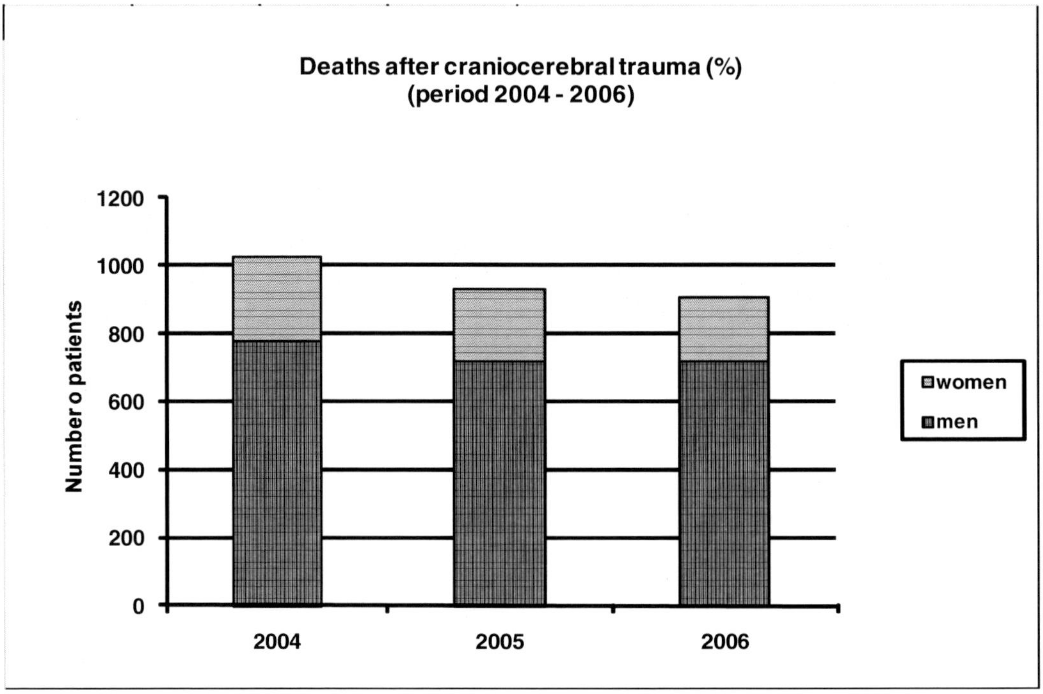

Diagram 3.

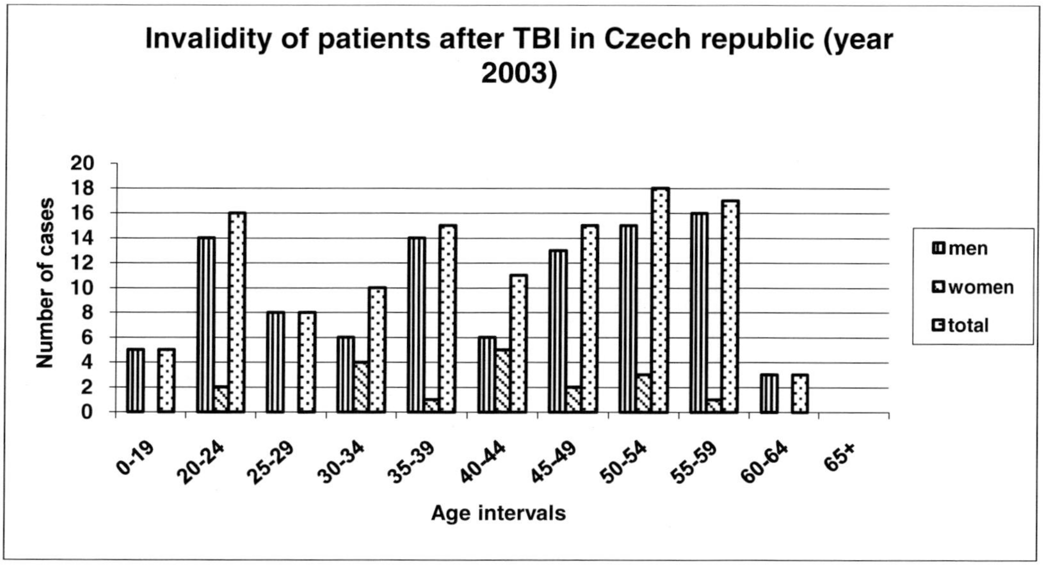

Diagram 4.

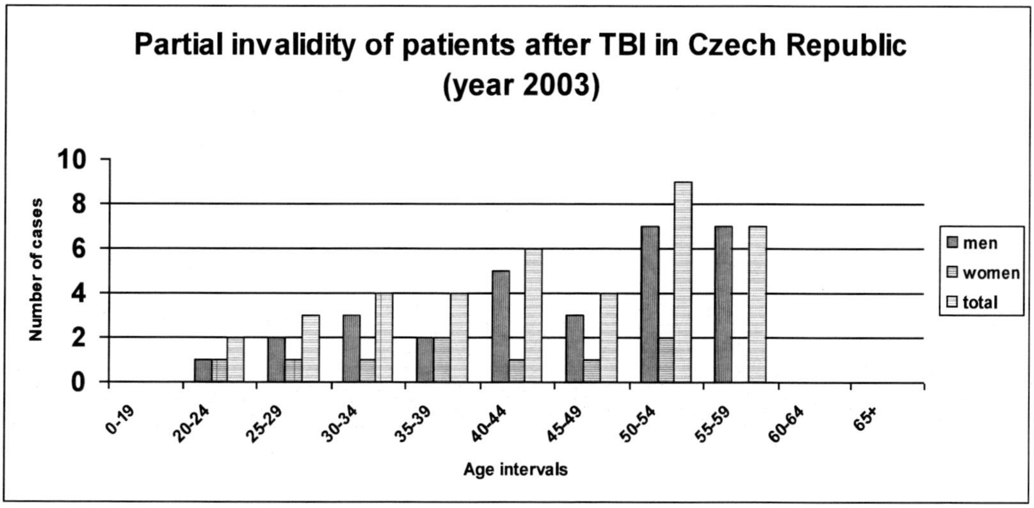

Diagram 5.

References

Angerová, Y.: Úrazy hlavy – TBI (Traumatic Brain Injuries). [Head injuries - TBI] In: Použitý mozek. Sborník referátů přednesených v centru neuropsychologické rehabilitace. [A used brain. A collection of papers presented in the Centre for Neuropsychological Rehabilitation] (edited by J. Šplíchal), Praha, Klinika rehabilitačního lékařství 1. LF UK, 1999.

Beneš, V.: Evaluation of disturbances of consciousness. *Acta Neurochirurgica* 55, 1981, pp. 265–271.

Beneš, V.: Some remarks to the evaluation of disturbances of consciouconsciousness. Zbl. *Neurochirurgie* 45, 1984, pp. 314–317.

Binder, L. M., Rohling, M. L., and Larrabee, G. J.: A review of mild head trauma. Part I: Meta-analytic review of neuropsychological studies. *Journal of Clinical and Experimental Neuropsychology* 19, 1997, pp. 421–431.

Brooks, N.: Cognitive deficits. In M. Rosenthal, E. Griffith, M. Bond, Miller, J. (Eds.), Rehabilitation of the adult and child with traumatic *brain injury*. Philadelphia, F. A. Davis, 1990, pp. 163–178.

Cooper, P. R.: (Ed.) Head injury. Baltimore/London, Williams and Wilkins, 1982.

Cooper, P. R.: (Ed.) Head injury. 3rd Edition. Baltimore, Williams and Wilkins, 1993.

Dikmen, S., Temkin, N., and Armsden, G.: Neuropsychological recovery: relationship to psychosocial functioning and postconcussional complaints. In: Levin, H.S., Eisenberg, H., and Benton, A. (Eds.), Mild Head Injury. New York: Oxford University Press, 1989, pp. 229–241.

Hagen, C., Malkmus, D., and Durham, P.: Rancho Los Amigos Scale of cognitive functioning. Rancho Los Amigos Hospital, Communication Disorders Service, 1972.

Kamen, D., LaVecchio, F., and Morse, P.: S.H.I.P.: a model program for community service. Presented at the Tufts UnivesrityUniversity and Greenery Rehabilitation Conference on Head Injury: an integrated approach to behavioral rehabilitation, Boston, MA, 1998.

Kaplan, E.: The process approach to neuropsychological assessment of psychiatric patients. *Journal of Neuropsychiat*ry 2, 1990, pp. 72–87.

Kaplan, E., Fein, D., Morris, R., and Delis, D. C.: WAIS-R as a Neuropsychological Instrument (WAIS-R NI). San Antonio, TX: *The Psychological Corporation*, 1991.

Kiernan, R. J., Mueller, J., and Langston, J. W.: Cognistat (Neurobehavioral Cognitive Status Examination). Odessa, FL, Psychological Assessment Resources 1995, (translation into Czech language by Kulišťák, P., 1996, Cognistat. Praha, internal print of IPVZ).

Klonoff, P. S. and Dawson, L. K.: Commentary – neuropsychological evaluation of patients with traumatic brain injury: polarization versus holistic integration. Archives of Clinical *Neuropsychology* 19, 2004, pp. 1095–1101.

Kondáš, O.: Príručka k testu obrázkovo-slovníková skúška [Pictorially-Lexical Test: the practitioner's handbook]. Bratislava, Psychodiagnostické a didaktické testy, 1970.

Kulišťák, P., Matecha, V., Kupka, K., and Kubicek, M.: Neuropsychological and SPECT assessment of patients with brain injury: long-term follow up study. Abstract der 14. Jahrestagung der GNP/NVN. *Zeitschrift für Neuropsychologie* 10, 1999, p. 246.

Levin, H. S.: Neurobehavioral sequelae of closed head injury. In: P. R. Cooper (Ed.), Head injury. 3rd Edition. Baltimore: Williams and Wilkins 1993, pp. 525–551.

Levin, H. S., Benton, A. L., and Grossman, R. G.: Neurobehavioral consequences of closed head injury. New York: Oxford University Press, 1982.

Lezak, M. D.: Assessment of psychosocial dysfunctions resulting from head trauma. In: M.D. Lezak (Ed.), Assessment of the behavioral consequences of head trauma. New York: Alan R. Liss, 1989, pp. 113–143.

Long, C. J. and Williams, J. M.: Neuropsychological assessment and treatment of head trauma patients. In: H.A. Whitaker (Ed.), Neuropsychological studies of nonfocal brain damages. New York, Springer-Verlag 1988, pp. 132–161.

Mangione, T., Potter, D., Kamen., and LaVecchio, F.: An analysis of the needs of people with traumatic head injuries: Commonwealth of Massachusetts. In: Massachusetts

Rehabilitation Commission Statewide Head Injury Program Report: The status of people with brain injuries in Massachusetts: epidemiological aspects and service needs. Boston: Massachusetts Rehabilitation Commission, 1988.

Matěcha, V., K. P., Roubíčková, J., Kubíček, M., and Šercl, M.: Rehabilitace chronického stádia stavů po těžkém kraniocerebrálním poranění [Rehabilitation of chronic stage of states after a severe craniocerebral injury]. *EuroReHab*, 1997, pp. 7-33.

Morse, P. A. and Montgomery, C. E.: Neuropsychological evaluation of traumatic brain injury. In: R. F. White (Ed.), Clinical syndromes in adult neuropsychology: the practitioner's handbook. Amsterdam: Elsevier, 1992, pp. 85–175.

Murray, G. D., Teasdale, G. M., Braakman, R., Cohadon, F., Dearden, M., Iannotti, F., Karimi, A., Lapierre, F., Maas, A., Ohman, J., Persson, L., Servadei, F., Stocchetti, N., Trojanowski, T., and Unterberg, A.: The European Brain Injury Consortium survey of head injuries. *Acta Neurochirurgica* (Wien) 141, 1999, pp. 223–236.

Nebudová, J.: Kraniocerebrální úrazy. [Craniocerebral injuries] Praha: Triton, 1998, p. 126.

Pang, D.: Physics and pathophysiology of closed head injury. In: M. D. Lezak (Ed.), Assessment of the behavioral consequences of head trauma. New York: Alan R. Liss, 1989, pp. 1–17.

Podell, K.: Sports concussion and adaptive and veridical decision making in the frontal lobes. Workshop on 8th Nordic Meeting in Neuropsychology, August 26–29, Turku, Finland, 2004.

Prigatano, G.: Personality and psychosocial consequences after brain injury. In: G. Prigatano, D. J. Fordyce, H. K. Zeiner, J. R. Roueche, M. Pepping, B. C. Wood (Eds.), Neuropsychological rehabilitation after brain injury. Baltimore: The Johns Hopkins University Press,1986, pp. 29–50.

Prigatano, G. and Fordyce, D.: Cognitive dysfunction and psychosocial adjustment after brain injury. In: G. Prigatano et al. (Eds.), Neuropsychological rehabilitation after brain injury. Baltimore: The Johns Hopkins University Press, 1986, pp. 1–17.

Savage, R. C. and Wolcott, G. F.: Overview of acquired brain injury. In: R. C. Savage, G. F. Wolcott (Eds.), Educational dimensions of acquired brain injury. Austin, TX: Pro-ed.

Smrčka, M. a kol. (2001) Poranění mozku. [Brain injuries] Praha: Grada Publishing, 1994, p. 272.

Stuss, D. T. and Gow, C. A.: „"Frontal dysfunction"" after traumatic brain injury. Neuropsychiatry, Neuropsychology, and Behavioral Neurology 5, 1992, pp. 272–282.

Varney, N. R. and Roberts, R. J.: (Eds.) The evaluation and treatment of mild traumatic brain injury. Mahwah, NJ: Lawerence Erlbaum Associates, Publ.,1999, 541 pp.

Wood, R.: Behaviour disorders following severe brain injury: their presentation and psychological management. In: Brooks, N. (Ed.), Closed head injury: psychological, social and family consequences. New York: Oxford, 1984, pp. 195–219.

Zakzanis, K. K., Leach, L., and Kaplan, E.: Neuropsychological differential diagnosis. Lisse: Swets and Zeitlinger Publishers, 1999.

http://www.cdc.gov/ncipc/pub-res/TBI_in_US_04/TBI-USA_Book-Oct1.pdf

In: Cognitive Deficit in Mental and Neurological Disorders ISBN: 978-1-60741-957-0
Editors: H. Kucerova, M. Preiss

Chapter XV

Vascular Dementia

Sabina Telecka

Abstract

Vascular dementia (VaD) is the second most common type of dementia in elderly people, just after Alzheimer's disease (AN). Nevertheless, it is often underestimated or even neglected. However, physicians still more often draw attention to the possible increase of incidence of this disease in the future—especially due to the growing incidence of cardiovascular diseases.

Generally, vascular dementia is defined as a cognitive deficit on the basis of vascular brain disease. In order to consider such a diagnosis, we need the following evidence: reduction of cognitive abilities (neuropsychological examination), signs of vascular brain disease (imaging methods) and a causal relationship. Other etiologies must also be excluded.

In contrast to Alzheimer's disease, VaD is not a disease with a uniform clinical picture and course. The term "vascular dementia" needs to be perceived as a broad spectrum of cognitive disorders associated with vascular brain disease, of which only a part meets the general criteria of dementia. Therefore, the current effort is to replace this term with a more comprehensive name *"vascular cognitive impairment"* (VCI).

Vascular cognitive impairment is a disease that is potentially "causally" curable if diagnosed in the early stages. Hence, the principle is the *causal* approach—focused on the cause of the disease. The anti-aggregation therapy, completed with a consistent therapy of underlying vascular risk factors (especially arterial hypertension, diabetes mellitus, and hypercholesterolemia), is mainly concerned.

The role of a psychologist, except for mapping the cognitive abilities and possible personality changes, will consist of psychotherapeutic and cognitive-rehabilitation care (in cooperation with other specialists, as needed).

1. Introduction

1.1. History

The term *"arteriosclerotic dementia"* (originally "arteriosclerotic psychosis") originated in 1910, when Emil Kraepelin separated a special group of dementias from the class of senile and presenile dementias. The terms such as "arteriosclerotic brain degeneration," "senile cortical atrophy," "periventricular white matter atrophy," "perivascular gliosis" appeared.

In 1974, Hachinski, Lassen, and Marshall correlated dementia with the volume of brain tissue impaired during infarctions; the concept of *multi-infarction dementia* was established. The first diagnostic criteria were designed—Hachinski ischemic score (HIS). It appeared capable of differentiating between the multi-infarction and Alzheimer's dementia but was not able to differentiate the mixed disorders (Román, 1999).

In the 1990s, new diagnostic criteria were prepared that, as an integral part, include the results of imaging and neuropsychological methods, such as the California criteria (State of California Alzheimer's Disease Diagnostic and Treatment Centers, CADDTC), MKN-10 and DSM-IV criteria and especially the NINDS-AIREN (National Institute of Neurological Disorders and Stroke-Association Internationale pour la Recherche et l´Enseignment en Neurosciences) criteria.

In 1994, the Consortium of Canadian Centres for Clinical Cognitive Research concluded that no one criteria was superior to the others (Chui et al., 2000); however, the NINDS-AIREN criteria are most often preferred.

1.2. Classification of Vascular Dementias

We can find various classifications of vascular dementias in the literature. Because of this, the situation does not make for an easy survey; various classifications often use various nomenclatures for the same clinical units. We build upon the works of Román (1999) and Erkinjuntti (2002). A picture of the cognitive deficit in single subtypes is described in the relevant subchapter.

According to localization, we classify vascular dementias as follows:

- *cortical*—strategically located infarction, multi-infarction dementia,
- *subcortical*—lacunary dementia, Binswanger's disease.

According to etiology:

- *ischemic*—disease of small or large arteries, cardioembolism, hypoxia,
- *hemorrhagic.*

According to clinical course:

- *acute:* up to three months after stroke
- *subacute:* with chronic-progressive course.

1.3. Risk Factors

We may prevent the development of vascular cognitive impairment (in contrast to the majority of cognitive deficits having different etiologies) by means of primary and secondary prevention of vascular brain disease.

Risk factors that *cannot* be therapeutically affected include: age (>45 years), male gender, genetic predisposition, previous cerebrovascular accident, low grade of achieved education.

Risk factors that *can* be therapeutically affected include: arterial hypertension, diabetes mellitus, hypercholesterolemia, coronary artery disease, arteriosclerosis, cardioembolism, overweight, smoking, excessive consumption of alcohol (adjusted, Román, 1999; Schmidt et al., 2000; Pohjasvaara et al., 2000).

1.4. Prevalence

Vascular dementia is the second most common cause of dementia in Europe and the United States, and it is generally the most common cause of dementia in some regions of Asia (Alagiakrishnan, 2007). Prevalence is 1.5% in the western countries and approximately 2.2% in Japan. Incidence and prevalence of vascular dementia is increases rapidly with age; prevalence is higher in males than females; there are differences in prevalence and incidence between countries (it accounts for 50%, 20%, 15% and 13% of all dementias in people above 65 years of age in Japan, Europe, Latin America and Australia, respectively).

Mortality is significantly increased in patients with dementia following stroke—the five-year survival rate is 39% for patients with vascular dementia compared to 75% in healthy individuals. Vascular dementia is associated with higher mortality compared to Alzheimer's disease—due to co-existence with other arteriosclerotic complications.

2. Major Domains of the Measurable Cognitive Abilities

In the literature on vascular dementia, we can find various batteries of tests for measurement of single cognitive domains. However, the trend to examine the patient on a complex level prevails, altogether with regard to a broad ethiopathogenetic basis and a varied picture of the syndrome of vascular dementia—the problems with single domains most often depend on the localization of particular neurological deficits.

2.1. Screening

The purpose of screening methods is a "rough" differentiation of the standard from the pathology. The patient often encounters these methods for the first time in the general practitioner's or specialist's (neurologist, psychiatrist) office. However, results of these methods must be followed with specialized neuropsychological examinations. There are a number of methods and, therefore, we cover only a few of them.

Domain	Symptom	Problems
Executive abilities	Decision-making, planning, problem-solving, prediction of results, focusing on goal, learning by learning, feedback ability, regulation of correct social behavior, control of vigilance, cognitive flexibility.	Problems from the beginning of the disease, especially in the subcortical impairment.
Psychomotor pace		Retardation, which is very often already in the initial phase
Vigilance	Targeted, maintained, distributed, and alternated.	Problems very often already from the beginning.
Symbolic abilities	Speech (apprehension, repetition, denomination, fluency). Reading, writing, calculating.	Aphasia, alexia, agraphia, acalculia—rather in the later phases or as an isolated deficit.
Memory	Visual-auditory-tactile-taste-olfactory/short-/long-term/declarative-(semantic-episodic)-non-declarative-procedural	Difficulties according to localization of the deficit
Visual-spatial and constructive-practical capabilities	Spatial orientation, determination of relations between the objects or with regard to the patient, assembling, formation, drawing	Difficulties rather in the later phases
Motor performance	Rough and fine motor functions, ability to cope with the sequences of tasks	Aphasia—rather in the later phases or as an isolated deficit (in strategically located infarction).

2.1.1. Mini-mental State Examination, MMSE (Folstein et al., 1975)

This method is by far the most common in studies that investigate the neuropsychological aspects of vascular dementia (due to its limited use, it is not described in detail). It helps to detect mental impairment especially in elderly people. It correlates highly with other screening methods, e.g., with the Dementia Rating Scale (Taussig et al., 1996). The advantage of this method is its conciseness and its ease of evaluation. However, without other tests, its predicative value is limited, from a psychologist's point of view.

2.1.2. Mattis Dementia Rating Scale, MDRS or only DRS (Mattis, 1988)

Another commonly used screening method; it was designed to discriminate types of dementia, especially Alzheimer's, Huntington's, and Parkinson's dementia (e.g., Salmon et al., 1989). However, it is also used during investigations of vascular dementia (e.g., Borson, Scanlan, 2003).

2.1.3. Cambridge Neuropsychological Test Automated Battery, Cantab (Robbins, 1994)

This method was developed especially for the diagnosis of cognitive deficits in patients with neurodegenerative diseases or cerebral impairment. It is sensitive for detection of the early stages of the disease. The test is computerized and is independent of language and cultural traditions.

2.1.4. Mini-Cog (Borson et al., 2000)

Mini-Cog is a rapid screening method for detection of dementia in elderly people. Borson et al. (2000) report higher sensitivity in comparison to the MMSE, its administration time is shorter and its diagnostic value is not affected by language or education.

According to some investigations (Borson, 2003), it appears that Mini-Cog can detect mild cognitive deficits as a pre-grade of dementia. However, in this case, there is some skepticism due to the brevity of the test; it is unlikely to be able to fully detect and evaluate cognitive deficits.

2.1.5. The 7-Minute Screen (Solomon et. al., 1998)

A screening tool designed originally for detection of Alzheimer's disease. The advantage is its short administration time (seven minutes).

2.2. Global Mental Status

Global mental status of a patient should be mapped in detail after a screening examination. Commonly used methods include the Wechsler intelligence tests—the most recent revision *WAIS-III (Wechsler Adult Intelligence Scale).*

Useful information from the tests focuses on the determination of the pre-morbid intellectual level.

2.2.1. The Ammons Quick Test (Ammons, Ammons, 1962)

A passive-response picture-vocabulary test; it can be administered even to physically challenged individuals. The results are comparable with the WAIS IQ scales.

2.2.2. The North American Adult Reading Test, Naart (Blair, Spreen, 1989)

A reading test used for determination of verbal intellectual ability. The results are also comparable with the WAIS scales.

2.2.3. The Wide Range Achievement Test, WRAT (Wilkinson, 1993)

This test focuses on performance in reading, spelling, and written arithmetic.

2.3. Executive Abilities

Problems with executive abilities (impairment in the frontal lobes) are often seen in patients with vascular dementias, especially in cases of subcortical vascular dementia. However, the tests for measurement of executive abilities are not designed specifically for this type of disease. Studies in vascular dementia often include the Trail Making Test, Stroop Color, and Word Test and Wisconsin Card Sorting Test.

2.3.1. Trail Making Test, TMT (Reitan, Wolfson, 1985)

The psychomotor pace (part A) and cognitive flexibility (part B) tests are concerned. Part B is especially sensitive for detection of executive abilities (e.g., Demakis, 2004).

2.3.2. Stroop Color and Word Test (Stroop, 1935)

This test measures the ability of shifting the vigilance; it is a measure of flexibility. It is sensitive for detection of brain damage, especially in the frontal areas (e.g., Perret, 1974, Demakis, 2004).

2.3.3. Wisconsin Card Sorting Test, WCST (Heaton, 1981)

This test is sensitive to brain dysfunctions in the area of the frontal lobe (more accurately, the dorsolateral area of the left frontal lobe).

2.3.4. Design Fluency Test (Jones-Gotman, 1991)

This test measures the ability to form new, abstract designs. It does not require any special aids. It was designed as a non-verbal analogy to verbal fluency tests. Its purpose is to create as many nonsensical designs as possible, which "cannot be denominated."

It appears that this test is sensitive in patients who suffer from dementia (Spreen, Strauss, 1998). It is generally classified among the tests that are sensitive to frontal lobe impairment.

2.3.5. Five-Point Test (Jones-Gotman, Milner, 1997)

This test was also designed as a non-verbal analogy to verbal fluency tests. It is sensitive for detection of brain damage in general and more specifically to areas in the frontal lobe (Spreen, Strauss, 1998).

2.3.6. Cognitive Estimation Test, CET (Shallice, Evans, 1978)

Patients with brain impairment, especially in the area of the frontal lobe, have problems with cognitive estimations (which are a part of executive abilities). This test includes questions, to which the respondents possibly do not know the exact answer. The ability to select the adequate plan and to check the probability of the estimation is used; exact calculations are not important (e.g., “What is the average length of human backbone?”). This test was originally designed for the British population; its advantages are easy administration, short time requirements and good predicative value.

2.4. Psychomotor Pace

As already stated, cognitive deficit often develops slowly, especially in cases of subcortical vascular dementia, and reduced cognitive flexibility or psychomotor pace may be one of the few warning signals. To examine it, we can use, for example, the **Symbols** subtest from the *WAIS* scale (this subtest can be found in a number of studies on vascular dementia) or *TMT, part A.*

Psychomotor pace is an integral part of other cognitive domains. Therefore, it can be monitored using other tests.

2.5. Vigilance

We should also focus on the quality of concentration of vigilance during the examination because vigilance disorders could, like psychomotor pace, be one of the first symptoms of cognitive deficit. The most frequently used tests are based on the principle of discrimination of shapes, provide information on the quality of focused vigilance, accuracy of perception, and psychomotor pace.

Except for short-term targeted concentration (measurable with a variety of tests), it is very important to monitor long-term concentration of vigilance of the patient over the course of the entire examination. We can monitor the quality of vigilance in many tests focused primarily on other cognitive domains. Again, no tests specifically designed for patients with vascular dementia are available..

TMT, part A and Repeating of numbers, the Stroop tests, as well as the *Symbols* from the Wechsler's tests are suitable because they can be used within the examination of other cognitive abilities; they are often a part of research studies as well.

2.6. Speech (Phatic) and other Symbol Abilities

Speech disorders may also be a part of the symptomatology of vascular dementia—therefore, it is reasonable to examine speech (ideally in cooperation with clinical logopedist).

Patients with impaired frontal lobes have problems with pace and fluency of speech. The tests aimed at these characteristics are, therefore, often classified in the group of methods that map executive abilities. The tests aimed at speech are part of more extensive test batteries.

2.6.1. Verbal Fluency Tests, VFT

There are a number verbal fluency tests available; they measure speed and flexibility of verbal-intellectual processes—e.g., Controlled Oral Word Association Test, Thurstone Verbal Fluency.

In cases of lexical fluency, the task is to create as many words as possible that start with the given letter, during one minute (first names, numbers and identical words with different suffixes are not valid). The letters F, A and S are used in English.

In case of semantic fluency, the task is to name as many words as possible that belong to a defined category during one minute—e.g., "animals" or "food."

2.6.2 Boston Naming Test (Kaplan et al., 1983)

This test is based on a high incidence of problems with naming in patients with aphasias and other neurological disorders. It measures the ability to name displayed objects. It is a good tool for differentiation between Alzheimer's and vascular dementia (Barr et al., 1992).

2.6.3 Token Test (De Renzi, Vignolo, 1962)

This test was designed to detect mild disorders of the receptive function of speech and comprehension of auditory instructions; it has been modified in various ways. Agnosia must be excluded prior to this test.

This test is often used in studies of vascular dementia.

2.6.4. Western Aphasia Battery, Wab (Kertesz, 1979)

This battery contains language subtests and tasks focused on reading, writing and non-verbal subtests. It may be used in differential diagnostics of speech disorders associated with Alzheimer's disease and cerebrovascular accidents (Horner et al., 1992).

2.7. Memory

Mnestic difficulties are not determinative in cases of vascular dementias. However memory must be examined. There are a number of memory tests—however, the scope of this work does not include discussing them in detail.

2.7.1. Wechsler Memory Scale-III, WMS-III (Wechsler, 1997)

This test maps visual and auditory-verbal modality; it is focused on immediate and delayed performance as well as on working memory. It is a frequently used battery.

2.7.2. Memory Assessment Scales, MAS (Williams, 1991)

This is another battery focused on testing of verbal and visual memory in adults. It provides information about immediate and delayed memory and the ability to recognize information and objects.

2.7.3. Verbal Learning Tests

These tests are focused on verbal learning, organization, and memory. The task is to remember a list of words (presented several times in sequence). A list-distracter (to divert the vigilance) can also be a part of this test as well as a section involving re-identification and recognition. These tests are also a part of more extensive test batteries.

E.g., *Rey Auditory Verbal Learning Test (Schmidt, 1996), California Verbal Learning Test (Delis et al., 1987).*

The *Rey-Osterrieth figur*e (see 3.6.2) can be used for testing of visual modality. The test is useful since it can be administered very quickly.

2.8. Constructive-Practical and Visual-Spatial Abilities

2.8.1 Clock Drawing Test (Sunderland Et Al., 1989)

There are various versions available that are slightly different from each other. Difficulty performing the task indicates constructive apraxia. This test is associated with temporo-parietal functions. It has been used in studies of vascular dementia; however, it does not specifically differentiate between Alzheimer's disease and vascular dementia (Spreen, Strauss, 1998).

2.8.2. Rey – Osterrieth Figure (Meyers, Meyers, 1996)

The aim is to draw a complex figure according to a model; when the model is removed the figure must be drawn (as accurately as possible); the test is repeated again in 30 minutes. Part "recall" can also be used; parts of the figure are presented to the patient, and they must decide if the parts were present in the original figure.

This test is frequently used by neuropsychologists. This test maps the visual-spatial constructive abilities and visual-motor control and vigilance and mnestic capacity (Spreen, Strauss, 1998).

This test is not used specifically for vascular dementias. However, it is suitable because of the relatively large amount of diagnostic data that can be obtained from it.

2.8.3. Assembly Tests and Block Designs from the Wechsler Tests

Apart from constructive-practical abilities, executive functions are a prerequisite for successful completion of this task.

2.9. Motor Abilities

Tests of motor performance are an integral part of neuropsychological examinations. The tests provide information about psychomotor pace, fine, and rough motor functions and evaluate the presence of possible apraxia—useful tests are listed in the previous subchapter.

2.9.1. Finger Tapping Test (Reitan, Wolfson, 1985)

The purpose of this test is to measure psychomotor pace. The performance of the right and left hand are monitored—the patient presses the key as quickly as possible. The test is part of the Halstead-Reitan battery.

2.10. Behavior

If dementia is suspected, the patient's behavior must also be monitored as well as how they cope with the activities of daily living. There are a large number of various scales regarding this topic; we state those that appear most often in the literature with regard to vascular dementia. It is very important to compare the data from the scale with personal patient observations (as with all other examinations of the abilities and functions) and observations and information provided by members of the patient's family.

2.10.1. Instrumental Activity of Daily Living, IADL (Lawton, Brody, 1969)

Apart from detection of a patient's cognitive level, a number of studies on vascular dementia have focused on the patient's ability to cope with normal daily activities.

One of the evaluated scales, IADL, evaluates a patient's ability to use a telephone, travel, do shopping, prepare meals, perform housework, take medicines, and manage money. Each of these activities has three grades—from trouble-free behavior to complete disability.

2.10.2. Neurobehavioral Rating Scale, NRS (Levin et al., 1987)

This scale was designed for patients who are able to provide valid answers using other methods (e.g., MMPI). The items concern cognition, metacognition, somatic areas/anxiety, and language areas.

Sultzer (1993) states that compared to patients with Alzheimer's disease, patients with vascular dementia have worse cognitive as well as depressive symptoms.

2.11. Personality and Emotivity

We should not focus only on cognitive abilities when making a diagnosis—information about the patient's personality is very important! Unfortunately, we often do not have enough time to get this information.

2.11.1. Rorschach test (Rorschach, 1921)

This complex method can provide information about the structure of the patient's personality, their current emotional status and possible organic brain damage; however, it does not provide specific information about vascular dementia.

2.11.2. MMPI (Butcher et al., 1989)

This well-known and accepted method is often used, together with the neuropsychological tests, for mapping personality and emotional status. It may also help in further understanding the reactions of patients with neurological damage.

2.11.3. Neuropsychiatric Inventory, NPI (Cummings et al., 1994)

This inventory concerns neuropsychiatric problems that are common in patients with dementia: hallucinations, agitation, dysphoria, anxiety, apathy, irritability, euphoria, disinhibition, aberrant behavior, problems with behavior during the night, and problems with food intake.

2.11.4. Beck Depression Inventory, BDI (Beck, 1993) and Others

The BDI involves a self-assessment scale that is used in clinical practice and research. Inventory items focus on the affective, cognitive, motivation, and physiological symptoms of depression. The questionnaire measures the current status and not depressivity as a feature of personality.

The following methods are used to assess depression in patients with post-stroke depression (e.g., Provinciali, Coccia, 2002): the *Hamilton evaluating depression scale—HAMD* (Hamilton, 1967), the *Zung objektive depression scale—SDS* (Zung, 1965), and the *Geriatric depression scale—GDS* (Yesavage et al., 1983).

3. Course of the Cognitive Deficit

3.1. Prodromal Phase

Multi-infarction dementia was considered to be the main type of vascular dementia. The opinion that sudden deterioration of cognitive abilities was related to clinically manifested cerebrovascular accident dominated. However, this would mean that there is no prodromal cognitive deficit similar to mild cognitive impairment described in Alzheimer's disease. However, today we know that in contrast to multi-infarction dementia (with dominating cortical deficit) subcortical dementia has a slow onset of difficulties often without a history of cerebrovascular accident, and reduced cognitive flexibility is one of a small number of signs (Garret, 2004).

The Canadian study of health and aging (Ingles, 2002) showed that the problems of some patients with vascular cognitive impairment had recovered spontaneously over a five-year period. This would mean that the occurrence of mild cognitive impairment does not have to cause a picture of dementia.

3.2. Multi-Infarction Dementia

This disease is caused by multiple territorial infarctions during closure or narrowing of main cerebral arteries. *Fast onset of cognitive difficulties and gradual worsening* (sometimes with transitional improvement) is a typical sign. *Unstable distribution* of single difficulties (mainly at the beginning) is substantial—depending on the areas in the brain that were affected. Some abilities may, therefore, deteriorate very early while others remain relatively intact.

3.3. Strategically Located Ictus

Depending on the location, a number of cognitive, mnestic and behavioral changes can be seen that do not always satisfy the criteria for dementia as a global impairment.

3.4. Subcortical Vascular Dementia

Subcortical ischemic vascular disease/dementia, SIVD (Erkinjunnti et al., 2000) is a disease of small arteries (arterioles) in the subcortical area with a characteristic chronic course, fluctuations, and progressive deterioration. Step-by-step deterioration, which is generally associated with vascular dementia, is often missing; therefore the difficulties may be misdiagnosed as Alzheimer's disease (Schmidtke, 2003).

The problems often start *very slowly. Impairment of executive abilities* together with reduced *cognitive flexibility and reduced psychomotor pace* are typical. Memory disorders (which may be mild), especially reduced recall, can appear sometimes from the beginning; therefore, hints are beneficial (Erkinjuntti, 2000). Apathy or depression also occurs frequently.

The lesions look like multiple lacunary infarctions or affections of the white matter. Objective neurological examination shows pyramidal and extrapyramidal symptoms, incontinence, pseudobulbar syndrome, and gait disorders. Most of the patients are treated for arterial hypertension. Hyperlipidemia, diabetes mellitus, and other diseases are common.

Subtypes: *lacunary dementia* (synonym: dementia with lacunary infarctions, status lacunaris) and *Binswanger's disease* (synonym: Binswanger's dementia, Binswanger's encephalopathy).

3.5. Late Stage

Cognitive deficits become *generalized* in the later stages of the disease—it cannot be easily determined which type or subtype of dementia is present in the patient.

Patients with vascular dementia are often well aware of their disability, which is one of the factors that cause high incidences of depression (up to 60% of cases).

4. Proposal of Standardized Examination of the Cognitive Functions

For planning, we must observe especially the purpose of the examination: The patient who is suspected of having cognitive deterioration must be examined in detail in order to map *a distribution of single abilities* (Tab. 1). More specific methods should be used in the next *differential diagnostic decision-making* on the particular type of dementia (Tab. 2). Another structure should be chosen when *planning research studies* (Tab. 3 and 4).

As for the tables, it must be noted that most of the tests are complex—they are focused on many cognitive domains at once; some tests may appear several times in the table (classification according to domains is somewhat artificial in this case).

Dialogue is an integral part of the examination— with the patient and with someone who has close personal contacts (to facilitate getting a complete history).

Single test methods are described in the relevant subchapter.

Table 1. Test methods suitable for detection of deterioration of the cognitive abilities

Global status	WAIS-III, CANTAB
Memory	WMS-III, R-O figure, Verbal learning tests
Executive abilities	TMT B, Stroop, CET
Speech abilities	Verbal fluency tests, Token Test, or WAB
Visual-spatial and constructive-practical abilities	R-O figure, Clock Test, Blocks, Jigsaw
Psychomotor pace	Symbols, TMT A
Vigilance	TMT A, repeating of numbers from the WAIS
Symbolic abilities - orientation	Reading, writing, calculation + drawing of a human figure
Emotivity-depression	BDI
Behavior	IADL, NPI, or. NRS

4.1. Deterioration of the Cognitive Abilities

It is difficult, if not impossible, to submit a test battery that could be used in all examinations. We must always take into account the circumstances of the patient—and this is particularly true in cases of cognitive deterioration. For example, drawing of a human figure, or a test of reading and writing ability, is for some patients, so difficult that a copy of an R-O figure would be almost impossible; moreover, having the patient confront these marked limitations could subsequently reduced their motivation, and reduce their willingness to continue cooperating, or it could increase their depressive status We must also take into account patient fatigue, and adapt the testing period accordingly. The examination should not leave the patient exhausted!

The list of examinations is rather informative.

4.2. Differential Diagnostics: Vascular Dementia X Alzheimer Disease

Neuropsychological differentiation between Alzheimer's disease and vascular dementia is often difficult, although these diseases have different etiologies. A number of studies (e.g., Erkinjuntti et al., 1986; Almkvist et al., 1999) have reported similar neuropsychological characteristics of both diseases. According to these studies, any efforts at differentiation would not be practical and of limited value. In addition, both diseases have similar risk factors. New studies have appeared that provide evidence of a positive effect when cognitive drugs (currently used only in case of Alzheimer's disease) are used for vascular dementia, and, therefore, it may be presumed that, in the future, therapeutic procedures for these diseases will converge.

On the contrary, some studies have found differences. Poorer memory and speech is usually reported in patients with Alzheimer's disease, while poorer executive abilities and an uneven distribution of the cognitive deficit is reported in patients with vascular dementia (e.g., Uzzel, 2000; Graham et al., 2004).

In Table 2, we propose methods that can be used to supplement diagnostic data. However, we make note that differentiation can be misleading.

Table 2. Differential diagnostics of vascular dementia and Alzheimer disease - supplement to the diagnostics of cognitive functions

Executive abilities	WCST, Design Fluency Test, or Five-Point Test
Speech abilities	BNT
Personality, emotivity	ROR, GDS

4.3. Research Studies

We must primarily follow the purpose of the study when planning its design. Psychological tests are most often used in combination with other medical methods (e.g., pharmacotherapy, imaging methods). The tendency to *reduce* the period of psychological testing is common; however, it is *arguable* to generalize the acquired information. If we have enough space, we can use any other method, e.g., from the list above.

The sets of proposed tests are just for orientation; tests that are frequently used in various studies are presented.

Table 3. Studies—proposal of basic battery of tests

Screening	Mini-Cog (including drawing of the clock)
Executive abilities	TMT or Stroop
Speech abilities	Verbal fluency tests
Emotivity	BDI, or HAMD

Table 3. Studies—proposal of more detailed battery of tests

Screening	MMSE, CANTAB
Executive abilities	TMT, Stroop
Memory	Repeating of figures from the WAIS-R, R-O figure, Verbal learning tests
Speech abilities	Verbal fluency tests
Visual-spatial and constructive abilities	R-O figure, or Clock Test
Emotivity - depression	BDI, or HAMD, SDS
Behavior	IADL, or NPI or NRS

As an illustration, the neuropsychological tests used for detection of cognitive deficits in the Canadian study of health and aging are presented (*www.csha.ca).* The study was performed in Canada from 1991 to 2001, and involved 10,263 people over 65 years of age.

Table 5. Battery of tests in the CSHA

Memory	WAIS-R—Information and repeating of figures, Benton's tests of visual retention, Rey Auditory-Verbal Learning Test, Working Memory, Buschke Cued Recall Test
Abstraction thinking	WAIS-R - similarities
Executive abilities	WAIS-R—symbols, Trail Making Test
Judgment	WAIS-R—understanding
Aphasia	Token Test, Boston Naming Test, Tests of verbal fluency
Apraxia	Clock test, Gesture Execution Test
Agnosia	Buschke Visual Identification Test
Construction	WAIS-R—blocks
Premorbid intellect	Wide Range Achievement Test - Reading

5. Rehabilitation and Psychotherapy of the Cognitive Deficit

5.1. Cognitive Rehabilitation

The patient with brain damage requires complex therapy with an emphasis on *cognitive and psychosocial functioning.* It is not possible to separate these aspects, although in some cases, affection in one of these areas may appear as more marked relative to the other area.

Wilson (1997) evaluated various methods of neuropsychological rehabilitation of which the most successful was considered to be a holistic model, which stresses integration of cognition and emotions. Of course, it is ideal to combine cognitive rehabilitation with psychotherapy.

Rehabilitation of patients with vascular dementia should generally include (Garrison, 2000):

- Compensation of cognitive deficits;
- Training of movement;
- Reduction of problematic behaviors (e.g., by means of supportive psychotherapy);
- Education of family and consideration of hiring a caregiver;
- Safety training (including fall prevention).

Due to its complexity, it should ideally be ensured by a *team of specialists:* neurologist, psychologist, psychiatrist, logopedist, social worker, physical therapist, dietary nurse, and, if needed, a legal consultant.

Cognitive rehabilitation (or cognitive training) should always be performed with a focus on the particular needs of the patient with regard to routine daily activities.

Rehabilitation is especially important in patients with initial cognitive deficits, as it can play an important role in increasing (or at least limiting the decline) in their quality of life. Some authors call attention to the fact that rehabilitation is most effective in those patients who experienced limited, especially focal impairment, in an otherwise intact terrain. Nevertheless, there are some authors (e.g., Clare, Woods, 2003) who state that there is no evidence for any positive benefit as a result of cognitive rehabilitation.

In cases of cognitive deficit, we can differentiate three main areas of dysfunctions: memory, language abilities, and visual-spatial abilities (Uzzel, 2000).

The following is used in *memory disorders*: drill and practice, visual imagination, system of cards with notices, programs based on residual abilities of learning. It is always necessary to find out which "type" of memory is impaired in a given case (e.g., semantic or episodic) and to individually select the optimal approach. It is important to take into account motivation: the patient wants to recall where they put their car keys and what to buy in the store; however, patients are not interested in recalling of the list of words that are unrelated to their daily needs. Therefore, an individual approach is needed when designing rehabilitation a plan. For example, some patients prefer to learn (or to repeat) the names of people they often meet, which helps them to engage in social activities again. Others want to focus on repeating generally known information; and others yet prefer working on developing practical skills.

Speech disorders cause marked difficulties in psychosocial functioning—either the expressive or receptive component is involved or, in some cases, both. They often cause social isolation and may persist for extended periods. Speech analysis of the patient makes the creation of an individual rehabilitation plan possible; something that is best handled by a logopedist.

Visual-spatial dysfunction may also be very devastating. It causes spatial confusion, disables reading or writing, use of tools at work; because of it, patients cannot leave their homes without the assistance of another. Many daily activities become impossible; and often it puts an end to personal independence (e.g., driving). Individual rehabilitation plans must therefore be emphasized—and training related to the daily activities of a particular patient should be stressed.

Proposal of particular topics in rehabilitation of patients with initial dementia (Clare et al., 2001)

- Practicing of the names of people the patient meets—in order not to feel uncomfortable in communication with people.
- Using aids such as a calendar or memo pad—instead of asking family members.
- Practicing information regarding the family—to better engage in the conversations.
- Coping with the operation of the household items, equipment and machines (washing machine)—to improve self-care activities e.g., hygiene.
- Recognition of coins and banknotes—to facilitate shopping.

Cognitive rehabilitation in combination with physical movement is often recommended. Some yoga elements are suitable—the patient should try to focus on his body and feelings during the training (this also allows the patient to work on concentration and vigilance at the same time). Walking outside is also suitable—with a focus on activities around the patient's home or to trying to recall events and experiences after returning home from a walk. Another useful activity that can be employed before going to bed is to have the patient try to recall the event of the passed day—with the focus on visual or auditory stimuli depending on which causes more problems for the patient. In cases of anatomic difficulties, it is useful for the patient to learn how to "describe" problematic terms—using a synonym or whole sentences; then speech fluency is not so markedly impaired.

It can also be very stimulating to play games with the patient—word soccer, finding a town or a well-known personality, fabrication of words that begin with a certain letter, composition of sentences from selected words, doing puzzles or playing cards. The advantage is that such play involves using many cognitive abilities at once; if the patient enjoys game-playing, it can motivate the patient and enhance his willingness to engage in similar activities again; also important is that no expensive aids are needed, and the patient can play the games at home—with his partner, children or grandchildren. Reading aloud is also an excellent rehabilitation method—either reading news from the newspaper, fairy tales or any subject of interest.

There are a number of computer games aimed at rehabilitating single abilities or more global tasks—e.g., Train the Brain, Rehabit, RehaCom, Cognition, PSS CogReHab, and others. Programs, which were originally intended for diagnostics of cognitive abilities, can also be used as well. Interactivity of such programs is a definite advantage—the patient may work alone (e.g., at home) while still getting motivational feedback.

Cognitive rehabilitation does not eliminate problems with memory and other problem areas for the patient, but it can teach his to cope with his problems better—to be self-supportive—and, therefore, it can markedly improve the quality of the patient's life.

Rehabilitation must present the patient with a realistic assessment and expectations; some setbacks are normal—not everything will go perfectly, but the patient should be encouraged not loose his motivation.

5.2. Changes of Personality and Defense Mechanisms

Patients with brain lesions of various etiologies often have *mental inefficiency* (fast mental exhaustion after modest mental activity); reduced self-confidence (in case of impairment of the right hemisphere), unrealistically increased self-assessment (in case of impairment of the left hemisphere); and premorbid "damped" personality features are accentuated.

Due to the multifaceted clinical picture of vascular cognitive impairment (and its broad ethological basis), it is impossible to unambiguously describe the changes that occur in personality structure.

According to the literature (see above) and in cases of strategically located infarctions, we can see, except for cognitive deficits, *loss of motivation and initiative, emotional lability*, or *disinhibition*; *apathia* and *depression* in cases of subcortical vascular impairment. However, rather than focus on the symptoms of a particular brain lesion, the authors are mostly focused on the more complex elements of the patient's personality and the changes the patient is going through (perhaps because physicians are mainly involved in the topic of vascular dementia).

It is generally accepted that a particular psychological reaction with subsequent changes in living and behavior always occur in response to any serious disease. In cases of vascular cognitive impairment, two factors occur at the same time—vascular problems and cognitive deficits. Patients after cerebrovascular accidents are very often fearful of a recurrence. They are preoccupied with imminent limitations (paralysis, aphasia) and the possibly of death. When cognitive deficits are combined with vascular problems, the situation becomes even more problematic.

Sometimes, a spontaneous *restructuring of the patient's value system* occurs, and consequential changes in lifestyle result; the patient has at least some active control over the situation. Ideally, this step is supported by the patient's surroundings.

Unfortunately, we can often see a *passive attitude*, associated with anxiety and depression. Passivity may be instinctively supported by physicians who often prescribe anxiolytic drugs or antidepressives without a detailed knowledge of the situation. It is the task of the psychologist to give the patient an outlet for negative emotions and allow the patient to talk about his fears and anxieties regarding the situation—however, not all patients can be motivated to cooperate with a psychologist. Focusing more and more on active coping should proceed gradually; therefore, it is important to start with cognitive rehabilitation as soon as possible—the patient then receives tools needed to cope with the new limitations associated with his condition.

Depreciation or even *negation* is another reaction to emerging limitations. This occurs frequently in patients with subcortical vascular dementia without obvious brain accident. The situation is made worse because the onset is often very slow and the patient's personal contacts (including some physicians) do not notice it. Of course, it is very difficult to work with the patient with such defense mechanisms. Some problems appear during the psychological examination; however the patient usually "forgets" them. Then, the patient is not motivated to participate in psychotherapy or cognitive rehabilitation; however, right in this phase of the disease, a lot can be done for increasing or at least maintaining the current quality of life.

Depression does not have to appear at the beginning the current disease. Because the feelings associated with the disease are often preserved in cases of vascular dementia, depression should be a generally expected and understandable condition that can occur anytime during the entire course of the disease.

The world of the patient often falls to ruin: at home and at work his performance is reduced; he has feelings of inadequacy and he realizes the consequences his impairment will have on his future (lifestyle, sports, hobbies, etc); and he may find that it is all more than he can cope with. He often has the feeling that his family and friends have turned away from him, are frightened by and do not understand him. Significant changes can also occur in relationship with a partner: he may feel that he has become a burden and that he no longer provide any benefit for his partner.

Patients resort to various defense mechanisms; *frustration, anger, anxiety, aggressiveness* or the converse, *sadness and apathy* may occur. Their personality characteristics may completely change.

Personality changes are one of the basic symptoms of advanced dementia (not only vascular). *Reduction of emotional control* or *motivation* or *changes of social behavior are* discussed most often. Emotional lability, irritation, apathy, or coarse social behavior can occur. Psychological help consists especially as support of the patient (assuming the patient is motivated for at least basic cooperation) and second, support of the patient's family.

5.3. Psychotherapy

Focusing on *the most active situational coping*, as stated above, has proven to be effective in psychotherapy for patients with vascular dementia (similar to other serious diseases). The feeling of *responsibility* for themselves and their surroundings should be strengthened at the same time. The goals set at the beginning or during therapy should be realistic in any case.

Unfortunately, in cases of dementia, the patient cannot be motivated by meeting other patients who overcame the disease (because, regrettably, we cannot treat dementia). It could be beneficial to *meet*—and to share problems—with other patients who are roughly at the same stage of the disease. According to various references in the literature, patient groups appear to be very useful in cognitive rehabilitation. Ideally, supportive groups involving family members of patients' should be arranged.

It is also important to provide *information* about the disease, its course and treatment possibilities to the patient (and the patient's relatives), including discussions of the proper lifestyle changes. Additionally the psychologist should work as an agent between the patient and his physician. Last but not least, practical information can be very useful: Contacts to daily social welfare institutions, caregiver service, spa, etc.

One of the main principles of psychotherapy is to emphasize to patients and help them understand how important it is to keep trying—and to live as active and as meaningful a life as possible.

Conclusion

Vascular dementia is the second most common type of dementia, after Alzheimer's disease. It is not a disease with a uniform clinical picture and course, but it consists of a *broad spectrum* of cognitive disorders linked to cerebrovascular disease, of which, only some fulfill the general criteria for dementia. Therefore, the current effort is to replace this term by a more comprehensive term "*vascular cognitive impairment*" (VCI).

Multi-infarction dementia (MID) is typically present with a sudden decline in cognitive abilities and followed by gradual deterioration. The character of the cognitive deficit depends on the extent and localization of the brain infarction. MID used to be considered to be a synonym of vascular dementia. In cases of *strategically located ictus,* the clinical picture depends on localization and extent of the lesion—cognitive deficits can be isolated and do not have to fulfill the criteria for dementia. *Subcortical vascular dementia* occurs very unobtrusively and progresses slowly (not "step by step"), and the condition may oscillate. Executive dysfunction is typical for the early stages of the disease. However it may present, for an extended period, as only psychomotor retardation or reduced cognitive flexibility; therefore, this type of vascular dementia may remain unrecognized for a long time.

We can often see so called *mixed dementia*—with the symptoms of both vascular brain disease and Alzheimer's disease. The risk factors and pathogenesis of these two disorders overlap; hence, some authors consider differentiation between them as misleading and counterproductive (especially in the elderly population).

Apathy and depression are also part of the clinical picture, since patients remain cognizant over time.

There are a *number of diagnostic criteria* with various sensitivity and specificity (e.g., NINDS-AIREN, HIS). There are no test methods designed specifically for vascular dementia—it is not a homogenous disease as mentioned previously. We should focus generally on cognitive abilities during *neuropsychological examinations;* in as much detail as possible regarding dysexecutive syndrome, phatic, visual-spatial, and constructive-practical abilities. Last but not least, we should map the extent of the patient's depression and possible changes in personality.

Psychological *rehabilitation* must be focused individually on the deficits that most affect the individual patient. We must always take into account the patient's ability to cope with *daily activities*—including cognitive and psychosocial aspects.

Many authors call attention to the fact that the incidence of vascular dementia will probably increase in the future, which is linked to an unfavorable trend in the prevalence of cardiovascular diseases. Therefore, going forward, it is very important to intensively focus on the problems associated with vascular dementia. Such a focus should result in *improvement of diagnostic methods* (especially early stages of the disease), formulation of a generally accepted *diagnostic criteria* or designing a criteria for the single subgroup of vascular dementia, development of new *therapeutic strategies,* and planning of future *research.*

In: Cognitive Deficit in Mental and Neurological Disorders
Editors: H. Kucerova, M. Preiss
ISBN: 978-1-60741-957-0

Chapter XVI

Neuropsychological Rehabilitation after Head Injuries in Czech Republic

Petr Kulistak

The aim of a medical stay of patients after traumatic head and brain injuries is their complex rehabilitation (a so-called integrative model). One of the components of such rehabilitation is represented by treatment of impaired cognitive functions. A structure of the model is situationally conditioned mainly by the size of a rehabilitation institution (here, situation in a particular institution—Army Rehabilitation Institute in Slapy nad Vltavou, Prague-West—is being described). The clinic is not primarily oriented only to the patients in question. The rehabilitation treatment is offered also to patients after other brain lesions, such as strokes, and to patients after brain operations due to various causes (tumors, aneurysms). However, the main portion of patients is represented by persons after orthopedic operations (joint replacements) and other skeleton injuries that require subsequent treatment.

It is typical for cranio-cerebral traumas to occur as a component of a poly-trauma, in which the head is only one of the affected parts of the body. Unfortunately, consequences of such cases are most painfully felt just after motor deficiencies are already improved, and when problems in the cognitive domain emerge. The length of the remedial stay is the most problematic issue in this area, since the treatment of brain injuries requires much longer time than mere orthopedic deficiencies. In this regard, the requirements of cognitive rehabilitation are usually not met in practice. At the same time, the patients in question cannot continue in such highly specialized rehabilitation (the clinic provides treatment for the whole Czech Republic) and almost nowhere in their place of residence. On the contrary, patients with motor problems are usually able to resume their rehabilitation process due to prevalent accessibility of related remedial departments in district towns or in larger villages. Unfortunately, the rehabilitation of cognitive functions is still not accepted as a specific domain of remedial medicine. A potential prolongation of the remedial stay due to such "insignificant" reasons is thus primarily dependent on the comprehension of an attending doctor, who is responsible for the decision. Although the duration of apparent improvement of a cognitive function is not exactly specified yet, some data (e.g., Thomsen, 1984; Brooks et al., 1986; Kulišťák et al., 1998, 2000, 2001, 2002) imply it may take years or even decades. During this period, "positive" changes in cognitive functions, as well as in emotions and personality, can be observed.

Rehabilitation Team

In addition to medical professions—internists, neurologists, and balneologists—mainly *physical therapists*, whose task lies predominantly in work with the body, belong to the team. They also engage in respiratory therapy, yoga, therapy on a posture-graphy platform (practicing control of posture and balance), as well as in many other standard remedial techniques. Furthermore, with regard to preparation for a job, occupational therapy, which is carried out in a very modern and practically equipped room, is especially significant. Tens of tools are present in the room, which help patients with motor deficiencies to restore or rebuild their motor patterns employed in routine household activities, such as preparation of food. In addition, an area equipped with basic tools for working with wood and metal is also part of the room, as well as a potter's wheel, a kiln for firing of ceramic handicrafts, and other tools and instruments that make various activities of a physically disabled person more pleasant. Moreover, the occupational therapy contributes significantly to restoration of impaired functions in many cognitive domains (see e.g., Faktorová, 1999a,b; 2003), such as perception, attention, visuo-spatial abilities, executive functions (planning, ability to finish a commenced activity, resumption of such activity, anticipation of subsequent steps when performing more sequences of a process), and short- and long-term memory related to the motor area (in most cases, implicit, procedural memory is activated; and since most patients in question suffer from amnesia, in which procedural memory does not tend to be impaired, the process of utilization of this non-declarative component of memory helps to restore their self-confidence in the area of operational abilities). The occupational therapy is based on an assumption that "a person's (patient's) involvement in a goal-oriented and subjectively meaningful activity encourages their mental and physical functions, as well as their overall well-being, and thus leads to improvement of the person's health" (Faktorová, 2003, p. 354).

In addition to the mentioned techniques of the occupational therapy, in our system, we attempt to continue—in the final phase—in the broad spectrum of partial auxiliary approaches by means of their integration in a so-called pre-occupational trial (if the profession of a patient and conditions in the institution are convenient—e.g., an accountant or an economist engaged in activities of their professions, and other specialists in related workrooms). Such trial represents a partial verification of achievement of complete reintegration of the affected person. Unfortunately, new "market" conditions of the Czech health service do not already allow such complete "simulation" of a patient's profession. Nowadays, the preparation in the area of activities of daily living (ADL) is terminated in the occupational therapy room, or in "field," i.e., in the course of occasional shopping, traveling by public transport, etc., in an assistant's presence.

Logopedic *(aphasiologic)* specialists *engage in reeducation of all types of communication disorders, which means both disorders of spoken language— aphasia— and impairments of graphic side of speech—written and read expression, voice disorders, various sensory disorders combined with speech impairments, and swallowing (see e.g., Škodová, Jedlička et al., 2003; Kulišťák et al., 1997).*

A clinical *rehabilitation psychologist* is responsible mainly for "mental" well-being of patients in a remedial institution. Their work consists of provision of short-term supportive psychotherapy and crisis intervention for patients and possibly also for their partners and other related persons who acutely require such care. The psychologist predominantly deals with relationship problems that either patients already "bring" with themselves or that emerge as delayed or prolonged reactions to the injury itself. However, the main reasons of such problems are usually difficulties associated with adaptation to changes in physical, as well as mental living, and emotional and behavioral disorders, which arise as a consequence of a cranio-cerebral trauma, a stroke, or other lesions of CNS. Another substantial issue, which requires intervention of an experienced clinical rehabilitation psychologist, is creation of a patient's further life perspective. Especially in the case of long-term rehabilitation of the cognitive component of an impairment, such perspective may seem to be very distant and indefinite. According to a well-known schema of reaction to a catastrophic event (sometimes called posttraumatic stress syndrome), a "delayed shock" accompanied by precipitate suicidal behavior may emerge right in the course of a rehabilitation process. However, one may prevent such behavior by both careful observation of clients' moods and by psychotherapeutic intervention (see e.g., Šplíchal, 1999). Sometimes, also difficulties in coping with demands of the rehabilitation complex are present—exhaustion, fatigue, overload caused by number of procedures, or by their unsatisfactory organization, wandering while trying to find a relevant department—which are also solved by the rehabilitation psychologist together with a client/patient (recommendation of suitable resting activities, relaxation, etc.), as well as with employees who are responsible for planning. Unfortunately, the clinic does not have facilities and capabilities comparable to those seen at a visit in a neurological rehabilitation clinic in Deggendorf, Bavaria, where a patient with multiple severe cognitive deficits has a rehabilitation assistant at his/her disposal for most of the day. The assistant helps the patient with various activities, walks him/her to relevant specialized departments, and assists in doing physical and cognitive "home-works." We solve this deficiency by means of training of an accompanying person (relative, partner, etc.), who is hospitalized together with the patient/client and who provides for the mentioned needs. However, the person has to get acquainted with all duties by specialized staff, which may represent a problem. In addition, the person's close relation to the patient may be considered as both an advantage and disadvantage. Furthermore, a person that would be willing to undergo the rehabilitation stay together with the patient is often hardly found in the client's environment. Therefore, the treatment tends to rest on the institution.

A *neuropsychologist* is another member of the rehabilitation team. His/her work consists of initial diagnostics, a check examination in the course of the rehabilitation stay, and evaluation of a patient's condition at the end of the stay. On the basis of input data on the patient's state of cognitive functions, the neuropsychologist develops a remedial plan of the patient's optimal restoration. The plan is then regularly monitored both by a classic neuropsychological examination and by results (usually diagrams, various indexes of errors, speed, etc., see below) gained from exercises on special rehabilitation computer programs. In the final evaluation, the neuropsychologist maps achieved successes/failures in detail (improvements, regressions, stagnations, plateaus) and on their basis recommends subsequent treatments, which, however, usually lacks. In Czech republic, there are no—apart from a few exceptions—successive outpatient departments that would take care of patients/clients after a stay in a rehabilitation institution focused on cognitive functions treatment. A so-called "tele-therapy" by means of a rehabilitation computer program NEUROP 2 (Gaál, 2002), which we have again seen during the visit in German rehabilitation institutions, has not been adopted yet, although all Czech materials are already prepared for it (author of this chapter; for more details see below). Moreover, the program enables to "tailor exercises to a patient's needs" by a possibility to adjust stimuli and to use materials from the domestic environment or from the client's interest area. In other words, the program has all characteristics that still do not offer any rehabilitation department together with their employees.

Computer-Assisted Neuro-Cognitive Rehabilitation

Nowadays, the main focus of work with patients after head/brain injuries lies in computer-assisted neuro-cognitive retraining. Since the situation was different in the past and computer rehabilitation programs were not yet available some 15 years ago—or they were too expensive—the "exercises" with particular cognitive domains were carried out with the help of amateurishly made visual aids, components of some of neuropsychological testing batteries (Lurija's neuropsychological examination—Czech version by Danish author Anne-Lise Christensen, 1974), various children's construction kits, puzzles, Pexeso games (also known as Concentration or Pairs), and other educational aids used in kindergartens or in lower grades of elementary schools. Similarly, Rehabit (Reitan evaluation of hemispheric ability and brain improvement training), a structured program for retraining of neuropsychological abilities, which comes from a neuropsychological laboratory of Ralph M. Reitan and Deborah Wolfson (Reitan, 1992), is still based on the mentioned principles— although, naturally, it already consists of specially and professionally made equipment. Sometimes, computer programs are criticized for their inability to provide tactile and proprioceptive feedback, which indeed may be restrictive in some cases. Therefore, the department of neuropsychological rehabilitation has launched an experimental program of training in virtual reality, which is able to supplement the older program with the previously absent sensory perceptions. Needless to say, obdurate objectors of computer-assisted rehabilitation of cognitive functions will surely introduce additional criticism. However, it would be more contributing if they bring out a constructive suggestion of how to ensure rational cognitive rehabilitation without enormously increasing expenses on individual therapist for every patient. They would have to solve also the safety of road transport, because the highest number of patients sustain an injury in road accidents. We use two professional computer rehabilitation programs—a German RehaCom (1997) and an American PSS CogReHab (1994). In case a client/patient is interested in it, we subsequently employ the "tele-therapy" (which consists of training of the person at his/her home and either sending the results on a portable medium by mail or handing them on at a visit to the neuropsychologist) with the help of the program NEUROP 2 (Gaál, 2002). So far as verbally presented stimuli in RehaCom are concerned, they were successfully translated into Czech language. Furthermore, instructions (written in English) are presented to the patient also in a verbal way (in Czech) by an examiner.

Two research projects with a complex design have been done to evaluate and compare effectiveness of the both programs and rehabilitation without the use of computers. However, an obstacle to systematic research work in the realm of cognitive functions rehabilitation is represented also by a system of receiving and releasing the patients to/from hospitals. Since only the patient's motor state of health is monitored and the requirements of the cognitive rehabilitation are not taken into account, it is not possible to study the effectiveness of the rehabilitation methodically. Predominantly, evaluations in a form of research with N=1 tend to be published, and they are usually the results of outpatient visits at other institutions.

Groups of Patients and of Accompanying Persons

At first, when the spatial conditions, as well as lower number of patients/clients enabled it, we were working with persons after head/brain injuries (and after strokes, too) also in the form of group therapies. The content of the meetings followed the requirements of neuro-psychotherapy (Kulišťák, 2003; Grawe, 2004), because classic forms of any of the psychotherapeutic schools were not shown to be suitable for patients with cognition impaired in such a way. For example, Šplíchal (1999, p. 46) writes about some "adaptation" of classic psychotherapy for this specific population, but he does not elaborate further what it should consist of. He states that "in most cases (not always), an attempt to commence psychotherapy is meaningful, but continuation in a long-lasting fruitless effort is not." Nevertheless, all psychologically-neuropsychological treatment is always carried out within the scope of a "psychotherapeutic" milieu. However, sometimes, it is difficult to ensure such approach also by other persons involved in the complex integrated rehabilitation system (nurses, physical therapists, etc.). Although the medical staff is being regularly familiarized with the issue of the persons with brain injuries, particularities of such patients are not always fully respected. We have had an opportunity to get acquainted with both the theoretical publications by main protagonists of psychotherapy for patients with brain injury (Prigatano, 1986), and practical demonstrations of particular forms of such work (Ben-Yishay, 2004a,b). We try to apply the experiences primarily in the individual approach to clients. Moreover, no Czech insurance company would probably cover the financial burden of such treatment. Gradually, since the groups were done in a so-called open form, this kind of therapy had to be abandoned. It was not possible to ensure absolute continuity for the participants and to accomplish the laboriously created program, which respected the mentioned principles of the neuro-psychotherapeutic work. A situation with groups for accompanying persons turned out in a similar manner. Nowadays, such persons are offered individual consultations, as well as introduction to main principles of the "neuro-psychotherapeutic" care about a patient (this happens within the scope of the previously mentioned rehabilitation instructions). An effort to provide a continuation of psychotherapeutic groups or individual therapy for the patients/clients after the release from an institution has meant a considerable disappointment for us. It has been found that a lot of private psychotherapists offer their services primarily to relatively "healthy" people. Consequently, if a "real patient" shows up—in this case a person after a brain injury—they are not capable of helping, because they are not familiar with the issue of neuro-psychotherapy. Patients/clients of this kind thus come back to our—neuropsychological—outpatient care shortly afterwards.

A short case study: When being abroad, a 32-year-old Czech woman sustained a severe poly-trauma (fractures of pelvis and thorax) in a car accident. A severe head and brain lesion (six-week-long coma) was also part of the trauma. From the beginning of her state of vigilance, she was being rehabilitated by means of a computer under supervision of a neuropsychologist. Later, a neuro-pedagogic and other specialists in motor rehabilitation took care of her. We saw her for the first time approximately 1.5 year after the injury—when she came to the rehabilitation clinic in order to finish her treatment. Since almost all her brain functions—except verbal memory—were already at that time at a high level, we employed visual support. After repeated movements, her state was improved practically "ad integrum" (except the memory). She found a part-time job in her field—health service—but a possibility to have a part-time job was soon cancelled. We managed to find her a place in a hotel, where she worked as a receptionist without any problems. However, relationship problems emerged: her husband started to go out with his secretary, he repudiated his wife, deprived her of their child, and forced her out of their house; consequently, she had a psychic breakdown. The psychotherapy that was being arranged for her in famous psychotherapeutic centers (every time when prodromal symptoms of infaust development of the relationship were present) did not have any effect. After her suicide attempt, a psychiatrist had to be consulted and antidepressant therapy by medicaments was initiated. Finally, the woman, who was indeed excellently neuropsychologically (with the help of neuro-psychotherapy) rehabilitated (in Germany) after an almost lethal brain injury, ended in a very unfortunate way owing to the insufficiency of the Czech psychotherapy.

Brain Trauma as a "Therapeutic Tool"

The irony is that severe brain injury may cause a "permanent cure" of addiction to the so-called hard drugs, which usually cannot be achieved by any psychotherapeutic method.

A short case study: A young man, a student of a university in his fourth year, was, at the age of 24 years, run down by a car when riding his mountain bike. He suffered a poly-trauma with a severe head/brain injury (CT examination has shown post-contusion centers temporo-occipital on the right side; subdural pallial haematoma). On the reception to the rehabilitation institution, the man's parents informed that their son had not already studied for a longer period of time, because he had been gravely addicted to hard drugs (cocaine, etc.). The initial examination showed that in addition to frequent impairment of attention/concentration, explicit memory (mainly the verbal component) was extensively damaged, and some emotional/behavioral disorders (irritability, indifference or even apathy) were present due to a right-side localization of the impairment. These personality discrepancies were gradually—in seven years—improved, although mild memory problems still remain to be present. Nevertheless, the man has not taken drugs anymore, and he has a stable relationship with his partner. He worked as a laic therapist, but he had to find a job in a foreign company due to financial provision of his arising family.

A short case study: A young, 19-year-old man, who worked as a car-mechanic, experienced a severe car accident on an access road, in which the other three passengers died owing to a bump into a machine used for refining road surface. He suffered a severe poly-trauma with multiple head/brain injuries, as well as injuries of lower limbs. Since the man was addicted to hard drugs, in the process of clarification of the accident, it was speculated whether the young people were driving under the influence of addictive substances. Although the man's premorbid intellectual level had been slightly lower than in the previously mentioned case, the state of cognitive functions and of self-care abilities was improved to such extent that he was able to live independently—and, at present, already with his girlfriend. Nowadays, he is certified fully disabled, but only because of orthopedic problems (so far, it was not possible to completely eliminate a defect on his lower limb by operation). For now, he has not resumed to take drugs.

Naturally, a similar form of "treatment" cannot be recommended for use in a wider extent. Nevertheless, a comparison of imaging techniques findings in addicted persons and findings in the two mentioned young men, who have unintentionally abandoned their addiction, would be very interesting. Maybe some conclusions that would be contributive to helping heavily addicted persons could be done on the basis of such comparisons.

Conclusion

Our system, which integrates neuropsychological rehabilitations (see Appendix), is based on an assumption that every person with a brain impairment suffers from unique physical, mental, or social problems in the process of rehabilitation. In order to enable the patient's optimal return to other relatively "integrated" people, we have to thoroughly apply the latest findings of neurosciences—which means also of the neuropsychology—which concern various forms of restoration of impaired or lost cognitive functions. The aim of the integrative program is not only the work with the cognitive functions, but also work with domains of emotions, behavior, and personality taken as particular components of a compact whole (neuro-psychotherapy). Such approach should facilitate a patient/client's process of searching for his/her own environment and for conditions that would support a fulfilling life with common troubles, as well as pleasures. However, it is a fact that many requirements of an ideal process of reintegration either still lack in our system or do not work as they should. Unfortunately, this is how our life, indeed, is—the life of relatively healthy people—and this unfortunate state affects the life of persons with impaired brain impairments even more.

References

Ben-Yishay, Y. (2004a), Holistic neuropsychological rehabilitation: conceptual foundations. 8th Nordic Meeting in Neuropsychology, Turku, Finland.

Ben-Yishay, Y. (2004b), Holistic neuropsychological rehabilitation: clinical illustrations. 8th Nordic Meeting in Neuropsychology, Turku, Finland.

Brooks, N., Campsie, L., Symington, C., Beattie, A., McKinlay, W. (1986), The five-year outcome of severe blunt head injury: a relative's view. *Journal of Neurology, Neurosurgery and Psychiatry* 49: pp. 764-770.

Faktorová, M. (1999a), Ergoterapie pacientů po poranění mozku. [Occupational therapy for patients after brain injury] In J. Šplíchal (Ed.), Použitý mozek. Sborník referátů přednesených v Centru neuropsychologické rehabilitace. Praha, Klinika rehabilitačního lékařství 1. LF UK, pp. 114-117.

Faktorová, M. (1999b), Metody a přístupy aplikované v ergoterapii. [Methods and approaches applied in occupational therapy] In J. Šplíchal (Ed.), Použitý mozek. Sborník referátů přednesených v Centru neuropsychologické rehabilitace. Praha, Klinika rehabilitačního lékařství 1. LF UK, pp. 118-121.

Faktorová, M. (2003), Vyšetření ergoterapeutem a terapie kognitivních a percepčních poruch u pacientů po poškození mozku. [Examination by an occupational therapist and therapy of cognitive and perceptional disorders in patients after brain impairment] In Neurologie 2003. Praha, Triton, pp. 353-377.

Gaál, L. (2002), NEUROP 2: počítačová diagnostika a rehabilitácia. Užívateľská príručka. [NEUROP 2: computer diagnostics and rehabilitation. A practitioner's handbook.] Bratislava.

Grawe, K. (2004), Neuropsychotherapie. Göttingen: Hogrefe Verlag GmbH, Co. KG, 509 pp.

Christensen, A.-L. (1977), Lurijovo neuropsychologické vyšetření. [Lurija's neuropsychological examination] Bratislava, Psychodiagnostické a didaktické testy.

Kulistak, P., Matecha, V., Kupka, K., Kubicek, M. (1998), Rehabilitation of cognitive functions in right cerebellar hemisphere hemorrhage: single-case follow-up study. Abstracts of II Mediterranean Congress of Physical Medicine and Rehabilitation, May 20-23, Valencia, Spain, 191.

Kulistak, P., Matecha, V., Kupka, K., Kubicek, M. (1999), Neuropsychological and SPECT assessment of patients with brain injury: long-term follow up study. Abstracts der 14. Jahrestagung der GNP/NVN. Zeitschrift für Neuropsychologie 10: 246.

Kulistak, P., Matecha, V., Kupka, K., Kubicek, M. (2000), Neuropsychological tests and rCBF (SPECT) results of neurocognitive retraining in patients with disease of brain: longitudinal study. Twenty-Third Annual INS Midyear Conference Abstracts. *Journal of the International Neuropsychological Society* 6: 381.

Kulistak, P., Matecha, V., Kupka, K., Bunocav, M., Kubicek, M. (2002), Long-term development of rCBF (SPECT) in cerebellum lesion: single-case study. Twenty-Fifth Annual INS Midyear Conference Abstracts. *Journal of the International Neuropsychological Society* 8: 505.

Kulišťák, P. (2003), Neuropsychologie [Neuropsychology]. Praha, Portál, 328 pp.

Kulišťák, P., Lehečková, H., Mimrová, M., Nebudová, J. (1997), Afázie [Aphasias]. Praha, Triton, 229 pp.

Prigatano, G.P., Fordyce, D.J., Zeiner, H.K., Roueche, J.R., Pepping, M., Wood, B.C. (1986), Neuropsychological rehabilitation after brain injury. Baltimore, The Johns Hopkins University Press.

PSS CogReHab. The ultimate multimedia cognitive rehabilitation software system (1994). Indianapolis, Psychological Software Services, Inc.

RehaCom. Computer-aided procedures for cognitive rehabilitation (1997). Mödling, Dr. G. Schuhfried GeS. M.b.H.

Reitan, R.M. (1992), REHABIT. A cognitive rehabilitation program. Tucson, Reitan Neuropsychology Laboratory.

Škodová, E., Jedlička, I. a kol. (2003), Klinická logopedie [Clinical logopedics]. Praha, Portál, 612 pp.

Šplíchal, J. (1999), Psychologické poradenství a psychoterapie u osob po poranění mozku [Psychological counseling and psychotherapy in persons after brain injury]. In J. Šplíchal (Ed.), Použitý mozek. Sborník referátů přednesených v Centru neuropsychologické rehabilitace. Praha, Klinika rehabilitačního lékařství 1. LF UK, 43-46.

Thomsen, I.V. (1984), Late outcome of very severe blunt head trauma: a 10-15 year second follow-up. *Journal of Neurology, Neurosurgery and Psychiatry* 47: 260-268.

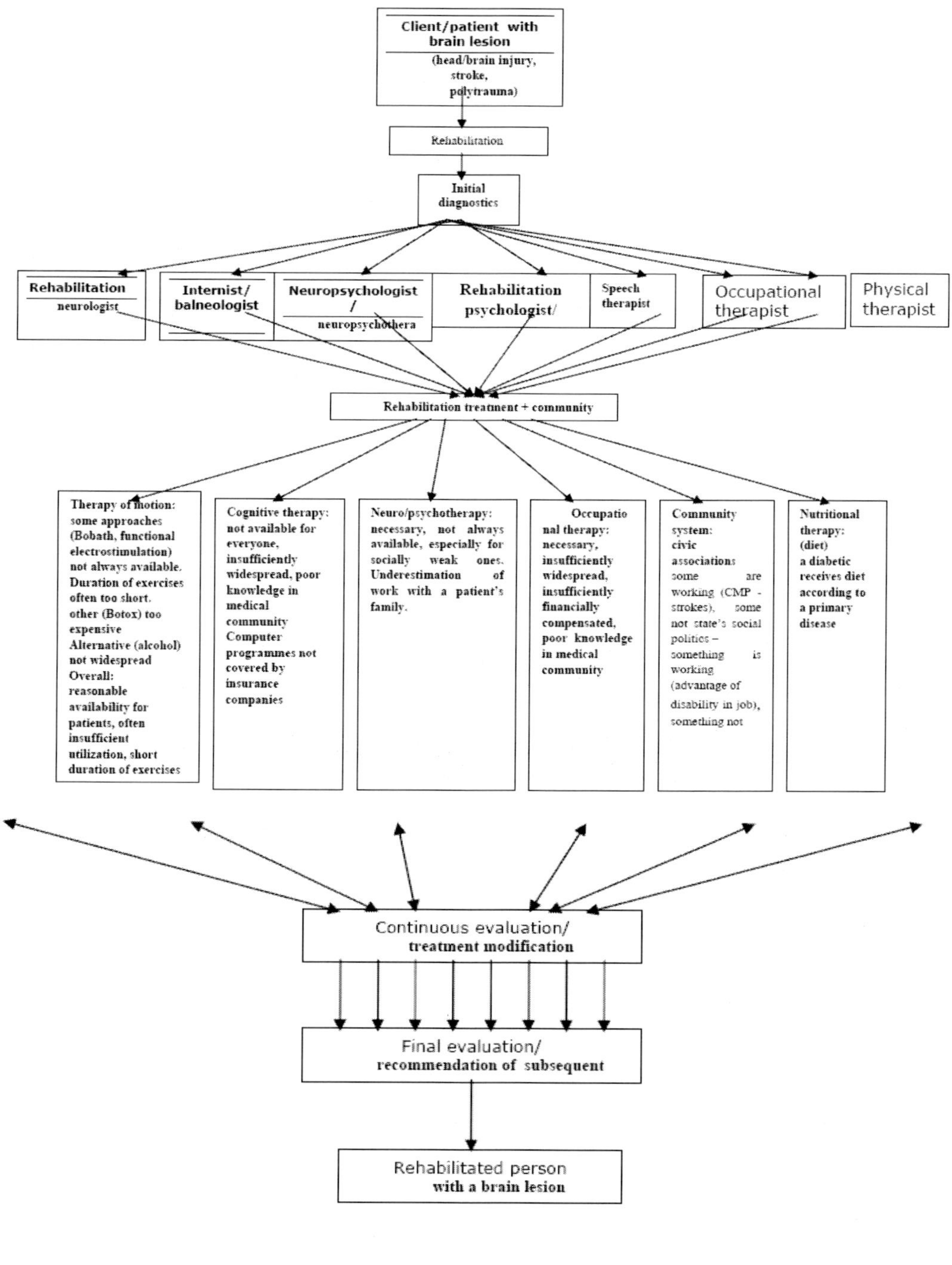

Author's List

Daniela Ripova, M.A., PhD
Miloslava Raisova, M.A., PhD
Ales Bartos, MD, PhD.
Jan Preiss, M.A.
Lenka Kramska, M.A., PhD.
Hana Kucerova, M.A., PhD.
Zuzana Rihova, M.A., PhD.
Radovan Prikryl, MD, PhD.
Petra Navratilova, M.A.
Prof. Eva Ceskova, MD, PhD.
Petr Kulistak, M.A., PhD.
Marek Preiss, M.A., PhD.
Lenka Miovska, M.A.
Michal Miovsky, M.A., PhD.
Danica Klempova, MD
Pavel Kubu, MD
Karel Nespor, MD, PhD.
Tomas Palenicek, MD, PhD.
Marketa Mohaplova, M.A.
Pavel Mohr, MD, PhD.
Prof. Hana Papezova, MD, PhD.
Svetlana Zuchova, MD
Miroslava Benesova, M.A.
Jan Roth, MD, PhD.
Jiri Klempir, MD, PhD.
Prof. Evzen Ruzicka, MD, D.Sc.
Olga Klempirova, M.A.
Natasa Spackova, M.A.
Sabina Telecka, M.A.

References

Airaksinen E, Wahlin Å, Forsell Y, Larsson M. Low episodic memory performance as a premorbid marker of depression: evidence from a 3-year follow-up. *Acta Psychiatr Scand* 2007;115(6):458-465.

Anders M, Uhrová T, Roth J, et al. Deprese v neurologické praxi (1st ed.) Praha: Galén 2001; 280.

Austin MP, Mitchell P, Goodwin GM. Cognitive deficits in depression. British Journal of Psychiatry *2001, 178: 200–206.*

Basso MR, Bornstein RA. Neuropsychological deficits in psychotic versus nonpsychotic depression. Neuropsychology *1999;13:69–75.*

Baštecký J, Kümpel Q, Vojtěchovský M (eds.). Gerontopsychiatrie. Praha: Grada 1994; 317.

Bierman EJM, Comics HC, Gundy CM et al. The effect of chronic benzodiazepine use on cognitive functioning in older persons: good, bad or indifferent? *Int. J. Geriatr. Psychiatry* 2007; 22: 1194–1200.

Biringer E, Lundervold A, Stordal K, Mykletun A, Egeland J, Bottlender R, Lund A. Executive function improvement upon remission of recurrent unipolar depression. *Eur Arch Psych Clin Neurosciences* 2005;255:373-380.

Block JH, Gjerde PF, Block JH. Personality antecedents of depressive tendencies in 18-year-olds: A prospective study. *J Personal Social Psychol* 1991;60:726-738.

Burton, R. The Anatomy of Melancholy. Philadelphia, New York: J. W. Moore, J. Wiley, 1850.

Butters MA, Becker JT, Nebes RD, Zmuda MD, Mulsant BH, Pollock BG, Reynolds ChF. Changes in cognitive functioning following treatment of late-life depression. *Am J Psychiatry* 2000;157:1949–1954.

Cervilla JA, Prince M, Joels S, Mann A. Does depression predict cognitive outcome 9 to 12 years later? Evidence from a prospective study of elderly hypersensives. *Psychological Medicine* 2000;30:1017-1023.

Chamberlain SR, Sahakian BJ. Cognition in Mania and Depression: Psychological Models and Clinical Implications. *Curr Psych Rep* 2004;6(6):451-458.

Chowdhury R, Ferrier IN, Thompson JM. Cognitive dysfunction in bipolar disorder. Curr Opin Psychiatry *2003;16:7–12.*

Christensen MV, Kyvik KO, Kessing LV. Cognitive function in unaffected twins discordant for affective disorder. Psychological Medicine *2006;36:1119-1129.*

Christensen H, Griffiths K, MacKinnon A. A quantitative review of cognitive deficits in depression and Alzheimer-type dementia. *JINS* (1997), 3 : 631-651.

Clark L, Iversen SD, Goodwin GM. A neuropsychological investigation of prefrontal cortex involvement in acute mania. Am J Psychiatry *2001;158:1605–1611.*

Clark L, Sarna A, Goodwin GM. Impairment of Executive Function But Not Memory in First-Degree Relatives of Patients With Bipolar I Disorder and in Euthymic Patients With Unipolar Depression. *Am J Psychiatry* 2005;162:1980-1982.

Cui X, Lyness JM, Tu X. Does Depression Precede or Follow Executive Dysfunction? Outcomes in Older Primary Care Patiens. Am J Psychiatry *2007;164:1221-1228.*

Deuschle M et al. Impaired declarative memory in depressed patients is slow to recover: -clinical experience. *Pharmacopsychiatry* 2004;37:147-151.

Elliot R. The neuropsychological profile in unipolar depression. Trends Cogn Sci *1998;2:447–454.*

Fava GA, Ruini C, Belaise C. The concept of recovery in major depression. *Psychological Medicine* 2007;37:307-317.

Fennig S, Mottes A, Ricter-Levin G, Treves I, Levkovitz Y. Everyday memory and laboratory memory tests: general function predictors in schizophrenia and remitted depression. *J Nerv Ment Dis* 2002;190:677-682.

Fleming SF, Blasey Ch, Schatzberg AF. Neuropsychological corralates of psychotic features in major depressive disorders: a review and meta-analysis. *J Psych Res* 2004;38:27-35.

Flynn JR. Massive IQ gains in 14 nations: What IQ test really mesasure. *Psychological Bulletin* 1987;101:171-97.

Gallagher P, Robinson LJ, Gray JM, Porter RJ, Young AH. Neurocognitive function following remission in major depressive disorder: potential objective marker of response? *Aust N Z J Psychiatry* 2007;41(1):54-61.

Haeffel GJ. Cognitive vulnerability to depression: Distinguishing between implicit and explicit cognitive processes. The University of Wisconsin – Madison 2005; 53.

Hamilton EW, Abramson LY. Cognitive patterns and major depressive disorder: a longitudinal study in a hospital setting. *J Abnorm Psychol* 1983;92(Suppl 2):173-84.

Hultsch DF, Hunter MA, MacDonald SWS, Strauss E (2005). Inconsistency in response time as an indicator of cognitive aging. In: Duncan J, Philips L, McLeod P, 2005. Measuring the mind: Speed, control, and age. Oxford University Press.

Judd LL, Schettler PJ, Solomon DA, Maser JD, Coryell W, Endicott J, Akiskal HS. Psychosocial disability and work role function compared across the long-term course of bipolar I, bipolar II and unipolar major depressive disorders. *J Affect Disord* 2008;108 (1-2):49-58.

Kessing LV. Cognitive impairment in the euthymic phase of affective disorder. *Psychol Med* 1998; 28:1027-1038.

Kopeček M. Kognitivní efekt antidepresiv. In Preiss M, Kučerová H, eds. Neuropsychologie v psychiatrii. 1st ed. Praha: Grada Publishing 2006;305-331.

Mahncke HW, Bronstone A, Merzenich MM. Brain plasticity and functional losses in the aged: scientific bases for a novel intervention. *Prog Brain Res* 2006;157:81-109.

Marcos T, Portella MJ, Navarro V, Gastó C, Rami L, Lázaro L, Salamero M. Neuropsychological prediction of recovery in late-onset major depression. *Int J Geriatr Psychiatry* 2005;20:790-795.

Marvel ChL, Paradiso S. Cognitive and neurological impairment in mood disorders. *Psychiatr Clin N Am* 2004;27:19-36.

Mulder RT. Personality pathology and treatment outcome in major depression: A review. *Am J Psychiatry* 2002;59:359-371.

Müller N. Mechanisms of relapse prevention in schizophrenia. Pharmacopsychiatry *2004;37(Suppl 2):141-7.*

Mundt C. Psychological Perspectives for the Development of Future Diagnostic Systems *Psychopathology* 2002;35:145-151.

Neu P, Bajbouj M, Schilling A, Godemann F, Berman RM, Schlattmann P. Cognitive function over the treatment course of depression in middle-aged patients: correlation with brain MRI signal hyperintensities. *J Psychiatry Res* 2005;39:129-135.

O´Brien JT, Lloyd A, McKeith I, Gholkar A, Ferrier N. A Longitudinal Study of Hippocampal Volume, Cortisol Levels, and Cognition in Older Depressed Subjects. *Am J Psychiatry 2004*;161(11):2081-2090.

Oldehinkel AJ, van den Berg MD, Bouhuys AL, Ormel J. Do Depressive Episodes Lead to Accumulation of Vulnerability in the Elderly? *Depress Anxiety* 2003;18:67-75.

O´Donovan. Achieving and Sustaining Remission in Depression and Anxiety Disorders: Introduction. Can J Psychiatry *2004;49(3 Suppl 1):5S-9S.*

Ormel J, Oldehinkel AJ, Nolen WA, Vollebergh W. Psychosocial disability before, during and after a major depressive episode. A 3-wave population-based study of state, scare, and trait effect. Arch Gen Psychiatry *2004;61:387–392.*

Paelecke-Habermann Y, Pohl J, Leplow B. Attention and executive functions in remitted major depression patients. *J Affect Dis* 2005;89:125-135.

Paradiso S, Lamberty GJ, Garvey MJ, Robinson RG. Cognitive impairment in the euthymic phase of chronic unipolar depression. *J Nerv Ment Dis* 1997;185:748-754.

Petersen, T.; Sordiny, C.; Neault, N. B.; Kornbluh, R.; Albert, J. E. et al.: A survey of prescribing practices in the treatment of depression. Prog Neuropsychopharmacol Biol Psychiatry *2002, 26: 177–187.*

Pardo J, Pardo P, Humes S, Posner MI. Neurocognitive dysfunction in antidepressant-free, non-elderly patients with unipolar depression: Alerting and covert orienting of visuospatial attention. *J Affect Dis* 2006;92(1):71–78.

Paykel ES, Weissman MM. Social adjustment and depression. A longitudinal study. *Arch Gen Psychiatry* 1973;28(5):659-663.

Porter RJ, Gallagher P, Thompson JM, Young AH. Neurocognitive impairment in drug-free patients with major depressive disorder. *Br J Psychiatry* 2003;182:214–220.

Preiss M, Kučerová H, Lukavský J, Stěpánková H, Šóš P, Kawaciukova R. Cognitive deficits in the euthymic phase of unipolar depression. *Psychiatry Research* 2009;169:235-239.

Purcell R, Maruff P, Kyrios M et al. Neuropsychological function in young patients with unipolar major depression. *Psychol Med* 1997;27:1277–1285.

Ravnkilde B, Videbech P, Clemmensen K, Egander A, Rasmussen NA, Rosenberg R. Cognitive deficits in depression. *Scand J Psychol* 2002;43:239-251.

Reppermund S, Zihl J, Lucae S et al. Persistent cognitive impairment in depression: the role of psychopatology and altered hypothalamic-pituitary-adrenocortical (HPA) system regulation. Biol Psychiatry *2007;62:400-406.*

Riso LP, Blandino JA, Penna S, Dacey S, Grant MM, du Toit PL, Duin JS, Pacoe EM, Ulmer ChS. Cognitive Aspects of Chronic Depression. *J Abnorm Psychol* 2003;112(Suppl 1):72-80.

Roiser JP, Rubinsztein JS, Sahakian BJ. Neuropsychology of mood disorders. Psychiatry *2006;5:158-162.*

Sheline YI. Consequences of depression in the hippocampus and other brain regions. In: Olié JP, Costa E, Silva JA, Macher JP (Eds.): Neuroplasticity. A new approach to the pathophysiology of depression. London: Science Press 2004.

Schatzberg AF, Podeber JA, DeBattista Ch. et al. Neuropsychological Deficits in Psychotic Versus Nonpsychotic Major Depression and No Mental Illness. *Am J Psychiatry* 2000;157:1095-1100.

Schotte CKW, Bossche BVD, Doncker DD, Clara S, Cosyns P. A biopsychosocial model as a guide for psychoeducation and treatment of depression. *Depress Anx* 2006;23:312-324.

Shenal BV, Harrison DW, Demaree HA. The neuropsychology of depression: A literature review and preliminary model. *Neuropsychology Review* 2003;13(1):33-42.

Smith A, Graham L, Senthinathan S. Mindfulness –based cognitive therapy for recurring depression in older people: A qualitative study. *Aging Ment Health* 2007;11:346-357.

Stewart WF, Ricci JA, Chee E, Hahn SR, Morganstein D. Cost of lost productive work time among US workers with depression. JAMA *2003, 23: 3135–3144.*

Tancer ME, Golden RN, Ekstrom RD, Evans DL. Use of electroconvulsive therapy at a university hospital: 1970 and 1980-81. *Hosp Community Psychiatry* 1989;40(1):64-8.

Tohen M, Hennen J, Zarate CM Jr. et al. Two-year syndromal and functional recovery in 219 cases of first-episode major affective disorder with psychotic features. Am J Psychiatry *2000;157:220–228.*

Vavrušová L. Depresia – spúšťací faktor narušenia neuroplasticity? Psychiatrie pro praxi *2004;1:20–22.*

Weiland-Fiedler P, Erickson K, Waldeck T, Luckenbaugh DA, Pike D, Bonne O, Charney DS, Neumeister A. Evidence for continuing neuropsychological impairments in depression. *J Affect Dis* 2004;82:253-258.

Williams RA, Hagerty BM, Cimprich B, Therrien B, Bay E, Oe H. Changes in directed attention and short-term memory in depression. *J Psychiatr Res* 2000;34(3):227-38.

Zammit S, Allebeck P, David AS, Dalman C, Hemmingsson T, Lundberg I, Lewis G. A longitudinal study of premorbid IQ score and risk of developing, schizophrenia, bipolar disorder, severe depression, and other nonaffective psychoses. Arch Gen Psychiatry *2004;61:354–360.*

Zimmerman M, McGlinchey JB, Posternak MA, Friedman M, Attiullah N, Boerescu D. How Should Remission From Depression Be Defined? The Depressed Patient's Perspective. *Am J Psychiatry* 2006;163:148-150.

Index

B

C

D

E

F

G

J

K

L

M

N

Q

R

S

T

U

V

W

Y

Z